Gabriel COSCAS

OCT in AMD

Optical Coherence Tomography in Age-Related Macular Degeneration

2nd Ed.

OPTICAL COHERENCE TOMOGRAPHY
in
AGE-RELATED MACULAR DEGENERATION

OCT in AMD

Gabriel COSCAS

2nd Ed.

Florence COSCAS, Sabrina VISMARA
and
Alain ZOURDANI and C. Iole Li CALZI
(Créteil and Paris)

With the participation of
Gisèle SOUBRANE (Créteil, France), Eric SOUIED (Créteil, France)
Cynthia TOTH (Durham, North Carolina, USA), Yasuo TANO (Osaka, Japan),
Marc De SMET (Amsterdam, The Netherlands),
Giovanni STAURENGHI (Milan, Italy), Bruno LUMBROSO (Rome, Italy)

and the help of
Giuseppe CARELLA (Piacenza, Italy), Michael REGENBOGEN (Tel Aviv, Israel), Joël UZZAN (Rouen, France)

ANNUAL REPORT OF THE FRENCH OPHTHALMIC SOCIETY
English-language translation and review were performed by Anthony Saul, Ricky Zolf, Jean Pierre Hubschman, and Irena Tsui. Editing was provided by Tina-Marie Gauthier.

Springer

Gabriel COSCAS
Professeur Emérite des Universités
Hôpital de Créteil. Département d'ophtalmologie de Créteil
Université Paris XII – Val de Marne
gabriel.coscas@gmail.com

ISBN 978-3-642-10181-6 Springer-Verlag Berlin Heidelberg New York

Bibliografische Information der Deutschen Bibliothek
The Deutsche Bibliothek lists this publication in Deutsche Nationalbibliographie;
detailed bibliographic data is available in the internet at http://dnb.ddb.de.

Springer Medizin
Springer-Verlag GmbH
ein Unternehmen von Springer Science+Business Media

springer.com

Planning: Hanna Hensler-Fritton, Heidelberg
Project management: Ulrike Dächert, Heidelberg
Design: deblik Berlin
Typesetting: TypoStudio Tobias Schaedla, Heidelberg
Printer: Stürtz GmbH, Würzburg

SPIN: 12873104

Printed on acid free paper 18/5135 – 5 4 3 2 1 0

To my grandson, Gabriel
To my wife and family
To Créteil

Preface for the Second Edition

Gabriel COSCAS

In recent years, examination of the posterior pole of the eye and the macular region by SD-OCT has taken on a more prominent role for diagnosis of age-related macular degeneration (AMD), monitoring the response to treatment, and for assessing future prognosis. This new imaging system allows more precise analysis of qualitative and quantitative alterations of the macula in AMD.

Although it is still vital to compare images obtained by SD-OCT to clinical data, angiographies, and functional investigations, the accuracy of the images obtained and their correlation to fundus photography can provide a better understanding of the therapeutic results.

Decisions regarding therapeutic indications, duration, and frequency will be based largely upon the analysis of this new imagery. Current SD-OCT exams are therefore indispensable in the framework of the comprehensive review of the patient and careful monitoring of ocular developments.

Continuous improvement of the different Eye Tracking software makes the comparison of images at different stages of the disease and its treatment easier. Better yet, it provides more accurate analysis of the outer layers of the retina allowing an indication of the state of photoreceptor cells themselves and the expected response to various therapeutic approaches.

Preface

Gisèle SOUBRANE

Over recent decades, as a result of progress in basic and clinical research, our knowledge on age-related macular degeneration (AMD) has been improved and refined, leading to a renewed interest in this disease.

However, the etiology, pathophysiology, clinical features, and natural history of AMD remain unclear. Until these unknowns can be elucidated, the primary objective for all ophthalmologists is to diagnose AMD as early as possible in order to optimize the use of new treatment options.

Gabriel COSCAS has trained a large number of ophthalmologists and whole generations of retinal specialists all over the world. He is renowned in France and worldwide for his remarkable clinical knowledge of AMD, which is based on his considerable personal experience.

This book provides precise and sometimes surprising answers to our questions. As an experienced, critical, and well-informed clinician, he provides us yet again with a book that illustrates his exceptional capacity for analysis, classification, and synthesis. All aspects that ophthalmologists need to understand are explained by rich imaging, based on all types of imaging modalities and supported by OCT.

A wide range of fundus imaging modalities are now available, and this book explains the respective value of each technique. The information provided by OCT is presented logically by comparison with plain films, autofluorescence, fluorescein angiography, or indocyanine green angiography. Meticulous biomicroscopic examination of macular changes and the essential value of fluorescein angiography for the detection of anatomical alterations of the macula and for precise evaluation of lesions and their course by indocyanine green angiography have naturally led Gabriel COSCAS to analyze the new data provided by OCT.

As a result of an original and often innovative approach combined with an acute sense of clinical observation, Gabriel COSCAS has described and classified new clinical signs.

The retina exerts a continuous fascination for clinicians who specialize in this field. In particular, the macula is the subject of intellectual curiosity reflected by an urgent desire to understand the physiological and pathological mechanisms and to continually develop new treatments.

Gabriel COSCAS has always expressed his passion for this tiny zone, which allows for the miracle of reading. This book should trigger a renewed interest in AMD, stimulated by the author's relevant comments and discussions.

Rapid or even dramatic progress has been made in the field of AMD over recent years, leading to a constant revision of our basic concepts. The research subtending this progress has also revealed unexpected aspects of this disease. The pathogenesis of AMD is being completely restructured, which will probably lead to a new definition of this disease.

Current treatment modalities for neovascularization have provided a definite advancement, but response to treatment is difficult to analyze. A large part of this book is therefore devoted to recent therapeutic approaches and assessment of response after the various treatments.

The meticulous analysis of a series of clinical cases will undoubtedly be highly appreciated, as it provides the reader with a real reflection of the author's extensive clinical experience. These new treatment modalities require particularly attentive and specific follow-up to determine the optimal strategy. Precise analysis of imaging signs guides the choice of first-line treatment and subsequent treatments in the case of relapse or recurrence. The ophthalmologist's clinical skills and experience are an essential part of this approach.

Today, all ophthalmologists are responsible for the diagnosis and choice of treatment for patients with AMD, which means that all practitioners must be familiar with the signs of the most recent or sophisticated morphological and functional examinations, including OCT, and with the most recent treatment modalities.

This book is both scientific, as it analyzes data concerning the most recent, more sophisticated OCT systems, and practical, as it provides the reader with a reasonable body of easily accessible knowledge. This book will allow each practitioner to understand, interpret, and adapt treatment in their patients' best interests.

Following his previous publications, Gabriel COSCAS once again shares his knowledge not only at the Créteil School but with all readers. The quality of the images and the text clearly reflect the extent of his skills and the precision of his knowledge, continuously refined by clinical observation.

Such books would be impossible without the serene enthusiasm, cheerful energy, and confident humanity of Gabriel COSCAS and his colleagues.

Foreword

Gabriel COSCAS

It is a great pleasure for me to address, in the context of this Annual Report, all of my French and international ophthalmology friends and all those who want to share the recently acquired information provided by optical coherence tomography.

These *Annual Reports* have become a French tradition, based on an in-depth study over several years to clarify the clinical results of a new method of investigation. A teamwork approach progressively collected the elements of a prolonged clinical experience, then analyzed and summarized these data to illustrate, by means of selected images, the main signs visualized by OCT that has rapidly become a field of major interest to ophthalmologists.

It is an even greater pleasure for me and for all of the Créteil School, in that we experienced and have tried to share, the clinical and scientific revolution of the era of angiography and laser, which allowed us to visualize retinal capillaries and choroidal neovascularization and attempt to halt the progression of these lesions by photocoagulation.

The "era" of OCT appears us to have evolved in three phases:

The first phase consisted of visualization of indirect signs: exudates and fluid accumulation, so inappropriately called "retinal" thickening.

The second phase was that which provided, by means of Spectral-Domain technology, much sharper images of lesions, detachments, and inflammatory reactions. In particular, this new imaging modality allows exact correlations with angiography on each examination and during follow-up.

The third phase has just begun, with analysis and monitoring of alterations of the outer layers and photoreceptor cell damage.

Major advancements have already been made, as OCT now combines the data of morphological imaging and functional imaging to provide real "*non-invasive optical biopsies*."

With this tradition and with this future, this book is therefore dedicated to all those who inspired me with my love for this field, all those who taught me, all those who have accompanied me for more than fifty years of ophthalmology, and of course, to all of the younger generations.

The tenderness, advice, and confidence of my mother and father are still very clear in my mind: they still help me, guide me, and accompany me with the same tenderness and same confidence as that of my parents-in-law.

My wife *Gisèle*, my daughters *Florence and Brigitte*, and each of my five *grandchildren* form my family circle. I compensate for my lack of time by my intense love and recognition for their tenderness and for the pride that they inspire in me. Each one leads his or her own life, but we are all united to overcome our difficulties and share our happiness. Their support, their affection, their understanding, and the interest that they have shown in this new project have been extremely valuable to me.

Créteil has remained at the center of my work. My continued participation in the work of the *Créteil School* that I love so much, and in the innovations provided by Gisèle Soubrane, has been a privilege and a source of happiness. This school is a place of permanent and daily enrichment, due to its warm and unending welcome, its original points of view, and our fascinating discussions. My friendly discussions with Eric Souïed, particularly on his recent studies, have highlighted the role of genetics and nutritional and environmental factors. Each new generation of associate professors, assistants, interns, and residents from all over the world has provided new points of view and all therefore participated in the elaboration of this book.

I would also like to thank the leading international experts who contributed to the prestige of this "Report" and the *Sociétés d'Ophthalmologie de France*, such as Professors *Cynthia Toth* from Durham, *Yasuo Tano** from Osaka, *Marc De Smet* from Amsterdam, *Giovanni Staurenghi* from Milan, *Bruno Lumbroso* from Rome, and *Giuseppe Carella* from Milan.

My four closest colleagues, *Florence Coscas, Sabrina Vismara, Alain Zourdani, and C. Iole Li Calzi*, accompanied me daily and contributed their youth, their effort, and their assistance to collect and select an immense amount of documentation. It was a true pleasure to work with them and nothing could have been done without them. I would also like to thank all of my colleagues at Créteil and at the Odéon Center, and all of the ophthalmologists who sent me their clinical cases or valuable comments.

Christian Lamy was an efficient, intelligent, and understanding publisher for the French edition of this book. For the English edition, I am thankful to have had the guidance and support of Hanna Hensler-Fritton and the rest of my colleagues at Springer Publishing, who worked so diligently to bring this book to fruition.

I would like to acknowledge the contribution of Ricky Zolf, Anthony Saul, Jean Pierre Hubschman, Irena Tsui, and Tina-Marie Gauthier, who assisted me in the preparation of this book, providing English-language translation, review, and editing.

The *Sociétés d'Ophthalmologie de France* and their presidents, and President Christophe Baudouin and Secretary-General Pierre Larricart in Paris, have once again entrusted me with this task and have provided me with continuing friendship and support. This tradition of Annual Reports will surely continue.

While writing this book, I thought of you dear Readers each day, and it is a great pleasure to dedicate this book to each of you!

---

*Professor Yasuo Tano passed away on January 31, 2009. In addition to his valuable contribution to this book, Professor Tano will be remembered for his leadership in the global advancement of ophthalmology.

Contents

INTRODUCTION – *G. COSCAS (France)* 1

IMAGING MODALITIES
CONTRIBUTION OF OCT
OPTICAL SECTIONS IN OCT
BASIS OF INTERPRETATION
RESPONSE TO TREATMENT
FUTURE DIRECTIONS
REFERENCES

CHAPTER 1 – *G. COSCAS (France)* 5

PRINCIPLES OF OCT – EXAMINATION TECHNIQUES – MAIN OCT SYSTEMS

PRINCIPLES OF TIME-DOMAIN AND SPECTRAL-DOMAIN OCT 6
CONVENTIONAL (TIME-DOMAIN) OCT 6
SPECTRAL-DOMAIN OCT 8
FUTURE DIRECTIONS 12
- Technological Parameters
- Ultrahigh-Resolution OCT
- Correlation Studies
- 3D OCT
- Segmentation
- Imaging of the Choroid
- Adaptive Optics
- Functional OCT

CONCLUSION 14
REFERENCES 14

CHAPTER 2 – *C. A. TOTH, S. FARSIU, A. KHANIFAR, G. CHONG (USA)* 15

APPLICATIONS OF SPECTRAL-DOMAIN OCT IN AMD

INTRODUCTION 17
- Time-Domain OCT
- Spectral-Domain OCT

ADVANTAGES OF SD-OCT IN AMD 20
- Macula
- Retinal Layer Segmentation
- Drusen
- Choroidal Neovascularization
- Geographic Atrophy

COMPARATIVE ANALYSIS 28
IMAGE PROCESSING 30
CHALLENGES AND FUTURE DIRECTIONS IN SD-OCT IMAGING 30
CONCLUSION 32
REFERENCES 32

CHAPTER 3 – *A. GIANI, M. CEREDA, G. STAURENGHI (Italy)* ... **35**

SPECTRAL-DOMAIN OCT – *SPECTRALIS HRA-OCT *and CIRRUS** ZEISS**

INTRODUCTION ... 37
*SPECTRALIS** HRA-OCT ... 38
Image Acquisition
Software
3D Visualization Mode
Thickness Measurement Mode
Follow-up
TruTrack™
IMPROVEMENT OF RETINAL AND CHOROIDAL VISUALIZATION ... 44
*CIRRUS** OCT ... 45
Technical Specifications of the *Cirrus** Zeiss
Wavelength
Software and Image Acquisition
Raster Mode
Cube Acquisition
Retinal Thickness
Follow-up
Advantages of the *Cirrus**

CHAPTER 4 – *M.D. de SMET, M.E.J. van VELTHOVEN (The Netherlands and USA)* ... **49**

COMBINED OPTICAL COHERENCE TOMOGRAPHY AND CONFOCAL OPHTHALMOSCOPY (OCT/SLO)

INTRODUCTION ... 51
PRINCIPLE OF THE OCT/SLO SYSTEM ... 52
C-SCAN AND B-SCAN ACQUISITION ... 52
OCT/SLO HARDWARE ... 52
CLINICAL USE OF OCT/SLO ... 54
EVALUATION OF THE NORMAL FUNDUS ... 56
OCT/SLO TOMOGRAPHY ... 60
Follow-up
Overlay with Angiography
CONCLUSION ... 64
REFERENCES ... 64

CHAPTER 5 – *T. WAKABAYASHI, Y. OSHIMA, F. GOMI, Y. TANO (Japan)* ... **67**

PRINCIPLES AND APPLICATIONS OF MODERN OPTICAL COHERENCE TOMOGRAPHY

INTRODUCTION ... 69
First Generation of OCT
Recent Advancement in OCT Technology
BASIC CONCEPTS: TD-OCT and SD-OCT ... 69
Time-Domain OCT
Ultrahigh-Resolution OCT (UHR-OCT)
Spectral-Domain OCT or SD-OCT

Imaging Advancements in SD-OCT
Improved Imaging Quality
INTERPRETATION OF THE NORMAL MACULA 70
3D Imaging
CLINICAL APPLICATIONS OF 3D SD-OCT........ 76
Registration
Image Segmentation
Measuring and Mapping Retinal Thickness
Current Applications of SD-OCT in AMD
SD-OCT Imaging and 3D Analysis in Vitreoretinal Diseases
CONCLUSION 78
REFERENCES 78

CHAPTER 6 – *B. LUMBROSO, R. ROSEN, M. RISPOLI (Rome and New York)*........ **85**

SPECTRAL-DOMAIN OCT/cSLO

INTRODUCTION 87
INTERPRETATION 87
TECHNOLOGY 87
Time-Domain versus Spectral-Domain
Time-Domain Analysis
Spectral-Domain Analysis
THE SPECTRAL B-SCAN 88
Presentation of the Results
Retinal Mapping
3D Reconstruction
C-SCAN 88
ADVANTAGES OF SD-OCT 92
Contrast
Artifacts
Microperimetry

CHAPTER 7 – *G. COSCAS, F. COSCAS, S. VISMARA, A. ZOURDANI, C.I. Li CALZI (Créteil and Paris)*........ **97**

OCT INTERPRETATION
Clinical Analysis and Interpretation of OCT Characteristics in AMD.
Comparison with Angiography.

INTRODUCTION 99
Interpretation of an OCT Image

RETINAL PIGMENT EPITHELIUM 101
In the Normal Eye 101
In Clinical Practice 104
Main Abnormalities of the RPE Band 106
Interruptions of the RPE

POSTERIOR TO THE RPE BAND 115

Accumulation of Material Posterior to the RPE: Drusen 115
Accumulation of Material Posterior to the RPE: Drusenoid PED 120
Posterior to the RPE: Serous and Fibrovascular PED 126
Posterior to the RPE: Shadowing or Hyper-Reflectivity 134

ANTERIOR TO THE RPE BAND 140

Fluid Accumulation Anterior to the RPE:
SUB-RETINAL DETACHMENTS (SRD) 140
Features of SRD and its Evolution 142
Cystoid Macular Edema 150
Bright Hyper-Reflective Spots and Dense Zones 159
External Limiting Membrane and IS/OS Interface
Bright Hyper-Reflective Spots
Hyper-Reflective Material
Response to Treatment
Retinal Hemorrhage 167

CHAPTER 8 – Part 01

G. COSCAS, F. COSCAS, S. VISMARA, A. ZOURDANI, C.I. Li CALZI (Créteil and Paris) **171**

CLINICAL FEATURES AND NATURAL HISTORY OF AMD

Part 01. AGE-RELATED MACULOPATHY

INTRODUCTION 173

New OCT Techniques
Imaging Modalities
Correlations
Clinical Practice

AGE-RELATED MACULOPATHY 174

Different types of Drusen 174

Diffuse Deposits
Hard Drusen
Soft Drusen
Natural History 180
Atrophy
Drusenoid PED
Neovascular Complications

CLINICAL CASE No. 01, Mixed Drusen and CNV 184
Clinical Signs
Follow-up
CONCLUSION 189
Deposits 190
Biomicroscopy
Changes in the Outer Retinal Layers
Complications

CHAPTER 8 – Part 02

G. COSCAS, F. COSCAS, S. VISMARA, A. ZOURDANI, C.I. Li CALZI (Créteil and Paris) **195**

CLINICAL FEATURES AND NATURAL HISTORY OF AMD

Part 02. AGE-RELATED MACULAR DEGENERATION (AMD):

Diagnosis, Observation, and Post Treatment Follow-up

INTRODUCTION 197

CLINICAL CLASSIFICATION 198
Clinical Features and Natural History on AMD 198
Treatment 198

OCCULT CHOROIDAL NEOVASCULARIZATION
VASCULARIZED PIGMENT EPITHELIAL DETACHMENT 201

Contribution of OCT 201
Exudative Reactions 201
Imaging Modalities (TD-OCT; SD-OCT) 202

CLINICAL CASES OF OCCULT CNV 203

Table of Clinical Cases 204

CLINICAL CASE No. 01: Occult CNV – Initial Stage, Asymptomatic 206
CLINICAL CASE No. 02: Occult CNV – Initial Stage, Symptomatic 210
CLINICAL CASE No. 03: Occult CNV – Early, Small 212
CLINICAL CASE No. 04: Occult CNV – Moderately Large 216
CLINICAL CASE No. 05: Occult CNV – Minimally Classic 222
CLINICAL CASE No. 06: Occult CNV – Minimally Classic 226
CLINICAL CASE No. 07: Occult CNV, Large 232
CLINICAL CASE No. 08: Mixed (Classic and Occult) CNV of Equal Dimensions 240
CLINICAL CASE No. 09: Progressive Proliferation of Occult CNV 246
CLINICAL CASE No. 10: Occult CNV with Serous PED 252
CLINICAL CASE No. 11: Occult CNV at the Edge of Serous PED 256
CLINICAL CASE No. 12: Large, Advanced Occult CNV 260
CLINICAL CASE No. 13: Hemorrhagic Complication of Occult CNV 264
CLINICAL CASE No. 14: Advanced CNV with Hemorrhagic Complications 266
CLINICAL CASE No. 15: Advanced Occult CNV 268

CONCLUSION 174

CHAPTER 9 – *G. COSCAS, F. COSCAS, S. VISMARA, A. ZOURDANI, C.I. Li CALZI (Créteil and Paris)* **275**

CHORIORETINAL ANASTOMOSES **275**

PATHOGENIC HYPOTHESES 277

CLINICAL FEATURES 278
- Fluorescein Angiography
- SLO-ICG Angiography
- Spectral-Domain OCT
- Complications
- Prognosis

TREATMENT MODALITIES 280
- Laser Photocoagulation
- Photodynamic Therapy
- Anti-Angiogenic Therapy
- Combined Therapy
- Protection of the Fellow Eye

Table of Clinical Cases 281

CLINICAL CASE No. 01: CHORIORETINAL ANASTOMOSIS 282
CLINICAL CASE No. 02: CHORIORETINAL ANASTOMOSIS 288
CLINICAL CASE No. 03: CHORIORETINAL ANASTOMOSIS 292
CLINICAL CASE No. 04: CHORIORETINAL ANASTOMOSIS 296
CLINICAL CASE No. 05: ADVANCED FORM 298

CONCLUSION 300

CHAPTER 10 – *G. COSCAS, F. COSCAS, S. VISMARA, A. ZOURDANI, C.I. Li CALZI (Créteil and Paris)* **301**

POLYPOIDAL CHOROIDAL VASCULOPATHY **302**

Clinical Features 302
- Polypoidal Formations
- Abnormal Choroidal Vessels
- Hyper-Fluorescent Plaque
- Choroidal Neovascularization

Contribution of OCT 304
Natural History 304
Treatment 304

Table of Clinical Cases 305

CLINICAL CASE No. 01: PCV with Serosanguineous PED 306
CLINICAL CASE No. 02: PCV with Fibrous Changes 314
CLINICAL CASE No. 03: PCV with Longstanding Course 318

CONCLUSION 322

CHAPTER 11 –

G. COSCAS, F. COSCAS, S. VISMARA, A. ZOURDANI , C.I. Li CALZI (Créteil and Paris) **323**

CLASSIC CHOROIDAL NEOVASCULARIZATION **325**

CLINICAL FEATURES **325**

Initial Definitions
Current Classification
Frequency

CONTRIBUTION OF OCT 325
Imaging Modalities 326

CLINICAL CASES OF CLASSIC CNV

CLINICAL CASE No. 01: SMALL CLASSIC CNV 328
CLINICAL CASE No. 02: LARGE CLASSIC CNV 334

CONCLUSION 339

CHAPTER 12 –

G. COSCAS, F. COSCAS, S. VISMARA, A. ZOURDANI, C.I. Li CALZI (Créteil and Paris) **341**

ATROPHIC FORMS (DRY AMD) **343**

INTRODUCTION 343
Definitions
Complications
Biomicroscopy
Fluorescein Angiography
Indocyanine Green Angiography

CONTRIBUTION OF OCT 344
Time-Domain OCT
Spectral-Domain OCT
PROGNOSIS 344

TABLE OF CLINICAL CASES OF ATROPHIC AMD 346
CLINICAL CASE No. 01: DRY AMD: INITIAL STAGE 348
CLINICAL CASE No. 02: DRY AMD: EARLY EXTRAFOVEAL FORM 352
CLINICAL CASE No. 03: DRY AMD: ADVANCED FORM 354
CLINICAL CASE No. 04: MACULAR ATROPHY FOLLOWING RPE TEAR 356
CLINICAL CASE No. 05: MACULAR ATROPHY DUE TO VITELLIFORM MACULAR DYSTROPHY 360

OCT AND DRY AMD 364

CHAPTER 13 – *G. COSCAS (France)* 365

THE CONTRIBUTION OF OCT 366

RECENT ADVANCES 366

Comparison of Fluorescein Angiography, ICG Angiography, and OCT 367

CONTRIBUTION OF TIME-DOMAIN OCT 367
- Different Types of Choroidal Neovascularization
- Fluid Accumulation
- Demonstration of retinal fluid
- Criteria of Stabilization or Scarring
- Limitations of TD-OCT

CONTRIBUTION OF SPECTRAL-DOMAIN OCT 369
- Technological Progress
- Clinical Applications
- Outer Retinal Layers
- Neovascularization
- Inflammatory Reactions
- Scarring, Fibrosis, and Atrophy
- Correlations

CONCLUSION 374

INTERPRETATION OF OCT EXAMINATIONS 376

OCT READING GRID/CHART OF EXUDATIVE AMD 377

APPENDIX – *G. COSCAS (France)* 379

COMMERCIALLY AVAILABLE SPECTRAL-DOMAIN OCT EQUIPMENT

SPECTRALIS™ HRA-OCT Heidelberg Engineering/SanoTek 380

TOPCON 3D OCT 382

RTVue, EBC MEDICAL 384

Spectral OCT/SLO – Ophthalmic Technologies, Inc. OTI 386

Cirrus™ HD-OCT-Carl Zeiss Meditec 388

Author

Gabriel COSCAS

Professeur Emérite des Universités
Hôpital de Créteil. Département d'ophtalmologie de Créteil
Université Paris XII, Val de Marne
gabriel.coscas@gmail.com

Co-Authors

Giuseppe CARELLA

Professore dipartimento di oftalmologia e sciense
Scienze della visione (HSR)
Universita di Milano, Italia
g.carella@alice.it

Gabriel CHONG

Resident in Ophthalmology
Duke University Medical Center
Durham, NC, 27710, USA
gabriel.chong@duke.edu

Florence COSCAS

Praticien hospitalier
Hôpital de Créteil. Département d'ophtalmologie de Créteil
Université Paris XII, Val de Marne
Centre d'exploration ophtalmologique de l'Odéon
coscas.f@wanadoo.fr

Marc De SMET

Professeur d'ophtalmologie
Département d'ophtalmologie de l'Université d'Amsterdam
Département d'ophtalmologie, ZNA campus Middelheim
Anvers, Belgique

Sina FARSIU

Research Associate in Ophthalmology
Duke University Medical Center
Durham, NC, 27710, USA
sina.farsiu@duke.edu

Andrea GIANI

Fellow Eye Clinic
Department of Clinical Science Luigi Sacco
Sacco Hospital, University of Milan, Italy
andreagiani@gmail.com

Fumi GOMI

Associate Professor
Department of Ophthalmology
Osaka University Medical School, Japan
fgomi@ophthal.med.osaka-u.ac.jp

Aziz KHANIFAR

Clinical Associate in Ophthalmology
Duke University Medical Center
Durham, NC, 27710, USA
azizkhanifar@gmail.com

C. Iole LI CALZI
Ophthalmologista
Dipartimento di Neuroscienze Cliniche
Sezione di Oftalmologia (Prof G. Lodato)
Università degli Studi di Palermo, Italia
yole2123@yahoo.it

Bruno LUMBROSO
Professore Libero Docente,
Università di Roma
Rome Eye Hospital, Italy
bruno.lumbroso@libero.it

Yusuke OSHIMA
Assistant Professor
Department of Ophthalmology
Osaka University Medical School, Japan
oshima@ophthal.med.osaka-u.ac.jp

Michael REGENBOGEN
Département d'ophtalmologie de Tel-Aviv
Sourasky Medical Center
Université de Tel Aviv. Israel
michelr.007@hotmail.com

Marco RISPOLI
Dirigente Medico,
Reparto Oculistico
Ospedale Eastman, Rome, Italy
Email: rispolimarco@yahoo.it

Richard ROSEN
Associate Professor of Clinical Ophthalmology,
New York Medical College, Dpt Ophthalmology,
Surgeon, Residency Program Director,
The New York Eye and Ear Infirmary, New York, N.Y.
rrosen@nyee.edu

Gisèle SOUBRANE
Professeur d'ophtalmologie, Chairperson
Département d'ophtalmologie de Créteil
Université de Créteil, Paris XII, Val de Marne
gisele.soubrane@chicreteil.fr

Eric SOUÏED
Professeur d'ophtalmologie
Département d'ophtalmologie de Créteil
Université de Créteil, Paris XII, Val de Marne
eric.souied@chicreteil.fr

Giovanni STAURENGHI
Professor and Chairman of Ophthalmology
Director II School of Ophthalmology
Department of Clinical Science Luigi Sacco,
Sacco Hospital, University of Milan, Italy
giovanni.staurenghi@unimi.it

Yasuo TANO
Professor and Chair
Department of Ophthalmology
Osaka University Medical School, Japan
tano@ophthal.med.osaka-u.ac.jp

Cynthia TOTH

Professor of Ophthalmology and Biomedical Engineering
Duke University Medical Center
Durham, NC, 27710, USA
toth0004@mc.duke.edu

Joël UZZAN

Praticien Attaché
Département d'ophtalmologie de Créteil
Université de Paris XII, Val de Marne
Département de rétine, Clinique Mathilde, Rouen
ophtalmo@uzzan.net

Sabrina VISMARA

Ancien Assistant Spécialiste d'Ophtalmologie
Praticien Attaché à la Fondation Rothschild, Paris
Praticien hospitalier, Montreuil
sabrinavismara@gmail.com

Taku WAKABAYASHI

Vitreoretinal Fellow
Department of Ophthalmology
Osaka University Medical School, Japan
twaka@ophthal.med.osaka-u.ac.jp

Alain ZOURDANI

Ancien Praticien Assistant-Hôpital de Créteil, Paris XII
Praticien Attaché-Hôpital universitaire St Roch de Nice
Centre d'Imagerie et Laser de Nice
alain.zourdani@yahoo.fr

Surreal Imaging

Giuseppe CARELLA
(Milan, Piacenza)

Real Imaging

Gabriel COSCAS
(Créteil and Paris)

Surreal Imaging

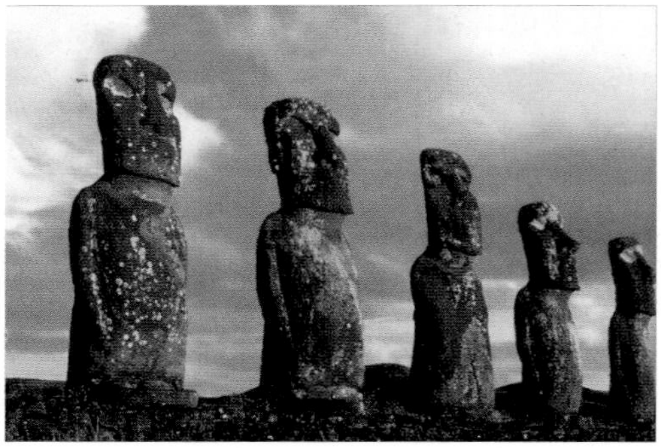

Witnesses

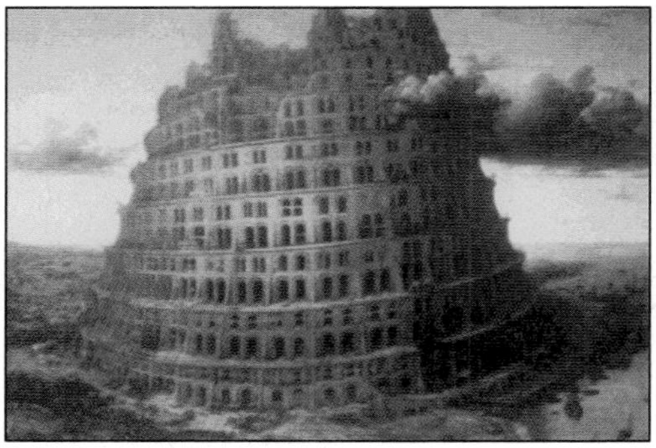

Languages

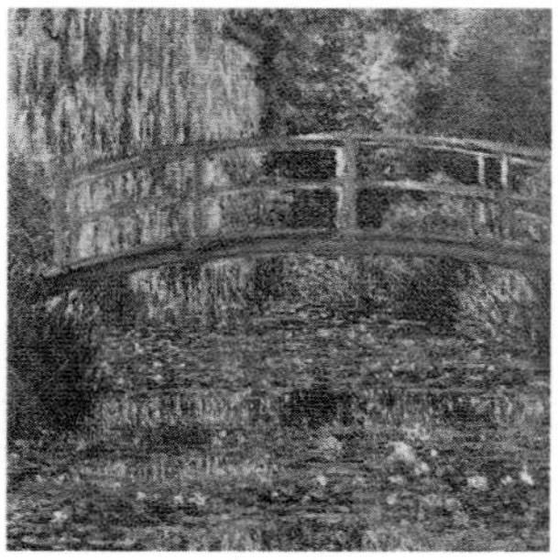

Before

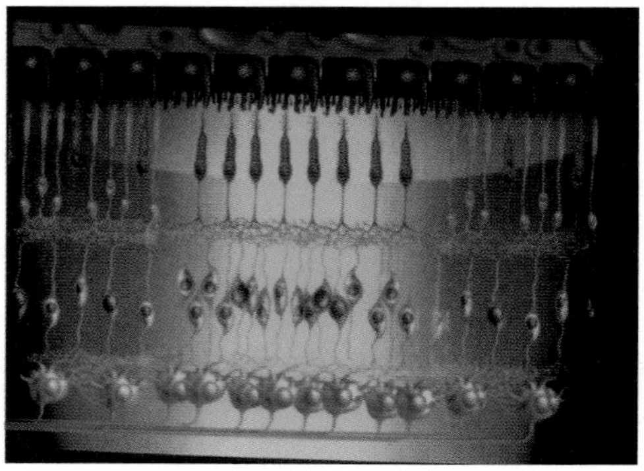

Receptors

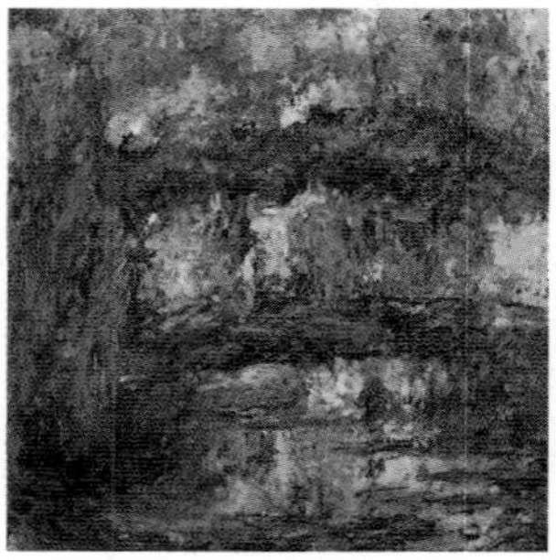

After

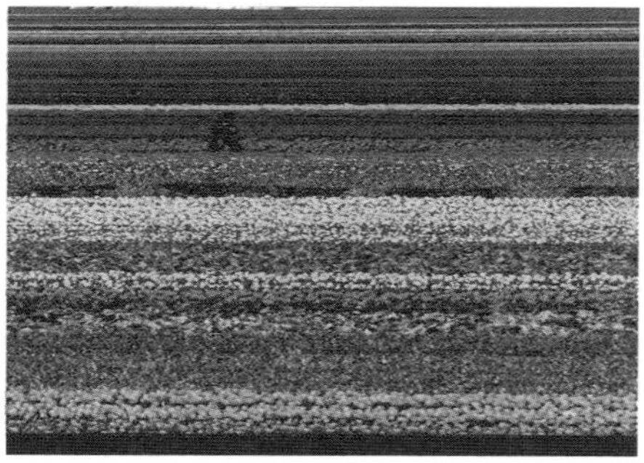

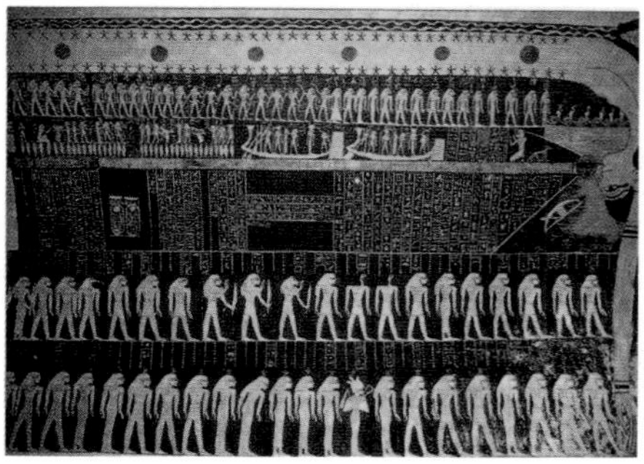

Retinal layers

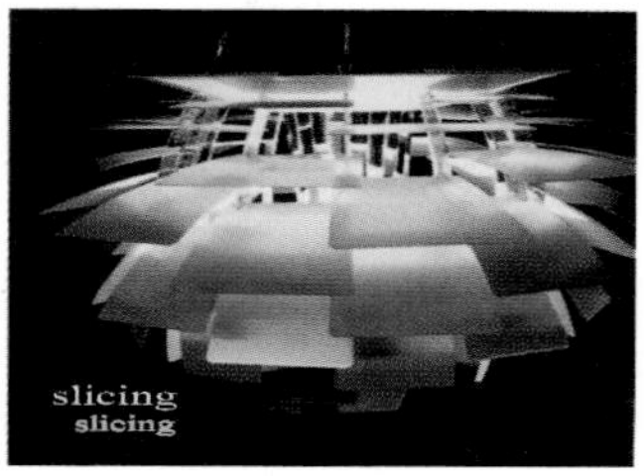

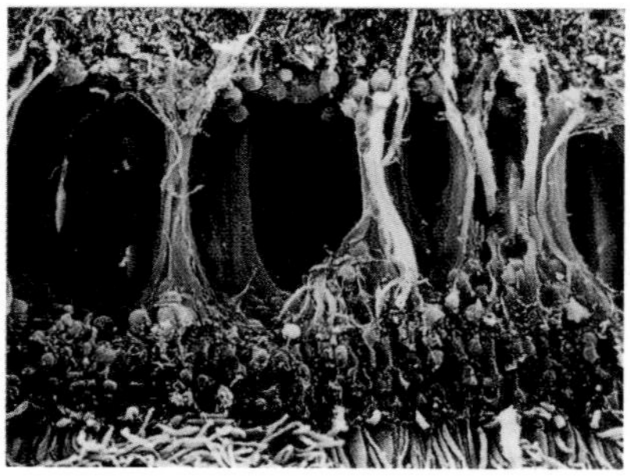

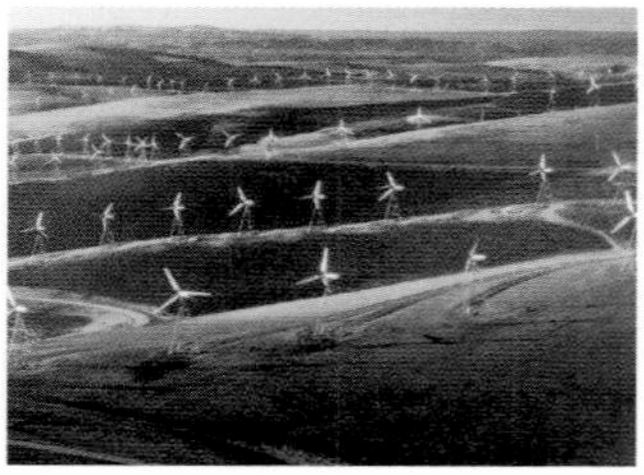

Disorders

Real Imaging

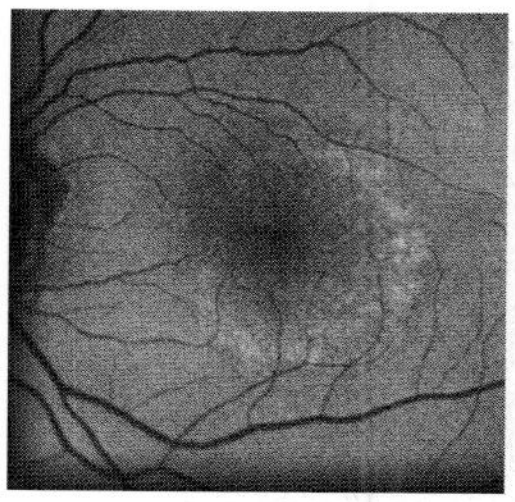
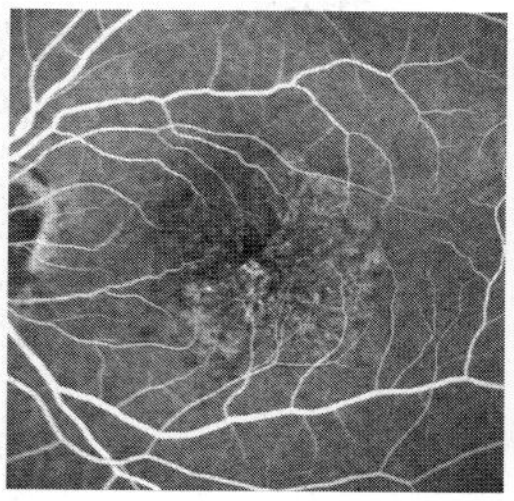

Witnesses

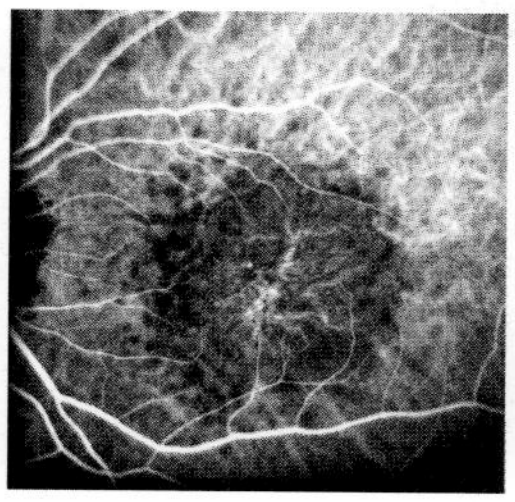
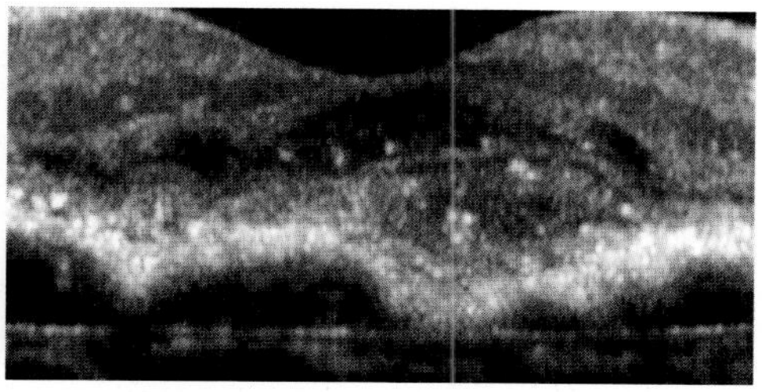

Languages

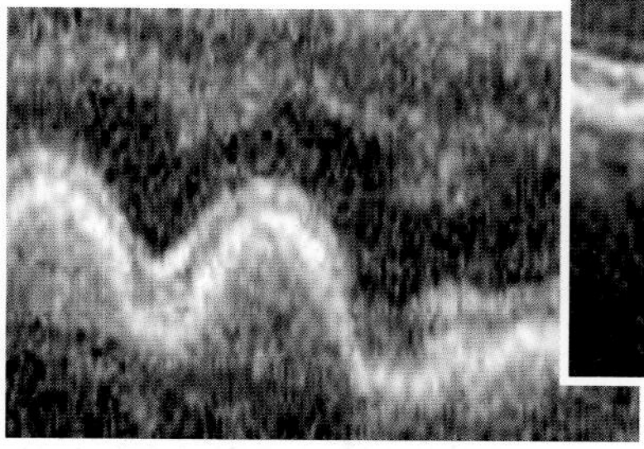

Before

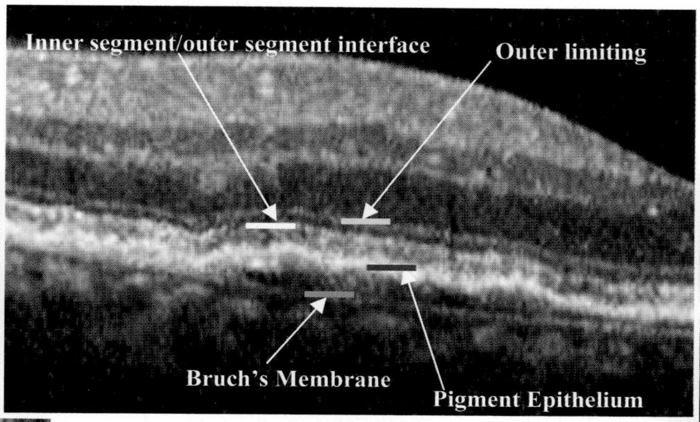

Receptors

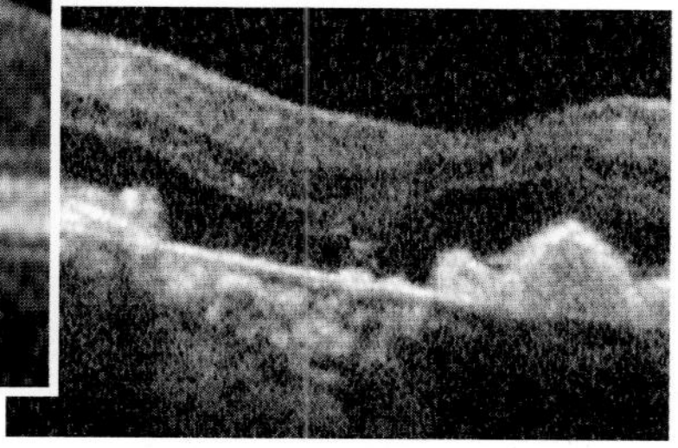

After

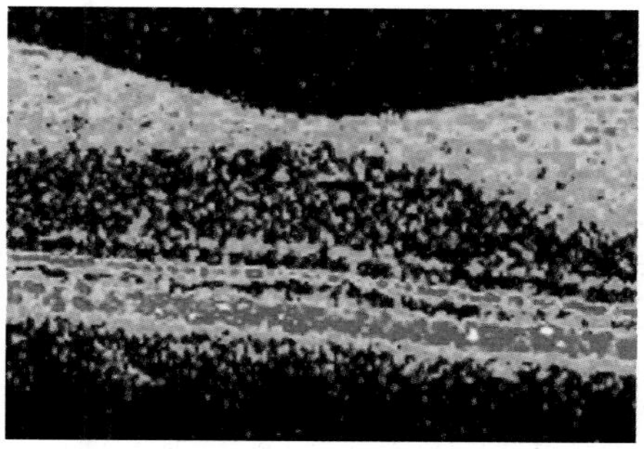
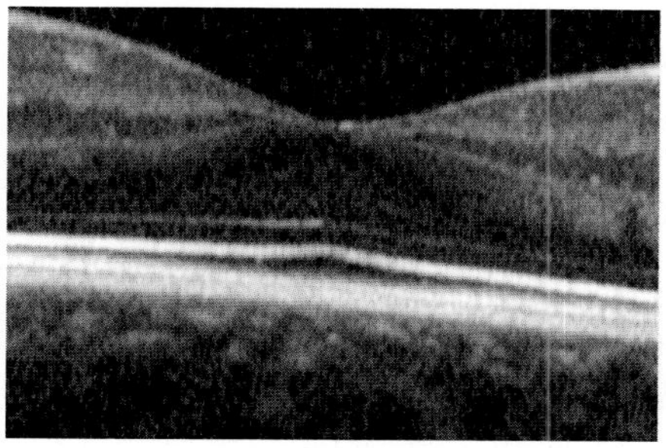

Retinal layers

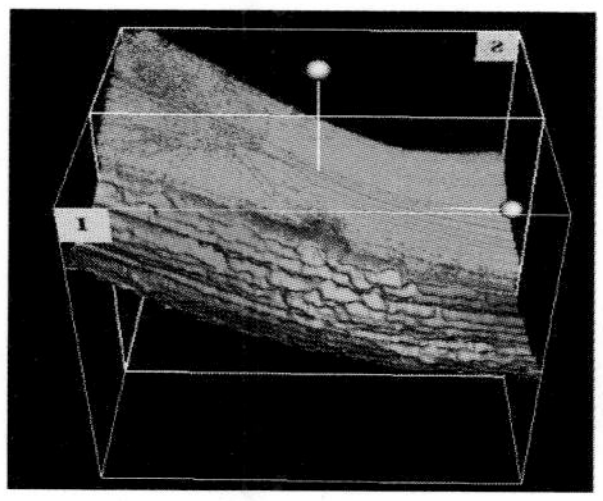
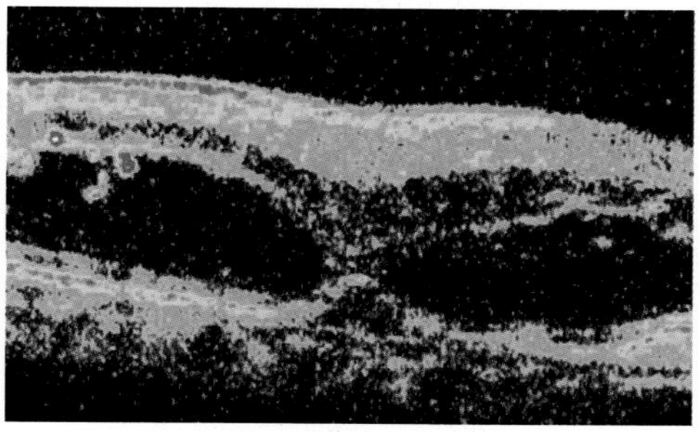
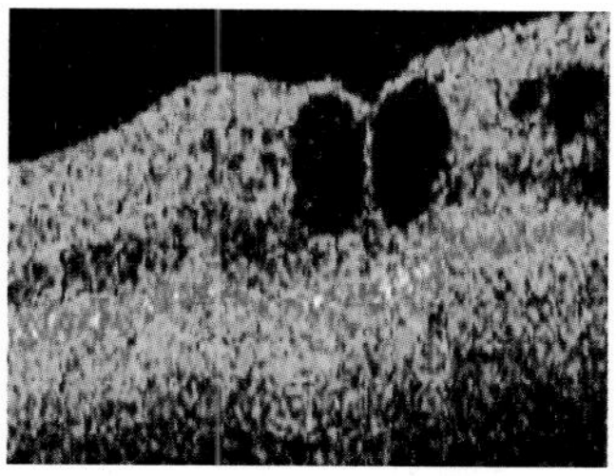

Disorders

Introduction

Optical coherence tomography (OCT) provides images of retinal structures that could not previously be obtained by any noninvasive diagnostic method.

Ocular media are essentially **transparent** and transmit light with only a minimal scatter and attenuation, allowing easy access for biomicroscopic examination and photography.

Fundus imaging has therefore been developed and improved by successive waves over the last forty years with the successive use of fluorescein and indocyanine green (ICG) angiography, scanning laser ophthalmoscope (SLO), and more recently, **optical coherence tomography (OCT)**.

Age-related macular degeneration (AMD) is undoubtedly one of the diseases having derived the greatest benefit from progress in these imaging modalities, allowing definition of its various clinical features, natural history, and assessment of response to treatment.

Imaging Modalities

Each imaging modality has had its hour of glory and each modality provides essential elements.

- *Fluorescein angiography*, for the first time, visualized the so-called "classic" subretinal choroidal neovascularization and the abnormal leakage of fluorescein across their walls. It is considered to be the gold standard clinical investigation for AMD.
- *Indocyanine green (ICG) angiography*, using the SLO, transformed deep, ill-defined so-called "occult" subretinal pigment epithelium (sub-RPE) choroidal neovascularization into a well-defined and well-delineated network.
- *Optical coherence tomography* (OCT) allows assessment and sometimes detection of subretinal and intraretinal fluid related to abnormal exudation from choroidal neovascularization.

However, no statistically significant **objective comparison** of these various methods has been published.

A masked study based on separate and then combined interpretations of these three imaging modalities is currently underway, at a sufficiently large scale to determine the optimal examination procedure and whether comparison of these various images is the essential and/or most effective method.

Contribution of OCT

OCT provides **anteroposterior images** by measuring the echo time and intensity of reflected or backscattered light from intraretinal microstructures.

These anteroposterior 2D or B-scan images (analogous to those of ultrasound), were demonstrated for the first time by Huang in 1991 and by Fercher and Swanson in human retina, in 1993.

Since that time, OCT has rapidly become a noninvasive **optical imaging modality for medical diagnosis** in ophthalmology, allowing *in vivo* visualization of the internal microstructures of the retina on these sections.

Its major clinical impact can also be evaluated by the large number of research studies and publications reflecting the immense progress already made in this field, followed by clinical applications and successive generations of OCT instruments.

Images are obtained in two or three dimensions and represent variations of these reflections (and backscatter) of light either in a plane of section or in a volume of tissue.

Evaluation of **variations of retinal thickness** by optical coherence tomography has been considerably developed over recent years, as this technique is noninvasive and easy to perform and interpret.

The outer layers of the retina can now be analyzed due to recent technological progress allowing high definition and especially high-speed and volume imaging.

This allows the analysis of certain structural changes, particularly affecting photoreceptors and their interface, thereby providing *functional information* on these tissues.

The possibility of **integrated structural imaging and functional imaging** will play an increasingly important role in clinical applications.

Optical Sections in OCT

Anteroposterior OCT optical sections visualize the succession of retinal layers and retinal pigment epithelium (RPE) and the presence of any spaces between these layers, allowing a first approach that is often almost intuitive.

This anteroposterior dimension of OCT provides a spectacular complement to angiographic data.

OCT scans can visualize exudative reactions with **fluid accumulation** (intraretinal, subretinal, and posterior to the RPE). Comparative quantitative evaluation of these images during the course of the disease is particularly useful. Sometimes it even allows their discovery at a stage, which is often difficult to assess by other imaging methods.

These scans are optical ultrasound scans based on the **principle of light interferometry**.

Real-time images of the **microscopic retinal tissues** closely reflect *histological sections* of the macula and fovea.

Increasingly, they resemble a real anatomical representation, especially with the development of **ultrahigh-resolution** techniques and the upcoming combination with **adaptive optics**.

Basis of Interpretation

1. Angiography

Angiography clearly provides the following basic concepts:

- *Visualization* of fundus blood vessels and their circulatory dynamics,
- Fluorescein *leakage* and therefore leakage of serum across the walls of active choroidal neovascularization,
- Slow and progressive *staining* of the fibrous tissue accompanying choroidal neovascularization, and
- Abnormal *transmission* across the altered pigment epithelium.

Angiography (FA and ICG) remains essential for demonstrating *choroidal neovascularization*, to confirm their presence, determine their site in relation to the center of the fovea, define their type as sub-RPE or subretinal, measure their dimensions, and identify their feeder vessels.

Some clinical forms of choroidal neovascularization were only identified as a result of angiography, for example, forms associated with *serous detachment* of the RPE, or *chorioretinal anastomoses*, or comprising polypoidal choroidal vasculopathy.

- Several fairly distinct clinical pictures and natural histories have been defined:

  – **Classic or type I subretinal choroidal neovascularization** (CNV) with a rapid growth, highly symptomatic, and sight threatening course. Fluorescein angiography remains essential to demonstrate classic or predominantly classic CNV.

Classic CNV, which is not the most frequent type (10% to 25%), was a major indication for laser photocoagulation and PDT.

  – **Occult or type II sub-RPE choroidal neovascularization** has a slow course and may often remain isolated and almost asymptomatic for a long time. The main indication for SLO-ICG angiography is to confirm and define the presence of this form of CNV, which is ill-defined or occult on fluorescein angiography.

Direct thermal laser photocoagulation and even PDT were often disappointing in these forms of sub-RPE occult CNV.

  – **Complex, mixed, or advanced** forms often comprising several types of neovascularization and pigment epithelial detachment (PED, [fibrovascular and/or serous]) and hematomas, fibrous tissue, and pigmented scars.

- The **indications for modern treatments** by intravitreous injections are based on this precise angiographic diagnosis.

This probably applies to the indications for each retreatment and for any decision to suspend treatment, especially when there is a doubt concerning the risks of progression and the results already obtained.

- Angiographies remain essential at all stages of diagnosis and follow-up to reliably interpret the abnormalities observed on OCT, to confirm the presence and degree of deterioration of CNV, and to assess their complications.

2. OCT Examinations

OCT undoubtedly provides remarkable, easily recognized and often simple, almost schematic information in AMD.

Whenever angiography is difficult to interpret, the OCT examination easily demonstrates, confirms, or sometimes even reveals signs that are particularly valuable, even for experienced ophthalmologists.

- **Retinal thickening** (measured between the inner limiting membrane and the RPE) whether or not it is confined to the center of the macula, related to abnormal exudation from choroidal neovascularization.
- The constant presence, in the case of occult subretinal CNV, of elevation or detachment of the RPE band.
- The presence of **subretinal fluid** (SRF), associated with diffuse fluid infiltration or accumulation within cystic spaces in the center of the macula forming cystoid edema.
- Zones of **relative hyper-reflectivity**, in contact with or away from the RPE, suggesting the presence of classic CNV. They must be distinguished from other highly reflective structures (pigment, fibrosis, exudate, pseudo-vitelliform material).
- **Alterations of the RPE** (irregularity, thickening or thinning, and fragmentation) frequently associated with occult CNV.
- **Alterations of outer retinal layers** (outer nuclear layer and external limiting membrane, interface between inner and outer segments [IS/OS] and **reactive signs** [bright hyper-reflective spots and zones of densification reflecting progression of the disease with a prognostic value]) can now be visualized.

These signs can now be analyzed as a result of the considerable improvement of the transverse resolution of OCT and volume imaging due to progress in spectral-domain detection.

Response to Treatment

OCT examinations appear to be particularly useful to define the **indications for modern treatments** by intravitreous injections and for analysis of the **response to treatment.**

The current strategy is now more and more clearly defined, as at each step of treatment, it is essential to evaluate variations of visual acuity and functional impairment together with precise biomicroscopic examination of the fundus completed by retinal photography.

The easy-to-perform OCT examination can then be used to demonstrate complete or partial resolution or persistence of subretinal and/or intraretinal fluid accumulation and cystoid edema and the various alterations of the outer retinal layers and signs in reaction to the presence and activity of CNV.

The indications for subsequent retreatment can also be based on and guided by these various signs.

When in doubt, and at regular intervals, angiographies should be obtained in order to interpret the favorable or unfavorable course and to confirm stabilization of the lesions and resolution of exudative reactions.

A **simple follow-up method** is often chosen:

- Visual acuity, biomicroscopy, and OCT before each injection, and
- Angiography, in case of doubt, and every three months.

The **duration of treatment** is still difficult to define, although the risk of recurrences appears to decrease with time.

Limits of OCT

Despite the importance of these various signs, it must be remembered that OCT cannot actually demonstrate a neovascular network or analyze whether it is an active growing CNV or pre-fibrotic CNV.

Any interpretation of an anteroposterior OCT section must be correlated with the corresponding fundus image, the direction of the scan, and its exact site in relation to landmarks visible on the red free fundus image or preferably on angiography.

Future Directions

The most recent improvements of OCT systems appear to facilitate this precise localization by simultaneously providing red free image, autofluorescence, or combining SLO-fluorescein or SLO-ICG angiography or even Eye-Tracking* systems.

Many other improvements include 3D images that can be easily adjusted by the operator and even the possibility of penetrating in various ways inside the entire studied tissue or eliminating certain layers and analyzing the various surfaces after segmentation.

The use of various wavelengths could allow deeper visualization of the choroid, and development of adaptive optics is very promising.

Linking with functional investigation modules, particularly *microperimetry* further completes the possibilities of these new modalities.

The various chapters of this book will schematically describe the optical principles of OCT and the various conventional interferometry (time-domain) and modern spectral-domain interferometry (Fourier-domain) systems used.

The examination procedure, with advice on how to avoid errors and artifacts and interpretation of the images obtained in normal subjects, will provide the basis for analysis of the OCT features of the main abnormalities observed in AMD.

In the last part of this atlas, the main clinical features of AMD on OCT will be successively analyzed and compared with angiography images.

References

Huang, D., Swanson, E.A., Lin, C.P., et al, Optical coherence tomography. *Science 1991.254,(5035), 1178–1181.*

Fercher, A.F., Hitzenberger, C.K., Drexler, et al, In-vivo optical coherence tomography *1993.116 (1), 113–15.*

Swanson, E.A., Izatt, J.A., Hee, et al, In-vivo retinal imaging by OCT. Optics Letters 1993.18 (21), 1864–1866.

Principles of OCT Examination Techniques Main OCT Systems

Gabriel COSCAS
(Créteil and Paris)

Principles of Time-Domain and Spectral-Domain OCT

Examination and imaging of the fundus, especially the macula, constitute an essential objective for diagnosis and follow-up.

Considerable progress has been made in this examination, based on ophthalmoscopy and color retinography. Fundus photographs obtained in monochromatic light are well known and easy to perform, and, more recently, **autofluorescence** photographs now constitute reference documents.

Due to the transparency of the intraocular media and the retina, *angiography* is able to visualize the vessels of the fundus and photograph the passage of certain dyes (fluorescein and indocyanine) after intravenous injection.

These imaging modalities have allowed considerable progress and remain the basis of our knowledge of retinal and choroidal vascular diseases. They also allow analysis of subretinal and intraretinal **detachable spaces**, demonstration of *macular edema*, and visualization of normal vascular networks and the various types of choroidal neovascularization.

However, in the absence of biopsies and therefore histopathological examination, useful information has been provided by OCT, which allows examination of the various layers of the retina on **anteroposterior scans** (*Huang 1991*[1], *Hee 1995*[2], *Puliafito 1995*[3], *and Toth 1997*[4]).

The Basic Principle of OCT

When a coherent light beam is projected onto the retina, the light crosses the transparent layers, is partly scattered and is then reflected from the vitreoretinal interface and the various layers of the retina and choroid, allowing the acquisition of images.

The light source is usually a superluminescent diode with a partially coherent beam composed of photons propagated in a straight line in the form of a wave front.

This beam undergoes changes as it crosses the various biological media: deviation of its path (*refraction phenomenon*) and *partial absorption* and a certain degree of *scatter* (when the medium is heterogeneous).

However, most of the light is reflected in the inverse direction to the incident beam. These reflected beams are recorded during OCT (**Figure 1**).

Acquisition of the OCT signal is based on splitting of the incident light beam into two fractions: a sample beam and a reference beam, which follow two different paths but with the same length.

When the reflected light beams (derived from each of these two paths) simultaneously reach the detector, they induce an interference signal. The amplitude of this interference signal is measured and is used to acquire the image.

The principle of OCT is based on the presence of **partial interference** between the light beam reflected by the retina and the other beam reflected by a reference mirror. The combination of a wavefront of several coherent light beams induces interference phenomena with amplitudes that are either cancelled or added, resulting in the formation of interference fringes.

Conventional (Time-Domain) OCT

Schematically, the light beam emitted by the superluminescent diode is split into two beams by a *beam splitter*: an incident beam enters the ocular media and is reflected by the various layers of the fundus; the other beam is reflected by a reference mirror (**Figure 2**).

As light is reflected back along the same path, these two beams meet and form interferences that are detected by a light detector.

Displacement of the mirror placed on the path of the reference light beam allows analysis of structures situated at various depths during each light echo acquisition, forming an A-scan (**Figure 2**).

An anteroposterior or **B-scan of retinal tissues**, composed by the various A-scan sequences, also requires **transverse scanning** of the retina in a predefined axis (horizontal, vertical, or oblique).

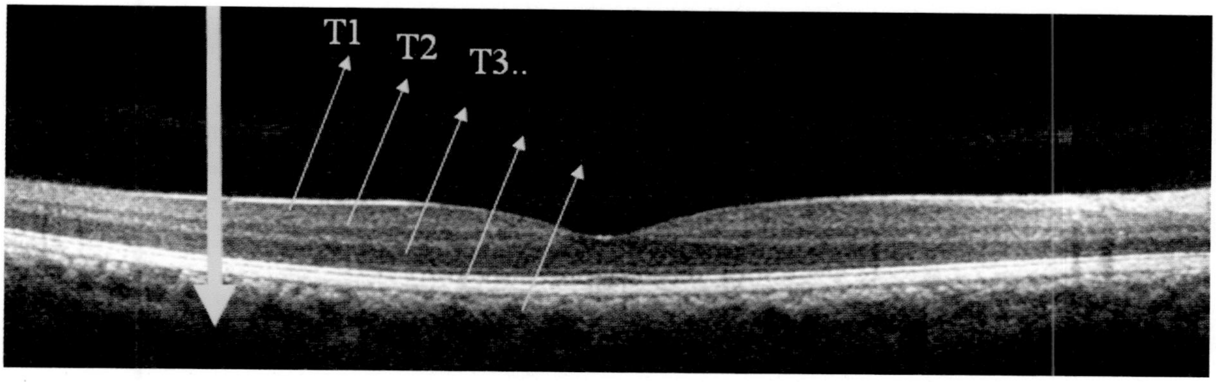

Figure 1: Basic principle of conventional Time-Domain OCT:
Each reflected light signal in T1, T2, T3..., is received at different times depending on the position of the mirror and the depth in the retina.

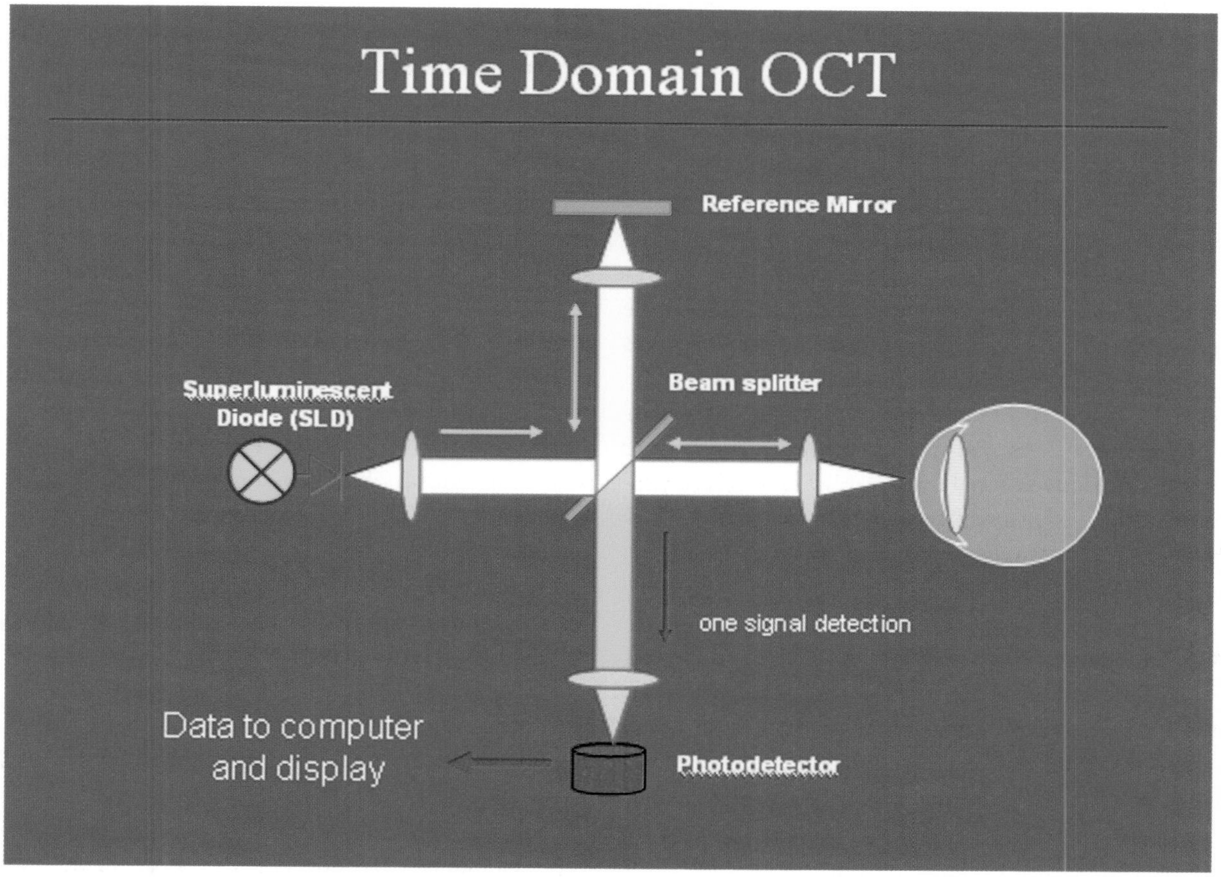

Figure 2: Diagram of the basic principle of conventional Time-Domain OCT:
- The light beam is split into 2 beams by a semi-reflecting mirror (beam splitter): a *reference beam* is received then reflected by a reference mirror that can be mechanically mobilized.
- The other *sample beam* continues along the same path and is reflected by the fundus.
- The 2 *reflected beams* are simultaneously directed onto the *photo detector*.

The combination of the wave front of each of these 2 beams results in the formation of interferences received by the detector and whose amplitude is measured to acquire the image. *(Courtesy of Dr. R. Weitz).*

The **precision of the image** obtained depends on the scan number of deep retinal zones. The signal obtained also partly depends on the *degree of absorption* of light by the various retinal and subretinal structures.

The time necessary for this scanning and for acquisition of these sections is the essential determinant of the quality of the signal, hence the name of Time-Domain given to conventional OCT or TD-OCT.

Spectral-Domain OCT

Further progress is underway with the development of Spectral-Domain OCT (SD-OCT), which allows much more rapid image acquisition.

A method based on the famous Fourier transform mathematical equation (1807) eliminates the need for a moving mirror in the path of the reference beam.

In Spectral-Domain OCT, the interferences between the sample beam and the reference beam are obtained in the entire spectrum, and all frequencies are analyzed simultaneously by a spectrometer (**Figure 3**).

In SD-OCT, the interference signal is a function of the wavelength, and all echoes of light from the various layers of the retina can be measured simultaneously (**Figure 4**).

SD-OCT image acquisition is therefore much more rapid than with the conventional system (TD-OCT) and provides excellent resolution. This property enables SD-OCT systems to capture a large number of high-resolution images.

SD-OCT imaging is 50 times faster than standard TD-OCT and 100 times faster than the first ultrahigh-resolution (UHR)-OCT. As the examination can be performed simultaneously in various planes, real high-speed 3D reconstructions can be obtained with hundreds of images per second.

Rapid scanning allows a large number of B-scans to be obtained in a very short time, with a marked reduction of artifacts related to patient movements (eye and respiratory movements) during the examination. This rapid scanning considerably increases the number and density of scans of the retina.

The use of **image processing systems** based on real-time *averaging* reduces the *signal-to-noise ratio* (SNR) and increases image definition and image quality.

Comparison

Comparison of images obtained with successive Time-Domain OCT systems (OCT 1; OCT 3, or Stratus) and those now obtained with Spectral-Domain systems demonstrates clearer images with higher resolution.

These SD-OCT systems have been more recently improved with the addition of various complementary functions (fundus photography, angiography, microperimetry, etc.) (**Figure 6**).

Various image fusion systems can be used to follow the natural history or response to treatment, sometimes even automatically by means of eye-tracking systems.

This book will discuss the applications and advantages of these systems for the diagnosis and treatment of the various forms of AMD.

The contribution of OCT is now widely recognized and applications of OCT are developing very rapidly in various fields (**Figure 6**).

The imaging of AMD has been considerably improved, not only for diagnosis but also for staging.

This imaging is also essential to guide the indications for current treatments and to assess the response to treatment.

OCT facilitates correlations with clinical data, angiographies, and functional investigations.

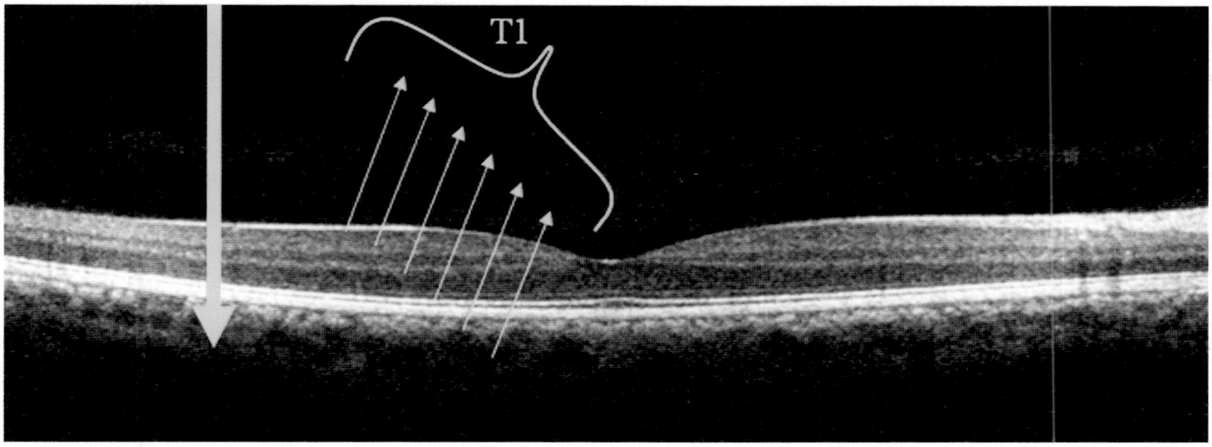

Figure 3: Basic principle of Spectral-Domain OCT based on Fast Fourier Transform.
All reflected light signals derived from the various layers are received simultaneously on the spectrometer.

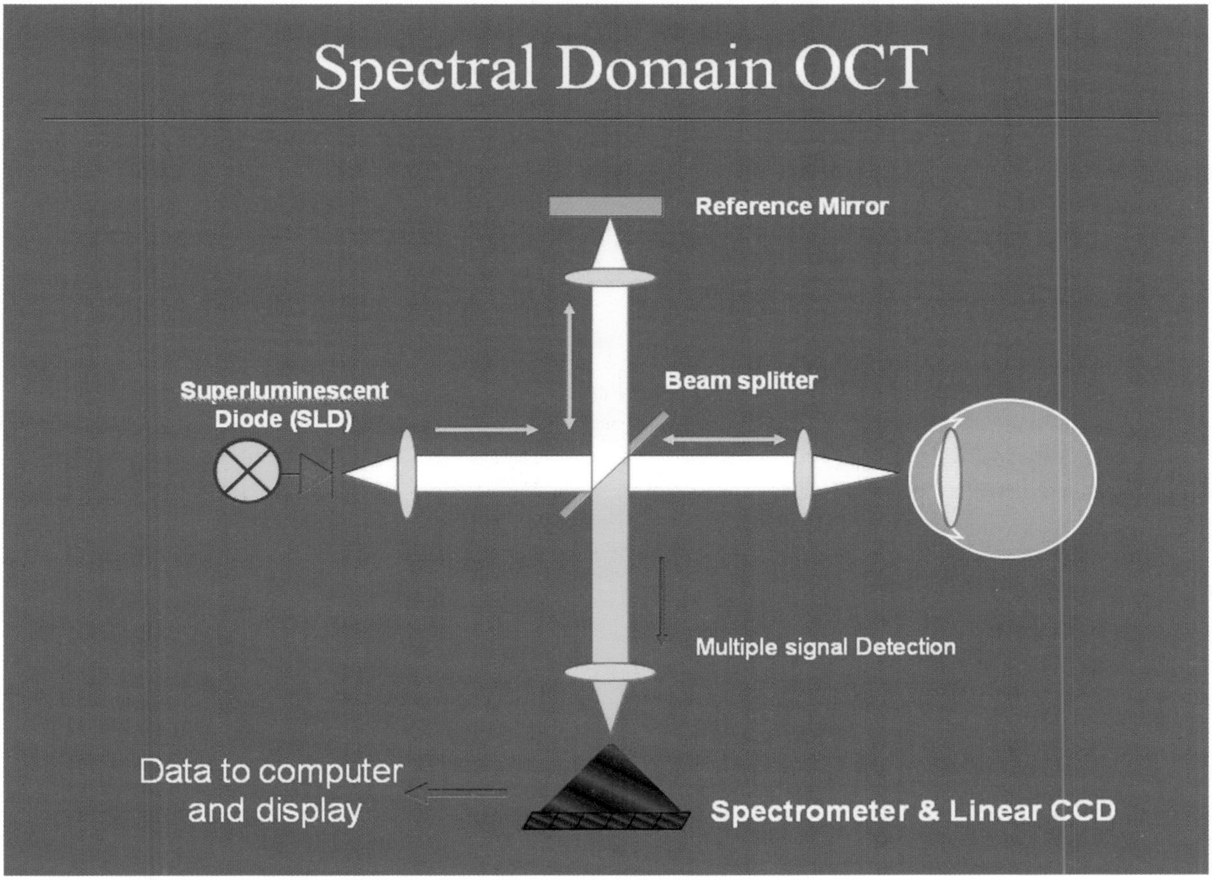

Figure 4: Diagram of the basic principle of Spectral-Domain OCT.
- The light beam is split into 2 beams by a beam splitter: the reference and sample beams are acquired simultaneously by a spectrometer
(which does not need to be mobilized). Signal analysis is based on Fast Fourier Transform.
(Courtesy of Richard Weitz, Toronto, Canada).

The higher resolution and more rapid scanning of SD-OCT provides advances in imaging (**Figure 5**).

The high resolution of SD-OCT images allows a **better discrimination** of retinal and subretinal layers.

SD-OCT imaging allows a reduction of **movement artifacts**, which cause distortion of the surface and the retina-RPE junction.

This more rapid image acquisition allows the creation of *3D images* and more precise *quantitative* measurements (total volume) of macular changes (fluids, drusen, CNV, edema), allowing follow-up after treatment.

The essential improvement that has yet to be made concerns very fine **interpretation** of the images obtained, associated with functional investigations and statistical analysis of data derived from large series of clinical cases.

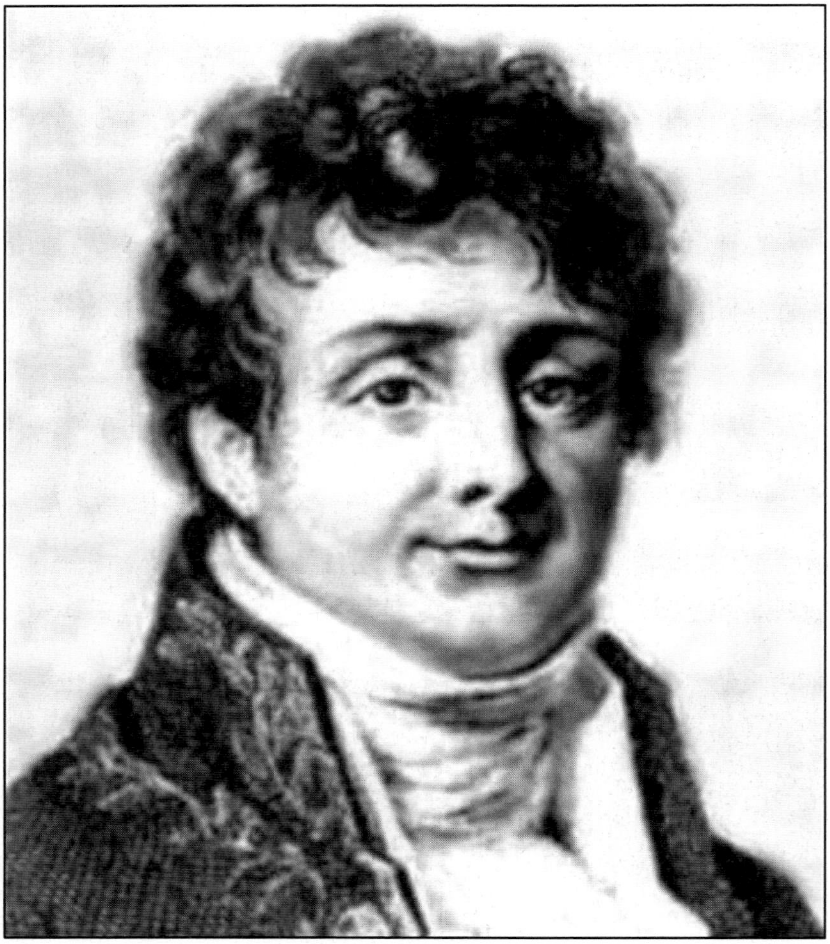

Figure 5. Jean-Baptiste Joseph FOURIER.
(Born in Auxerre, France on 21 March 1768, died in Paris, France on 16 May 1830).
After participating in the Napoleonic expeditions in Egypt, Fourier was appointed Prefect of the Empire, Professor at the Ecole Polytechnique, and Member of the French Academy of Science.
He published his mathematical studies and his famous equation to resolve problems of propagation of heat and on celestial and planetary temperatures between 1802 and 1807.
His work is universally known by the name of Fast Fourier Transform.

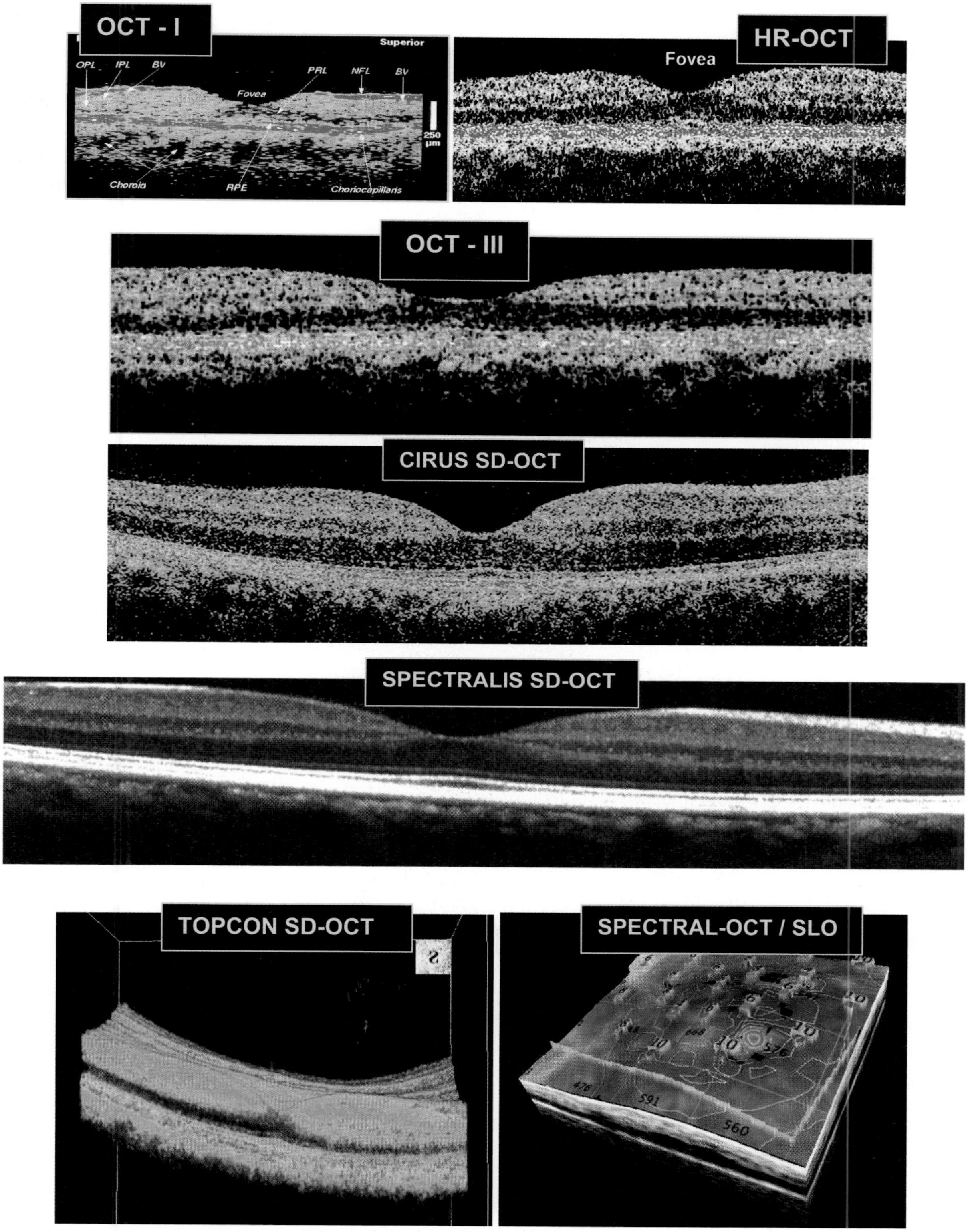

Figure 6. Images obtained with successive OCT systems
Time-Domain: (OCT 1; OCT 3 or Stratus) and the high-resolution images currently obtained *with Spectral-Domain OCT systems.*

Future Directions

The various technological parameters have been considerably improved over recent years, allowing substantial progress in the performances of OCT imaging.

Technological Parameters

Parameters that significantly influence the research and clinical value of these imaging modalities are:

- **Axial resolution** (or **depth**), which allows visualization of the morphological architecture of each retinal layer by means of the *ultrahigh-resolution* technique (*broadband light source*).
- **Transverse resolution of the image**, limited by *ocular aberrations*, but which, with the development of *adaptive optics*, could reach a sufficient level to distinguish cells themselves.
- The **data acquisition time** determines the *number of transverse pixels* of the OCT image (and the number of OCT images or the dimension of 3D data that can be acquired) has been improved by spectral domain techniques and progress in *CCD cameras*.
- The **sensitivity of detection** determines the ease with which good quality OCT images can be acquired (particularly in the case of ocular opacities). However, rapid acquisition limits this improvement of sensitivity.
- The **depth of penetration** into the tissues is essentially determined by the *optical properties of the tissues* (ie, it is highly dependent on the tissue studied and the imaging wavelength).

Studies are underway to visualize the choroid with different wavelengths.

- Image **contrast** to improve visualization of morphological structures as an additional diagnostic parameter.
- **Functional extensions of OCT** are currently under development to obtain functional retinal imaging including Doppler studies of blood flow, birefringence, spectroscopic properties, or retinal activity in response to light stimuli.

This technological progress may enable OCT to visualize tissue morphology at the cellular level, which would allow optical biopsy while providing physiological and metabolic information about the tissues.

All these image improvements obtained by these new techniques will probably have an important role in clinical applications (Drexler 2008[6]).

Ultrahigh-Resolution OCT

The axial resolution of OCT imaging is essentially determined by the **bandwidth** for the low coherence light source used for this imaging.

Ultrahigh-resolution OCT (**UHR-OCT**) allows an *in vivo* axial resolution of the image of the order of 2 μm to 3 μm compared to the standard resolution of 10 μm.

This almost cellular resolution allows visualization of each retinal layer similar to the level of resolution obtained by histopathology (Drexler 2003[7]).

Correlation Studies

Correlation studies have been conducted between UHR-OCT retinal sections in pigs and monkeys with histological sections from the same animals.

They have demonstrated the good correlation of the ten histological intraretinal layers with the corresponding features on UHR-OCT.

Clinical studies have demonstrated alterations of the photoreceptor layer in various macular diseases, and one study has even demonstrated a direct correlation with functional disorders in patients with Stargardt's disease (Ergun 2005[8]).

These studies appear to confirm the potential of UHR-OCT:

- To improve early diagnosis,
- Guide interpretation of images from the OCT systems already used in clinical practice,
- Guide treatment, and
- Contribute to a better knowledge of the pathogenesis of AMD.

3D OCT

In clinical practice, the acquisition of 3D volume information constitutes a major progress, as it provides structural information.

This information can then be used to generate anteroposterior images, fundus images, and measurements of retinal thickness by mapping and volume images of retinal structures, analogous to those of MRI images.

The essential parameter to obtain 3D imaging (3D-OCT) is **more rapid acquisition**.

A remarkable improvement of OCT image acquisition has been obtained by spectral domain detection based on Fast Fourier Transform, with a significant gain in sensitivity and speed, as all A-scan signals are measured simultaneously rather than successively (de Boer 2003[9]).

This much **faster acquisition** speed not only decreases eye movement artifacts on B-scans and therefore preserves the natural contours of the posterior segment, but it also allows better delineation of intraretinal layers as a result of improved axial resolution and an increased transverse pixel number (A-scan).

A series of closely spaced horizontal B-scans can be obtained to cover a volume of retina. Pilot clinical studies have been conducted with 3D UHR-OCT using the SD-OCT system (Schmidt-Erfurth 2005[11]).

Another important aspect of 3D-OCT is that it can generate a **virtual image** of the fundus, similar to that of fundus photography. This image of the posterior pole demonstrates the entire *retinal vascular network*, similar to that visualized by angiography, without the use of a contrast agent, but based on detection of the shadow projected by vessels onto the fundus image.

These 3D images allow **subtraction** of various parts of the retina to reveal information concerning *deeper structures* of the volume, which would be promising for the study of photoreceptor changes.

Segmentation

Another advantage of UHR-OCT would be objective and quantitative morphometric measurements and clearer **differentiation of retinal layers** at early stages of disease.

It is now possible to visualize not only the total thickness of the retina and/or nerve fiber layers, but also the **thickness of other retinal layers**, thereby providing previously unknown information.

Similarly, the **total volume** of intraretinal fluid can be demonstrated, quantified, and monitored, allowing objective assessment of the course of the disease.

Imaging of the Choroid

Although OCT imaging generally uses a wavelength of 800 nm, this wavelength has the disadvantage of limited penetration beyond the RPE due to absorption and backscatter accentuated by melanin or opacities of the media. These absorption properties are much lower at longer wavelengths.
Imaging at a wavelength of 1050 nm would allow better penetration and better visualization of choroidal structures, facilitating earlier and more precise diagnosis (Povaz 2007[12]).
Imaging of the choroid requires numerous technical improvements (high speed, light source, spectrometers, and adapted CCD cameras), allowing better visualization of the choriocapillaris and some choroidal vessels.

Adaptive Optics

Adaptive optics (AO) appears to be a promising approach to correct ocular optical aberrations in order to improve transverse resolution.

Over recent decades, AO is no longer confined to astronomy but is now applied in ocular optics with the use of deformable mirrors.

The combination of AO and SD-OCT can allow an axial resolution of 3 μm and a transverse resolution of 3 μm with decreased diffraction, raising hopes for resolution at the cellular level.

Numerous studies combining several technical improvements have allowed visualization of the interface, inner and outer segments, and the cone mosaic (Fernandez 2005[13], Zawadzki 2005[14], Zhang 2006[15]). The preliminary results show that the combination of AO and 3D UHR-OCT could achieve cellular resolution despite its marked technical complexity.

1

Functional OCT

Many approaches have already been investigated in the field of functional OCT, particularly **Doppler OCT** (measuring blood flow rates) (Leitgeb 2004[16]).

Clinical *in vivo* Color Doppler OCT (CD-OCT), has allowed 3D visualization of the retinal blood supply that some authors call "optical coherence angiography" (Makita 2006[17]).

Conclusion

The addition of techniques able to facilitate early diagnosis would allow more effective treatment in order to delay, stop, or even reverse disease progression. OCT will therefore play a considerable role by providing high-resolution images of the fundus.

The development of Spectral-Domain OCT and all of its subsequent refinements has considerably improved the quality of information concerning retinal structures and provides many new markers for follow-up of disease.

Many diseases, especially AMD, already benefit from this intense research designed to visualize the outer layers, more clearly understand and predict the various stages of the disease and its complications, and to adapt treatments accordingly.

As a result of multiple technological advances and interpretation of changes of architecture and cellular organization, morphological imaging will be completed by functional data.

Progress in OCT is a remarkable example of the advancement that can be achieved by collaboration between research scientists and clinicians for the benefit of our patients.

References

1. **Huang D, Swanson EA, Lin CP, Schuman JS, Stinson WG, Chang W, Hee MR, Flotte T, Gregory K, Puliafito CA.** Optical coherence tomography. *Science 1991;254:1178-1181.*
2. **Hee MR, Izatt JA, Swanson EA, Huang D, Schuman JS, Lin CP, Puliafito CA, Fujimoto JG.** Optical coherence tomography of the human retina. *Arch Ophthalmol 1995;113:325-332.*
3. **Puliafito CA, Hee MR, Lin CP, Reichel E, Schuman JS, Duker JS, Izatt JA, Swanson EA, Fujimoto JG.** Imaging of macular diseases with optical coherence tomography. *Ophthalmology 1995;102:217-229.*
4. **Toth CA, Narayan DG, Boppart SA, Hee MR, Fujimoto JG, Birngruber R, Cain CP, DiCarlo CD, Roach WP.** A comparison of retinal morphology viewed by optical coherence tomography and by light microscopy. *Arch Ophthalmol 1997;115: 1425-1428.*
5. **Pieroni CG, Witkin AJ, Ko TH, Fujimoto JG, Chan A, Schuman JS, Ishikawa H, Reichel E, Duker JS.** Ultrahigh resolution optical coherence tomography in non-exudative age related macular degeneration. *Br J Ophthalmol 2006;90:191-197.*
6. **Drexler, W., Fujimoto, J.G.,** State of the art in retinal optical coherence tomography. *Progress in Retinal Eye Research, 2008, 27, 1, 45-88.*
7. **Drexler, W., Sattmarin, H., Hermann, B., et al,** Enhanced visualization of macular pathology with the use of ultrahigh-resolution OCT. *Arch Ophthalmol 2003;121:695–706.*
8. **Ergun, E., Hermann, B., Wirtitsch, M., Unterhuber, A., Ko, T.H.,Sattmann, H., Scholda, C., Fujimoto, J.G., Stur, M., Drexler, W.,** Assessment of central visual function in Stargardt's disease/ fundus flavimaculatus with ultrahigh-resolution optical coherencetomography. *Investigative Ophthalmology & Visual Science 2005;46:310–316.*
9. **de Boer, J.F., Cense, B., Park, B.H., Pierce, C., Tearney, G.J., Bouma, B.E.,** Improved signal-to-noise ratio in spectral-domain compared with time-domain optical coherence tomography. *Optics Letters2003;28:2067–2069.*
10. **Monson, B.K., Greenberg, P.B., Greenberg, E., Fujimoto, J.G., Srinivasan, V.J., Duker, J.S.,** High-speed, ultra-high-resolution optical coherence tomography of acute macular neuroretinopathy. *Br. J.Ophthalmol. 2007;91:119–120.*
11. **Schmidt-Erfurth, U., Leitgeb, R.A., Michels, S., Povazay, B., Sacu, S., Hermann, B., Ahlers, C., Sattmann, H., Scholda, C., Fercher, F., Drexler, W.,** Three-dimensional ultrahigh-resolution optical coherence tomography of macular diseases. *Invest. Ophthalmol. Vis. Sci. 2005;46:3393–3402.*
12. **Považay, B., Hermann, B., Unterhuber, A.H.S., Zeiler, F., Morgan, J.E., Falkner-Radler, C., Glittenberg, C., Binder, S., Drexler, W.,** Three-dimensional optical coherence tomography at 1050nm vs. 800nm in retinal pathologies: enhanced performance and choroidal penetration in cataract patients. *Journal of Biomedical Optics2007, in press.*
13. **Fernandez, E.J., Drexler, W.,** Influence of ocular chromatic aberration and pupil size on transverse resolution in ophthalmic adaptive optics optical coherence tomography. *Optics Express 2005;13:8184–8197.*
14. **Zawadzki, R.J., Jones, S.M., Olivier, S.S., Zhao, M.T., Bower, B.A., Izatt, J.A., Choi, S., Laut, S., Werner, J.S.,** Adaptive-optics optical coherence tomography for high-resolution and high-speed 3D retinal in vivo imaging. *Optics Express 2005;13:8532–8546.*
15. **Zhang, Y., Cense, B., Rha, J., Jonnal, R.S., Gao, W., Zawadzki, R.J., Werner, J.S., Jones, S., Olivier, S., Miller, D.T.,** High-speed volumetric imaging of cone photoreceptors with adaptive optics spectral-domain optical coherence tomography. *Optics Express 2006;14:4380–4394.*

Applications of Spectral-Domain OCT in AMD

Cynthia A. TOTH,
Sina FARSIU, Aziz KHANIFAR, Gabriel CHONG

Duke University Eye Center
Durham, North Carolina 27710, USA

Introduction

High-resolution optical imaging of objects hidden in scattering media such as the human eye is a challenging and important problem with many industrial and medical applications.

To achieve this goal and create virtually blur-free images, several imaging systems have been developed that separate photons travelling through the scattering medium in a straight line from scattered photons (*Farsiu 2007*[1]).

Optical Coherence Tomography (OCT) first described in 1991 (*Huang 1991*[2]), used this type of system and was rapidly adopted for medical applications, especially for ophthalmic imaging.

Principle

OCT imaging systems are based on the principle of **low coherence interferometry** (*Dunsby 2003*[3], *Fercher 2003*[4]).

In this modality, a broadband light beam (or a very short wavelength coherent pulse) is split into two identical copies (**Figure 1**).

One copy travels through a predetermined distance in the free space (*reference beam*).

The other is directed into the eye and reflected back by the fundus (*sample beam*).

Interferometer

These two reflected beams are then incident on an **interferometer**, which generates a signal if the distances travelled by both the reference and sample beams are approximately equal.

This is the fundamental property of OCT systems, in which, although light is reflected back from all layers of the eye, only the photons from a preselected layer contribute to the interferometric signal.

To create axial images, the conventional **time-domain** OCT systems (TD-OCT) use a *moving mirror* in the reference beam path.

As the mirror is *mechanically moved* back and forth, the reference path is shortened or lengthened, creating interference images from shallower (towards vitreous cavity) or deeper (towards choroid) layers, respectively (*Huang 1991*[2], *Wojtkowski 2005*[6]).

A widely used clinical *Time-Domain* (TD) OCT system (marketed as the *Stratus** OCT, Carl Zeiss Meditec, Dublin, CA) acquires 512 axial scans (A-scans) of 8 to 10 micron axial resolution in 1.28 seconds (*Srinivasan 2006*[5]).

A more recent technology called **ultrahigh-resolution OCT** (UHR-OCT) employs femto-second lasers as the light source.

This source provides images with axial resolutions of 2 µm to 3 µm, demonstrating retinal morphology in much greater detail (*Pieroni 2006*[7]).

However, these systems are often slower than the TD-OCT systems (approximately 150 to 250 axial scans per second). The use of femto-second lasers in a commercial OCT system is complex and expensive.

Time-Domain OCT

Optical coherence tomography imaging has improved the visualization of vitreal, retinal, and subretinal structures.

These new data have allowed considerable progress in our understanding of pathological processes (*Huang 1991*[2], *Hee 1995*[8], *Puliafito 1995*[9], *Toth 1997*[10], *Toth 1997*[11], *Gallemore 2000*[12], *Ting 2002*[13]).

Time-Domain OCT (TD-OCT) has been used for evaluation and monitoring of *retinal diseases*.

It has also been used for evaluation of the optic nerve and nerve fiber layer, particularly in *glaucoma*, and for imaging of the *cornea* and *anterior chamber* (*Radhakrishnan 2001*[14], *Nolan 2007*[15], *Hess 2005*[16]).

However, the relatively unsatisfactory *signal-to-noise ratio* (SNR), and the slow image acquisition have limited the applications of these systems.

2

Involuntary patient eye movement during the image acquisition period also reduces image quality.

This remains a drawback even despite the use of algorithms that automatically align adjacent axial scans or eye-tracking protocols (*Srinivasan 2006*[5]).

Spectral-Domain OCT

Fortunately, spectral-domain OCT (**SD-OCT**) is now able to acquire images much more rapidly than the classic TD-OCT systems.

This progress has been achieved by the development and utilization of a new imaging technique based on (**Fast**) **Fourier Transformation** (Paris, 1807), providing higher resolution and better SNR (*de Boer 2003*[17]).

With the SD-OCT system, the interference signal is a **function of optical wavelength**, simultaneously measuring all echoes of light from *different layers*.

This property eliminates the need for a mechanically "moving" mirror.

This enables the state-of-the-art SD-OCT imaging systems to capture tens of high-resolution and high SNR frames, with an **axial resolution of less than 5 microns** in less than one second.

SD-OCT imaging is 50 times faster than standard TD-OCT and 100 times faster than previous UHR-OCT imaging systems (*Srinivasan 2006*[5]).

Future SD-OCT systems will go even further, acquiring *3D scans* at a speed of hundreds of high-resolution frames per second.

The use of compact, relatively inexpensive, robust, and low maintenance *super-luminescent diodes* (SLD) as the light source has significantly reduced the manufacturing cost and maintenance of SD-OCT systems and has made them much easier to use (*Chen 2005*[18], *Costa 2006*[19]).

Speed

When examining a human eye with a scanning technique, *speed* is important because patients blink, breathe, pulsate, and move their eyes.

This limits acquisition of images within the time constraints of the device and may require adjustments for eye movements.

The **rapid scanning of** SD-OCT allows the number and density of axial scans on the retina to be dramatically increased (*Chen 2005*[18], *Costa 2006*[19], *Leitgeb 2005*[20]).

Comparison

Comparison of a conventional TD-OCT scan and an SD-OCT scan (**Figures 2A, 2B, and 2C**) shows a clearer image with higher resolution.

In the time required to capture the TD-OCT image, tens of SD-OCT scans can be recorded, registered, and averaged creating an image with much better SNR.

In this chapter, we will successively study the **applications of SD-OCT**:

- For the *diagnosis and treatment of AMD*,
- By describing the *advantages* of this imaging system,
- The *specific features of various clinical forms of AMD*, and
- The *possibility of combining SD-OCT imaging with other imaging modalities.*

The development of automatic image processing systems for SD-OCT and future research for the *detection* and *prognosis* of AMD will then be discussed.

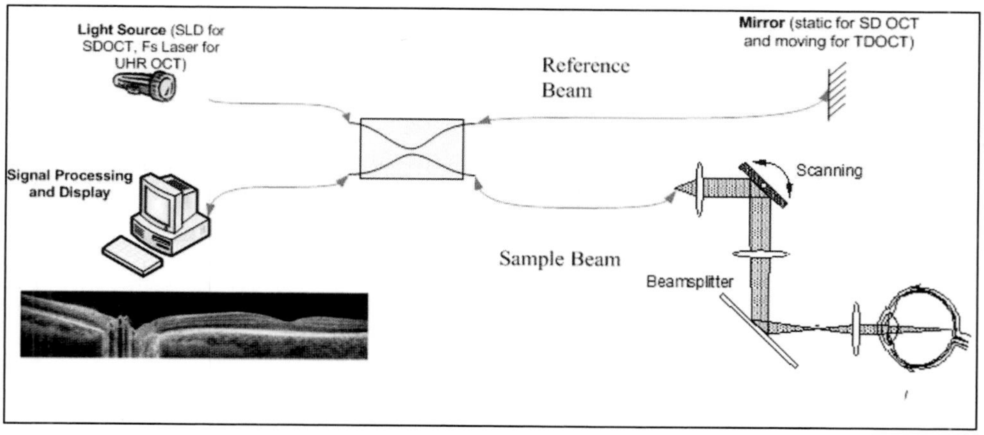

Figure 1: Diagram of an OCT imaging system: light source, mirror, and interferometer.

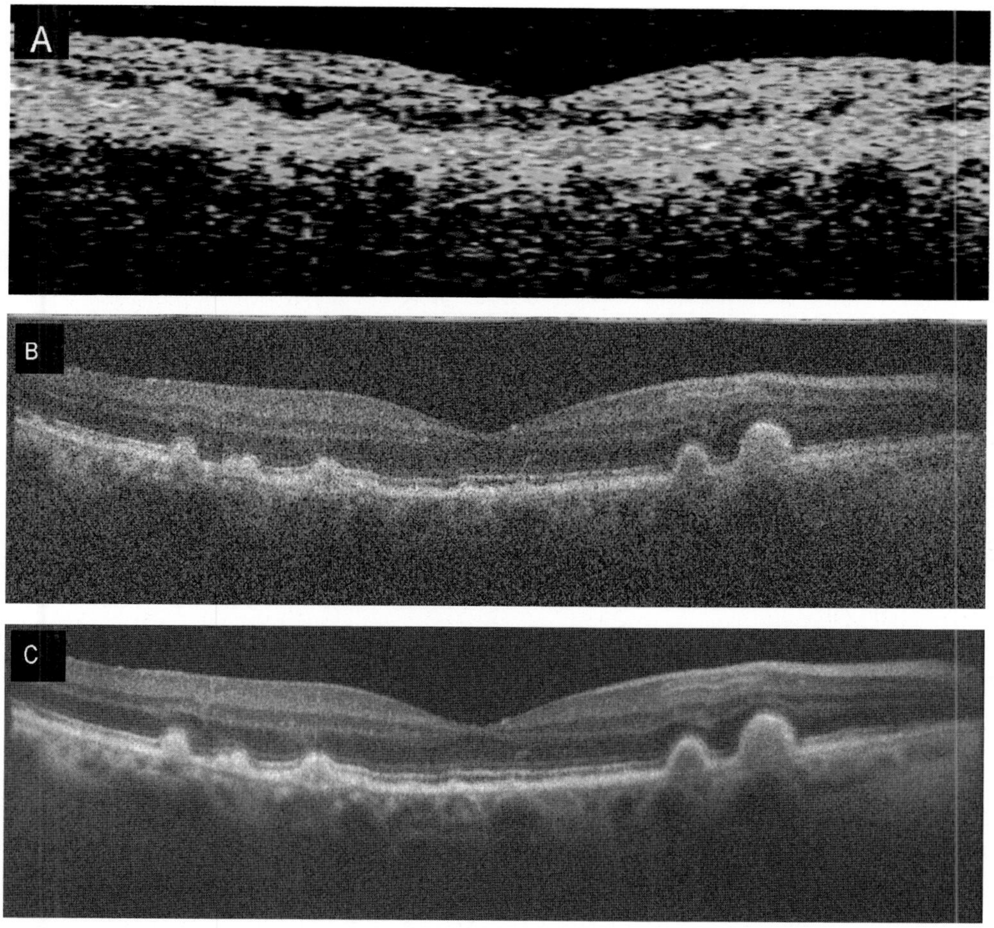

Figure 2: Comparison of images obtained in the same subject using different imaging systems.
A): Color-coded TD-OCT.
B): SD-OCT *(Prof. J.A. Yzatt's research prototype system).* Note the better resolution and SNR of the SD-OCT image.
Image acquisition in image B was obtained in a fraction of the time required for acquisition of image A, and image acquisition can be repeated many times.
C): To improve the SNR, the acquired image can be registered and averaged, providing the image shown in (image **C**).

2

Advantages of SD-OCT in AMD

As a result of its improved resolution and scanning speed, SD-OCT has several advantages for imaging of AMD, particularly preservation of retinal topography, larger field-of-view of the retina, greater scan density, and improved correlation of the image set to fundus features.

The **high-resolution** SD-OCT image quality results in *finer discrimination of retinal and subretinal layers.* For example, small drusen are readily differentiated from normal retinal pigment epithelial (RPE) architecture (**Figure 2C**).

The **scan density** of SD-OCT systems can be improved by the increased scanning speed during the same acquisition time. The *distance between consecutive images* is reduced to tens of microns compared to hundreds or even thousands of microns spacing in TD-OCT (*Leitgeb 2003*[20], *Choma 2003*[21]). Small lesions are therefore more likely to be detected on SD-OCT imaging.

Imaging may also extend across a **larger field-of-view** during the same acquisition time as a result of this high scanning speed.

Motion artifacts causing distortion of the retinal surface and retinal-RPE junction are decreased, avoiding errors of measurement of lesion dimensions, which is particularly important for imaging of small structures at the level of the retinal pigment epithelium (**Figures 2A and 2B**) (*Stopa 2007*[22]).

Improved retinal topographic imaging enhances the evaluation of structural changes caused by epiretinal membranes, fluid accumulation, RPE elevations, and RPE detachments (*Srinivasan 2006*[5]).

Quantitative measurements (eg, total volume) of macular changes such as subretinal fluid, drusen, CNV, and macular edema are more precise, facilitating analysis of response to therapy (**Figure 14**).

The higher imaging speed of SD-OCT also allows for **3D imaging** (**Figures 3A, 3B, and 3C**).

By summation of all pixels on an axial line, a two-dimensional image analogous to a fundus image, called the *Summed Voxel Projection* (SVP), is created (*Jiao 2005*[23]) (**Figure 3C**).

This technique allows the *simultaneous creation of fundus images and OCT images.* SVPs show features such as the macula, optic disc, and blood vessels and can be used to correlate OCT findings with fundus photographs or fluorescein angiograms (**Figures 4 and 5**).

1. Macula

Measurement and monitoring of **retinal thickness** is probably the most frequently used application of OCT in retinal disease, *especially AMD, macular edema, diabetic retinopathy, and epiretinal membrane.*

The ***Stratus* OCT system** can be used to calculate a **map of macular thickness** from 6 radial B-scans crossing at the fovea. The average thickness in 9 subfields centered on the fovea is calculated by interpolating data from these scans. Total macular *volume* is calculated in a similar way (**Figure 6**).

Spectral Domain OCT (SD-OCT) provides much higher resolution images (**Figure 7**).

However, algorithms are necessary to *establish correlations* with *Stratus** measurements.

Thickness measurements may appear to be different from those obtained by TD-OCT. In TD-OCT imaging, the photoreceptor outer segments are often not differentiated from the RPE and are therefore excluded from the retinal thickness calculation (**Figure 2A**).

The SD-OCT system acquires higher resolution images of the multiple hyper-reflective layers that comprise the photoreceptor-RPE-choriocapillaris complex.

SD-OCT retinal thickness measurements may include the photoreceptor outer segment layer, which is visibly separate from the RPE in these high-resolution scans (**Figure 2B**).

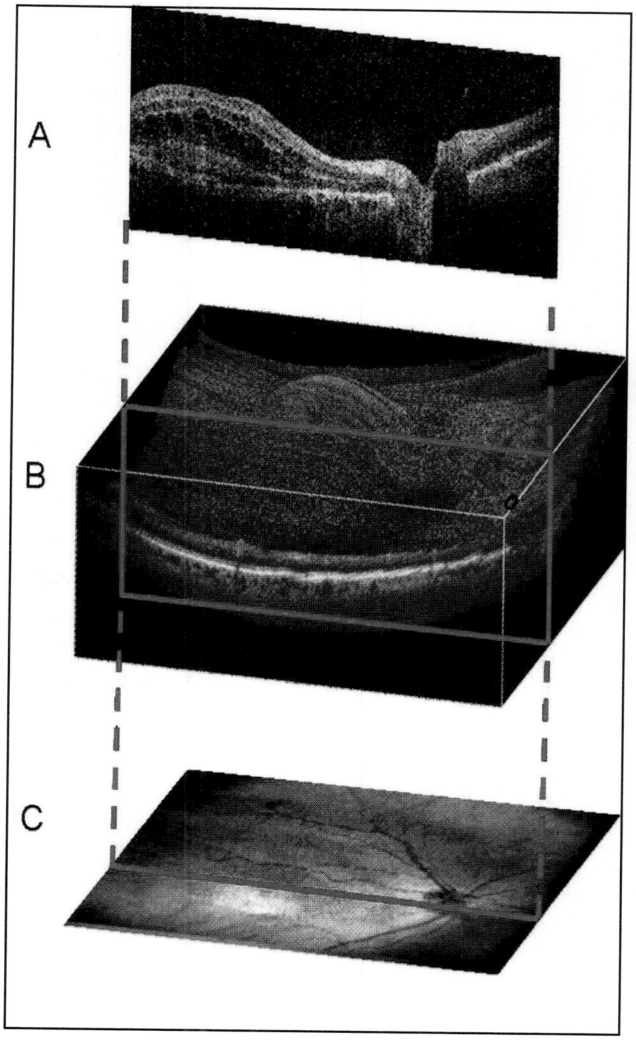

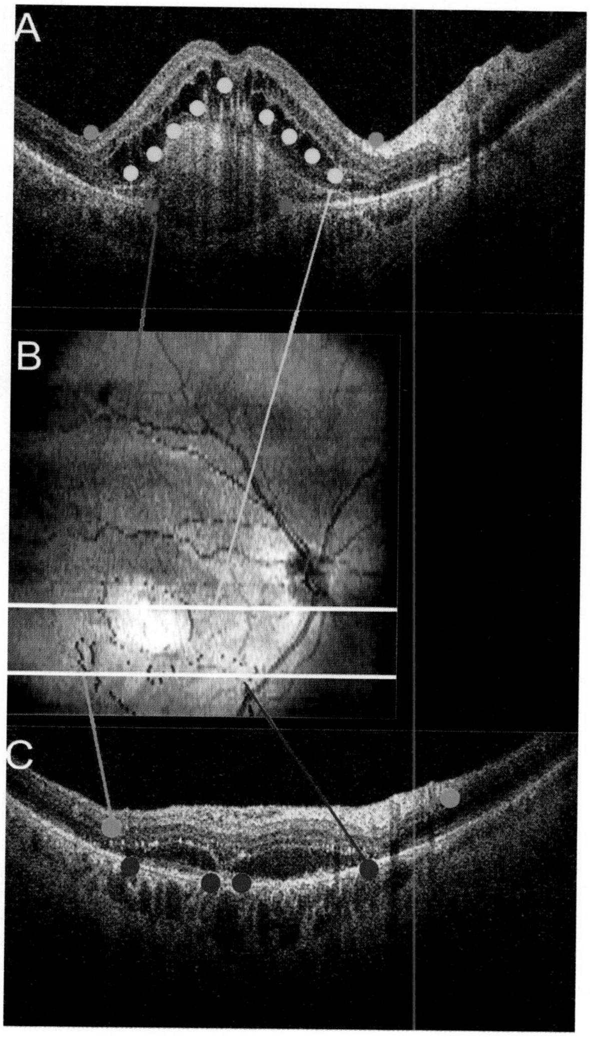

Figure 3: Generation of 3D images.

A): Example of a single B-Scan (*Prof. J.A. Yzatt's research prototype system)*.

B): 3D representation of 100 B-scan images after axial registration.

C): SVP (summed voxel projection) 2D image.
This image was created by summation of all B-scans in an axial direction.

Figure 4: SD-OCT B-scan *(Prof. J.A. Yzatt's research prototype system).*

A): Through the fovea: the edges of the CNV (red), cystoid macular edema (yellow), diffuse macular edema (green), and subretinal fluid (blue) are highlighted on each scan.

B): SVP (summed voxel projection) on OCT and color coding delineate the various lesions on an *en face* image (Nolan 2007[15]).

C): B-scan through subretinal fluid.

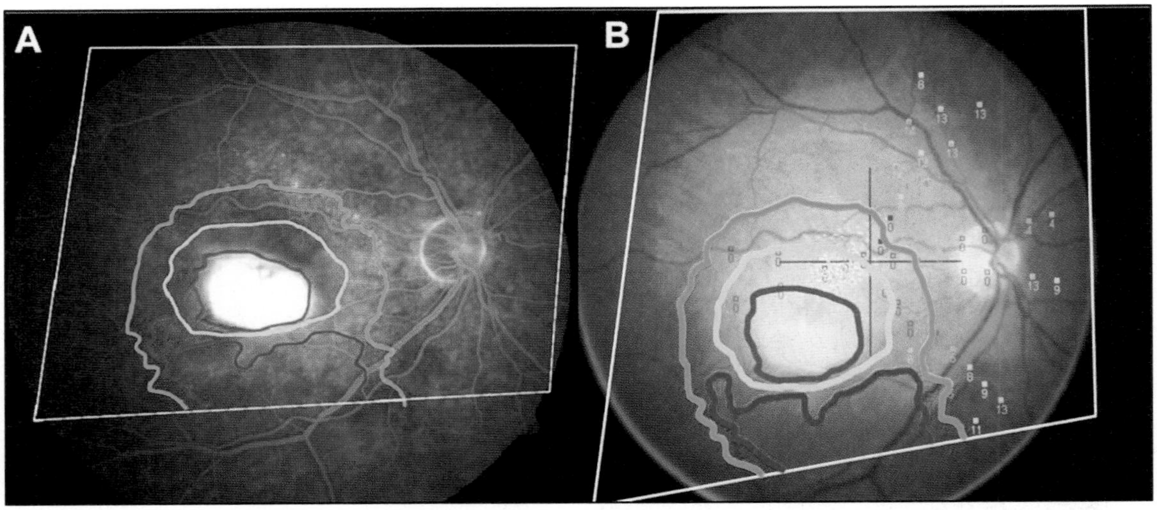

Figure 5: Color-coded SVP image (*right eye of patient shown in Figure 4*), co-registered with fluorescein angiography (**A**) and a microperimetry image (**B**).

A): Co-registered *en face* image showing the extent of the CNV (red), cystoid macular edema (yellow), diffuse macular edema (green), and subretinal fluid (blue), related to hyper-fluorescence on the angiogram. In this case, early hyper-fluorescence on fluorescein angiography corresponds to the zone of CNV on the *en face* SD-OCT image.

Subretinal fluid was barely visible on angiography after 6 minutes.

B): On microperimetry and on the co-registered angiographic image, macular edema on SD-OCT extends for about one disc diameter beyond the limits of the CNV and exactly corresponds to the zone of non-response on microperimetry (**B**). (*The frame shows the limits of the zone of investigation on SD-OCT.*)

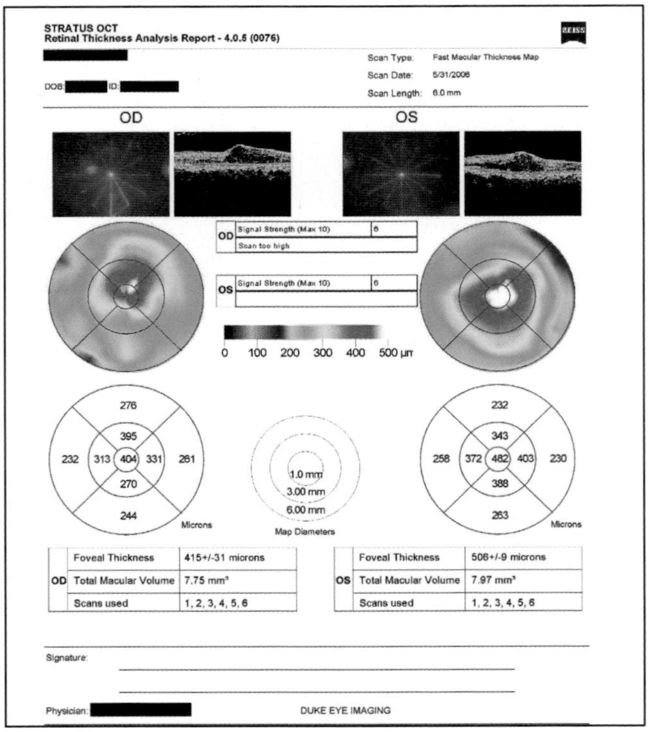

Figure 6: Example of a macular thickness map obtained with *Stratus* TD-OCT.*

The thickness of each field and color representations are extrapolated from 6 radial scans.

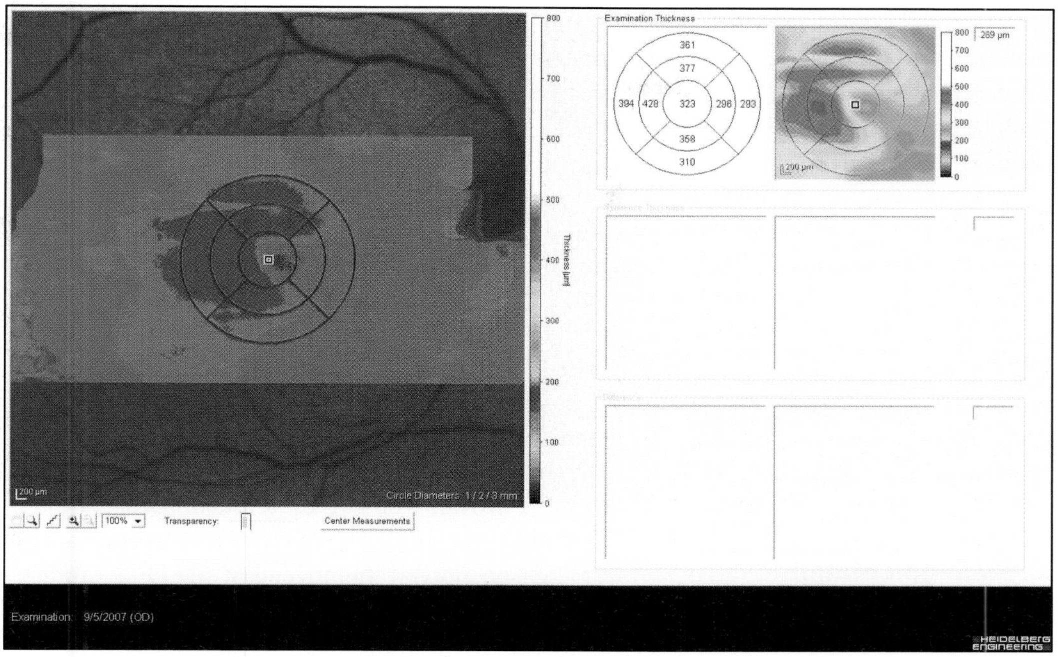

Figure 7: Example of a macular thickness map obtained with *Spectralis** (Heidelberg Engineering, GmbH) (The right eye of the patient is shown in Figure 6.)
The user can shift the frames to measure retinal thickness in all zones studied. The map is also recorded and co-registered on the green images generated by the SLO.

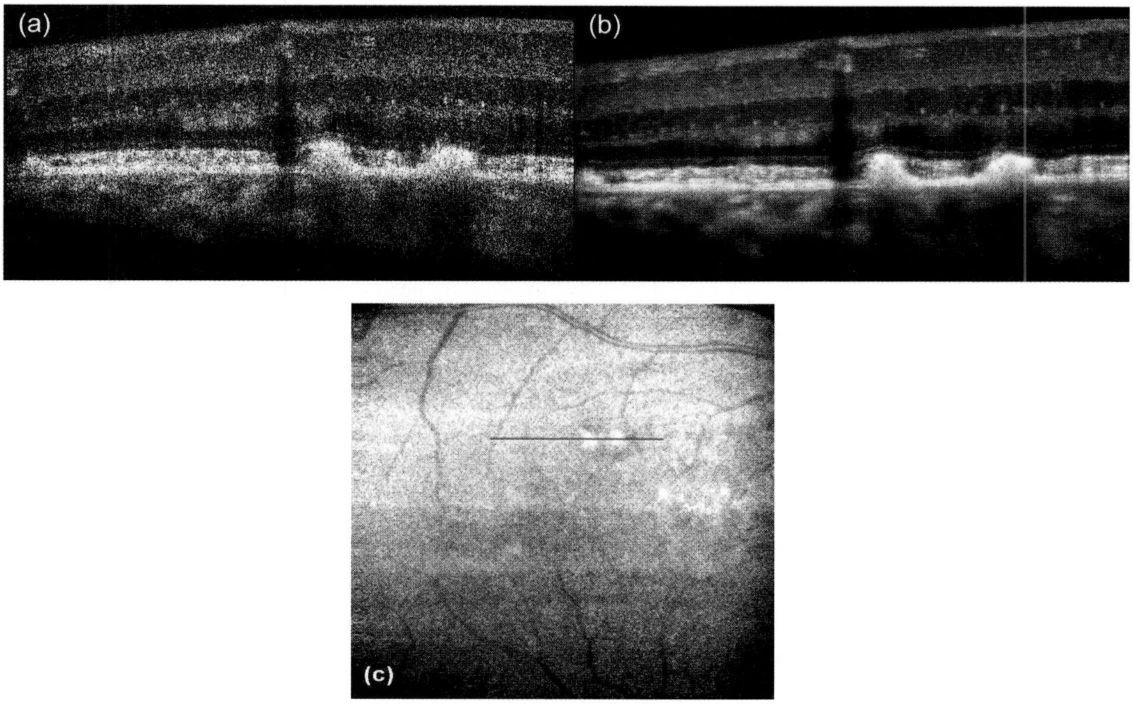

Figure 8: Application of *Adaptive Optics-OCT for the detection of drusen (Farsiu 2008**[43]) [*Courtesy of Dr D.X. Hammer*].
a): Single high- resolution *Adaptive Optics-OCT* image.
b): Summation of 11 aligned images.
c): Approximate localization of this scan on the SLO image, indicated by a red line.

The short acquisition time also allows imaging of the *entire macular region* and non-interpolated thickness and volumetric analysis based on images acquired simultaneously and co-registered with the fundus image (**Figures 5, 7, and 8**), thereby allowing measurement of retinal thickness at any point on the macula.

This allows a reduction of "erroneous" foveal thickness measurements due to decentration of macular images on TD-OCT.

With SD-OCT, the *center of the fovea* can be identified manually or automatically. Images in 3D can be obtained to analyze drusen, pigment epithelial detachments (PEDs), and choroidal neovascular complexes.

2. Retinal Layer Segmentation

Time-domain OCT can be used to measure the thickness of the nerve fiber layer or the entire retina from the vitreoretinal interface to the RPE. However, changes external to the RPE, such as PEDs or CNV, are not measured with conventional software.

OCT Reading Centers for clinical studies of AMD use custom programs or manual measurement, as conventional TD-OCT is unable to isolate a specific layer of the posterior segment other than the nerve fiber layer (*Zhang 2007*[24]).

Consequently, the volume of a PED or the subretinal space cannot be calculated in the context of long-term follow-up.

SD-OCT facilitates image segmentation by improved boundary identification: it is now possible to distinguish certain layers of the retina such as the *plexiform layer*, *subretinal space*, and *subretinal pigment epithelial space* (**Figures 9 and 10**).

These segmented layers can be used for further analysis, such as measuring the thickness and volume of individual retinal layers and monitoring these changes over time (*Farsiu 2005*[25], *Haeker 2007*[26]).

Segmentation of retinal layers into a *neurosensory component* and a *subretinal space component* is also a promising new option to monitor the course of the disease.

3. Drusen

For decades, *in vivo* imaging of drusen was based on **color fundus photography**. Epidemiologic studies use this modality to evaluate the distinctness, area, and number of drusen.

This assessment is used to predict the risk of AMD progression, despite the limited agreement between observers (*AREDS 2001*[27]).

Imaging of drusen remains limited on **TD-OCT** due to various artifacts.

With SD-OCT (or UHR-OCT), improved **imaging of drusen** constitutes a major progress (*Pieroni 2006*[7]). While color photography may suggest a certain degree of phenotypic homogeneity, SD-OCT studies demonstrate the **detailed structure of drusen** (**Figure 11**).

In vivo evaluation of drusen composition is important in view of recent *histopathologic* and *genetic* findings demonstrating phenotypic variability related to the *presence of* **various components** such as amyloid β (*Anderson 2004*[28]), activated complement products (*Anderson 2002*[29]), glycoproteins, and choroidal dendritic cell processes (*Hageman 2001*[30]). However, the correlation between these findings and genetic markers and the risk of progression is unknown at the present time.

Segmentation techniques can precisely identify areas of RPE elevation (**Figures 9A and 9B**) and variability in drusen structure (**Figures 2, 10, 11, 12, and 13**), taking into account differences in shape, internal reflectivity, and homogeneity, which provide considerable precision to the analysis of drusen (*Khanifar 2007*[31]).

Imaging of the **internal structure of drusen** is now possible and could be an indirect measurement of complement-related activity (**Figure 13**). However, this work has not yet been validated by clinical studies.

These segmentation techniques can also be used to measure **total drusen volume** in the context of monitoring of disease progression and to assess the risk of progression (**Figure 14**). Computer-assisted analysis can be used to automate these studies.

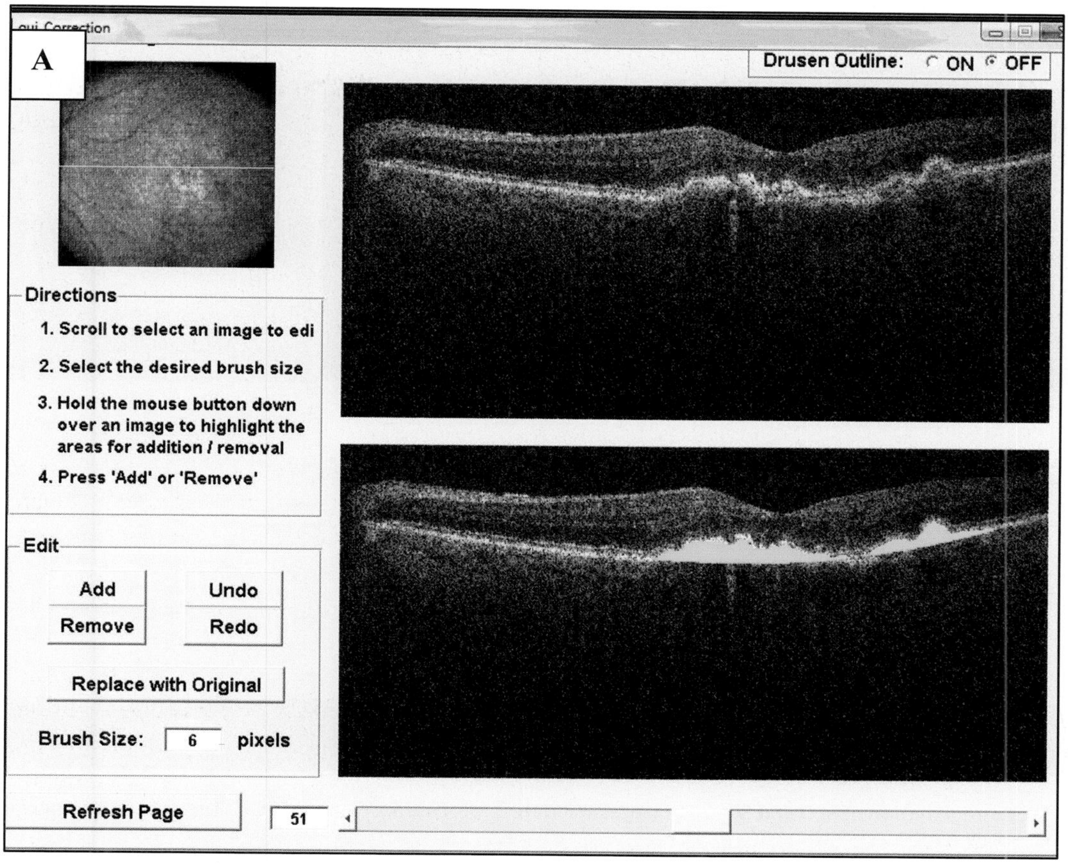

Figure 9A): Screenshot of the Duke OCT Retinal Analysis Program (DOCTRAP) and the Main Graphical User Interface (GUI).

With this equipment, the user can visualize and modify the automatic segmentation algorithm.

The area of drusen, obtained with the *Bioptigen Inc System** SD-OCT image (top right), is yellow on the bottom right image. The corresponding site of the B-scan on SVP is indicated on the top left section of the GUI.

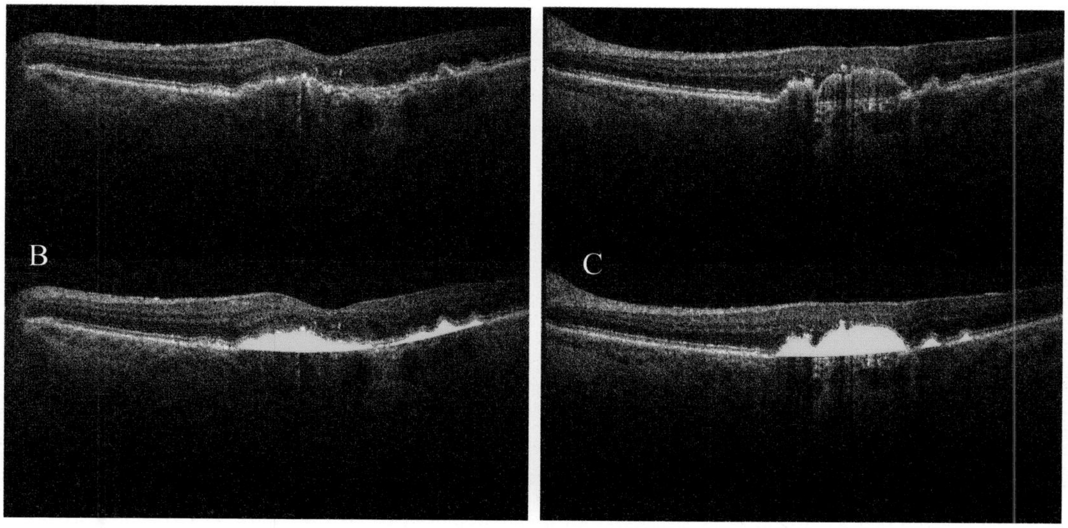

Figure 9B): and **C): Another example of segmentation of drusen.**

The original SD-OCT image is shown above with the automatically segmented image of the drusen below.

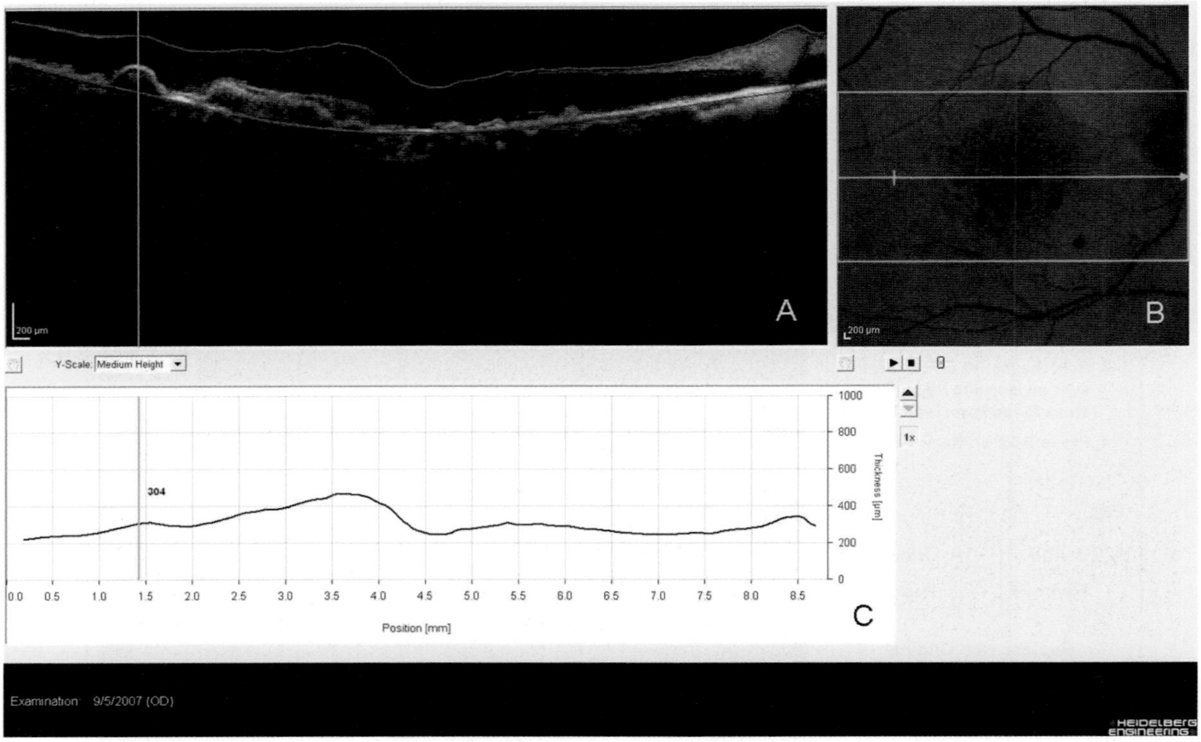

Figure 10: Co-registration of SLO and SD-OCT images using the prototype *Spectralis** SD-OCT (Heidelberg Engineering, GmbH).

A): SD-OCT image with segmentation of the neurosensory retina (red line). Note that the drusen are included in the area of the neurosensory retina.

B): The limits of the volumetric scan corresponding to the *en face* SLO image are indicated by green lines. The green line with a landmark shows the site of the scan shown in **A**.

C): The estimated retinal thickness is shown in **C**.

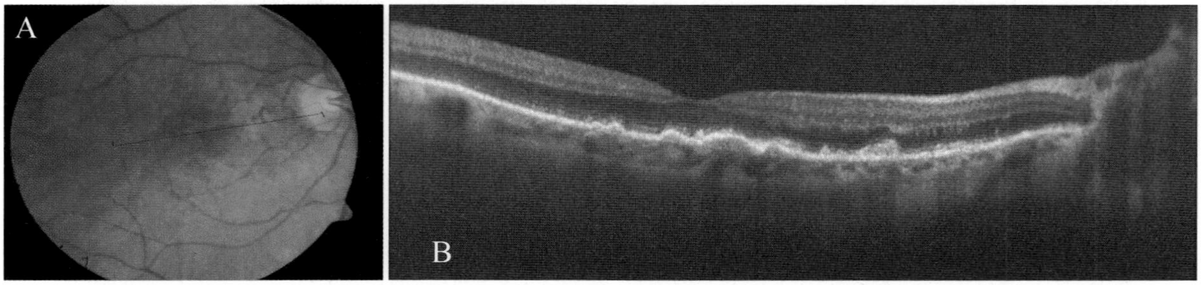

Figure 11: Comparison of the value of color photography. A): compared to **SD-OCT imaging. B): to localize drusen.** The black line on the color photograph corresponds to the plane of the SD-OCT scan (*Bioptigen Corporation System**).

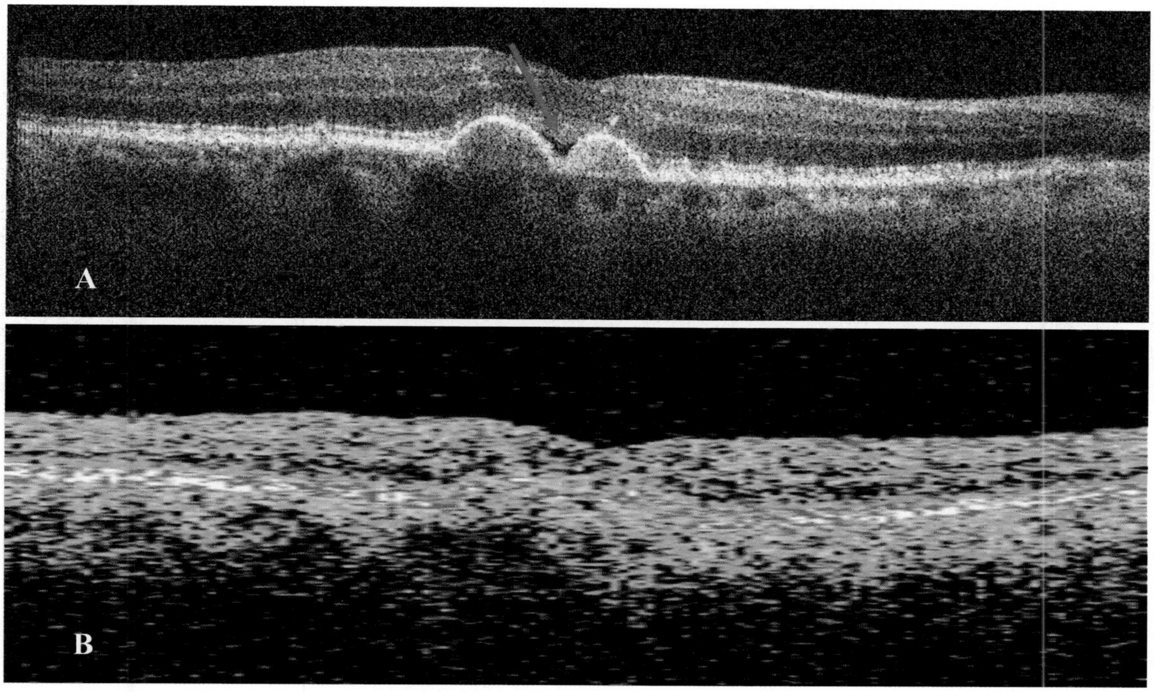

Figure 12: Comparison of detection of drusen with:
A): SD-OCT, *Bioptigen Inc System** and
B): *Stratus TD-OCT** System. Note the small zone of hypo-reflectivity (red arrow) suggestive of subretinal fluid on the SD-OCT image.

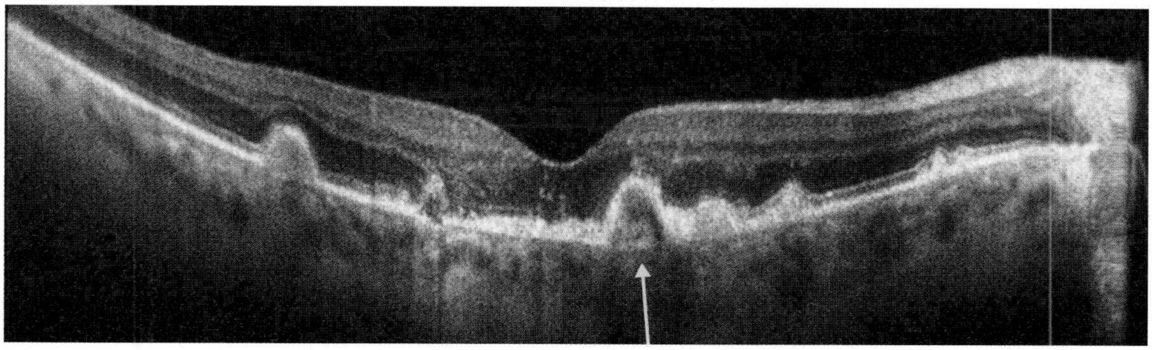

Figure 13: Example of an SD-OCT B-scan (*Bioptigen, Inc. System**) showing variable appearances of drusen. The arrow shows a drusen with an apparent nucleus.

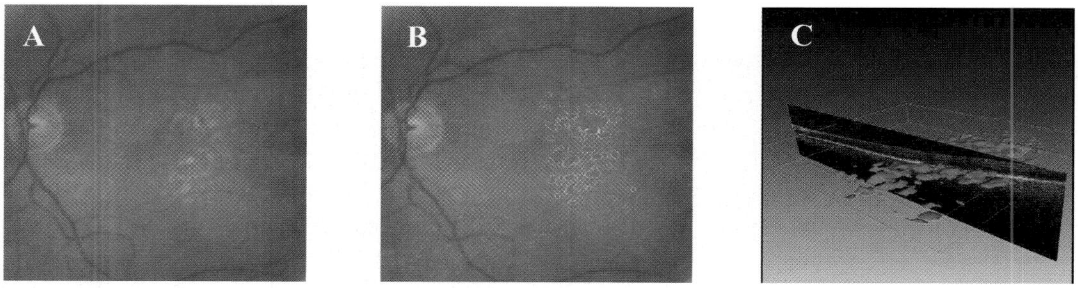

Figure 14: Volumetric representation of an SD-OCT image, which facilitates detection and analysis of drusen (*Prof J.A. Yzatt's research prototype system*).
A): Classic fundus photograph.
B): Apparent site of the drusen, shown on 2D image (fuchsia color).
C): With SD-OCT, it is possible to register and interpolate the sequence of B-scans, creating a 3D representation of the zone of drusen, their shape, and their volume (measured at 0.323 mm^3).

4. Choroidal Neovascularization

Conventional TD-OCT imaging revolutionized the assessment of retinal response to CNV by visualizing the frequent appearances of *macular edema* and **subretinal fluid**.

These images also established a correlation between visual acuity and the presence of cystoid macular edema, and between OCT measurements and response to therapy (Ting 2002[13]).

TD-OCT can also demonstrate the presence of **fibrovascular complexes** in the subretinal and sub-RPE space.

SD-OCT appears to be more easily quantifiable and more reliable to monitor **response to treatment** (**Figure 4**).

With SD-OCT, it is easier to differentiate between *type 1* and *type 2* membranes and to create a three-dimensional reconstruction of the neovascular complex and associated retinal lesions (*Schmidt-Erfurth 2005*[32]).

These relationships can be projected onto SVP images and correlated with fluorescein angiography or microperimetry for long-term follow-up (**Figure 3**).

Small foci of PED, CNV, or subretinal fluid are also more easily detected (*Stopa 2007*[22]).

This is particularly useful for the diagnosis of **chorioretinal anastomoses** or retinal angiomatous proliferation.

SLO SD-OCT will also be particularly useful to generate 3D datasets incorporating both angiographic data and high-resolution SD-OCT imaging (**Figure 15**).

Co-registration of SD-OCT with the fundus image, fluorescein angiography, and indocyanine green angiography facilitates precise identification of the site of CNV and changes in CNV over time.

This new imaging modality and these volume studies will allow more precise clinical studies.

5. Geographic Atrophy

Clinical studies are currently based on color photographs or, more recently, *autofluorescence* (Holz 2007[33], Bindewald 2005[34]).

Areas of atrophy can sometimes be demonstrated: RPE atrophy induces increased choroidal hyper-reflectivity.

The improved **transverse resolution** of SD-OCT more clearly delineates the borders between normal and abnormal RPE (**Figure 16**) and associated lesions (drusen, pigment changes, and photoreceptors).

As OCT measures **changes of tissue reflectivity** rather than physiologic changes (eg, lipofuscin deposition visible on autofluorescence), it provides a different method for identifying these atrophic areas.

The optimal method would be to **fuse the information** derived from these two imaging modalities, as with the *Heidelberg SLO-OCT*, which captures autofluorescent imaging integrated with 3D SD-OCT volume.

Once again, segmentation techniques allow correlation of RPE changes with changes of the overlying photoreceptor layer (**Figure 16**).

Comparative Analysis

Integrating data from different imaging sources is often very challenging, but certainly very useful for diagnostic and prognostic purposes, especially to identify the location relative to a specific retinal landmark, of an abnormality found on a 3D OCT image set.

This is made possible by **co-registration** of OCT and fundus images and the eye-tracking system (**Figures 4, 5, and 10**) *(Srinivasan 2006*[5]*)*.

Clinicians are currently able to define pathology on anteroposterior OCT scans based on previous clinicopathologic correlation studies (Toth 1997[10,11]).

However, this information is not sufficiently precise to define the **margins of the lesion,** and SD-OCT data are not integrated with conventional fundus imaging.

SVP images can be used to orient SD-OCT data in relation to a fundus image. It would also be very useful to combine *en face* images with OCT images.

Most communication still uses **printed documents** and therefore translation of 3D images into smaller 2D images that are easier to use in clinical practice than video sequences.

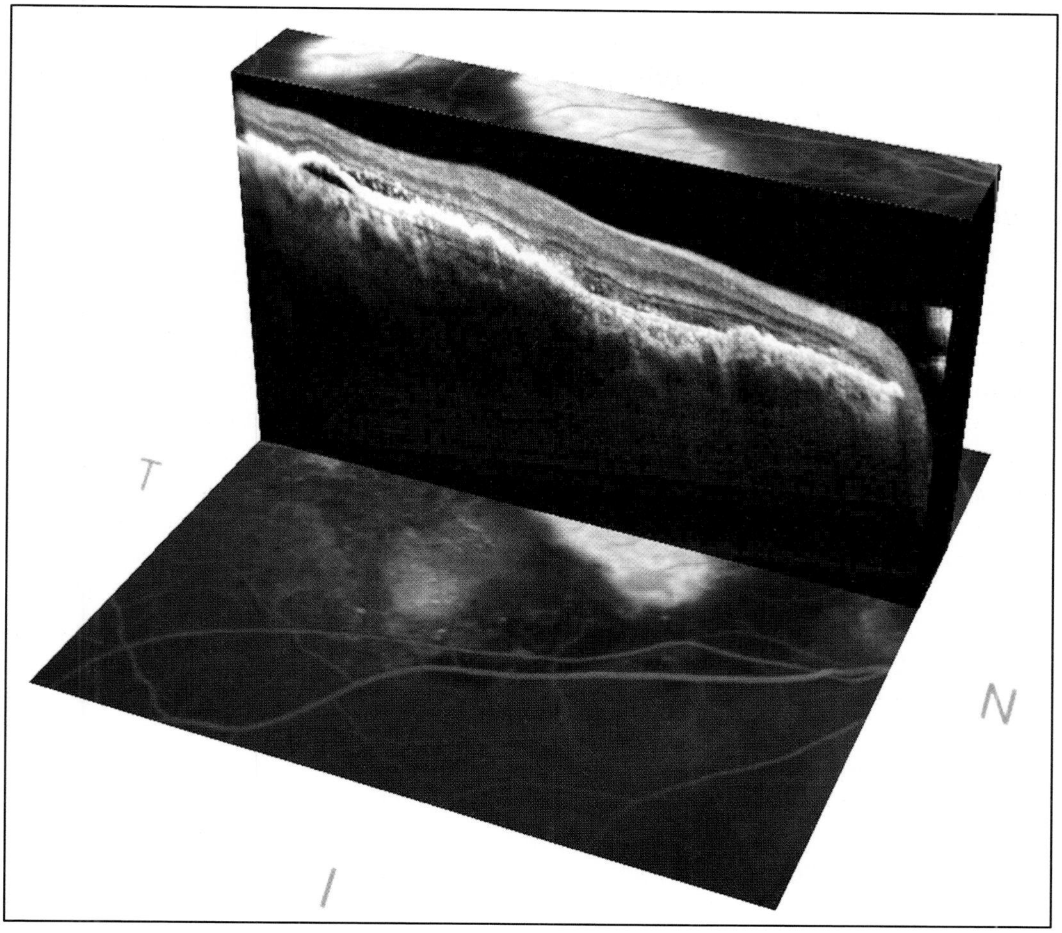

Figure 15: 3D image, *Spectralis SD-OCT (Heidelberg Engineering, GmbH).**
The bottom surface is a representation of fluorescein angiography after simultaneous acquisition by the SLO. Point by point correspondence between OCT and angiography.

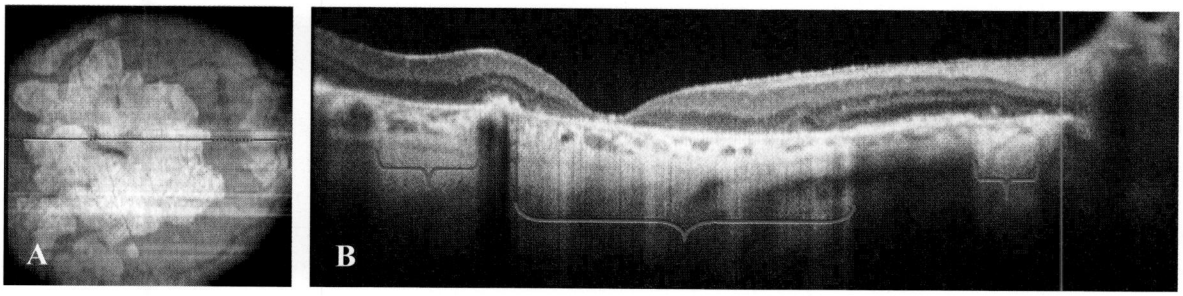

Figure 16: Value of SD-OCT for the detection of geographic atrophy *(SD-OCT, Bioptigen, Inc. System*)*.
A): SVP of an eye with geographic atrophy. The zone of atrophy appears pale and well-delineated on the SVP image. The red line shows the approximate site of the B-scan.
B): B-scan: The brackets in (B) correspond to the red line in (A), and emphasize the increased choroidal hyper-reflectivity characteristic of geographic atrophy.

It also remains difficult to correlate SD-OCT images with **microperimetry** data or fundus photographs captured in another session.

Current developments are designed to allow visualization of the extent of retinal lesions and to integrate these data into *en face* images to be used as a reference point (**Figures 4 and 5**) *(Stopa 2007[22])*.

Image Processing

In many practical cases, including studies of large patient cohorts, the large volume of information generated by the SD-OCT system is often too large and time-consuming to be fully analyzed and interpreted.

The development of *automatic or semiautomatic analysis systems* is therefore essential.

New image enhancement and image analysis algorithms are being developed for this purpose.

Image enhancement comprises denoising, deblurring, and contrast enhancement.

Image analysis uses computer-aided diagnosis and measurement algorithms.

The most important algorithm for image enhancement uses a computer to increase the SNR of the image.

Noise removal algorithms are essentially based on averaging of multiple images *(ImageJ–Rasband 2007[35] or MATLAB)*.

Special digital filters can be applied to reduce the noise level *(Ozcan 2007[36])*. While these filtering techniques reduce image sharpness, they can still provide very useful results (**Figures 17A, 17B, and 17C**) *(Farsius 2005[25], Thévenas 1998[38], Takeda 2007[39])*.

Semiautomatic segmentation techniques for **fluid-filled regions** have been developed for OCT images of AMD *(Fernandez 2005[40], Perona 1990[41], Xu 1998[42])*.

Automatic or semiautomatic **thickness measurements** of the various layers of the retina in AMD have been developed to allow separation of the retina into 5 layers on 3D images *(Fernandez 2005[37])*.

A fully automated method has been recently proposed to detect and segment drusen in retinal images captured by SD-OCT systems *(Graphical User Interface)* (**Figures 9 and 10**) *(Fernandez 2005[40], Perona 1990[41])*.

These studies can also be performed with the Heidelberg SD-OCT.

Challenges and Future Directions in SD-OCT Imaging

3D imaging using SD-OCT allows more detailed analysis of pathologic changes in the retina.

In particular, identification of very early changes in the various layers of the retina should be possible despite the inherent limitations of new software *(van Velthoven 2007[44])*.

Adaptive Optics

Integration of the **adaptive optics** into SD-OCT systems could be one of the most exciting advances *(Zawadzki 2005[45], Hammer 2007[46])*.

Adaptive optics uses a deformable mirror for wavefront estimation and correction of optical aberrations and even complex forms of astigmatism called coma or trefoil astigmatism.

The first laboratory applications of this system for detection of drusen appear to be very promising.

Registration and averaging of these images can improve their quality by demonstrating RPE abnormalities and all retinal layers (**Figures 8A and 8B**) *(Hammer 2007[46])*.

Biomarkers

SD-OCT techniques can now identify **biomarkers** to evaluate and possibly predict progression of AMD and measure changes in volume or extent.

A logical next step would be integration of methods able to measure *Doppler shifts* due to blood flow, *tissue oxygenation* based on spectroscopy, and intraretinal physiological responses by *birefringence* (*Yazdanfar 2003[47], Cense 2006[48]*).

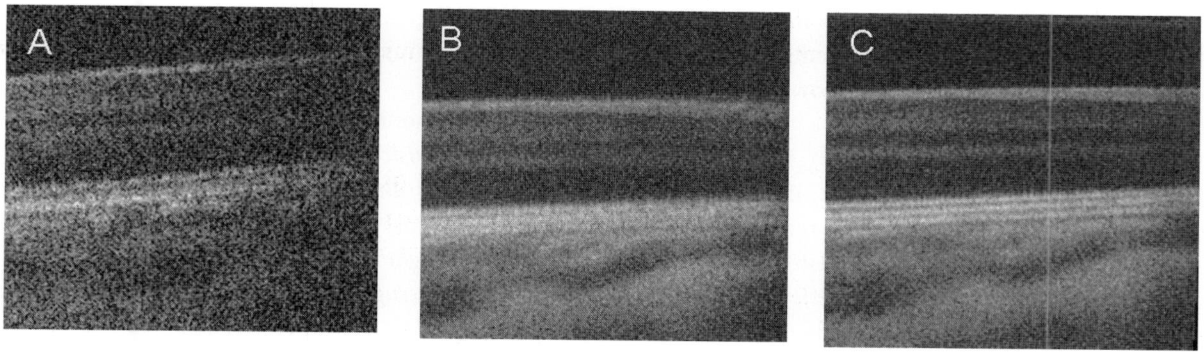

Figure 17: Effect of precise registration of averaged images:

A): Original B-scan.

B): B-scan after ImageJ registration.

C): B-scan after more robust image registration and filtering techniques.

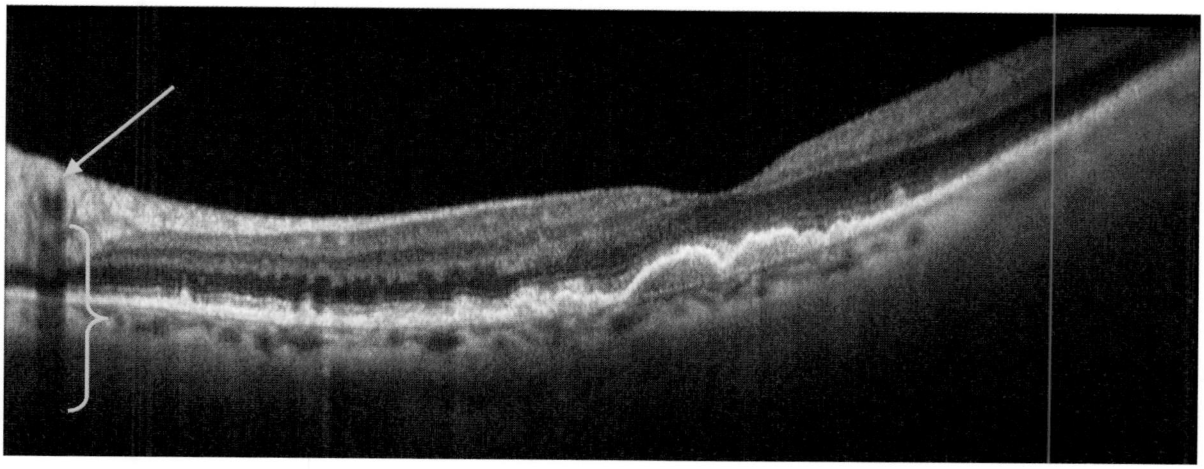

Figure 18: SD-OCT B-scan (*Bioptigen, Inc. System**)
Shadowing by a large vessel (arrow) in the peri-papillary region is clearly visible.

SD-OCT imaging may improve *phenotype-genotype correlations* and analysis of the course of the disease in clinical studies.

SD-OCT imaging is based on the location and differences in reflectance, and proximal hyper-reflective structures such as retinal vessels therefore shadow the underlying structures (**Figure 18**).

However, despite improved resolution, if a cell or tissue structure of interest does not differ in reflectivity relative to surrounding tissue, it cannot be isolated by OCT.

Future progress could include methods to **enhance contrast in reflectivity** of structures of interest.

The *sensitivity* and *specificity* of SD-OCT detection of lesions such as drusen or neovascularization have not been clearly established at the present time and will also depend on image processing and interpretation of these scans, which could become automated and reproducible.

Registration

Another challenge concerns the **registration** and accessibility of very large 3D datasets, and the development of data compression and transfer systems *(Wojtkowski 2005[6])*.

Eye motion artifacts could be corrected by eye-tracking systems and integration of SLO and SD-OCT systems.

Finally, the great variety of commercially available SD-OCT systems have created a highly competitive market as well as problems of compatibility and comparability of the images acquired by these systems, which can only be resolved by the development of **consensus standards**.

Conclusion

Spectral-Domain OCT provides several advantages compared to Time-Domain OCT, essentially shorter **acquisition times** and improved **axial resolution**.

Modern techniques allow *volumetric imaging* and B-scan co-registration with other types of fundus imaging, such as color photography and fluorescein and ICG angiography.

Denoising and **layer segmentation** also improve image quality, particularly for imaging of drusen and the consequences of CNV or geographic atrophy.

Trials of **quantification** and long-term **follow-up** will contribute to the prognostic assessment and treatment follow-up of AMD.

This technological progress will considerably improve the noninvasive study of retinal disease processes.

Acknowledgments

The authors wish to thank Dr. Daniel X. Hammer, Prof. Joseph A. Izatt, Bradley Bower, Dr. Neeru Sarin, Michelle McCall, Katrina Winter, and Anjum Koreishi for providing invaluable insight and data throughout this project.

This work was supported in part by National Institutes of Health Grant R21EY017393, National Institutes of Health Small Business Investigational Grant Subcontract from Bioptigen Inc., and by North Carolina Biotechnology Center Collaborative Funding Grant 2007-CFG-8005, entitled "Improving Imaging of Phenotypes in Age-Related Macular Degeneration."

References

1. **Farsiu S, Christofferson J, Eriksson B, Milanfar P, Friedlander B, Shakouri A, Nowak R.** Statistical detection and imaging of objects hidden in turbid media using ballistic photons. *Applied Opt 2007;46:5805-5822.*
2. **Huang D, Swanson EA, Lin CP, Schuman JS, Stinson WG, Chang W, Hee MR, Flotte T, Gregory K, Puliafito CA.** Optical coherence tomography. *Science 1991;254:1178-1181.*
3. **Dunsby C, French PMW.** Techniques for depth-resolved imaging through turbid media including coherence-gated imaging. *J Phys D:Appl Phys 2003;36:207-227.*
4. **Fercher AF, Drexler W, Hitzenberger CK, Lasser T.** Optical coherence tomography-principles and applications. *Rep Prog Phys 2003;66:239-303.*
5. **Srinivasan VJ, Wojtkowski M, Witkin AJ, Duker JS, Ko TH, Carvalho M, Schuman JS, Kowalczyk A, Fujimoto JG.** High-definition and 3-dimensional imaging of macular pathologies with high-speed ultrahigh-resolution optical coherence tomography. *Ophthalmology 2006;113:2054-2065.*
6. **Wojtkowski M, Srinivasan V, Fujimoto JG, Ko T, Schuman JS, Kowalczyk A, Duker JS.** Three-dimensional retinal imaging with high-speed ultrahigh-resolution optical coherence tomography. *Ophthalmology 2005;112:1734-1746.*
7. **Pieroni CG, Witkin AJ, Ko TH, Fujimoto JG, Chan A, Schuman JS, Ishikawa H, Reichel E, Duker JS.** Ultrahigh resolution optical coherence tomography in non-exudative age related macular degeneration. *Br J Ophthalmol 2006;90:191-197.*
8. **Hee MR, Izatt JA, Swanson EA, Huang D, Schuman JS, Lin CP, Puliafito CA, Fujimoto JG.** Optical coherence tomography of the human retina. *Arch Ophthalmol 1995;113:325-332.*
9. **Puliafito CA, Hee MR, Lin CP, Reichel E, Schuman JS, Duker JS, Izatt JA, Swanson EA, Fujimoto JG.** Imaging of macular

diseases with optical coherence tomography. *Ophthalmology 1995;102:217-229.*
10. **Toth CA, Birngruber R, Boppart SA, Hee MR, Fujimoto JG, DiCarlo CD, Swanson EA, Cain CP, Narayan DG, Noojin GD, Roach WP.** Argon laser retinal lesions evaluated in vivo by optical coherence tomography. *Am J Ophthalmol 1997;123:188-198.*
11. **Toth CA, Narayan DG, Boppart SA, Hee MR, Fujimoto JG, Birngruber R, Cain CP, DiCarlo CD, Roach WP.** A comparison of retinal morphology viewed by optical coherence tomography and by light microscopy. *Arch Ophthalmol 1997;115:1425-1428.*
12. **Gallemore RP, Jumper JM, McCuen II BW, Jaffe GJ, Postel EA, Toth CA.** Diagnosis of vitreoretinal adhesions in macular disease with optical coherence tomography. *Retina 2000;20:115-120.*
13. **Ting TD, Oh M, Cox TA, Meyer CH, Toth CA.** Decreased visual acuity associated with cystoid macular edema in neovascular age-related macular degeneration. *Arch Ophthalmol 2002;120:731-737.*
14. **Radhakrishnan S, Rollins AM, Roth JE, Yazdanfar S, Westphal V, Bardenstein DS, Izatt JA.** Real-time optical coherence tomography of the anterior segment at 1310 nm. Arch Ophthalmol 2001;119:1179-1185.
15. **Nolan WP, See JL, Chew PT, Friedman DS, Smith SD, Radhakrishnan S, Zheng C, Foster PJ, Aung T.** Detection of primary angle closure using anterior segment optical coherence tomography in Asian eyes. *Ophthalmology 2007;114:33-39.*
16. **Hess DB, Asrani SG, Bhide MG, Enyedi LB, Stinnett SS, Freedman SF.** Macular and retinal nerve fiber layer analysis of normal and glaucomatous eyes in children using optical coherence tomography. *Am J Ophthalmol. 2005;139:509-17.*
17. **de Boer JF, Cense B, Park BH, Pierce MC, Tearney GJ, Bouma BE.** Improved signal-to-noise ratio in spectral-domain compared with time-domain optical coherence tomography. *Opt Lett 2003;28:2067-2069.*
18. **Chen TC, Cense B, Pierce MC, Nassif N, Park BH, Yun SH, White BR, Bouma BE, Tearney GJ, de Boer JF.** Spectral domain optical coherence tomography: ultra-high speed, ultra-high resolution ophthalmic imaging. *Arch Ophthalmol 2005;123:1715-1720.*
19. **Costa RA, Skaf M, Melo LA, Calucci D, Cardillo JA, Castro JC, Huang D, Wojtkowski M.** Retinal assessment using optical coherence tomography. *Prog Retin Eye Res 2006;25:325-353.*
20. **Leitgeb R, Hitzenberger CK, Fercher AF.** Performance of Fourier domain vs. time domain optical coherence tomography. *Opt Express 2005;11:889-894.*
21. **Choma MA, Sarunic MV, Yang C, Izatt, JA.** Sensitivity advantage of swept-source and fourier-domain optical coherence tomography. *Opt Express 2003;11:2183-2189.*
22. **Stopa M, Bower BA, Davies E, Izatt JA, Toth CA.** Correlation of pathologic features in spectral domain OCT imaging with conventional retinal studies. *Retina 2008;28:298-308.*
23. **Jiao S, Knighton R, Huang X, Gregori G, Puliafito C.** Simultaneous acquisition of sectional and fundus ophthalmic images with spectral-domain optical coherence tomography. Opt Express 2005;13:444-452.
24. **Zhang N, Hoffmeyer GC, Young ES, Burns RE, Winter KP, Stinnett SS, Toth CA, Jaffe GJ.** Optical coherence tomography reader agreement in neovascular age-related macular degeneration. *Am J Ophthalmol 2007;144:37-44.*
25. **Farsiu S, Elad M, Milanfar P.** Constrained, globally optimal, multi-frame motion estimation. *Proc IEEE Workshop on Statistical Signal Processing 2005;July:1396-1401.*
26. **Haeker M, Sonka M, Kardon R, Shah VA, Wu X, Abràmoff MD.** Automated segmentation of intraretinal layers from macular optical coherence tomography images. *Proc SPIE 2007;6512:651214-1 to 651214-11.*
27. **Age-related eye disease study research group.** The age-related eye disease study system for classifying age-related macular degeneration from stereoscopic color fundus photographs: the age-related eye disease study report number 6. *Am J Ophthalmol 2001;132:668-681*
28. **Anderson DH, Talaga KC, Rivest AJ, Barron E, Hageman GS, Johnson LV.** Characterization of β amyloid assemblies in drusen: the deposits associated with aging and age-related macular degeneration. *Exp Eye Res 2004;78:243-256.*
29. **Anderson DH, Mullins RF, Hageman GS, Johnson LV.** A role for local inflammation in the formation of drusen in the aging eye. *Am J Ophthalmol 2002;134:411-431.*
30. **Hageman GS, Luthert PJ, Victor Chong NH, Johnson LV, Anderson DH, Mullin RF.** An integrated hypothesis that considers drusen as biomarkers of immune-mediated processes at the RPE-Bruch's membrane interface in aging and age-related macular degeneration. *Prog Retin Eye Res 2001;20: 705-732.*
31. **Khanifar AA, Koreishi AF, Izatt JA, Toth CA.** Drusen ultrastructure imaging with spectral domain optical coherence tomography in age-related macular degeneration. *Retina Society, October 2007, Boston, MA, USA.*
32. **Schmidt-Erfurth U, Leitgeb RA, Michels S, Povazay B, Sacu S, Hermann B, Ahlers C, Sattmann H, Scholda C, Fercher AF, Drexler W.** Three-dimensional ultrahigh-resolution optical coherence tomography of macular diseases. *Invest Ophthalmol Vis Sci. 2005;46:3393-402.*
33. **Holz FG, Bindewald-Wittich A, Fleckenstein M, Dreyhaupt J, Scholl HP, Schmitz-Valckenberg S.** Progression of geographic atrophy and impact of fundus autofluorescence patterns in age-related macular degeneration. *Am J Ophthalmol 2007;143:463-472.*
34. **Bindewald A, Schmitz-Valckenberg S, Jorzik JJ, Dolar-Szczasny J, Sieber H, Keilhauer C, Weinberger AWA, Dithmar S, Pauleikhoff D, Mansmann U, Wolf S, Holz FG.** Classification of abnormal fundus autofluorescence patterns in the junctional zone of geographic atrophy in patients with age related macular degeneration, *Br J Ophthalmol 2005;89: 874-878*
35. **Rasband WS, ImageJ,** *U. S. National Institutes of Health, Bethesda, Maryland, USA, 1997-2007, http://rsb.info.nih.gov/ij/.*
36. **Ozcan A, Bilenca A, Desjardins AE, Bouma BE, Tearney GJ.** Speckle reduction in optical coherence tomography images using digital filtering. *J Opt Soc Am 2007;24:1901-1910.*
37. **Fernandez DC, Salinas HM, Puliafito CA.** Automated detection of retinal layer structures on optical coherence tomography images. *Opt Express 2005;13:10200–10216.*
38. **Thévenaz P, Ruttimann UE, Unser M.** A pyramid approach to sub pixel registration based on intensity. *IEEE Trans Image Process 1998;7:27-41.*

39. **Takeda H, Farsiu S, Milanfar P.** Kernel regression for image processing and reconstruction. *IEEE Trans Image Process 2007;16:349-366.*
40. **Fernández DC.** Delineating fluid-filled region boundaries in optical coherence tomography images of the retina. *IEEE transactions on medical imaging 2005;24:929-945.*
41. **Perona P, Malik J.** Scale-space and edge detection using anisotropic diffusion. *IEEE Trans Pattern Anal Mach Intell 1990;12:629-639.*
42. **Xu C, Prince JL.** Generalized gradient vector flow external forces for active contours. *Signal Process, 1998;71:131-139.*
43. **Farsiu S, Chiu JC, Izatt JA, Toth CA.** Fast detection and segmentation of drusen in retinal optical coherence tomography images. *Proc SPIE Photonics West, San Jose, CA, 2008.*
44. **van Velthoven ME, Faber DJ, Verbraak FD, van Leeuwen TG, de Smet MD.** Recent developments in optical coherence tomography for imaging the retina. *Prog Retin Eye Res 2007;26:57-77.*
45. **Zawadzki R, Jones S, Olivier S, Zhao M, Bower B, Izatt J, Choi S, Laut S, Werner J.** Adaptive-optics optical coherence tomography for high-resolution and high-speed 3D retinal in vivo imaging. *Opt Express 2005;13:8532-8546.*
46. **Hammer DX, Iftimia NV, Bigelow CE, Ustun TE, Bloom B, Ferguson RD, Burns SA.** High resolution retinal imaging with a compact adaptive optics spectral domain optical coherence tomography system. *Proc SPIE 2007;Volume 6426.*
47. **Yazdanfar S, Rollins AM, Izatt JA.** In vivo imaging of human retinal flow dynamics by color Doppler optical coherence tomography. *Arch Ophthalmol 2003;121:235-239.*
48. **Cense B, Chen TC, Nassif N, Pierce MC, Yun SH, Park BH, Bouma BE, Tearney GJ, de Boer JF.** Ultra-high speed and ultra-high resolution spectral-domain optical coherence tomography and optical Doppler tomography in ophthalmology. *Bull Soc Belge Ophthalmol 2006;302:123-132.*

SPECTRAL-DOMAIN OCT
*Spectralis** HRA-OCT and *Cirrus** Zeiss

Andrea GIANI, Matteo CEREDA,
Giovanni STAURENGHI

Clinica Oculistica-Ospedale Luigi Sacco
Milan, Italy

Introduction

Optical coherence tomography (OCT) is a technology that allows noninvasive, almost histological tomographs of the retinal layers and anterior chamber structures.

Over recent years, the capacities of OCT for retinal diagnosis and follow-up have been improved, especially in vitreoretinal diseases, age-related macular degeneration, diabetic retinopathy, and macular dystrophies.

Principles

OCT is based on *low-coherence interferometry*, in which light is produced by a superluminescent diode (*high-resolution OCT*) or a femto-second laser (*ultra-high-resolution OCT*).

This light is split into two paths by optic fibers. The first, called *reference arm*, has a mirror that reflects light, while the second, called *sample arm*, is directed into the eye.

When light reflected from the two arms arrives simultaneously on the detector, it gives an **inteferometric signal**, and its amplitude is measured.

Time-Domain Technology

The first OCT systems were based on **time-domain technology** (TD-OCT), in which depth information (reflectance signal) is obtained by mechanical shifting of the mirror in the reference arm during each A-scan acquisition.

This helps to provide a graph of reflectance as a function of depth.

This technology is limited by the **time required to acquire** each **B-scan** (anteroposterior scan constituted by the various A-scan sequences). For example, it takes about 1 second to obtain a 512 A-scan tomogram, leading to possible artifacts due to eye movement.

Spectral Domain Technology

In **Spectral-Domain** OCT (SD-OCT), shifting of the mirror in the reference arm is not required, as the entire reflectance signal from the retina is acquired *simultaneously*.

Depth information is obtained by a *spectrometer* and analyzed by ***Fast Fourier Transformation.***

This allows a considerable reduction of the acquisition time and therefore enables a reduction of motion artifacts and the possibility of acquiring multiple B-scans within a very short time. This increased acquisition speed constitutes a **major progress** and has led to important new features.

- First, scans of an entire area can be obtained by acquiring successive adjacent B-scans. This area can then be studied point by point with no loss of information.

The examination can be performed simultaneously in various axes, allowing real 3D reconstruction.

- Second, real-time *image enhancement* (image averaging) systems can be developed to reduce *signal-to-noise ratio* (SNR) and improve the definition of single images.

3

*Spectralis** HRA-OCT

The **Spectralis*** is one of the newest OCTs based on spectral-domain technology and manufactured by *Heidelberg Engineering**. All features of spectral-domain technology are present with the possibility of simultaneous OCT examination and retinal imaging.

The **Scanning Laser Ophthalmoscope** *(SLO)* allows simultaneous acquisition of infrared, red-free, autofluorescence, and fluorescein and indocyanine green angiography.

The **technical specifications** are shown in the following table (**Table 1**).

Table 1. Spectralis* *Heidelberg Engineering** technical specifications.

Fluorescein angiography wavelength	488 nanometers
IR reflectance wavelength	760 nanometers
OCT wavelength	870 nanometers
OCT optical depth resolution	7 micrometers
OCT digital depth resolution	3.5 micrometers
OCT A-scan rate	40,000/second

Image Acquisition

*Spectralis** is an SLO-HRA angiography machine linked to a Spectral-Domain OCT module that can be used to obtain SLO fluorescein and/or indocyanine angiography or simultaneous acquisition of retinal images and OCT (**Figure 1**).

Software

The database *software and touchpad*, which allows selection of various laser filters and acquisition modalities, is identical to that of the conventional HRA.

When *acquiring simultaneous* SLO and OCT images, the operator can choose the position of the OCT scan line by clicking with the mouse on the SLO image and obtaining tomographic information on the most clinically relevant zones on the angiography or on retinal images.

The system is equipped with *Automatic Real Time mean function* (**ART software**) allowing real-time speckle noise reduction of images and **eye-tracking** technology (TruTrack™).

Single images or series of images can be obtained, allowing volume definition.

Single images can be produced by a *simple acquisition* of one B-scan and simultaneous retinal imaging.

Images can also be obtained by real time mean image *reconstruction* averaged in real time and calculated on a variable number of single scans.

The operator can choose the number of frames used, varying from 2 to 100 images, to achieve excellent definition.

The more the patient remains immobile, the more the software is able to use these images to reconstruct an averaged image, *thereby increasing definition and decreasing noise*.

The ***scan line position*** can be moved on the SLO image during acquisition.

Various OCT color presentations can be selected:
- Black for hyper-reflective zones and white for hypo-reflective zones, or vice versa, or
- Two *different color patterns* (normalized or customized).

The best presentation pattern to visualize fine structures is probably *black and white*, but this likely depends on the operator's usual practice and tends to be subjective (**Figure 2**).

A consecutive series of single B-scans (single or averaged) can be acquired on a 180° axis to ***reconstruct a volume***.

A grid can be displayed on the SLO image showing the position of each of the single B-scans. The operator can then move the camera to the center of the lesion or to an area of interest.

The density of scan lines and the dimensions of the zone examined can be selected on the grid.

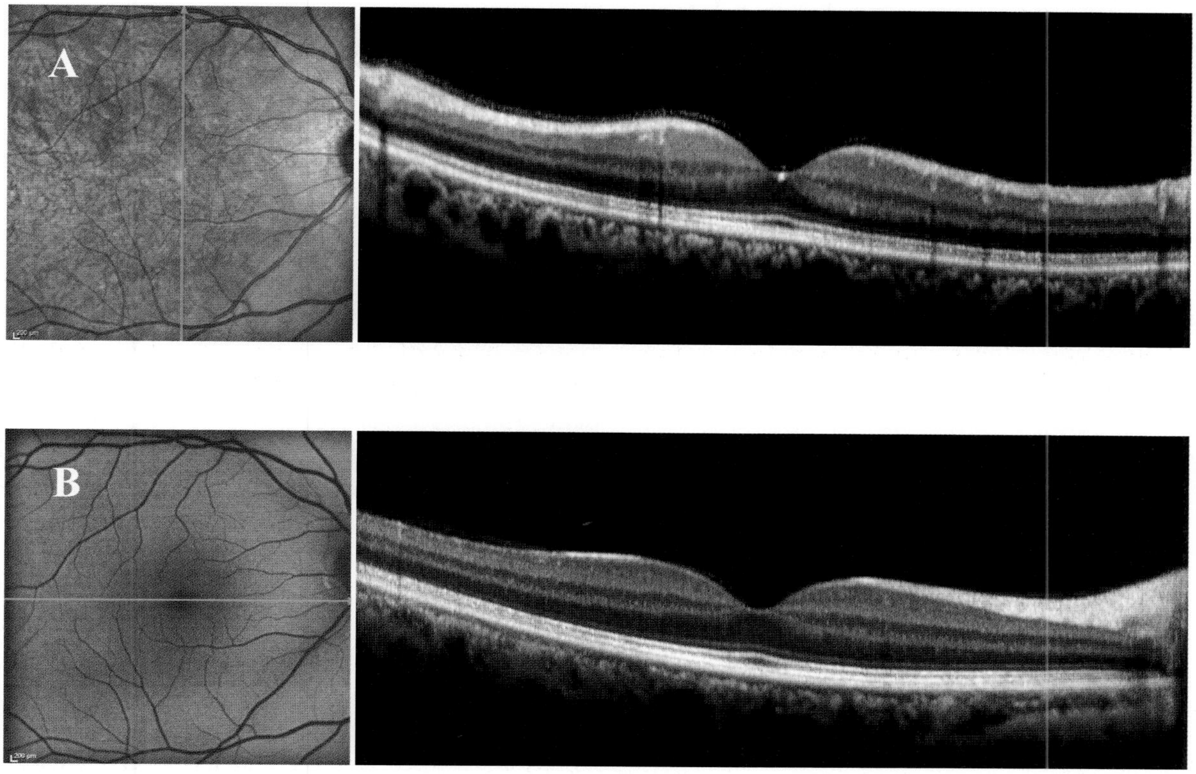

◘ Figure 1: Modern imaging of a normal retina (*Spectralis* Heidelberg Engineering).**
A): Infrared fundus photograph and horizontal OCT scan.
B): Autofluorescence fundus photograph and vertical OCT scan.

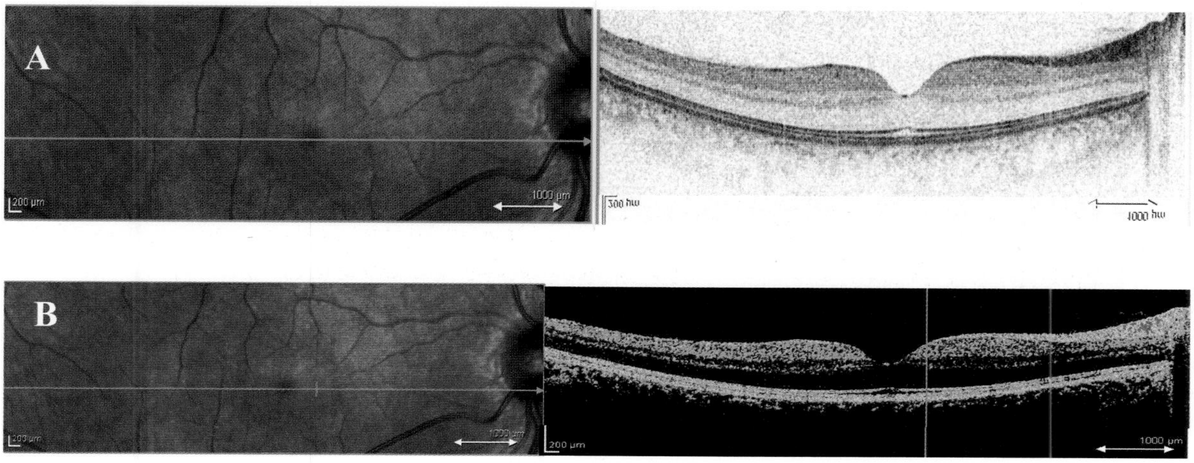

◘ Figure 2: Two different presentations of a linear OCT scan with *Spectralis* (Heidelberg Engineering*)* in the same normal subject.
A): Black and white: black for hyper-reflective structures and white for hypo-reflective structures.
B): Normal color fundus photograph and simple "false-color" OCT.

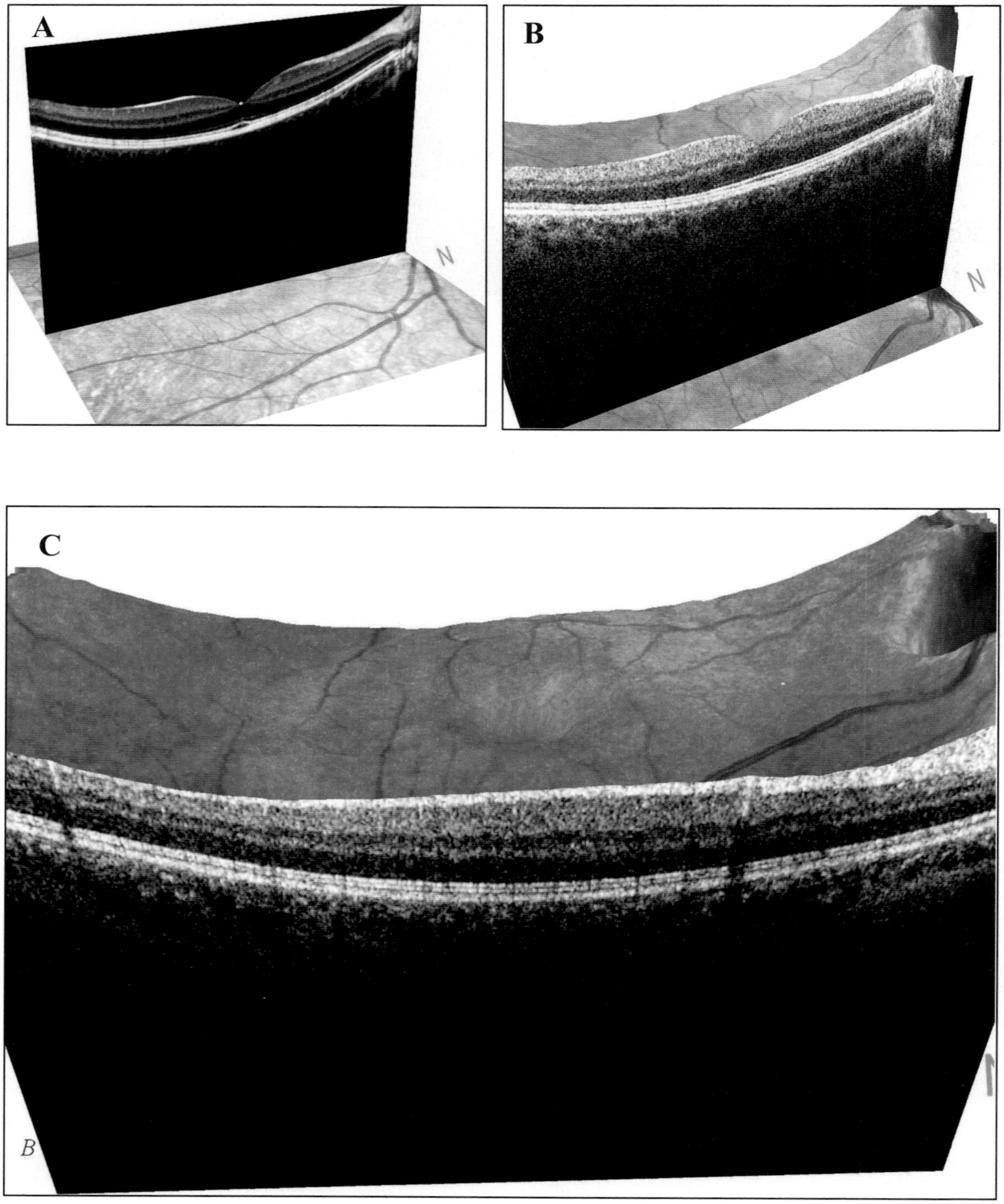

Figure 3: 3D reconstruction of OCT examinations.

A): Overlay of a single OCT scan of the fovea onto the infrared image.

B): Overlay of the OCT image and SLO funduscopy.

C): Overlay of infrared images and OCT, aligned to visualize the center of the fovea.

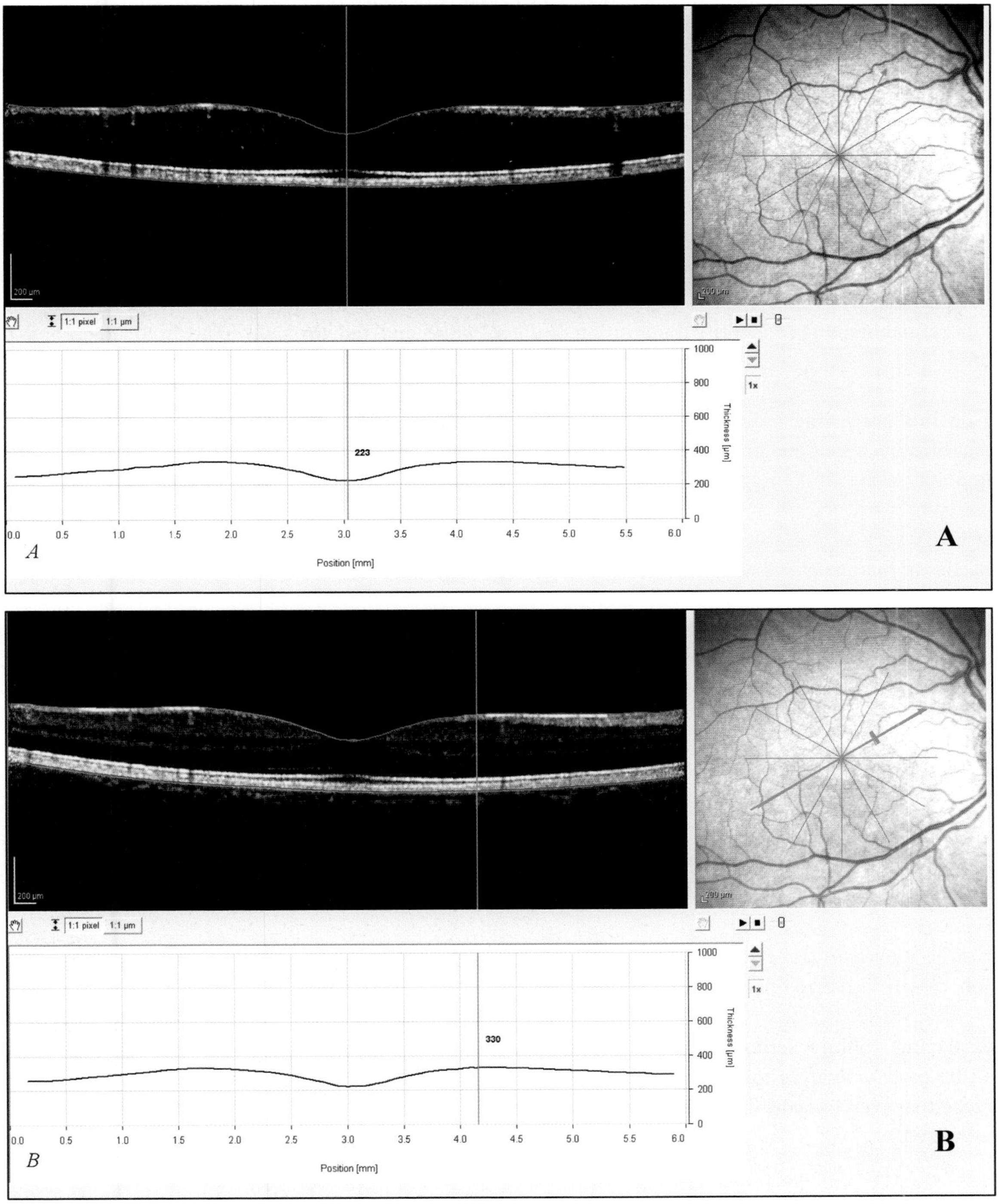

Figure 4: Simultaneous infrared and OCT images of the same normal retina showing how to identify the point of interest, visualize it on the OCT, and simultaneously see and measure the corresponding retinal thickness:

A): At the center of the fovea on the oblique line at 1 clock hour scan line.

B): At a point situated half a disc diameter from the fovea on the oblique line at 2 clock hours scan line.

Note the inner and outer boundaries of the retina, visible on the images (*red lines*).

The **acquisition speed** depends on the *dimensions* of the zone examined and especially on activation of the *ART system*.

All *images can be saved* and shown in Heidelberg software on completion of the acquisition session.

The Heidelberg **Eye Explorer software** allows visualization of each image already obtained.

Opening the selected image, SLO and OCT images appear in display mode, with a *green line* (horizontal or vertical) on retinal imaging to identify the position of the OCT scan.

Clicking on this green line indicates and visualizes the OCT scan line by a calliper and visualizes the corresponding point on the OCT image and vice versa.

This feature is very useful to investigate tomographic characteristics of *fine structures* within the image.

Acquisition of a star with variable position, size, and density allows not only vertical and horizontal sections, but also oblique sections always centered on the fovea.

3D Visualization Mode

In 3D visualization mode, SLO and OCT images are overlapped to more clearly visualize the various scans and tomography position.

Images can be moved in three axes and zoomed in and out to more clearly visualize fine structures (**Figure 3**).

When displaying volume series, the 3D visualization mode can be used to analyze tomographs in three axes: x, y, and z, so that even C-scans (**frontal or coronal** plane) can be visualized.

Thickness Measurement Mode

In thickness measurement mode, the software defines the inner and outer limits of the retina, **including the RPE**, on OCT images.

For each position of the A-scan, retinal thickness is calculated and displayed on a *graph* (**Figure 4**).

The segmentation line can be **displaced manually** (inferiorly or superiorly) to improve the precision of retinal thickness measurements and to correct certain errors related to hyper-reflectivity or hypo-reflectivity not corresponding to the limiting membranes or retinal pigment epithelium (RPE).

The software elaborates a **thickness** (and *volume*) map based on the ETDRS chart, with the typical color scale (white and red for thicker areas to green and blue for thinner areas).

This mapping can be *reproduced on corresponding fundus images* with adjustment of its transparency, topography, and dimensions.

Follow-up

The *Spectralis** apparatus uses an automatic ***eye-tracking system***.

*Spectralis** can set scan line position automatically using the follow up feature.

The images acquired at the first examination can be used as *reference images* for subsequent follow-up examinations.

TruTrack™

When the operator acquires follow-up images, *Spectralis** is able to track eye movements and perfectly sets the OCT scan line at the same position on fundus images (either reference images or SLO fluorescein or ICG-A images). This system is called **TruTrack**™.

This could dramatically improve the capability of **identification of minimal changes** on consecutive examinations.

It allows evaluation of *any changes* due to therapy or to the natural course of various retinal diseases (**Figure 5**).

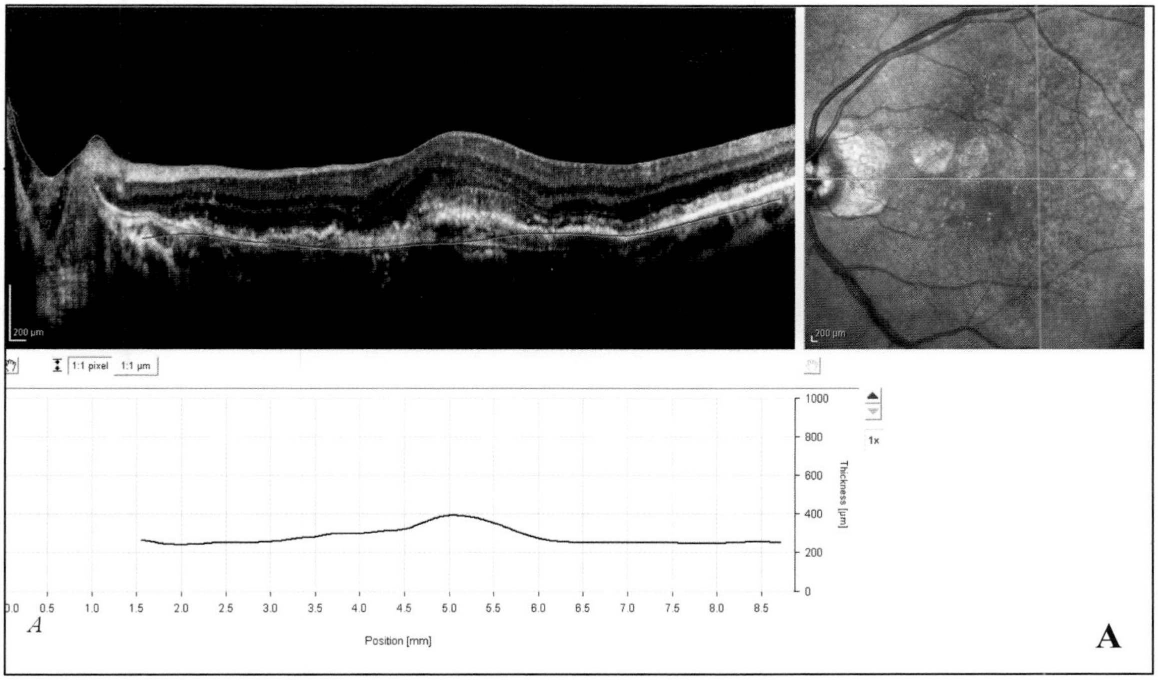

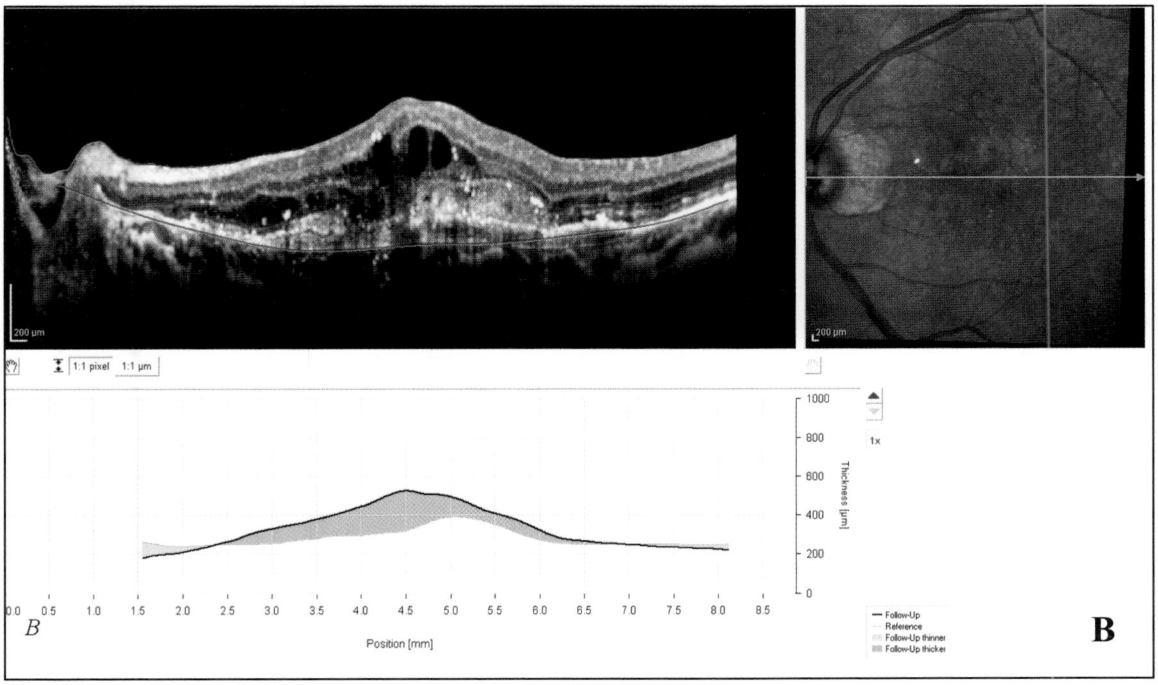

Figure 5: Two scan lines in the same patient at an interval of three months.

A): Reference image.

B): The image obtained three months later during follow-up.

The software overlays SLO images to obtain an OCT scan at exactly the same point.
Note the comparative diagram of retinal thickness on (B).

Improvement of Retinal and Choroidal Visualization

SD-OCT images provide high-definition visualization of *retinal layers* and clear discrimination of the *interfaces* between different reflectance structures.

Noise reduction provides a marked increase in contrast with improved discrimination of fine structures.

Stratified retinal structures can be seen on TD-OCT, but the margins of layers with different reflectance characteristics are not clearly delineated, and it is difficult to identify interfaces between these elements.

*Spectralis** images provide clear visualization and differentiation of each single layer, with sharper definition.

These images therefore show, starting from the surface:

- The *hyper-reflective* points at the margin of the fovea and at the surface of the avascular clivus correspond to the adherence of the vitreous onto the inner limiting membrane (ILM). This hyper-reflectance is due to the perpendicularity of the single A-scan in relation to the vitreous. This is only visible with *Spectralis** OCT.

- The following *five retinal layers* (nerve fibers, ganglion cells, inner plexiform layer, inner nuclear layer, and outer plexiform layer) can be easily discriminated.

In particular, the margins of the *nerve fiber layer* are sharper, and its characteristics are more clearly visible.

In the *ganglion cell layer*, individual cells are almost visible, while Time-Domain OCT is unable to identify single hyper-reflective spots as corresponding to cells.

Intraretinal vessels are identified not simply as hyper-reflective structures with a posterior shadowing effect into the retina, but with *Spectralis**, vessel shape is clearly shown, and it is often possible to identify the vessel wall and lumen.

The *outer nuclear layer* is visible as a hypo-reflectance structure very similar in TD-OCT and in SD-OCT.

The ***external limiting membrane*** can always be identified with *Spectralis**, while it is often difficult to assess with TD-OCT.

The first hyper-reflective band underneath the outer nuclear layer corresponds to the ***inner/outer segment interface*** of photoreceptors.

With *Spectralis**, it is possible to study photoreceptor layers in a incomparable way, in particular in dystrophies and in degenerative pathologies as dry and wet AMD. In these cases, the photoreceptor layer appears homogeneous with hyper-reflective fine deposits, and it is often possible to identify a jagged and irregular margin shape as an indirect sign of suffering.

The *RPE* layer is composed of two distinct hyper-reflective bands separated by a fine hypo-reflective strip. This feature has already been observed with ultrahigh-resolution systems. They differ from results using normal high-resolution TD-OCT images in which the RPE layer appears as a unique hyper-reflective band.

The hyper-reflective *outer band* may correspond to RPE cells, but the origin of the inner band remains unclear.

Many studies suggest that this band corresponds to *Verhoef's membrane*, constituted of tight junctions of RPE cells. According to another hypothesis, this band corresponds to basal infoldings and apical processes that enclose photoreceptor outer segments.

OCT images obtained with Spectral-Domain technology provide good visualization of the main vessels of the ***choroid***, possibly due to the longer OCT wavelength and the decreased absorption by the RPE.

In addition, *real-time averaging* results in a sharper image with fewer artifacts derived from structures underneath the pigment epithelium.

Finally, the *outermost layer* visible on *Spectralis** OCT is a moderately reflective structure that corresponds to sclera not detected by TD-OCT.

*Cirrus** OCT

The *Cirrus** apparatus is a Spectral-Domain OCT marketed by ***Carl Zeiss*** *(Meditec, Dublin, CA)*.

This equipment constitutes a new generation after the *Stratus** apparatus (the first and currently the most widely used Time-Domain OCT apparatus in clinical practice).

Like the other Spectral-Domain OCTs, the greatest improvement provided by *Cirrus** is the increased **acquisition speed**, allowing very fast B-scan image acquisition and a larger number of A-scans for each single B-scan **(Figure 6)**.

The *acquisition speed* of the *Cirrus** is about 100 times faster than that of the *Stratus**.

Technical specifications of the Cirrus *Zeiss (Table 2).**

Table 2. *Cirrus** technical specifications.

	*Cirrus** Spectral-Domain	*Stratus** Time-Domain
OCT wavelength	840 nanometers	820 nanometers
OCT optical depth resolution	5 to 7 micrometers	10 micrometers
Maximum A-scans per B-scan	4,000 to 8,000	512
OCT A-scan rate	18 to 40,000/second	400/second

Wavelength

The OCT wavelength is slightly longer than that of the *Stratus**, allowing greater penetration into the tissues and clearer visualization of subretinal elements.

Software and Image Acquisition

The current software version allows OCT acquisition in *3 different modes*.

The first mode consists of taking 5 consecutive raster horizontal scan lines in high-resolution definition. The operator can move the position of the five lines during the examination by analyzing SLO-red free fundus images.

Each raster scan line is constructed with single A-scans, which considerably increases the horizontal resolution.

In the other two modes, *Cirrus** acquires **retinal cube** sections.

This cube is formed by 512 (vertical) x 128 (horizontal) A-scans for macular studies, or 200 x 200 A-scans for optic nerve head studies.

The **acquisition time** in each mode is about one second or a little more. This reduces the possibility of motion artifacts, making the presence of poor fixation–observed in many patients–less problematic.

*Cirrus** has a powerful auto-regulation system for polarization and Z axis position, which facilitates acquisition. It generally provides very good examination quality, even for the higher bandwidth that reduces the importance of media opacity, such as in the case of cataract.

Raster Mode

In analysis mode, the operator can visualize all the different acquisitions. After raster acquisition, it is possible to examine each of the five consecutive B-scans, while clearly identifying the corresponding position on retinal imaging.

The position of the scan lines can be moved directly on retinal imaging and images can be zoomed on horizontal or vertical scans on the most relevant scan.

Cube Acquisition

Post-processing of cubes is more versatile and current software now allows **segmentation** of the various layers to study any lesions.

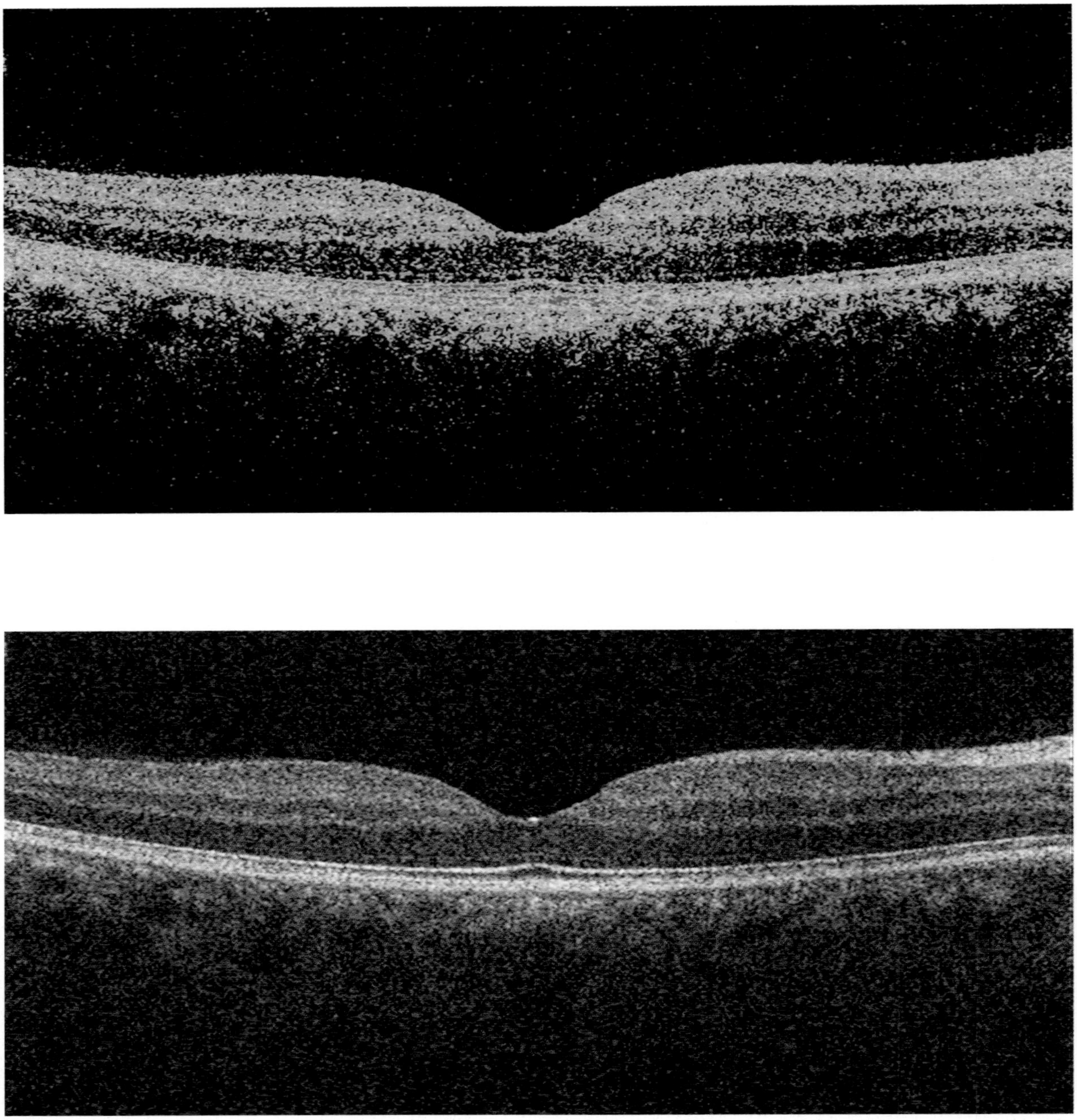

Figure 6: Single A-scan obtained with the Cirrus* *Zeiss OCT* apparatus.

Normal retina: note the detailed visualization of the profile, the fovea, the various retinal layers, and in particular, the interface and the external limiting membrane.

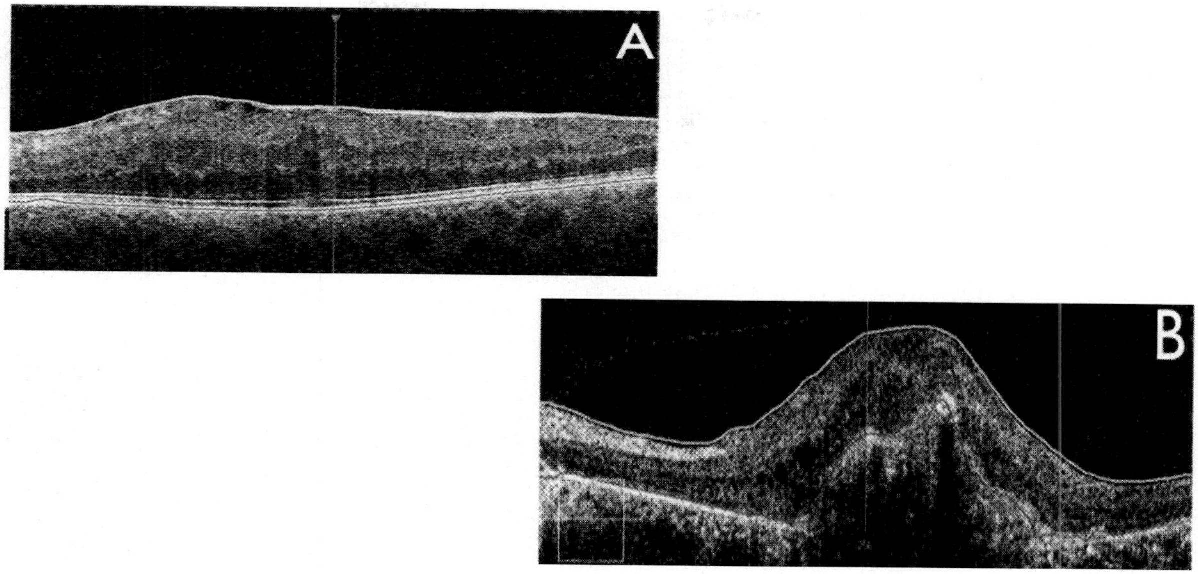

Figure 7. Identification of inner and outer boundaries *(Cirrus** OCT).
Precise identification even when pathological changes induce marked alterations of the normal shape of retinal layers, such as epiretinal membrane with edema (A) and choroidal neovascularization (B).

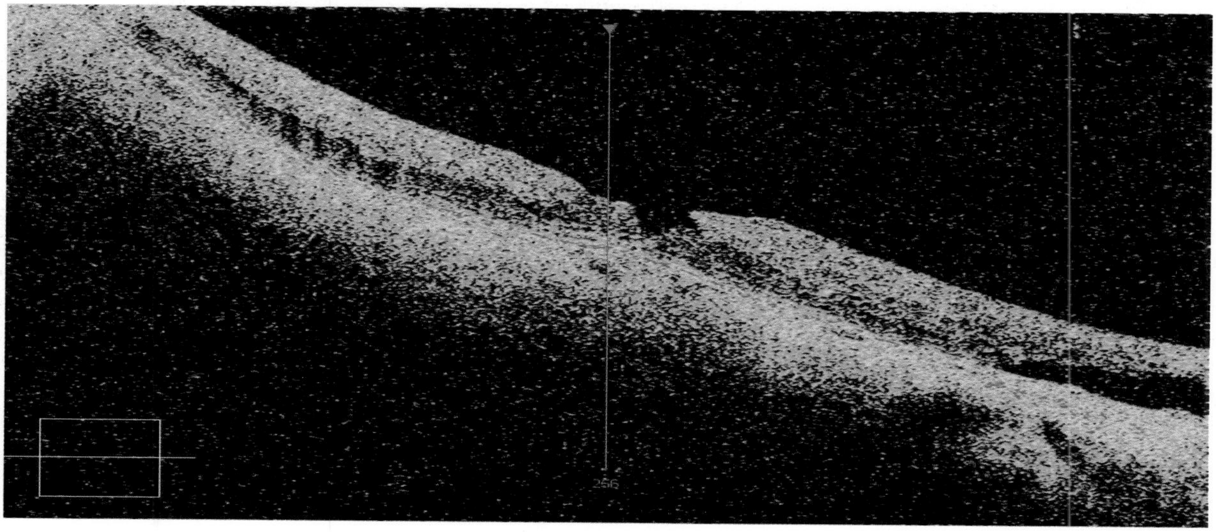

Figure 8. ***Cirrus*** **OCT in a case of severe myopia.**
Note the good quality of the image and good visualization of the pseudo-hole.
A serous neuro-epithelial detachment due to extra foveal choroidal neovascularization is visible in the temporal part of the image.

3

In normal visualization, it is shown the retinal SLO image with vertical and horizontal scan lines and correspondent tomographies.

It is possible to move this position directly on retinal imaging or to zoom in horizontal or vertical tomography series and choose the most relevant image.

Retinal Thickness

Retinal thickness can be determined on a *classical map* based on ETDRS zones or on a graph (**Figure 7**).

A *3D* map can also be obtained with white and red color coding for thicker areas and green and blue color coding for thinner areas.

Retinal Layers

The current software version is able to **isolate** the various layers of the retina. In particular, the profile of the *RPE* and the *ILM* are automatically identified and traced.

Analysis of retinal cube acquisition demonstrates the RPE and ILM, isolated from all other retinal layers, allowing separate visualization of either the single RPE or the ILM shape.

The software can also isolate RPE and ILM profiles and provide coronal (or frontal or *en face)* sections.

These sections are not only perpendicular to the laser beam, but also follow the shape of the retina facilitating quantification of a serous accumulation underneath the RPE or neuro-epithelium.

All **cube acquisitions** (512 x 128 or 200 x 200) can also be analyzed subsequently in advanced mode. The software simultaneously shows the tomographies in three axes (horizontal, vertical, and coronal) as well as the SLO retinal image.

Each single tomographic series can be analyzed more accurately, with a **zooming** effect and color coding or black and white visualization, adjusting contrast, and brightness.

By pointing and clicking on retinal images, the software shows the corresponding tomographies on vertical and horizontal axes.

Again, software can *isolate RPE and ILM profiles,* so that coronal tomographies visualization are not just perpendicular to laser direction, but they follow retinal shape making easier, for example, the quantification of a serous accumulation under RPE or under the neuro-epithelium

Follow-up

With the *Cirrus** apparatus, it is possible to set the position of the cube on the reference examination as a basis for subsequent follow-up, with automatic *repositioning* of the cube on the same retinal area on each examination.

Advantages of the *Cirrus**

The greatest improvement provided by the *Cirrus** (and Spectral-Domain technology in general) is the high *acquisition speed* and, consequently, the greater number of A-scans for each B-scan. A very large volume of information is therefore acquired in a single examination.

In clinical practice, comparison between *Cirrus** and *Stratus** also demonstrates other major advantages.

*Cirrus** allows **ease of acquisition**, even in the presence of media opacities. This feature is probably due to the higher wavelength used by *Cirrus** allowing deeper penetration in the case of early cataract.

It is not uncommon to obtain good images with *Cirrus** in patients who cannot be fully examined by *Stratus**. This is also the case in **myopic patients**, who are so difficult to examine (**Figure 8**).

Combined Optical Coherence Tomography and Confocal Ophthalmoscopy (OCT/SLO)

Marc D. de Smet, MDCM, PhD[1]
Mirjam E.J. van Velthoven, MD, PhD[2]

[1]*Department of Ophthalmology, Academic Medical Centre, Amsterdam, The Netherlands*

[2]*Advanced Retinal Imaging Laboratory, New York Eye and Ear Infirmary, New York, USA*

Introduction

Shortly after Optical Coherence Tomography (OCT) was introduced to ophthalmology, Podoleanu *et al* pioneered an OCT technique, which compiles scans along the Z (depth) axis, while fast scanning in the x-y plane (*Podoleanu 1997*[1]).

In this system, the high-resolution OCT images are **combined** with the surface imaging capability of a scanning laser ophthalmoscope (SLO), produced simultaneously through splitting of the light beam at its source (OCT/SLO) (*Podoleanu 1998*[2], *Podoleanu 1999*[3], *Podoleanu 2000*[4], *Podoleanu 2004*[5], *van Velthoven 2006*[6]) **(Figure 1)**.

This scanning technique produces longitudinal OCT scans, similar to those obtained with other OCT machines, but it is based on a different scanning strategy **(Figure 2)**.

Coronal Scans

In addition, two-dimensional images are generated as *coronal* scans (ie, parallel to the retinal surface).

However, although these coronal scans are generated in a plane familiar to ophthalmologists, their highly magnified nature make them initially, more difficult to interpret (*van Velthoven 2006*[6]).

Nevertheless, these images allow for three-dimensional visualization of the area under investigation, either mentally or by software rendering.

This **coronal** scanning can compensate for some of the limitations of conventional OCT, particularly precise localization of the OCT scan and extent of any longitudinal OCT scan and elimination of eye movement artifacts during image acquisition.

Both limitations make it hard to appreciate the extent of any pathological change within the area that is presumably scanned.

Exact Localization of each Scan

One of the **advantages** of simultaneously acquiring an SLO image and an OCT image is to determine the exact location of each scan.

The designers of the conventional OCT tried to overcome this problem by providing the operator with an infrared fundus video image displaying the scan line.

It is impossible, however, to determine the *exact location of the scan*, as the images are acquired sequentially and not simultaneously.

The conventional OCT also ignores any lateral eye movement occurring during the 2 seconds required to register the 512 A-scans that form a single line.

Lateral eye movements and saccadic movements occurring during image acquisition, and fixation problems can induce major *artifacts*. As the speed of *saccadic movements* can exceed 900 degrees per second, if this eye movement occurs during image acquisition, the scan's second section can be imaging a different retinal area than the first.

Fixation problems are more common with macular pathology, potentially magnifying the degrees of micro-saccadic eye movements as is evident during clinical examination. *Axial movement* (due to breathing, changes in muscular tension, and pulsatile blood flow in the retina and choroid) can also lead to acquisition shifts.

Within the conventional OCT, post-acquisition processing using a technique called auto-correlation provides some degree of compensation (*Schuman 2004*[7]).

The *quality of the OCT/SLO system* is due to its ability to display the **location and extent of any lesion** in the central retinal area. This may provide anatomical clues to understand the underlying pathophysiology (*Velthoven 2006*[6]).

The *high quality fundus image* provided by the ***confocal system*** is therefore better able to indicate the location of the longitudinal scan line.

Pixel-to-pixel correspondence between the OCT and confocal images ensures that all axial or lateral movements during image acquisition are recorded and visualized on the confocal image as a line shift or blurring.

This system has recently been commercialized by ***Ophthalmic Technology Inc.*** *(OTI Toronto, Canada)*. The OCT/SLO is also referred to in the literature as OCT-Ophthalmoscope, *en face* OCT, or transversal OCT.

Principle of the OCT/SLO System

A schematic diagram of the OCT/SLO is shown (**Figure 1**) (*Podoleanu 1999*[8], *Podoleanu 2002*[9]).

Major differences with conventional OCT concern *coronal scanning approach* and simultaneous acquisition of *confocal images.*

Two mirrors are used in the sample arm to acquire the OCT images in the x-y plane, which resembles the set-up of a confocal scanning laser ophthalmoscope (SLO).

Like conventional OCT, the OCT/SLO system uses a *superluminescent diode* with a central wavelength of 820 nm and a bandwidth of 20 nm (*Podoleanu 1998*[2], *Podoleanu 1999*[3], *Podoleanu 2000*[4], *Podoleanu 2004*[5], *van Velthoven 2006*[6]).

The light beam is split, directing one arm to the patient's eye (*sample arm*) and the other arm to a mirror (*reference arm*).

The returning light beams from the patient's eye and the reference arm are simultaneously collected through an **interferometer** to produce the OCT signal.

A fraction of the light returning from the patient's eye is directed through a pinhole to another detector to produce a **confocal signal**.

The images are produced simultaneously at the same scanning rate, and the images in the confocal and the OCT channels therefore present *strict pixel-to-pixel correspondence (Podoleanu 1999*[8], *Podoleanu 2002*[9], *Rogers 2001*[10], *Podoleanu 1998*[11]*).*

Depth (Z-axis) Resolution

Depth (Z-axis) resolution is about 10 µm and **transverse** (x-y plane) **resolution** is about 15 µm in the OCT channel (*Rogers 2001*[10]).

The confocal channel provides a depth resolution of about 3 mm (*Podoleanu 1999*[8]).

The focus in the confocal channel is not adjusted when changing the depth value in the OCT channel, and the confocal image therefore has the same appearance in all the pairs collected in the stack.

However, slight variations in the confocal images may be observed as a result of eye movements, and frame-to-frame variations can subsequently be used to correct the stack (*Rogers 2000*[12]).

C-Scan and B-Scan Acquisition

Longitudinal OCT scans (also called OCT **B-scans** in conventional OCT) are generated from successive in-depth reflectivity profiles acquired along the Z-axis in the x-z or y-z plane (A-scans) (*Schuman 2004*[7], *Hee 1995*[13], *Huang 1991*[14]).

The OCT/SLO produces *coronal* OCT scans (**C-scans**) in the x-y plane at a fixed Z-coordinate using *en face* flying-spot T-scan lines (**Figure 2**) (*Podoleanu 2000*[4]).

By changing the Z-coordinate in the OCT channel, OCT C-scans can be acquired at different depths in the retina.

The OCT/SLO can also produce *longitudinal B-scans* along a fixed axis in the x-y plane by continuously changing the depth (**Figure 2**).

OCT C-scans are acquired at a rate of 2 frames per second. B-scans are acquired in one second.

The scan depth along the Z-axis is set at 1.125 mm, but can be adjusted to more than 2 mm. The acquisition rate can also be increased but at the cost of decreased image resolution.

In the current system, each scan covers an area of 24° x 24°, roughly equivalent to an area of 8 mm x 8 mm.

Confocal images and coronal OCT images are simultaneously displayed on the computer as a pair, and each part is displayed as an array of 512 x 512 pixels. The images are visualized on a personal computer in gray scale, but can also be displayed in false color.

OCT/SLO Hardware

The **commercial version** of the OCT/SLO is similar to conventional OCT: the operator faces the patient and the computer screen during acquisition. The patient module comprises an adjustable chin rest.

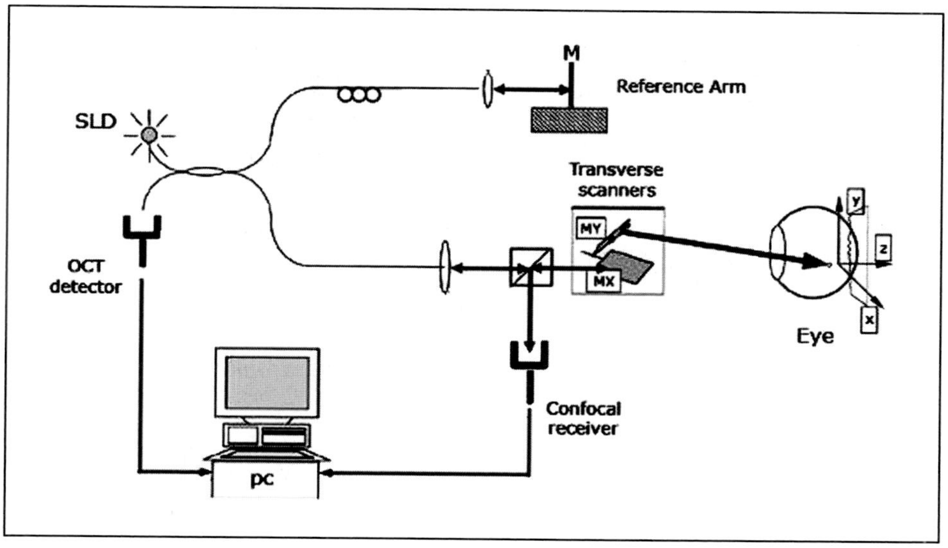

Figure 1: Schematic representation of the OCT/SLO device.
From the superluminescent diode light source (SLD) with a central wavelength of 820 nm, and a bandwidth of 20 nm, the light bundle travels to a Michelson interferometer where the light is split to a reference arm or to the eye. Light emanating from the eye is directed both to a confocal receiver and to the OCT detector. Both images are received by the computer for processing in pixel-to-pixel correspondence.

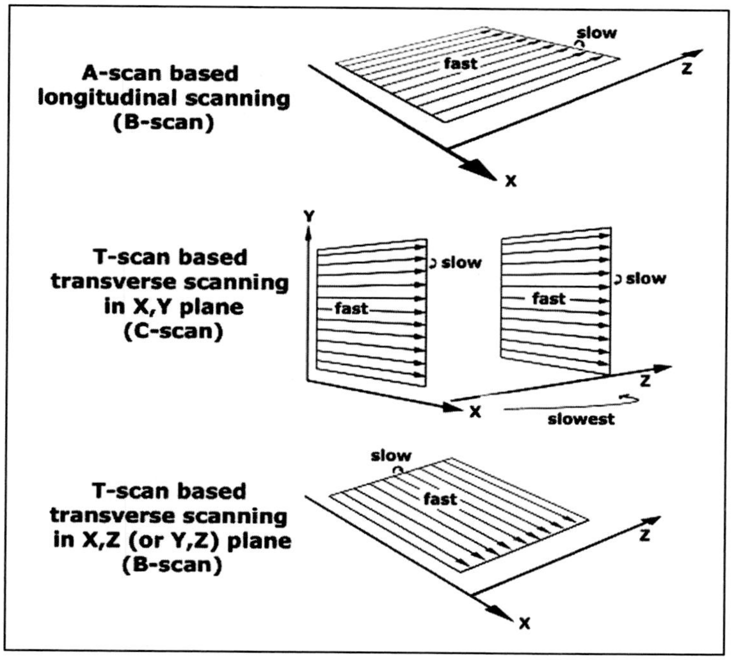

Figure 2: Schematic of existing OCT scanning protocols.
A): B-scans are acquired by accumulating a series of A-scans along the vertical Z-axis, with a rapid sweep along the axis of the retina (X-axis).
B): In OCT/SLO, B-scans are acquired by accumulation of transverse scans (T-scans) in a plane parallel to the retina, with a rapid sweep in the vertical axis.
C): C-scans are a reconstruction of these rapid B-scans (in spectral mode).

The device is mounted on a motorized table and consists of the OCT/SLO system with a joystick to move the machine vertically and horizontally, a PC, a flat screen monitor, and a foot pedal to operate the acquisition program.

The *acquisition program* is preinstalled, and starts up automatically when the system is turned on.

The patient's pupil does not need to be dilated before scanning, although a dilated pupil facilitates scan acquisition, especially in patients with very small pupils.

Clinical use of OCT/SLO

Compared to the Stratus* OCT, this system appears to require slightly more effort from both the operator and the patient, although the examination procedure is fairly similar.

The operator must understand the combination of **coronal OCT images** and **confocal images** to take full advantage of this scanning technique.

The Confocal Image

The confocal image provides the operator with a high quality fundus image, which may reveal areas affected by a change in *surface reflectivity*. These areas therefore require further attention.

Scanning a patient is only slightly longer than with conventional OCT, as the scanning rate is fairly similar to single scan acquisition rates.

With the OCT/SLO, all captured images are saved, while for the *Stratus**, only one image at a time is saved.

A single topographic stack of the OCT/SLO images is acquired in two seconds (similar to the time taken by the *Stratus** OCT fast macular thickness protocol, which takes 1.9 seconds).

Although the OCT/SLO software offers various scan modalities, only those suitable for scanning the majority of patients are generally used.

The best option is the "***Freeform Acquisition***" program, which allows the operator to switch back and forth from OCT C-scanning to OCT B-scanning, as necessary.

C-Scan

Images are initially captured as **C-scans** and, by moving the device back and forth, the operator can sweep through the macula or optic nerve head and analyze the pathology in real-time.

By clicking the foot pedal, the operator can switch to OCT **B-scan** mode.

The OCT B-scan line can be placed at any given position along the *horizontal* or *vertical* axis by dragging the center of the line using the mouse.

Radial lines can also be acquired by dragging the edge of the line to the preferred angle.

During OCT B-scanning, the coronal confocal image is refreshed every 2 seconds, ensuring accurate estimation of the position of the scan line. About 100 successive scans can be saved.

Alternatively, a "*Detailed Stack*" can be used, which captures 50 consecutive C-scans over an operator-selected fixed distance.

The default distance for this detailed stack is 1.125 mm, with each frame separated by an interval of approximately 20 μm.

Retinal Thickness

The "*Retinal Topographic Stack*" can be used to evaluate retinal thickness. This program allows acquisition of either macular or optic nerve head topography maps.

It acquires a stack of 100 consecutive C-scans over a fixed distance and an area of 15° x 15° in two seconds.

The operator can choose to examine the macula at a distance of 1.125 mm, retinal thickness at 1.5 mm, or the optic nerve head at 2.0 mm, but for each option the scan depth of the stack can be adjusted from 1 mm to 6 mm.

The scan area can be modified by the operator by dragging the square to the desired position on the fundus.

The *current software* allows post-acquisition analysis by providing the option to localize areas of interest by either encircling the area or marking a specific point **(Figure 3)**.

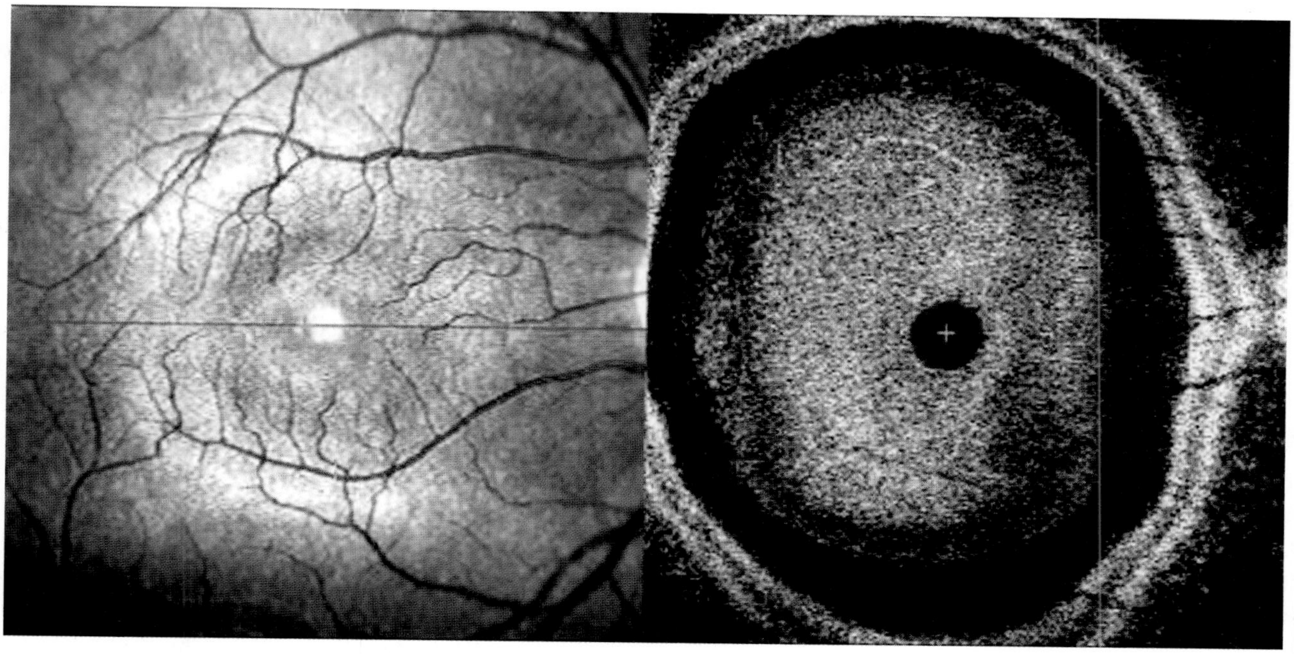

Figure 3: Time-Domain OCT/SLO images (SLO image on the left, *en face* OCT image on the right).
Strict pixel-to-pixel correspondence of the images outlined in green on each image.

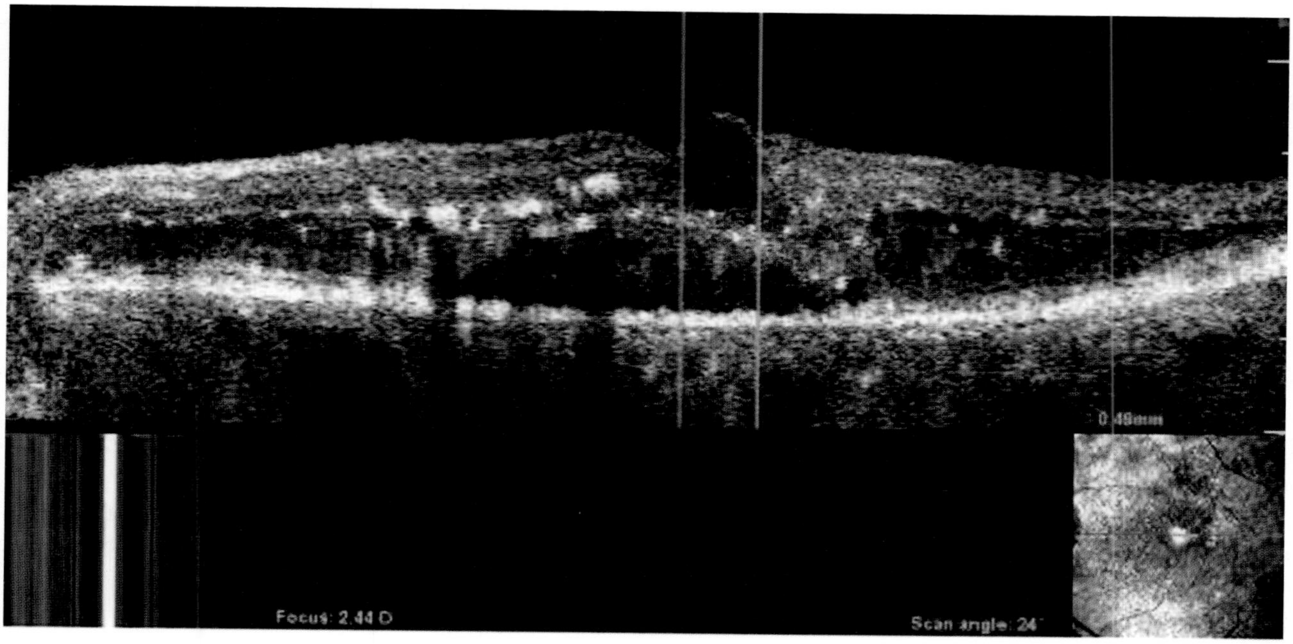

Figure 4: OCT B-scan.
A calliper function allows measurement of the distance between two vertical lines.

Whether the outline is made on the OCT or the confocal image, the corresponding area will be outlined in the fellow image.
On B-scans, a **calliper** function can be used to measure the distance between two vertical or horizontal lines (**Figure 4**).

Retinal Thickness

Retinal thickness can also be measured in the topographic stack and is displayed as a two-dimensional square showing either contour lines indicating various heights.

Retinal thickness can also be measured as a grid giving 16 averaged thickness measurements as areas expressed as X by X mm (**Figure 5**).

Retinal thickness is defined as the thickness between the *vitreoretinal interface* and the *retinal pigment epithelium* (ie, the second hyper-reflective layer at the outer retina).

The confocal image provides a good quality reference image for aligning consecutive topographic stacks and monitoring changes over time.

Evaluation of the Normal Fundus

To the uninitiated, individual OCT C-scans can be difficult to interpret. As with all diagnostic imaging techniques, however, it is a matter of pattern recognition and repetition.

OCT/SLO imaging is a *dynamic investigation* like fluoroscopy.

When acquiring OCT C-scans, abnormal or unusual areas are often seen.

The operator must recognize these areas and capture longitudinal B-scans in these areas of interest.
The operator must be familiar with normal anatomy visualized by OCT C-scans before analyzing pathological changes.

Normal Anatomy

Therefore, the normal anatomy as visualized by the OCT C-scans must first be discussed, before disease-related OCT images are introduced.

The images shown in **Figure 6** are part of a stack of OCT C-scans from the right macular area of a healthy subject. Numerous retinal layers become visible at different depths, from the *vitreoretinal interface* to the *choroid*. Due to the curvature of the eye, the edge of the scan images the **various retinal layers** arranged inside out, with the inner and outer retinal layers visible in a manner similar to "onion rings."

Retinal Vessels

Retinal vessels are easily recognized in the ganglion and inner plexiform layers.

They initially appear white in the more superficial layer (on the OCT C-scan) and then progressively appear darker (shadowing) on OCT C-scans of deeper layers of the retina.

As the **foveal pit** is the deepest part of the retina, the optically translucent vitreous remains visible as a small central dark circle.

The Retinal Layers

The following layers are progressively visualized in the macular region, around the foveal pit:
- The highly reflective **nerve fiber** layer (RNFL),
- The less reflective **inner and outer plexiform** and **nuclear layers,**
- The second highly reflective signal represents the interface of inner/outer segments of the photoreceptors,
- The following hyper-reflective layer is thought to be the **interface** with the **retinal pigment epithelium (RPE)** and **choriocapillaris.**

Taken through the central fovea, the OCT B-scan of the same subject, has a more familiar appearance (**Figure 7**).

As previously mentioned, the confocal part of the OCT C-scan demonstrates **possible movements** in the coronal and longitudinal sections.

The most obvious **motion artifact** is blinking, which is easily recognized (**Figure 8**).

Rapid (*saccadic*) eye movements during coronal scanning are seen as an unusual "tear" or "rip" in the confocal image (**Figure 9**).

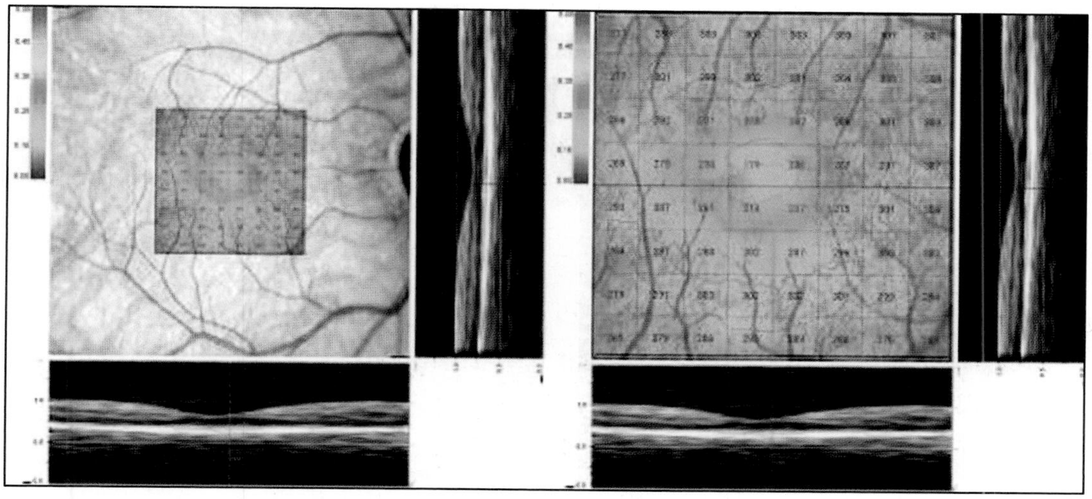

Figure 5: Measurement of retinal thickness.
Demonstration on a 2D square showing either the contour lines of different thickness measurements or a grid indicating mean measurements in the various zones of the grid.

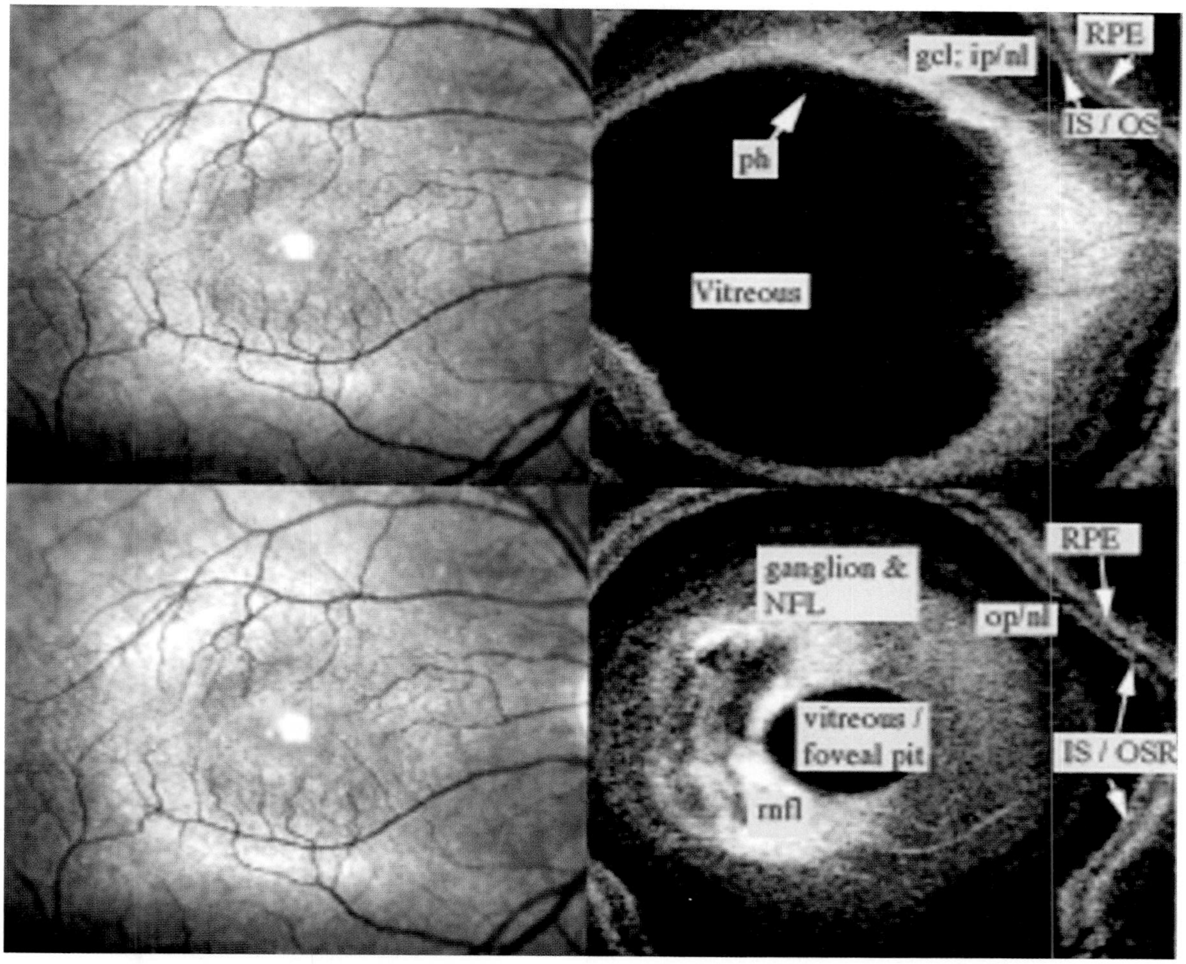

Figure 6: Comparison between a series of 5 C-scans and a B-scan indicating the various layers encountered at different depths along the Z-axis.
elm: external limiting membrane; **glc**: ganglion cell layer; **ilm**: inner limiting membrane; **ip/nl**: inner plexiform/nuclear layer; **IS/OS**: inner/outer segments; **op/nl**: outer plexiform/nuclear layer; **ph**: posterior hyaloid; **RPE**: retinal pigment epithelium.

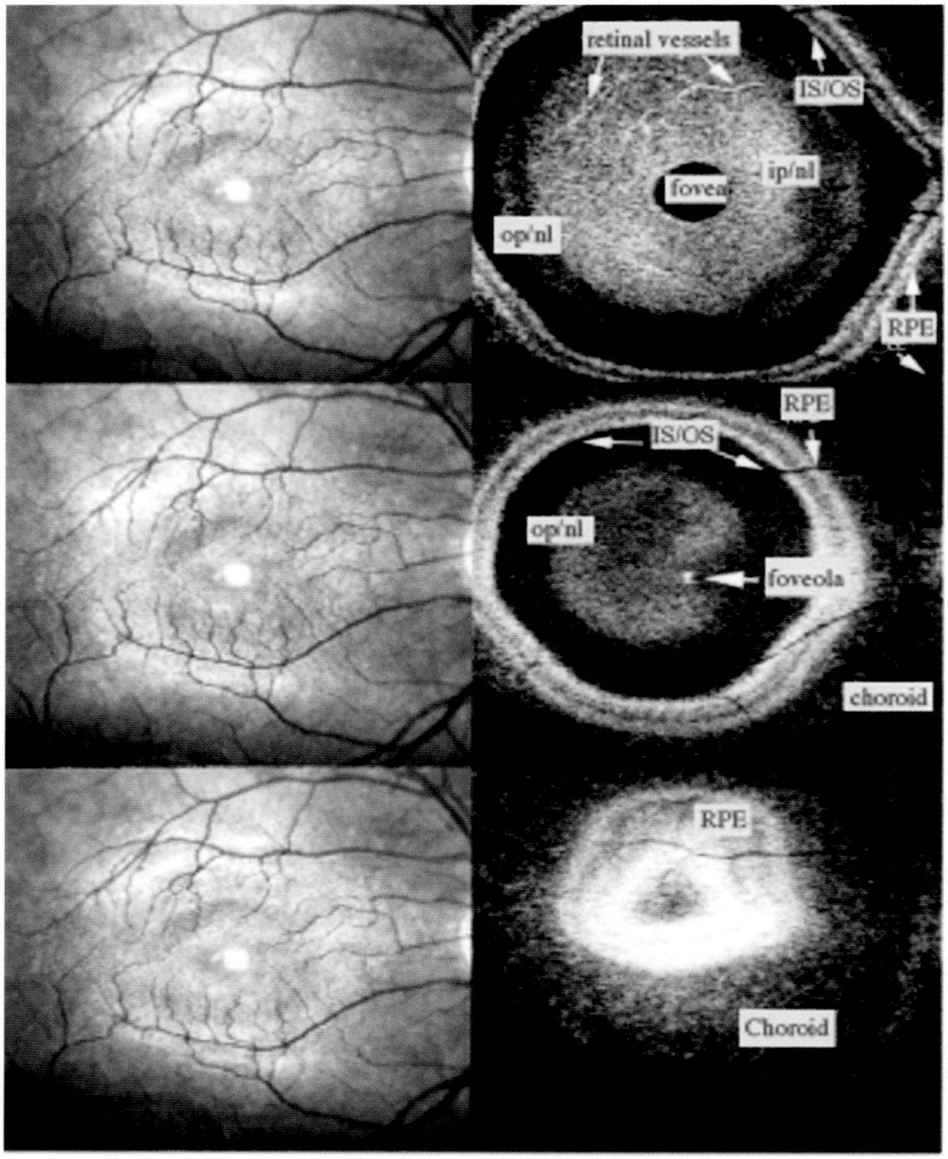

Figure 6 (continued): Comparison between a series of 5 C-scans and a B-scan indicating the various layers encountered at different depths along the Z-axis.

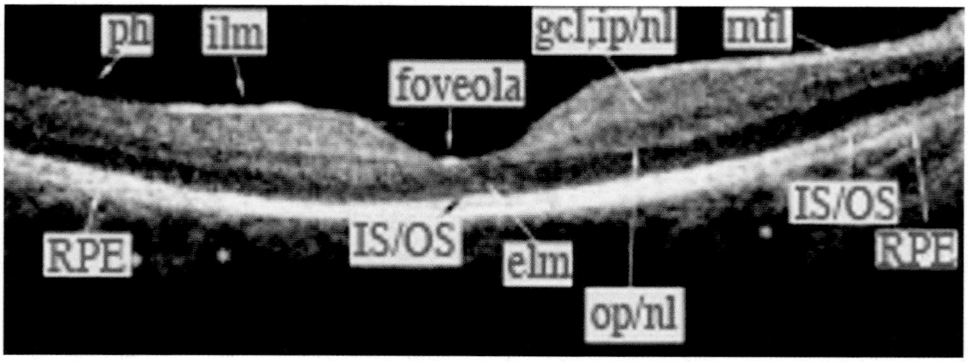

Figure 7: B-scan through the center of the fovea (same patient as in Figure 6).

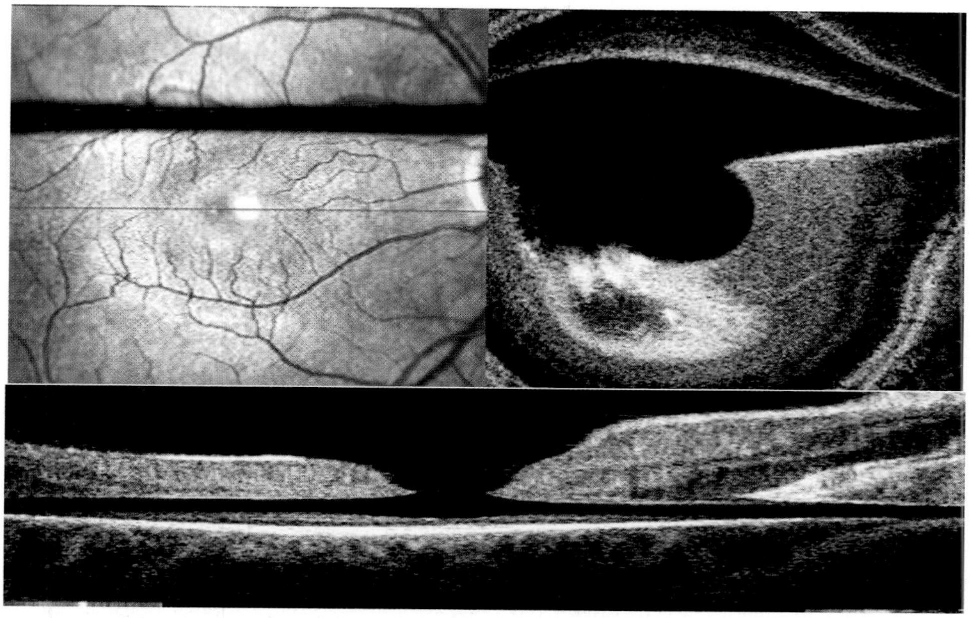

Figure 8: Blink artifact, visible as black bands on the C-scan or sliding distortion on the B-scan.

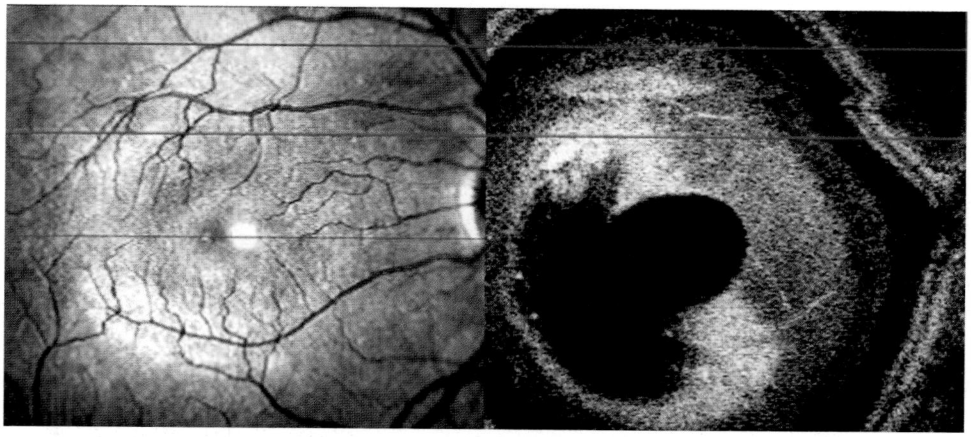

Figure 9: Pseudo-tear artifact due to saccadic movements.

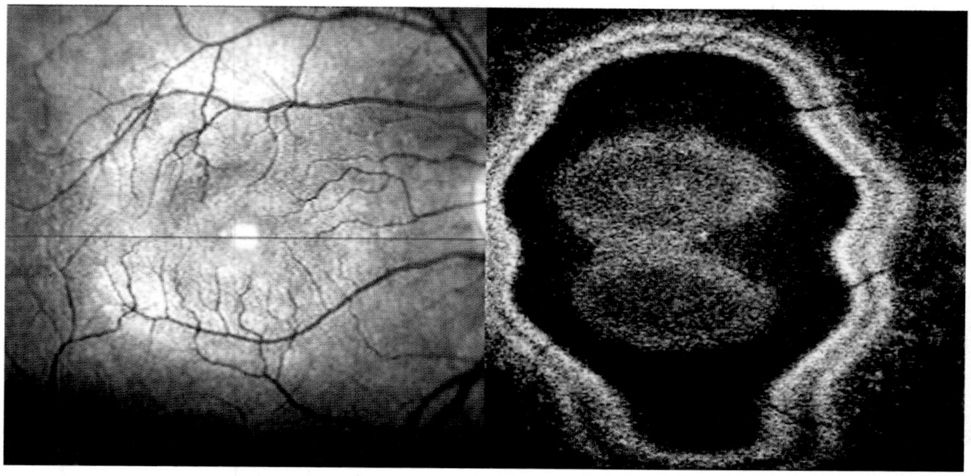

Figure 10: Breathing artifact with distortion of the coronal image.

Axial movements caused by breathing or change in muscular tension can be seen as distortions in the coronal scan, with complete loss of the circular outline of the globe (**Figure 10**).

Any *lateral movement* during scan acquisition causes displacement of these lines, corresponding to displacement of the B-scan.

These displacements can be marked on the confocal image to reveal the corresponding movement in the B-scan.

Axial movement in the B-scan can be seen as partial or complete elongations in certain layers of the retina, which can be either subtle or obvious.

Recognition of these **motion artifacts** on C-scan images allows full use of all captured images to reveal objective information about real changes in the retina.

Example: Cystoid Macular Edema (CME)

For example, the *appearance of CME* on longitudinal scans is well known (**Figure 11A**). It can also be easily recognized on C-scans.

Two successive frames in a patient with early CME are shown (**Figure 11B and C**).

Since the foveal contour has changed from a depression in the macular surface to a *fluid-filled mound* above the retinal surface, its crest is now seen before any of the retinal layers are visualized in the C-scan.

The area affected by cystoid changes is clearly visualized and even the separate cystoid spaces can be distinguished.

C-scans also allow recognition of more limited macular edema with small cystoid spaces, as in this case of Birdshot retinopathy (*van Velthoven 2005*[15]).

The retinal layers at the border of the C-scan (**Figure 12**) have an irregular shape, indicative of subtle retinal edema.

At the temporal side of the C-scan, small cystic changes are visible and their presence is confirmed on the usual longitudinal B-scan.

OCT/SLO Tomography

Follow-up

The only objective way to evaluate retinal thickness is to measure it on OCT scans.

Based on a stack of 100 consecutive fast OCT C-scans, the OCT/SLO provides a 3D rendering of an area of interest, such as in the macula (**Figure 13**).

B-scans are generated from this 3D stack. Although these B-scans show less detailed images than the regular OCT B-scans, the outer borders of the retina and fovea are clearly visible.

They are particularly useful to identify possible misalignment in a stack. A stack is topped with the confocal image and overlaid with a false-color scheme indicating the thickness.

Topographic images (**Figure 12**) are shown of the patient with CME (**Figure 11**).

Images were taken at the next visit following treatment (**Figure 14**).

The B-scan and the C-scan (**Figure 14**, top) still show obvious CME, and it is difficult to accurately assess the thickness.

The topographic image (**Figure 17**, bottom) shows a marked decrease in retinal thickness, clearly visible in the color profile.

Topographic comparison between two different visits is also possible (**Figure 15**).

These comparisons are generated by first selecting both stacks, and aligning them on a larger confocal image.

This process allows comparison of exactly the same areas.

After both images are satisfactorily aligned, a comparison is given as a subtraction image.

On one side, a 2D image using a different false-color scheme is shown to indicate the loss or gain in thickness, and on the other side, a 3D contour plot showing the change in retinal thickness is generated.

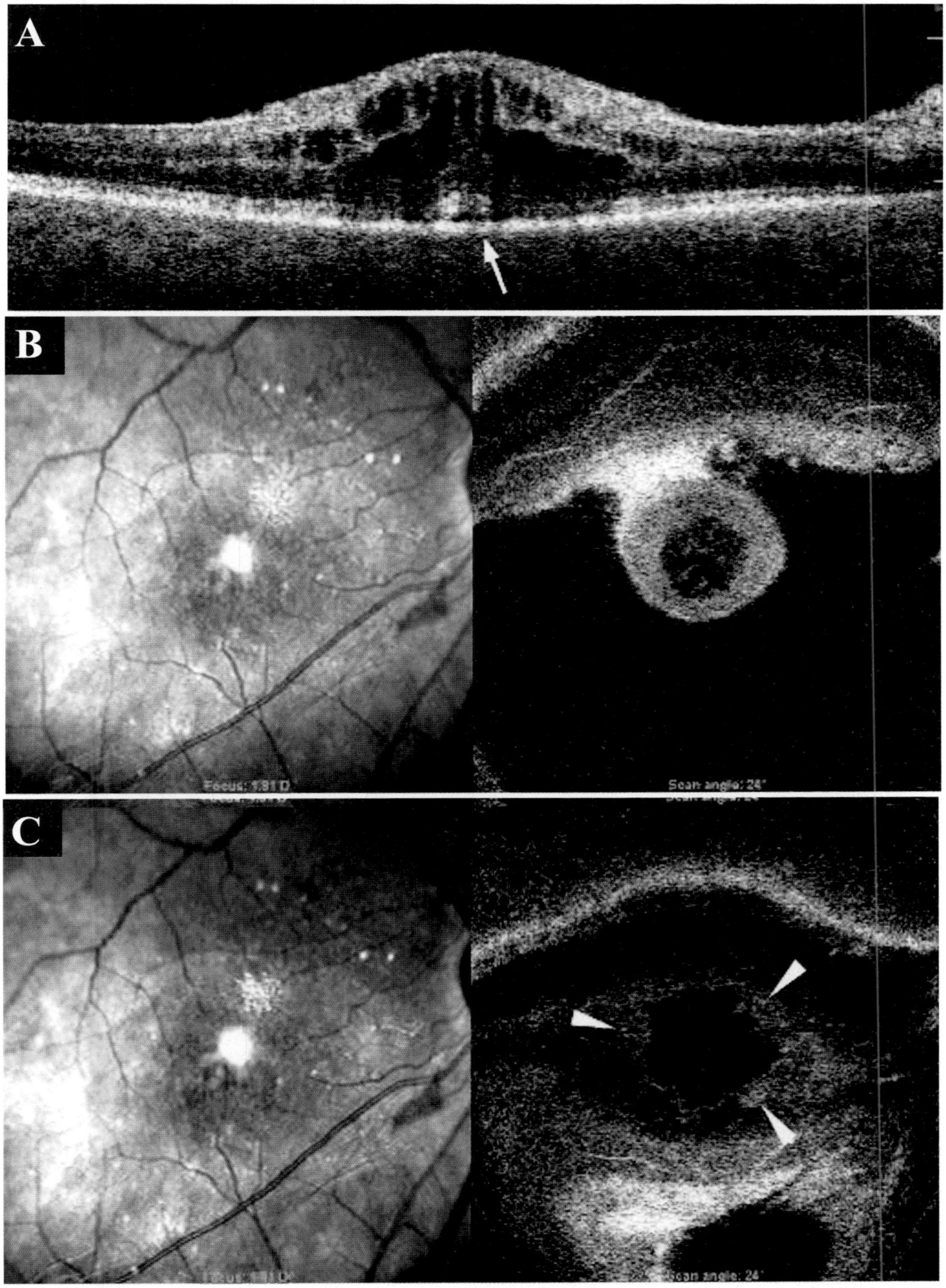

Figure 11: CME in a patient with uveitis.

A): Appearance on longitudinal B-scan

B and C): Appearance on C-scan: 2 successive views of severe CME.

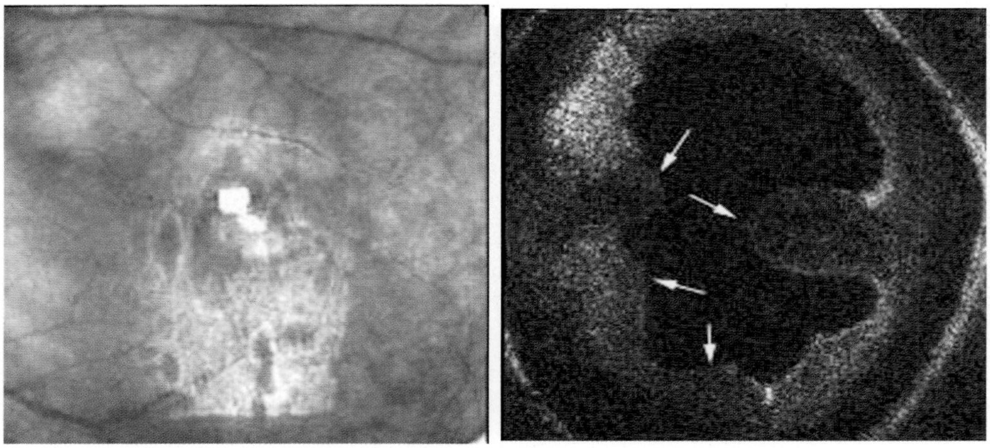

Figure 12: OCT C-scan appearance of early CME in a patient with Birdshot retinopathy.

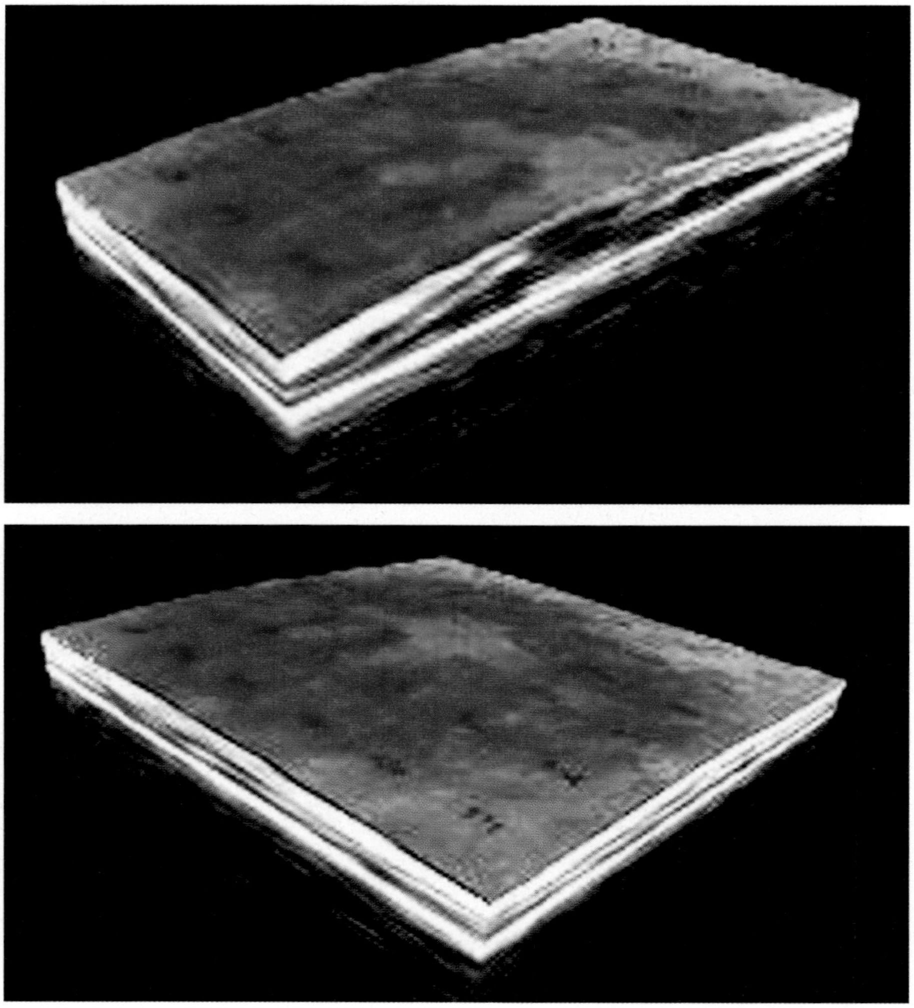

Figure 13: OCT/SLO topography: same patient as in Figure 12.

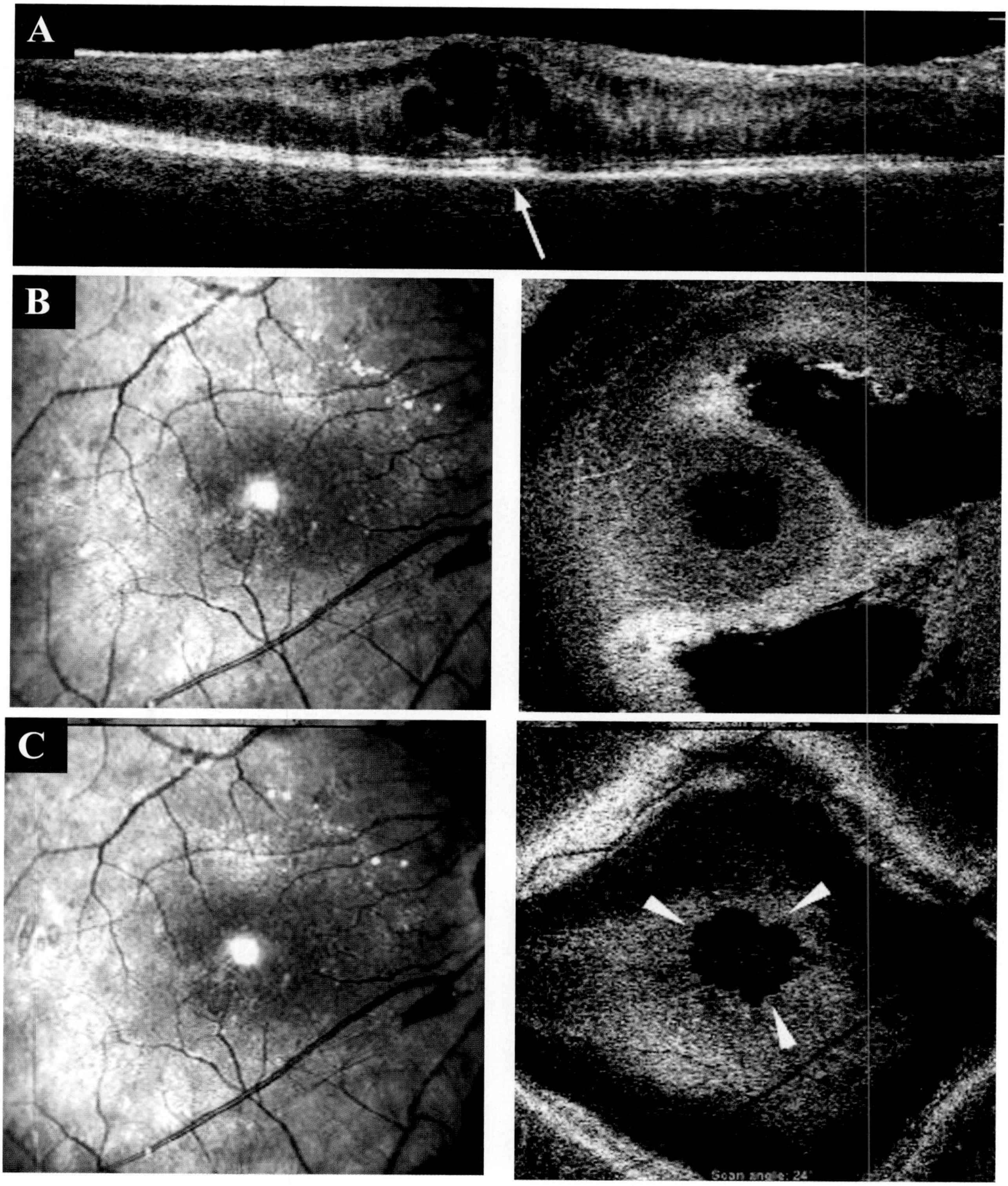

Figure 14: Images before and after treatment.

A): Top: Conventional B-scan showing CME.

B): Middle: C-scan, confirming edema, but it is difficult to accurately measure retinal thickness.

C): Bottom: C-scan, the next examination, after treatment, shows a marked reduction of retinal thickness.

4

Overlay with Angiography

The high quality fundus image obtained by the confocal channel can be used as a reliable **reference** to make software-inferred overlay images from more conventional diagnostic techniques as fluorescein angiography (FA) onto the OCT part of the C-scans.

With appropriate stand-alone software, conventional angiographic images can be spatially transformed and superimposed over the confocal image (van Velthoven 2005[15]).

The pixel-to-pixel correspondence between confocal and OCT images allows image overlay.

The late FA image of a Birdshot patient (**Figure 12**) shows leakage along the vascular arcades and in the fovea (**Figure 15**).

An overlay image of this FA and the C-scan is shown (**Figure 16**).

This image shows that the temporal area of retinal thickening on the OCT exactly matches the temporal, parafoveal area of leakage on the angiographic image.

Closer examination of these overlay images shows the **correlation** between the smaller areas of leakage at the nasal side of the fovea, along the vascular arcades on the angiographic image, and the irregular retinal contour on the C-scans.[15]

In the case of unexplained leakage on an angiographic image or an unexplained patchy surface on OCT, this overlay feature can be used to combine the functional and morphological information provided separately by the two imaging techniques and help elucidate the findings in either one or both.

A similar feature as described above is available in the system's acquisition program.

Conclusion

The advantage of the OCT/SLO is based on its ability to provide a real-time **overview** of the area of interest.

This allows rapid localization of abnormal areas and assessment of the extent of any pathology in the central retinal area.

The pixel-to-pixel correspondence between OCT and SLO images allows more accurate follow-up over time.

Accurate overlays between angiographic images and OCT can also be obtained. SLO combined with this OCT technology provides new anatomical data to understand the pathophysiology of retinal diseases.

The only major difficulty, is learning to interpret coronal images and evaluation of the new features displayed by this technology.

This new approach **will soon become self-evident**.

References

1. **Podoleanu AG, Dobre GM, Webb DJ *et al.*** Simultaneous en-face imaging of two layers in the human retina by low-coherence reflectometry. *Optics Letters* 1997;**22**:1039-41.
2. **Podoleanu AG, Seeger M, Dobre GM *et al.*** Transversal and longitudinal images from the retina of the living eye using low coherence reflectometry. *J Biomed Opt* 1998;**3**:12-20.
3. **Podoleanu AG, Rogers JA, Webb DJ *et al.*** Compatibility of transversal OCT imaging with confocal imaging of the retina in vivo. *SPIE* 1999;**3598**:61-7.
4. **Podoleanu AG, Rogers JA, Jackson DA.** 3D OCT Images from retina and skin. *Optics Express* 2000;**7**:292-8.
5. **Podoleanu AG, Dobre GM, Cucu RG *et al.*** Combined multiplanar optical coherence tomography and confocal scanning ophthalmoscopy. *J Biomed.Opt* 2004;**9**:86-93.
6. **van Velthoven ME, Verbraak FD, Yannuzzi LA *et al.*** Imaging the Retina by *en-face* Optical Coherence Tomography. *Retina* 2006;**26**:129-36.
7. **Schuman JS, Puliafito CA, Fujimoto JG.** *Optical Coherence Tomography of Ocular Diseases (2nd edition)*. 2 ed. Thorofare (USA): SLACK Inc., 2004.
8. **Podoleanu AG, Jackson DA.** Noise analysis of a combined optical coherence tomograph and a confocal scanning ophthalmoscope. *Applied Optics* 1999;**38**:2116-27.
9. **Podoleanu AG, Jackson DA.** Combined optical coherence tomography and scanning laser ophthalmoscopy. *Electronics Letters* 2002;**34**:1088-90.
10. **Rogers JA, Podoleanu AG, Dobre GM *et al.*** Topography and volume measurements of the optic nerve using *en-face* optical coherence tomography. *Optics Express* 2001;**9**:533-45.
11. **Podoleanu AG, Dobre GM, Seeger M *et al.*** Low coherence interferometry for *en-face* imaging of the retina. *Lasers and Light* 1998;**8**:187-92.
12. **Rogers JA, Podoleanu AG, Fitzke FW *et al.*** Visualisation and measurement methods using transversal OCT images of the eye fundus. *SPIE* 2000;**4160**:16-23.
13. **Hee MR, Izatt JA, Swanson EA *et al.*** Optical coherence tomography of the human retina. *Arch.Ophthalmol.* 1995;**113**:325-32.
14. **Huang D, Swanson EA, Lin CP *et al.*** Optical coherence tomography. *Science* 1991;**254**:1178-81.
15. **van Velthoven ME, de Vos K, Verbraak FD *et al.*** Overlay of conventional angiographic and en-face OCT images enhances their interpretation. *BMC.Ophthalmol* 2005;**5**:12.

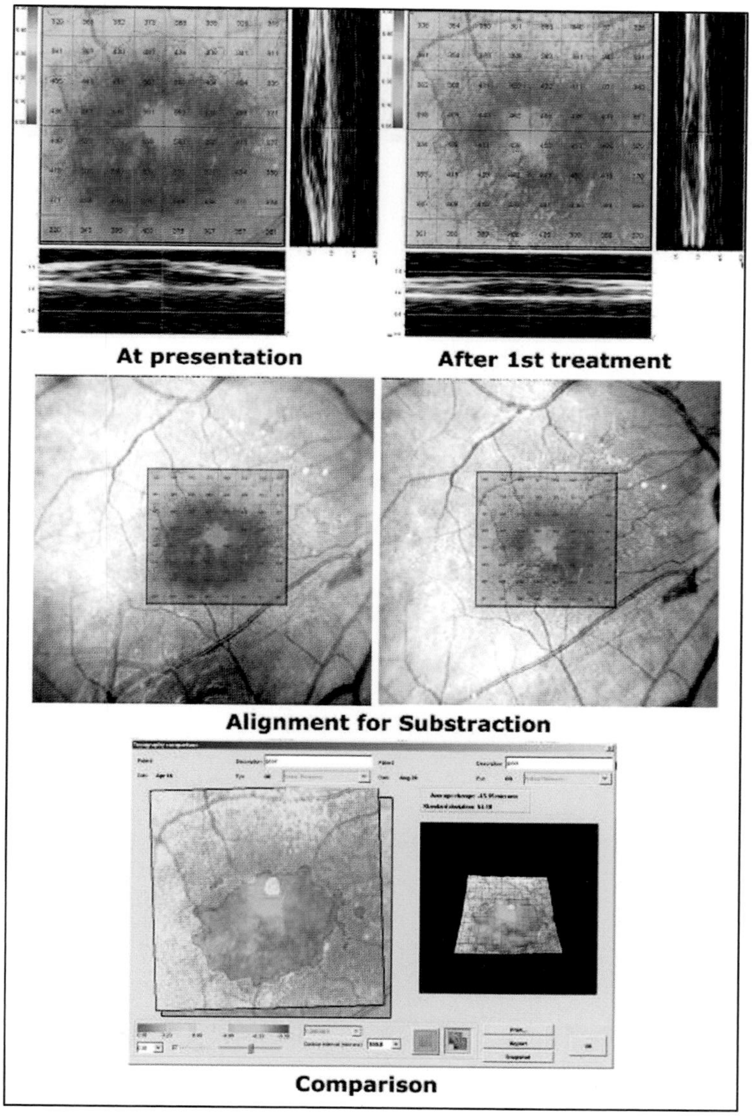

Figure 15: Images before and after treatment.

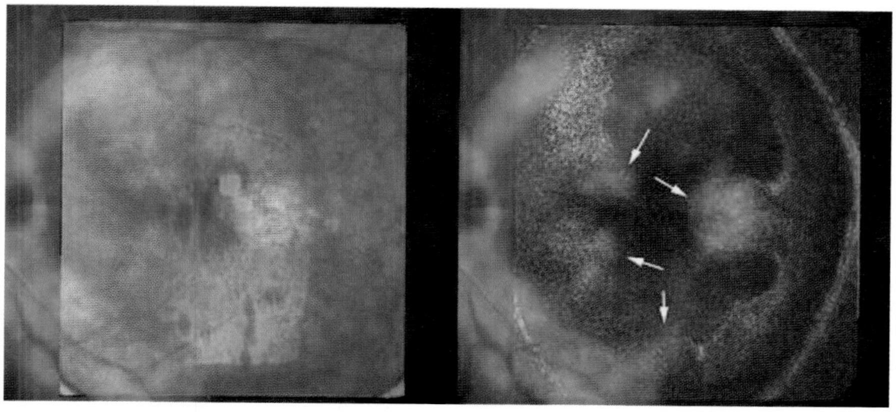

Figure 16: Overlay image of fluorescein angiography and OCT C-scan in a patient with Birdshot retinopathy (see **figure 12**). Leakage along the vascular arcades and in the fovea is visible on both images.

Principles and Applications of Modern Optical Coherence Tomography

Taku WAKABAYASHI, MD, Yusuke OSHIMA MD,
Fumi GOMI, MD, and
Yasuo TANO, MD

Department of Ophthalmology, Osaka University Medical School
Osaka, Japan

Introduction

Optical coherence tomography (OCT) is a noninvasive imaging technology that provides high-resolution cross-sectional images of tissue microstructures *in vivo*.

OCT imaging is useful for the evaluation of retinal anatomy (ie, to elucidate subtle **microstructural abnormalities** of the retina and to explore the adhesion of the vitreoretinal interface).

OCT is now one of the most useful modalities for evaluating and managing a variety of vitreoretinal diseases, such as *idiopathic macular hole*, *macular edema*, and *age-related macular degeneration* (AMD).

The principle of OCT was reported for the first time in 1991 (*Huang 1991*[1]). The first commercially available OCT (*OCT 1*^{TM} or System 2000 Humphrey Instruments, Inc.) was introduced in the mid-1990s.

First Generation of OCT

This *first generation of OCT* had an axial resolution of about 15 µm and a transverse resolution of 20 µm in tissue. The data acquisition rate was 100 A-scans per second.

The ***Stratus*** **OCT** (OCT 3000™, Carl *Zeiss Meditec, Dublin, CA*), a **Time-Domain** OCT (TD-OCT) apparatus, was introduced in 2002 and is now the most widely used OCT system.

This system provides axial resolution of up to 10 µm and a higher acquisition rate of 400 A-scans per second by using a high-speed scanning system, thus allowing a 4-fold increase in imaging speed compared with OCT-1.

The increased *axial* and *transverse* pixel counts of the *Stratus** OCT provides improved imaging quality.

Intraretinal as well as subretinal and subretinal pigment epithelium lesions can be clearly analyzed.

The *Stratus** OCT has therefore become a standard imaging modality for the diagnosis and assessment of AMD (*Salinas-Alamán 2005*[2], *Coscas 2007*[3]).

Retinal thickness analysis by OCT, which allows quantitative assessment of changes in retinal morphology, has become one of the critical parameters for various clinical trials (*Avery 2006*[4], *Michels 2005*[5], *Fung 2007*[6]).

Recent Advancement in OCT Technology

Spectral-Domain OCT (SD-OCT), also known as **Fourier-Domain OCT (FD-OCT)**, is a recent advancement in OCT technology.

This technology has considerably improved imaging quality with axial resolution of less than 5 µm and a 50-fold higher acquisition speed compared to conventional OCT (*Iam 2006*[7]).

The enhanced imaging capabilities of FD-OCT have the potential to improve the visualization of retinal morphology and provides **additional information** compared to *Stratus** to elucidate the pathogenesis of macular disease.

The increased scan speed also allows comprehensive 3D information, not previously available with *Stratus** (*Hangai 2007*[8]).

This chapter presents an overview of the principles of FD-OCT and demonstrates the high definition of this new generation of OCT on retinal morphology in normal subjects.

Basic Concepts: TD-OCT and SD-OCT

OCT performs cross-sectional imaging by directing a beam of light onto tissue and measuring the **echo time delay** and **intensity of backscattered light** from different tissue structures at varying axial distances in the eye.

Since OCT imaging uses light rather than sound, it is not possible to directly measure echo time delays.

Correlation techniques, known as **low-coherence interferometry**, are required (*Podoleanu 1997*[9], *Schuman 2004*[10]).

To measure echoes of light by low-coherence interferometry, a beam of broadband, low-coherence light is generated by a superluminescent diode.

The interferometer has a superluminescent diode (SLD) light source, sample (eye), reference mirror, and detector arms.

The output of the SLD light source is launched into the source arm and split by the coupler into the beam focused on the eye and then directed at a reference mirror.

The reflected light beam from the eye, consisting of *multiple echoes* of different intraocular structures, and the reference beam reflected from a reference mirror and consisting of a *single echo* at a known delay, is recombined by the *interferometer* and produces interference.

Time-Domain OCT

In TD-OCT, the reference mirror is moved to match the delay in various layers of the sample because interference is only observed when the reference delay matches the echo delay in the signal light (**Figure 1**).

The resulting interference signal is processed to give the **axial scan.** The reference mirror must move one cycle for each axial scan.

The need for this mechanical movement limits the image acquisition speed.

The single detector detects the output signal from the interferometer, which is then processed and displayed on a computer.

Ultrahigh-Resolution OCT (UHR-OCT)

A new generation of Time-Domain OCT has been developed, known as *ultrahigh-resolution OCT* (UHR-OCT).

This *ultrahigh-resolution OCT* will provide **axial image resolution of 3µm.**

UHR-OCT is not widely used in clinical practice, however, due to the need for a special light source (femto-second titanium-sapphire laser) and the long data acquisition time.

Spectral-Domain OCT or SD-OCT

In SD-OCT, the reference mirror is kept stationary (**Figure 2**).

The interference between the subject and reference reflections is split into a spectrum and captured by a **spectrometer** instead of a single detector.

The spectral interferogram is Fourier-transformed to provide an axial scan. The absence of moving parts allows the image to be acquired very rapidly.

The **comparison** of TD-OCT and SD-OCT is summarized (**Table 1**). Several types of SD-OCT are now commercially available (**Table 2**).

Imaging Advancements in SD-OCT

High Resolution

The **axial resolution** of OCT is essentially determined by the coherence length of the light source, which is inversely proportional to the bandwidth (*Wojtkowski 2007*[11], *Huang 2005*[12]).

Time-Domain OCT uses SLD sources emitting a wavelength of about 820 nm over a bandwidth of 20 nm with an axial resolution of about **10 µm** in tissue.

The *first* FDA-approved SD-OCT (***RTVue™ system***), uses SLD light sources with an 840 nm center wavelength over a bandwidth of 45 nm with an axial resolution of less than **5 µm**, (ie, 2-fold higher than that of Time-Domain OCT).

High-Speed Acquisition

*RTVue** can capture 2048 pixels (entire A-scan) simultaneously without any mechanical motion, while Time-Domain OCT captures one pixel at a time.

In the time it takes Time-Domain OCT to form a single axial scan, SD-OCT can capture an entire image.

The *RTVue** provides scan speed of ***26,000 A-scans per second***, 65 times faster than the conventional Time-Domain OCT system.

Improved Imaging Quality

Interpretation of the normal macula as a result of improved imaging quality

The shortened image acquisition time minimizes motion **artifacts**. In addition, the higher acquisition speed of SD-OCT can increase the number of transverse pixels per image to yield **high-definition** images with further improved image quality.

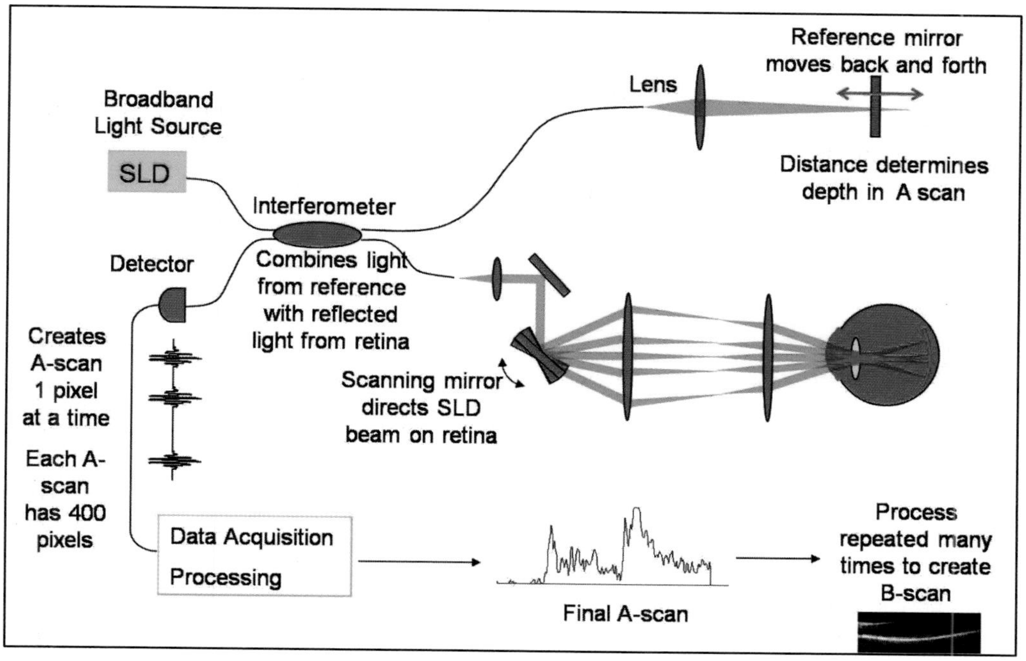

Figure 1. Diagram of Time-Domain optical coherence tomography.
The position of the reference mirror must be moved mechanically to measure the time delays of light echoes from different structures in the eye.

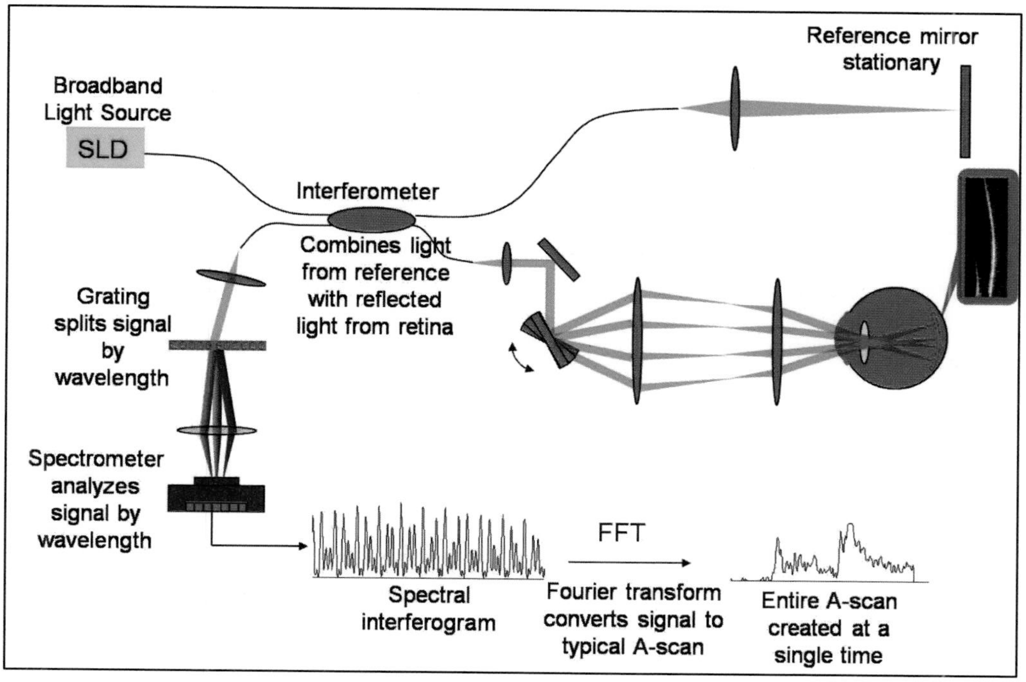

Figure 2. Diagram of Spectral-Domain optical coherence tomography.
The reference mirror is kept stationary. The interference between the sample and reference reflections is captured by a camera and analyzed as a function of wavelength. The spectral interferogram is Fourier-transformed to provide an axial scan. Thus, spectral domain detection measures all echoes of light simultaneously.

Table 1. Comparison of *Stratus** TD-OCT and SD-OCT specifications

	*Stratus** TD-OCT (OCT-3000™)	FD-OCT (RTVue™)
Light source	Superluminescent diode (SLD)	Superluminescent diode
Scan beam wavelength	λ=820 nm, ⊠λ=20 nm	λ=840 nm, ⊠λ=45 nm
Detector	Single detector	Spectrometer
Axial resolution	10 µm	~5 µm
Transverse resolution	20 µm	10-20 µm
Maximum A-scans per B-scan	512	4096
Acquisition time per one line scan	1.28 seconds	0.038 seconds
Scan depth	2 mm	2-2.3 mm
Scanning speed A-scans per second	400 A-scans/second	26,000 A-scans/second

Table 2. Available SD-OCT systems

Company	Name	Axial resolution (µm)	Acquisition speed (A-scans/second)	Features
Optovue	**RTVue-100**	~5	26,000	The first SD-OCT in the U.S.A.
Carl Zeiss	**Cirrus HD-OCT**	~5	27,000	Advanced software
Heidelberg	**Spectralis**	~7	40,000	Combines OCT with angiography
OTI	**Spectral CT/SLO**	~5-6	27,000	Microperimetry compatible
Topcon	**3D OCT 1000**	~5	20,000	
Optopol	**Copernicus**	~6	25,000	
Bioptigen	**3D SDOCT**	~6	20,000	

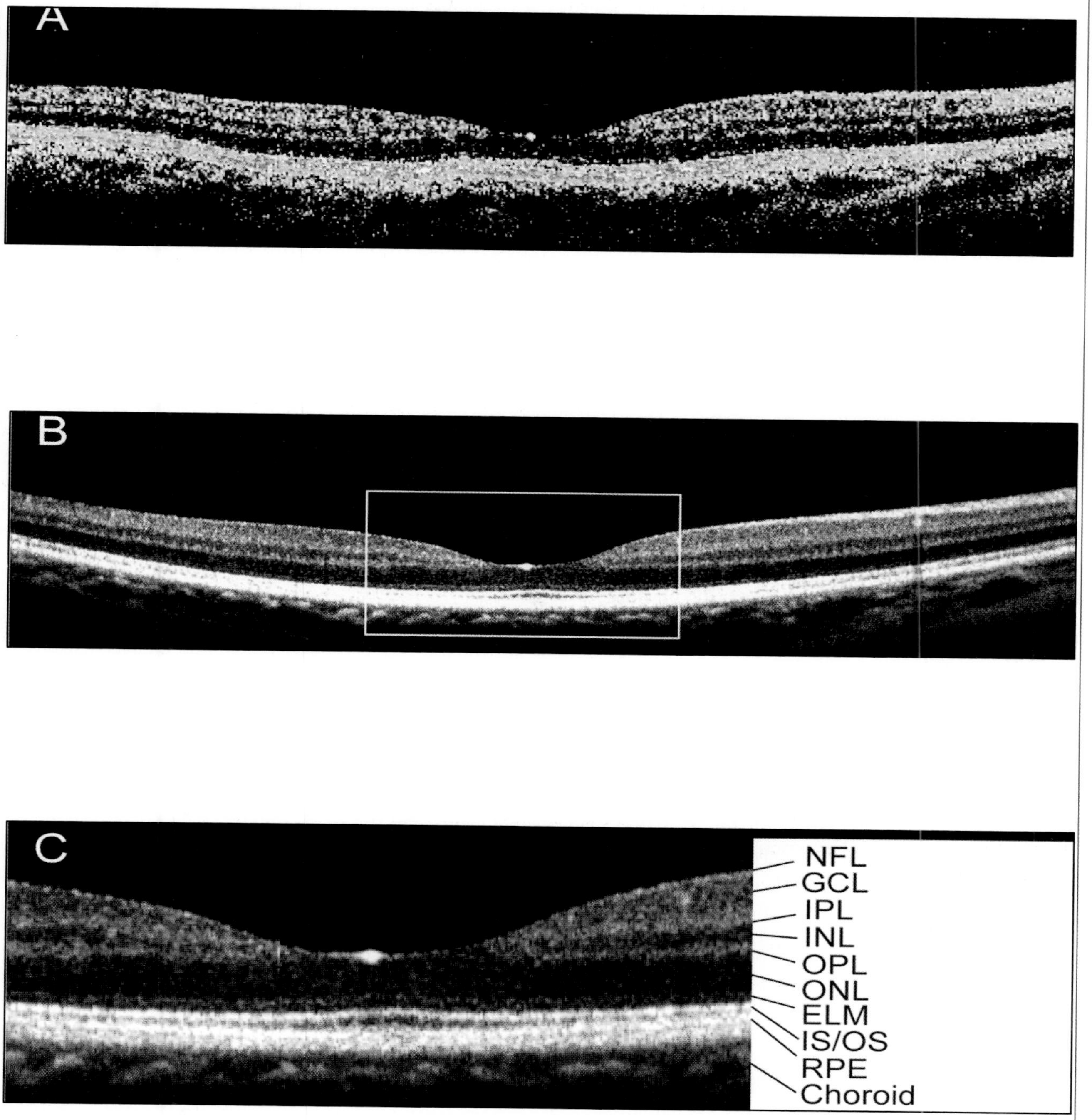

Figure 3. Stratus OCT (A) and Spectral-Domain OCT images (B, C) of the normal human macula. *(RTVue*^{TM} *Optovue*, Inc.).* Image acquisition time: 0.038 seconds. *NFL=nerve fiber layer; GCL=ganglion cell layer; IPL=inner plexiform layer; INL=inner nuclear layer; OPL=outer plexiform layer; ONL=outer nuclear layer; ELM=external limiting membrane; IS/OS=inner segments/outer segments; RPE=retinal pigment epithelium.*

Horizontal, cross-sectional images of the **normal human macula** taken by conventional TD-OCT (Stratus *OCT*) and Spectral-Domain system (*RTVue OCT*) are shown (**Figure 3**).

Most intraretinal layers can be visualized with *Stratus** (**Figure 3A**). However, SD-OCT (with *RTVue**) provides enhanced visualization of the intraretinal layers (**Figure 3B and 3C**).

The intraretinal layers

- The **first hyper-reflective layer** is the *nerve fiber layer* (NFL).
- **Low-backscattering intraretinal layers** are then visible: *Ganglion Cell Layer* (GCL), *Inner Nuclear Layer* (INL), and *Outer Nuclear Layer* (ONL).
- **Less reflective layers** are adjacent to these nuclear layers: the *Inner Plexiform Layer* (IPL) and the *Outer Plexiform Layer* (OPL).
- A **thin hyper-reflective layer above** the OPL corresponds to the *External Limiting Membrane* (ELM).

The ELM is not a physical membrane but is thought to be an alignment of structures between the photoreceptor cells and the Müller cells representing the inner border of the photoreceptor inner segment.

- **The hyper-reflective layer** below the ELM corresponds to the ***Interface*** between photoreceptor inner segments and outer segments (IS/OS).

The back reflection signal arising from IS/OS junction is thought to originate from the abrupt boundary between structures of the IS and highly organized OS, which contains stacks of membranous discs that are rich in the visual pigment rhodopsin (*Gloesmann 2003*[13]).

- The **bright backscattering layer** below the IS/OS interface corresponds to the *retinal pigment epithelium* (RPE).

The **distance** between the RPE and the IS/OS interface *is* consistent with the increase in length of the cone OS in this region.

- **Bruch's membrane** is not clearly visualized as an independent structure, as it is included in the highly reflective RPE.
- A **distal region of high reflectivity** corresponds to the *choroid*. The choroidal vessels induce shadowing effects that limit OCT imaging of deeper structures.

These interpretations are supported by studies comparing ultrahigh-resolution OCT images, and to histology, as well as the known optical properties of retinal layers in the animal retina (*Huang 2005*[12], *Gloesmann 2003*[13]).

Three-Dimensional OCT Imaging

Improved resolution and scan speed provide comprehensive three-dimensional information that could not be previously obtained with conventional TD-OCT systems.

Three-dimensional OCT (3D-OCT) data taken with *RTVue** consist of 101 B-scan images each associated with 512 A-scans equally spaced in a rectangular area with an axial length of 2 mm. Volume data acquisition of 4 x 4 x 2 mm can be completed in 2 seconds.

3D-OCT images of the normal retina provide a comprehensive view of the morphology of the entire foveal depression (**Figure 4**).

In addition to this 3D representation, a single cross-sectional image can be extracted and analyzed separately to identify a specific site of interest.

All of these cross-sectional images can be used to analyze various pathologies in three dimensions or to detect more localized pathologies without missing any important retinal features in the zone studied.

Three-dimensional imaging consequently allows better evaluation of the entire retina. Thus, the 3D-OCT imaging protocol achieves improved retinal coverage.

A cross-sectional image of the center of the 3D image, demonstrating the *central foveal depression* is shown (**Figure 4B**).

Characteristic features of this central foveal area are the high hyper-reflective *foveal pit* at the deepest location of the depression and a focal elevation of the OLM and the IS/OS interface (IS/OS junction).

The retinal vasculature can be visualized due to the detection of reflectance shadows by overlying vessels.

3D-OCT can also reconstruct the various retinal layers in the *en face* system.

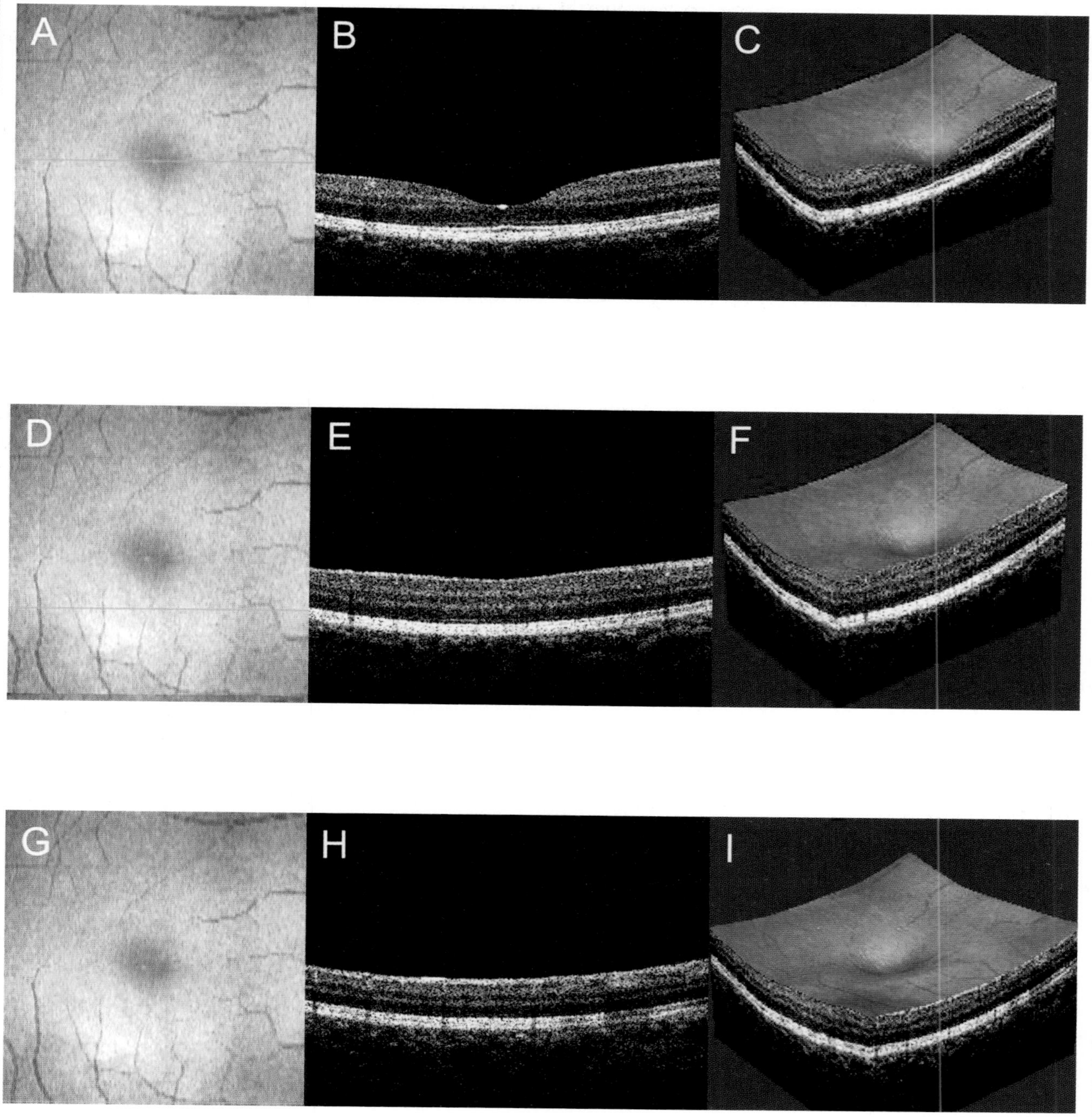

Figure 4. OCT fundus images (*RTVue™*).

A, D, and G): OCT fundus images.

B, E, and H): Anteroposterior images.

C, F, and I): 3D-OCT images.

Green lines indicate the exact locations of anteroposterior sections.

Clinical Applications of 3D SD-OCT

3D-OCT imaging data is useful for registration of OCT images of the fundus or to obtain features of segmentation of the various retinal layers, and to measure retinal thickness.

Registration

The 3D-OCT data obtained with SD-OCT can be used to create *virtual fundus images* that are similar to those obtained with fundus photography.

This OCT fundus image enables precise registration of each cross-sectional OCT image of specific features of the fundus.

OCT fundus images consequently enable direct comparison of OCT data and clinical findings, such as fundus photographs, fluorescein angiography, fundus autofluorescence, and microperimetry.

An example of an OCT fundus image obtained with *RT-Vue*™ is shown (**Figure 5**). This OCT fundus image can be directly correlated to a fundus photograph.

The white arrow indicates the retinal vessels identified:

- On the fundus photograph (**Figure 5A**), and
- On the OCT fundus image (**Figure 5B**),
- Corresponding to cross-sectional images (**Figure 5C**), and
- Corresponding to 3D images, respectively (**Figure 5D**).

This example demonstrates the ability to *precisely localize* a specific lesion and to directly correlate this lesion with the finding on the fundus photograph and OCT images.

These OCT fundus images can be used for tracking of subtle or focal pathologic changes in retinal disease.

Image Segmentation

3D images allow automatic segmentation of the different retinal layers.

An automatic segmentation of the OLM and the RPE at the same time as retinal thickness mapping obtained by the *Cirrus*™ HD-OCT (Carl-Zeiss-Meditec) in a normal human macula is shown (**Figure 6**).

Segmentation can be performed using the software developed for the *Cirrus**, designed to automatically delineate retinal and RPE layers.

This technique can provide **realistic identification** and delineation of choroidal neovascularization (CNV) and associated exudative changes in AMD.

In addition, automatic segmentation allows detailed quantitative and topographic analysis of CNV, RPE, and the overlying retina.

These various findings may improve the understanding of the pathophysiology of AMD and allow better follow-up of treatment.

Measuring and Mapping Retinal Thickness

The *Stratus** OCT measures retinal thickness by radial scans (6 mm in length) centered on the fovea (*Chan 2006*[14]). However, the majority of the macular surface is represented by *extrapolation* of the 6 sections obtained.

*Stratus** OCT also measures retinal thickness by identifying the most highly reflective anterior and posterior layers just anterior to the retinal RPE. *Stratus** OCT may therefore underestimate true retinal thickness.

In contrast, *RTVue** SD-OCT allows **more comprehensive analysis** of the retina with 11 horizontal and vertical lines (5 mm scan length and 0.5 mm interval) and 6 horizontal lines (3 mm scan length and 0.5 mm interval) (**Figure 7**).

SD-OCT is also able to differentiate the **IS/OS interface** as a distinct feature from the RPE.

*RTVue** shows **retinal thickness mapping** that measures retinal thickness as the distance from the inner surface (corresponding to the RPE) to the vitreoretinal interface.

These measurements correspond more closely to the real anatomical retinal thickness.

The inner retinal thickness is also measured from the vitreoretinal interface to the inner plexiform layer.

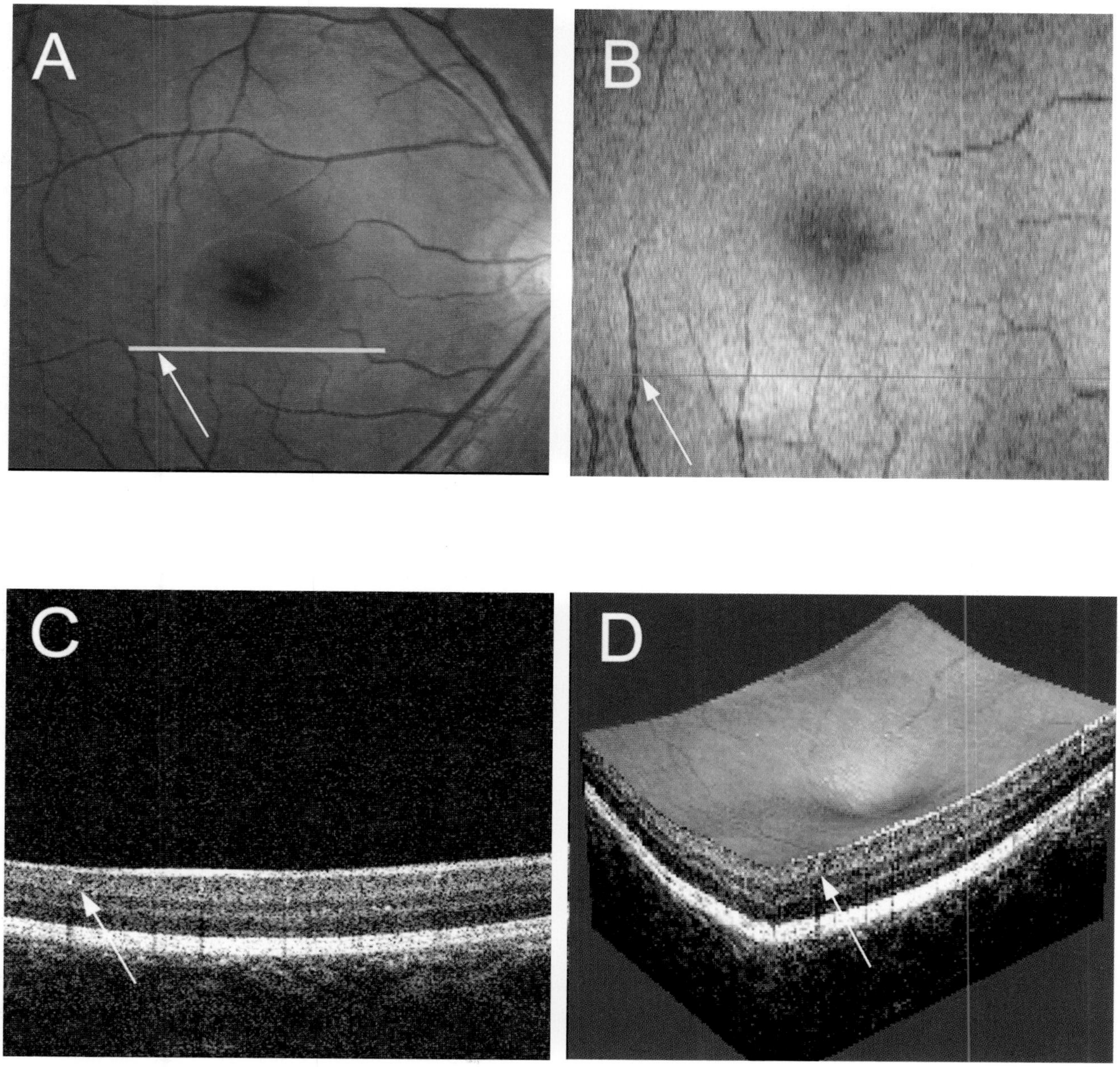

Figure 5. ***RTVue**** **OCT fundus images can be used for registration of cross-sectional images.**

A): Fundus photograph. Retinal vessels are indicated by a white arrow.

B): OCT fundus image.

C): Corresponding cross-sectional image.

D): 3D image.

Current Applications of SD-OCT in AMD

OCT analysis of AMD has become very useful in relation with PDT and anti-VEGF therapy.

Retinal thickness is an important parameter to analyze exudation, and the acquisition speed and *high resolution* obtained with SD-OCT *allows* new methods of visualization, mapping, and measurement of retinal thickness.

Precise clinical measurements and measurements of various **volumes** such as CNV, cystoid spaces, subretinal fluid, and lesions underneath the RPE, are also possible.

Evaluation of the photoreceptor layer and its integrity is possible. These advances offer more sensitive diagnostic indicators of disease and methods to assess disease progression.

SD-OCT may become an essential tool for diagnosis and to guide treatment decisions.

SD-OCT Imaging and 3D Analysis in Vitreoretinal Diseases

This chapter has described the basic concepts of TD-OCT and the more recently developed SD-OCT.

Several examples of imaging in vitreoretinal diseases are demonstrated by various clinical cases, such as:
- Idiopathic macular hole (**Figure 8**),
- Vitreoretinal traction syndrome (**Figure 9**),
- CNV in AMD (**Figure 10**),
- Polypoidal choroidal vasculopathy (**Figure 11**)
- Chorioretinal anastomosis (**Figure 12**).

Conclusion

TD-OCT provides useful information for the diagnosis of many vitreoretinal diseases. It has become a standard diagnostic instrument for vitreoretinal diseases, including AMD.

SD-OCT, a new generation of OCT, provides further progress and can be used to document even subtle changes in **chorioretinal microstructures**. In particular, the clinical use of SD-OCT will provide a wealth of information for the diagnosis and evaluation of AMD.

References

1. **Huang D, Swanson EA, Lin CP, et al.** Optical coherence tomography. Science. 1991;254:1178-81.
2. **Salinas-Alamán A, García-Layana A, Maldonado MJ, et al.** Using optical coherence tomography to monitor photodynamic therapy in age related macular degeneration. *Am J Ophthalmol. 2005; 140:23-8.*
3. **Coscas F, Coscas G, Souied E, et al.** Optical coherence tomography identification of occult choroidal neovascularization in age-related macular degeneration. *Am J Ophthalmol. 2007; 144:592-9.*
4. **Avery RL, Pieramici DJ, Rabena MD, et al.** Intravitreal bevacizumab (Avastin) for neovascular age-related macular degeneration. *Ophthalmology. 2006 Mar;113(3):363-372.*
5. **Michels S, Rosenfeld PJ, Puliafito CA, et al.** Systemic bevacizumab (Avastin) therapy for neovascular age-related macular degeneration twelve-week results of an uncontrolled open-label clinical study. Ophthalmology. 2005;112:1035-47.
6. **Fung AE, Lalwani GA, Rosenfeld PJ, et al.** An optical coherence tomography-guided, variable dosing regimen with intravitreal ranibizumab (Lucentis) for neovascular age-related macular degeneration. Am J Ophthalmol. 2007;143:566-83.
7. **Iam S, Zawadzki RJ, Choi S, et al.** Clinical application of rapid serial Fourier-domain optical coherence tomography for macular imaging. *Ophthalmology. 2006; 113:1425-31.*
8. **Hangai M, Ojima Y, Gotoh N, et al.** Three-dimensional imaging of macular holes with high-speed optical coherence tomography. *Ophthalmology. 2007; 114:763-73.*
9. **Podoleanu AG, Dobre GM, Webb DJ, et al.** Simultaneous en-face imaging of two layers in the human retina by low coherence reflectometry. *Opt Lett.* 1997;22:1039-41.
10. **Schuman JS, Puliafito CA, Fujimoto JG.** Optical Coherence Tomography of Ocular Disease. 2nd ed. SLACK Inc, 2004;3-19.
11. **Wojtkowski M, Leitgeb R, Kowalczyk A, et al.** In vivo human retinal imaging by Fourier domain optical coherence tomography. J Biomed Opt. 2002;7:457-63.
12. **Huang D, Kaiser PK, Lowder CY, et al.** Retinal Imaging. 1st ed. *Elsevier Mosby;2005:47-65.*
13. **Gloesmann M, Hermann B, Schubert C, et al.** Histologic correlation of pig retina radial stratification with ultrahigh-resolution optical coherence tomography. Invest Ophthalmol Vis Sci 2003;44:1696-703.
14. **Chan A, Duker JS, Ko TH, et al.** Normal macular thickness measurements in healthy eyes using Stratus optical coherence tomography. *Arch Ophthalmol. 2006;124:193-8.*

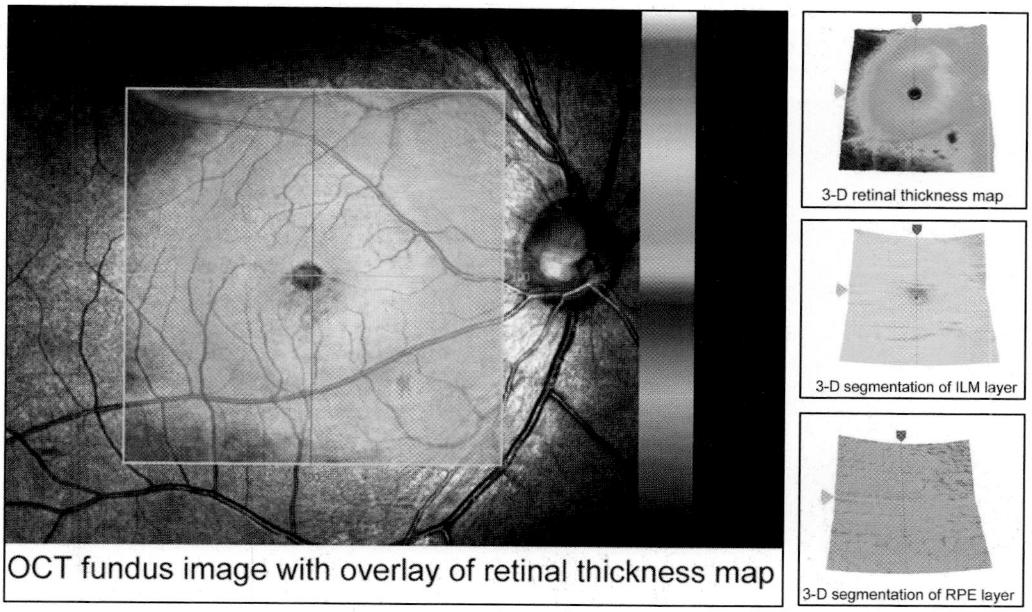

Figure 6. 3D segmentation of the ILM and RPE.
3D retinal thickness map of the normal human retina (*Cirrus** HD-OCT).

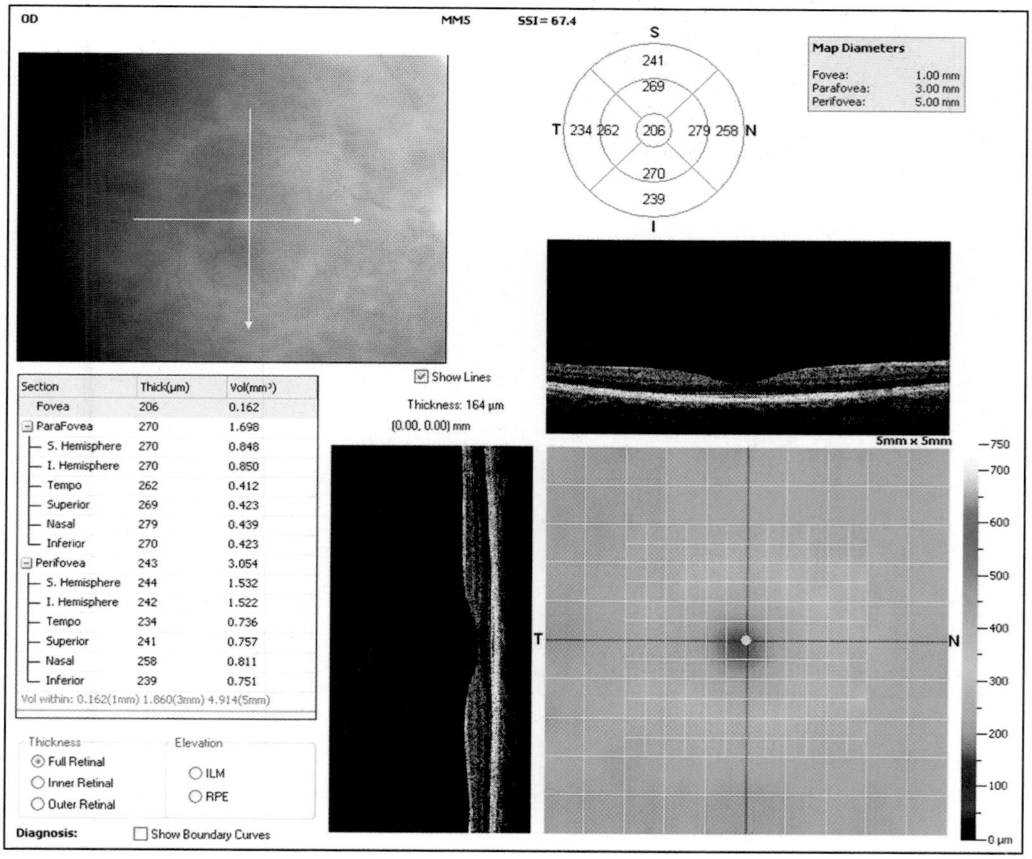

Figure 7. Retinal thickness measurement in a 5 mm x 5 mm area of the central macula (*MM5 protocol - RTVue**). The thickness of the inner and outer retinal layers can be measured separately or the entire retinal thickness can be measured.

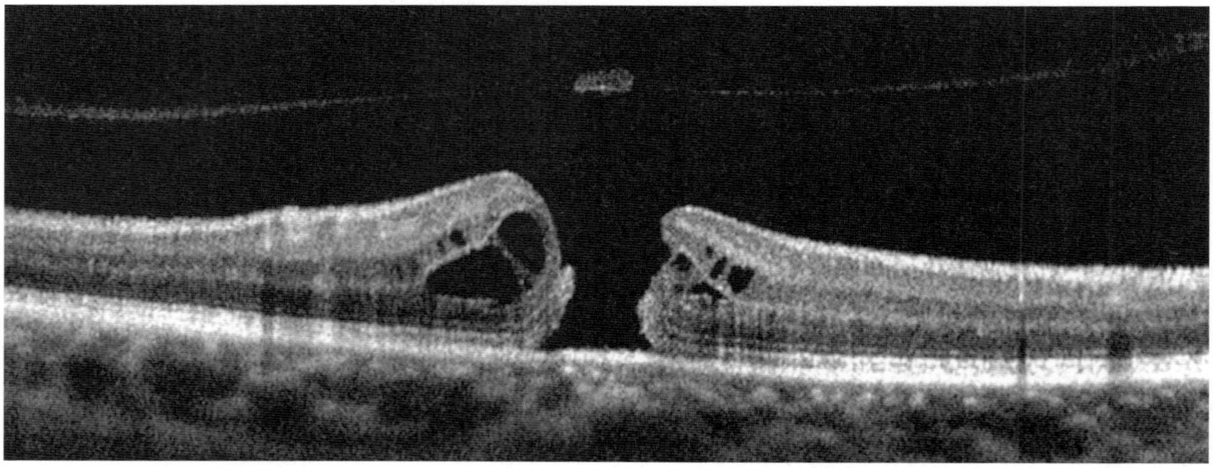

Figure 8. Idiopathic macular hole (*RTVue** SD-OCT).
The posterior hyaloid membrane is clearly visible with an operculum in front of the macular hole.
Multiple intraretinal cysts are clearly observed.

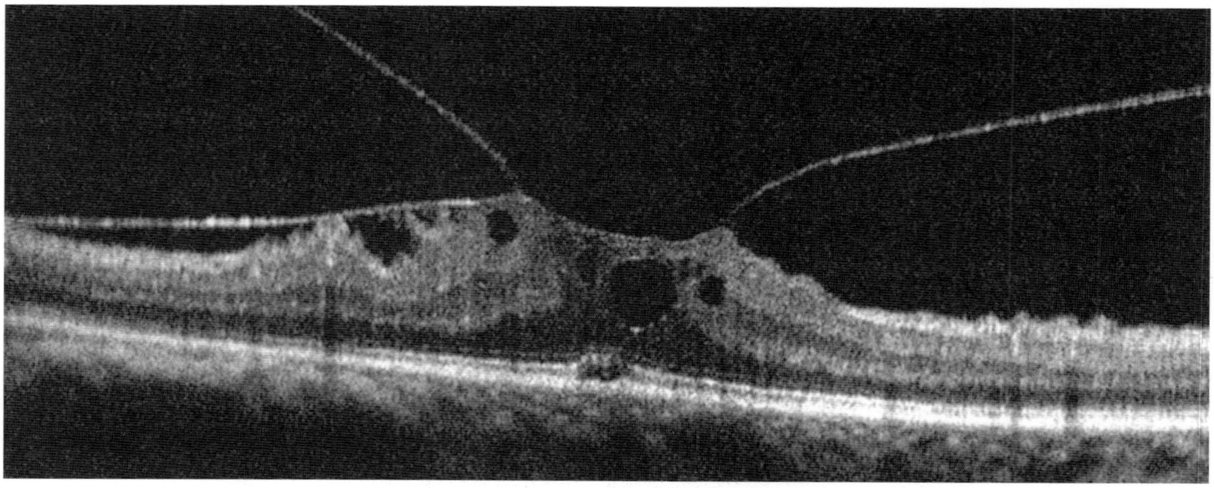

Figure 9. Macular traction syndrome (*RTVue** SD-OCT).
Adhesion of the posterior hyaloid to the macula, generating an inward tractional force causing macular edema with multiple intraretinal cysts.
The IS/OS interface is partially disrupted, but the ELM remains intact.

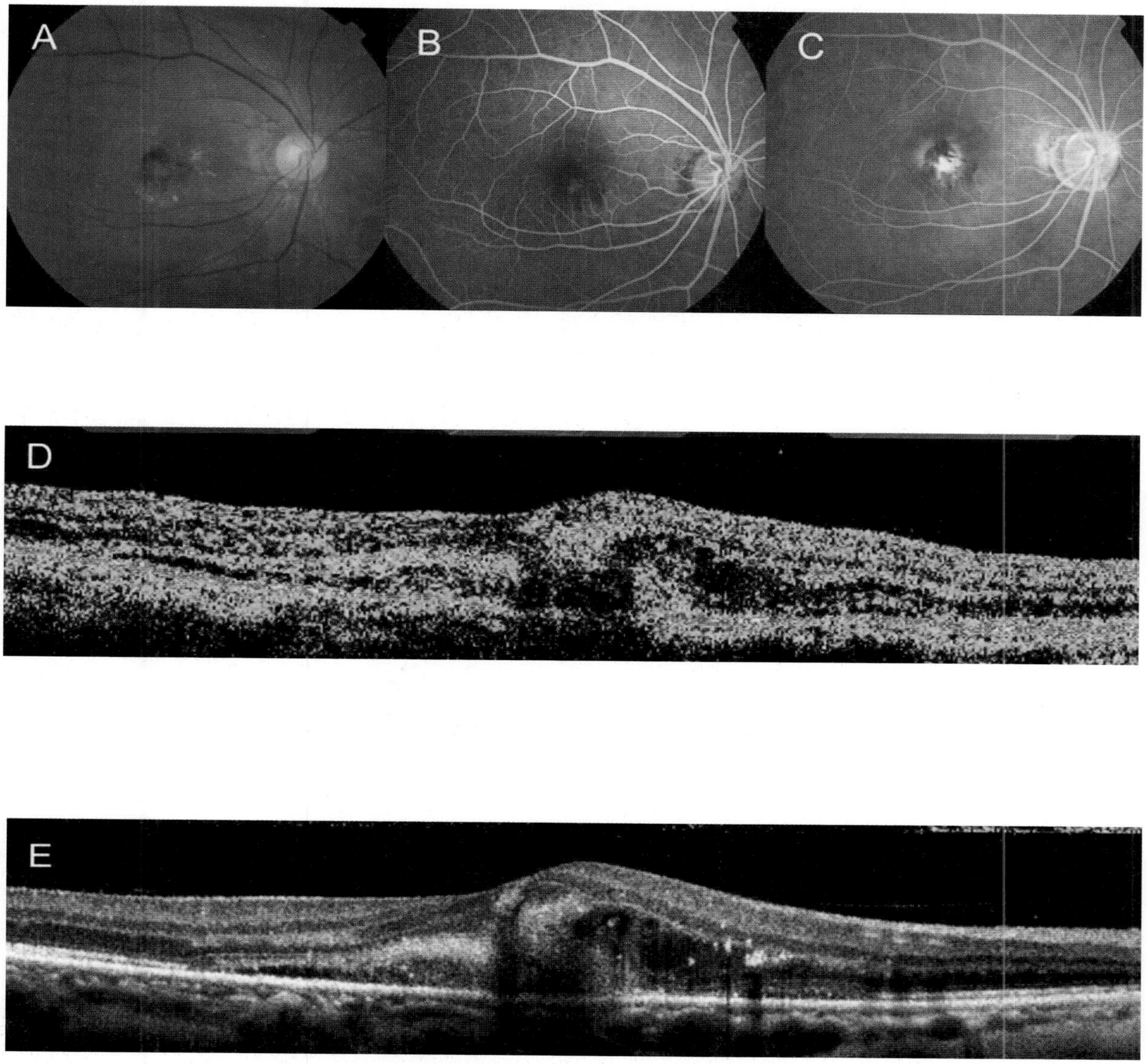

Figure 10. CNV in AMD.

A): Fundus photograph.

B and C): Early and late-phase fluorescein angiography: small classic CNV.

D): Horizontal section of the fovea on *Stratus** OCT: subretinal CNV and diffuse retinal thickening.

E): SD-OCT (*RTVue**): Protrusion of CNV and intraretinal cystic changes.

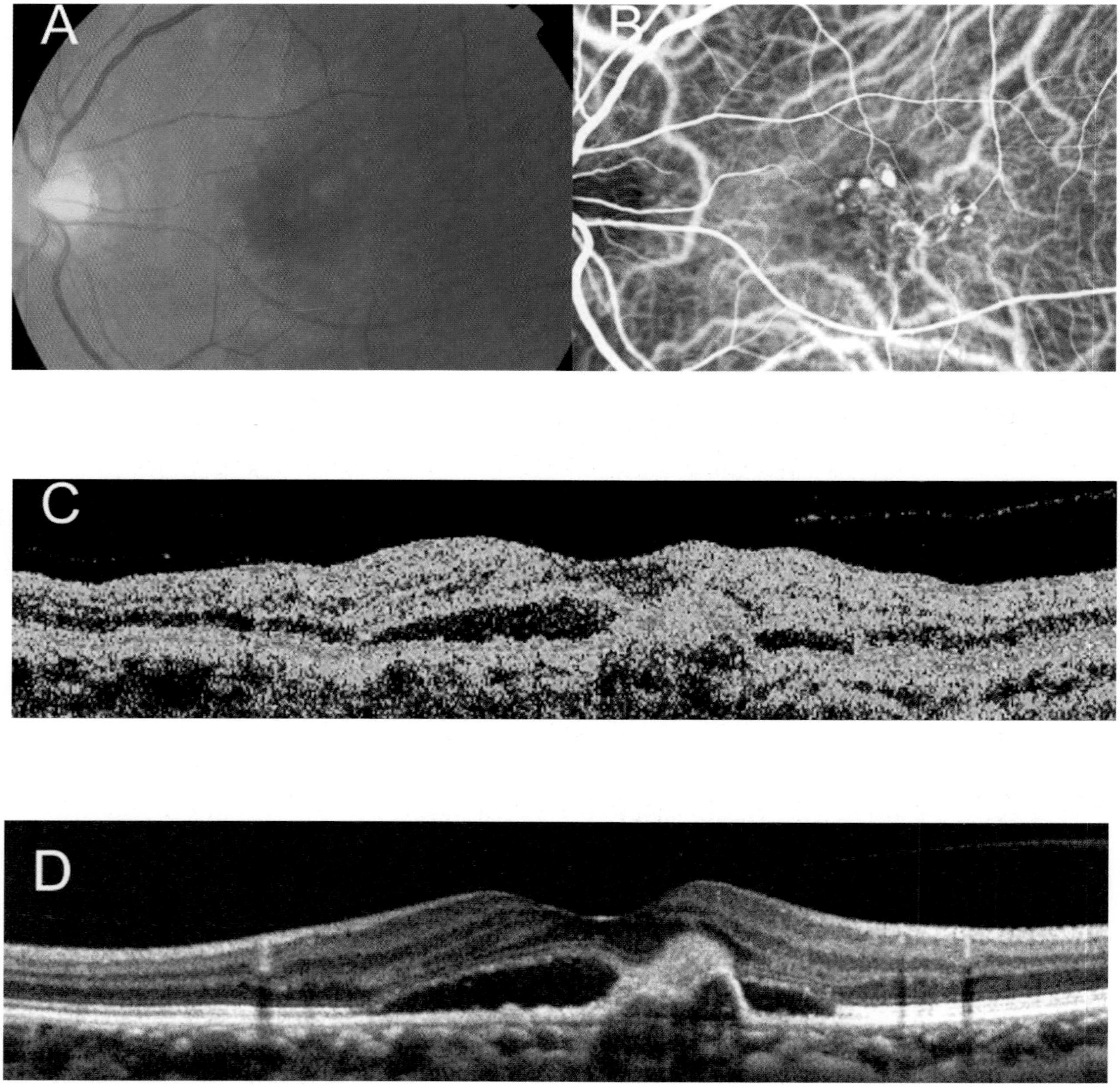

Figure 11. Polypoidal choroidal vasculopathy.

A): Fundus photograph.

B): ICG angiography: subfoveal polypoidal lesions in an abnormal choroidal vascular network.

C): *Stratus** OCT: protrusion of the RPE corresponding to the polypoidal lesions with increased tissue reflectivity and subretinal fluid.

D): SD-OCT (*RTVue**): subretinal fibrinous exudation and protrusion of the RPE, which is irregularly raised.

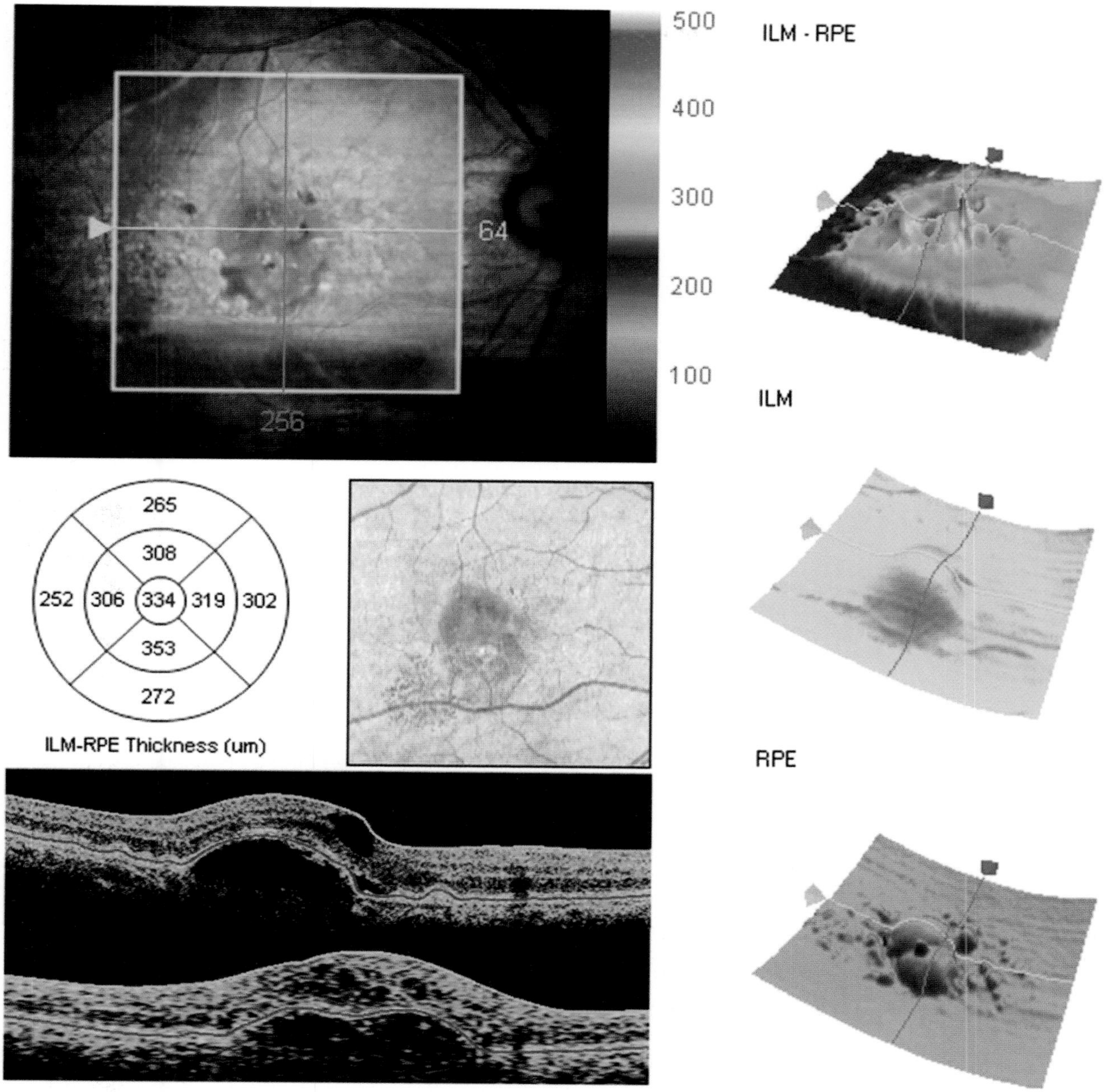

Figure 12: Automated segmentation of the RPE and ILM in a case of probable chorioretinal anastomosis (*Cirrus * HD-OCT*).

Spectral-Domain OCT/cSLO

Bruno LUMBROSO (Rome), Richard ROSEN (New York),
Marco RISPOLI (Rome)

Introduction

Spectral-Domain OCT (SD-OCT) instruments provide ophthalmologists with a significant amount of **new information**.

The images obtained with SD-OCT are much sharper and more precise that those obtained with Time-Domain OCT (TD-OCT).

With SD-OCT, so much information is provided in a single scan that interpretation of this data must be based on clearly defined logical criteria.

Interpretation

Interpretation of these new images is less intuitive than that of TD-OCT.

Normal or physiological images contain many structures and additional characteristics, some of which remain difficult to interpret.

Images obtained in **pathological** situations are not only more detailed, but often demonstrate structures and features not recently visualized by other modalities.

Some structures visualized as segmented and heterogeneous on TD-OCT may appear dense and homogeneous on SD-OCT.

It is still difficult to know whether these new features really correspond to pathological lesions or are simply related to optical and electronic phenomena.

For example, the external limiting membrane is much more clearly visualized on SD-OCT than on light microscopy histological preparations.

Similarly, the structure of the retinal pigment epithelium (RPE) appears to be stratified and has a different optical density from the appearance known up until now.

A good knowledge of anatomy and histology is essential to more clearly understand these new images.

In vivo layer-by-layer optical segmentation images of the retina are also entirely new and their interpretation requires a learning process.

Technology

Time-Domain versus Spectral-Domain

Time-Domain analysis consists of measuring the various times taken by the semi-coherent light beam to travel in the sample arm and the reference arm.

In contrast, Spectral-Domain analysis uses the basic harmonies of the light reaching the detector.

Time-Domain Analysis

Time-Domain OCT instruments have two acquisition strategies.

- *Point-by-point acquisition on the longitudinal axis:* with a series of A-scans over a defined distance (***Zeiss OCT 1, 2, and 3 Stratus****).

B-scans are constructed by a series of vertical segments of A-scans. The reference mirror is moved continuously to detect the plane of analysis.

- *Acquisition in a coronal plane*
(Ophthalmic Technologies, Inc. [OTI*] OCT/SLO).

The instrument uses a second low-frequency galvanometric mirror in the axis perpendicular to the A-scan to obtain segmental scanning.

The B-scan is constructed with a stack of horizontal scans.

Spectral-Domain Analysis

Spectral-Domain analysis uses the first acquisition strategy except that the galvanometric mirror is fixed.

This results in a very large number of A-scans per second (more than 25,000), associated with complete elimination of artifacts.

This **rapid scanning** rate allows acquisition of:
- A stack of closely spaced horizontal (**raster** sections),
- *3D reconstruction* of the retina,
- *In vivo* optical dissection.

The Spectral B-Scan

The resolution of SD-OCT systems is about 4 to 5 microns, although this resolution is not demonstrated *in vivo*.

SD-OCT scanning is objectively superior to that of previous systems and reveals different appearances in terms of reflectivity and structure.

SD-OCT systems also allow the acquisition of about 100 serial scans, from above downwards of the posterior pole, providing a **dynamic tomographic image** of the macular region (at a visual angle of about 25 degrees).

As a result of this technology, SD-OCT can be compared to ultrasound or a dynamic imaging technique assessing alterations of the various structures of the posterior pole and collecting the most significant images.

Presentation of the Results

The use of a grayscale for OCT images has two consequences (**Figures 1 and 2**):

- Evaluation of **black and white scans** appears to provide clearer information on alterations of retinal tissue and the IS/OS interface and changes of the neuro epithelium (high sensitivity).

This can be explained theoretically by the fact that the human eye has a higher sensitivity for grayscale discrimination than for the chromatic scale.

- However, **false-color** imaging highlights the presence of more marked alterations, allowing better definition of simple constituents (relative increase of the specificity of the technique).

The *retinal specialist* plays an essential role in **dynamic study** of retinal tissue and in selecting the most effective mode of visualization to demonstrate a specific disease.

For all of these structures, the *technician's role* must be limited to simple, routine acquisition, under the ophthalmologist's supervision.

OCT examinations conducted **without any clinical information** about the eye examined, may acquire sections that do not comprise the pathological zone, leading to false-negative results.

Retinal Mapping

Retinal mapping can be obtained in two ways:

- *Very rapid acquisition* (about one second) with a grid comprising relatively distant segments;

- Or a *slower method* (about two seconds) but with higher resolution on the vertical axis and closely spaced serial scans.

3D Reconstruction

Three-dimensional reconstruction is based on about 50 to 150 B-scans per second (**Figures 2 and 3**).

The software allows automatic subtraction of the various iso-reflective layers and manual dissection of the 3D cube.

Retinal mapping is precise and comprises very few artifacts, as it is acquired rapidly with a large number of scans (**Figure 4**).

Any artifacts can be eliminated manually on the individual scans constituting the map, by slightly altering the scan lines defined automatically by the software.

C-Scan

C-scans correspond to *coronal* reconstruction of the stack of B-scans.

This method results in a marked reduction of resolution and induces several artifacts, as B-scans may not always be perfectly aligned.

However, this type of C-scan has the advantage of demonstrating certain features by allowing examination of the retina in a plane that is not parallel to the tissue.

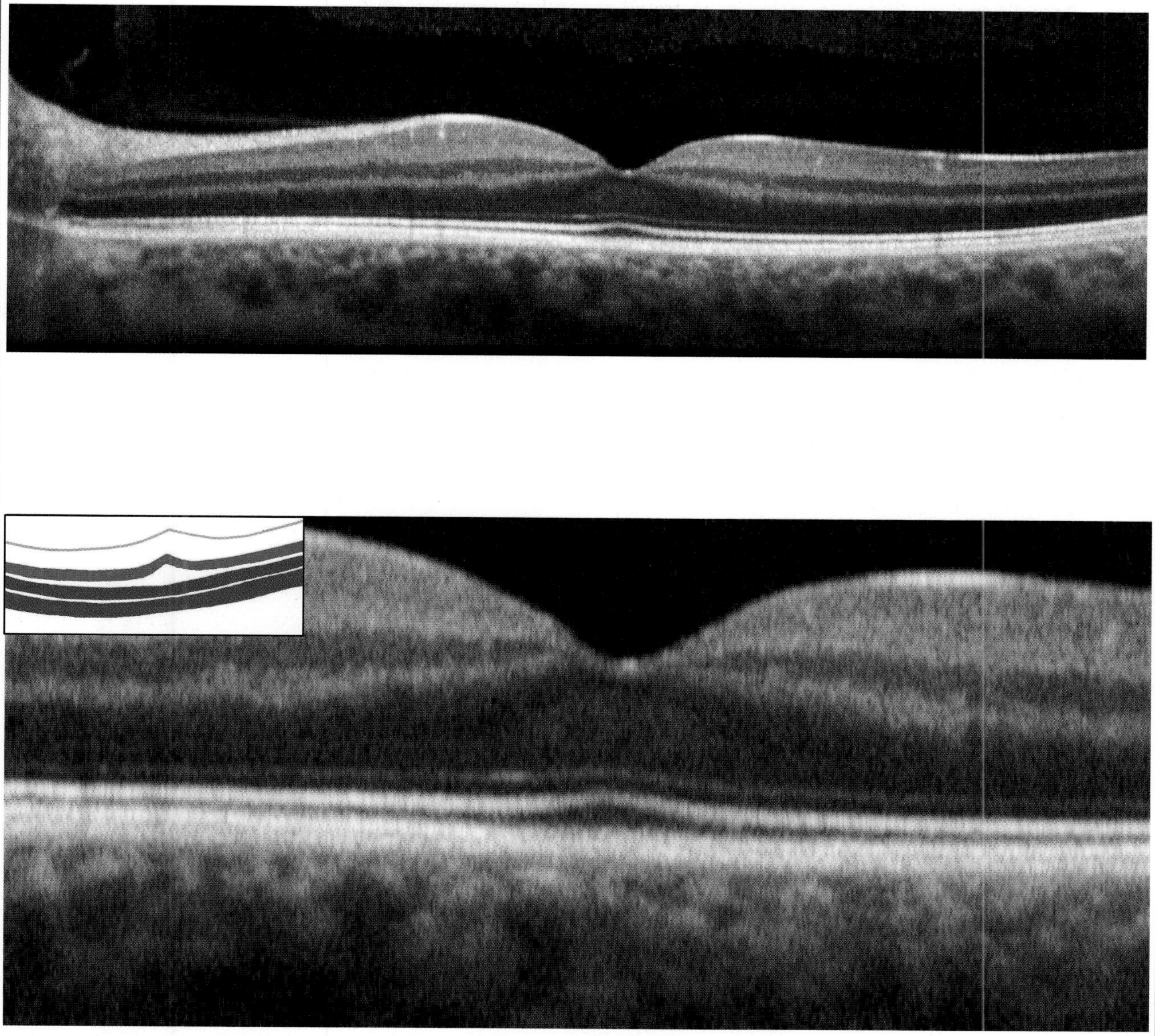

Figure 1. *OTI-OCT/SLO* B-scan.*

The most important feature is the line between the photoreceptor inner segments and outer segments. This interface, barely perceptible on histological sections, is clearly visualized on SD-OCT.

Another clearly visible structure is the *external limiting membrane*, between the outer nuclear layer and the cell bodies.

In the fovea, these two lines are situated further away from the RPE forming a small peak due to the increased length of photoreceptors in this zone (*diagram*).

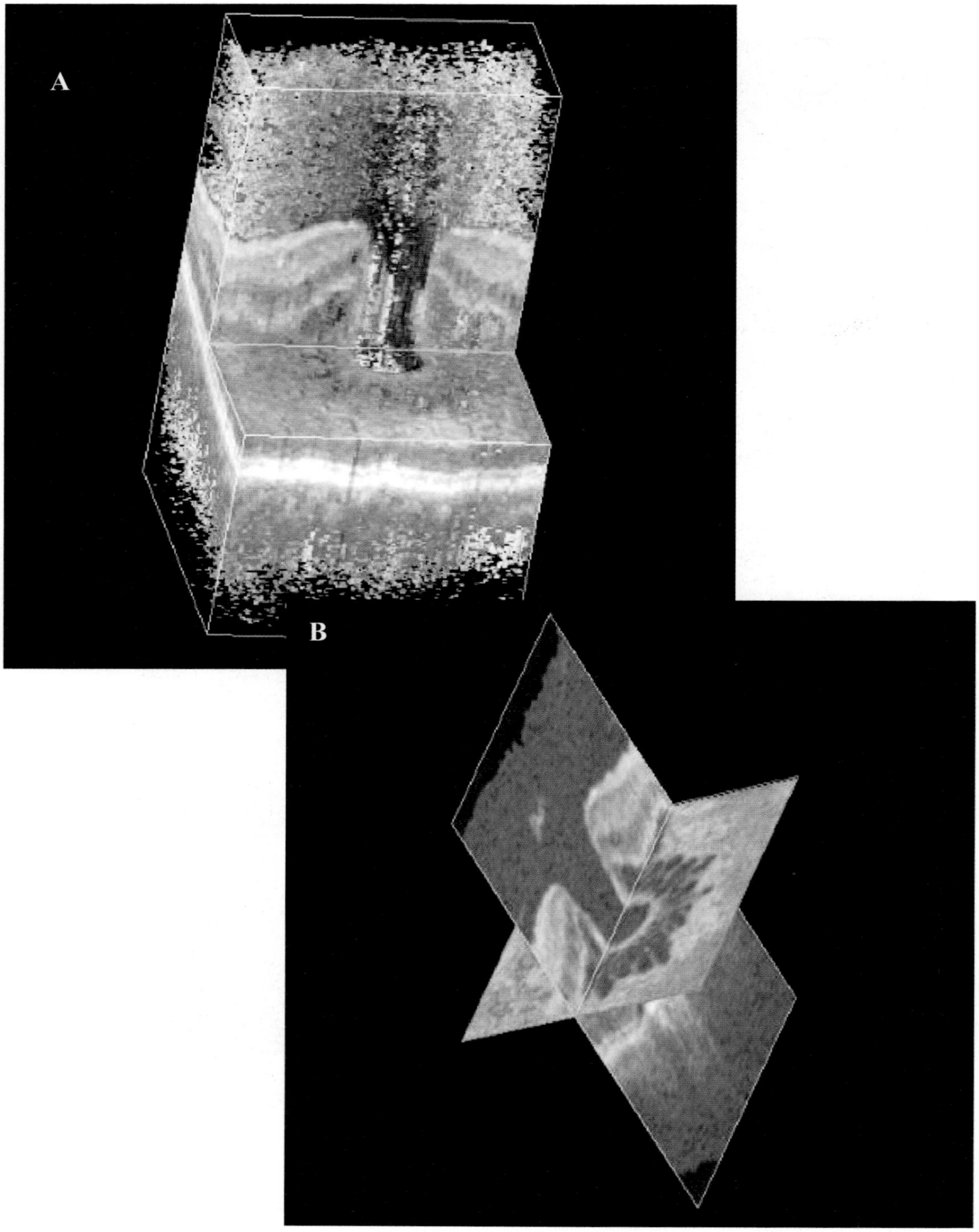

Figure 2. Volume representations.

A): Demonstration of the cube with export of a retinal segment demonstrating a full-thickness macular hole.

B): Demonstration of the intersection between the B-scan and the C-scan.

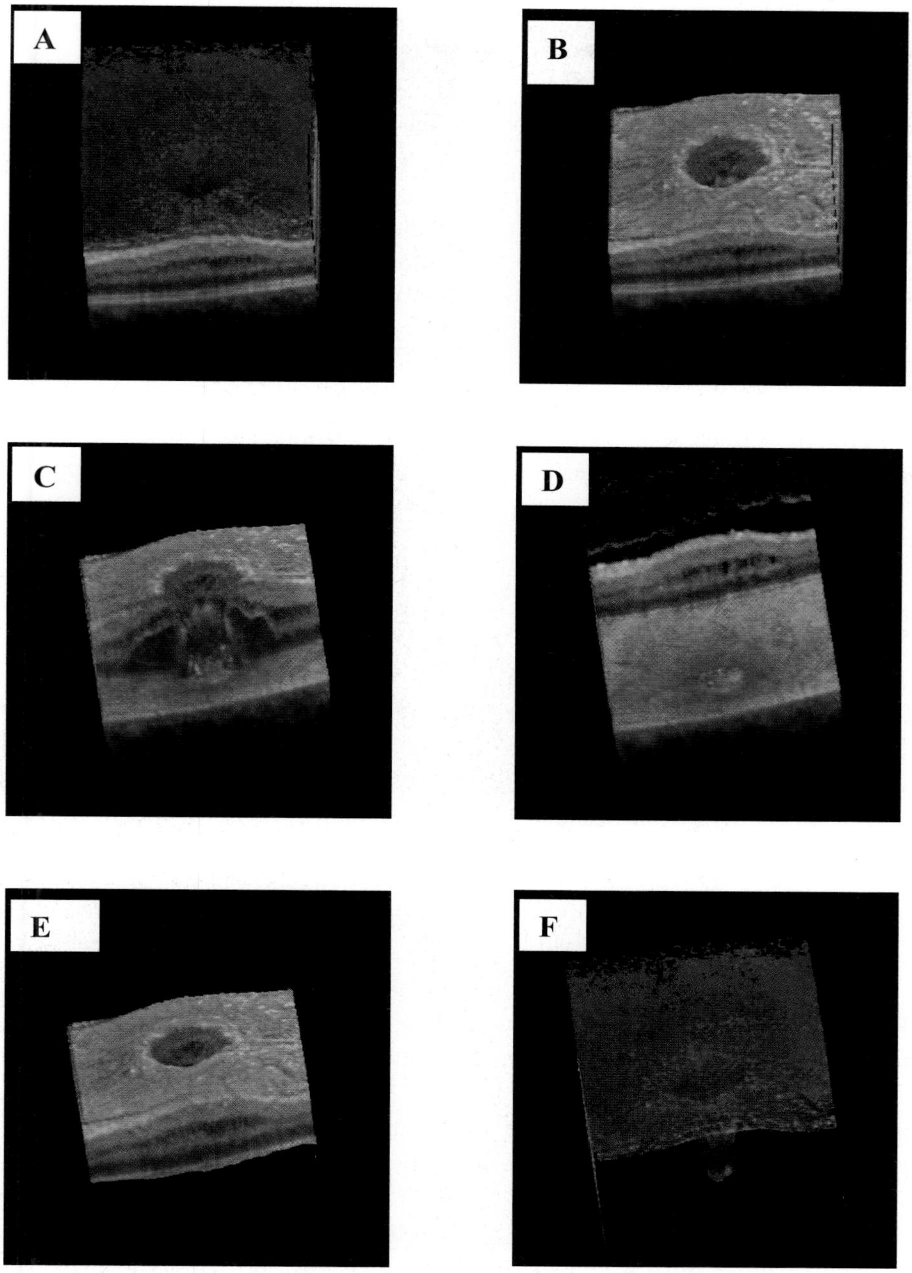

Figure 3. Appearance of the retinal cube with conventional color-coding.

A): Note the relative transparency of the vitreous allowing visualization of alterations of the vitreoretinal interface.

B): Segmentation: the vitreous has been subtracted, demonstrating the surface of the retina.

C): Partial export of the retina above the RPE.

D): Subtraction of the retinal cube to demonstrate the surface of the RPE.

E): Demonstration of the retinal cube with displacement of the vitreous from the RPE.

F): Demonstration of the isolated retinal cube.

Advantages of SD-OCT

SD-OCT visualizes certain layers that have not yet been clearly identified.

The reflectivity of lesions and known physiological structures varies with their depth and their density.

The **choroid**, for example, is clearly visualized by SD-OCT but is difficult to visualize with TD-OCT.

SD-OCT technology clearly visualizes deeper structures, allowing precise analysis of the choroidal plane.

SD-OCT also appears to be more suitable to examine a structure or a lesion with a particular density in the **vertical axis**.

Contrast

Overall, SD-OCT images can be considered to have a lower contrast than TD-OCT images, making it more difficult to examine hypo-reflective structures, such as the vitreous, vitreoretinal interface, intraretinal fluid, and elements situated close to the RPE-choriocapillaris complex.

Artifacts

Analysis of SD-OCT examinations reveals an almost complete absence of artifacts on the various sections.

A minor difficulty concerns **calibration of the reference plane** (the focal analysis plane), as two tissue images are acquired.

This analysis is easy to perform on the normal retina but can be more difficult on the pathological retina.

Microperimetry

In AMD, microperimetry can be used to evaluate the extent and density of scotomas and precisely record the presence of micro scotomas that are difficult to identify by other methods.

It can also be used to localize the fixation point, evaluate its stability, and localize this point in relation to the scotoma.

*OTI** SD-OCT allows immediate and simultaneous evaluation of retinal function and morphological data concerning retinal thickness and edema.

The apparatus software allows a combination of these functional tests and visualization of morphological abnormalities.

Conclusion

In summary, the OCT/SLO-OTI appears to be particularly useful in two fields.

First, it can be used to acquire 3D images that provide important information for diagnosis and which are very useful for teaching purposes.

Second, and possibly even more useful, OCT/SLO-OTI allows a combination of microperimetry and OCT to overlay retinal thickness mapping and functional studies of the retina.

Microperimetry provides an exact point-by-point correspondence between fundus images and perimetry results.

Microperimetry combined with OCT allows real-time retinal function studies with ophthalmoscopic control of the retinal surface (Menke 2006[1]).

An important field of application is the study of retinal sensitivity in various macular diseases.

Many studies are in process in different diseases such as diabetic retinopathy (before and after treatment) (*Carpineto 2007*[2], *Vujosevic 2006*[3], *Okada 2006*[4]), and other diseases (*Carpineto 2005*[5], *Ojima 2008*[6], *Charbel 2008*[7]), as well as definition of the fixation point in patients with low vision.

This easy-to-use instrumentation combining OCT and microperimetry can therefore provide detailed analysis of fixation and correlations between anatomical lesions and retinal dysfunction.

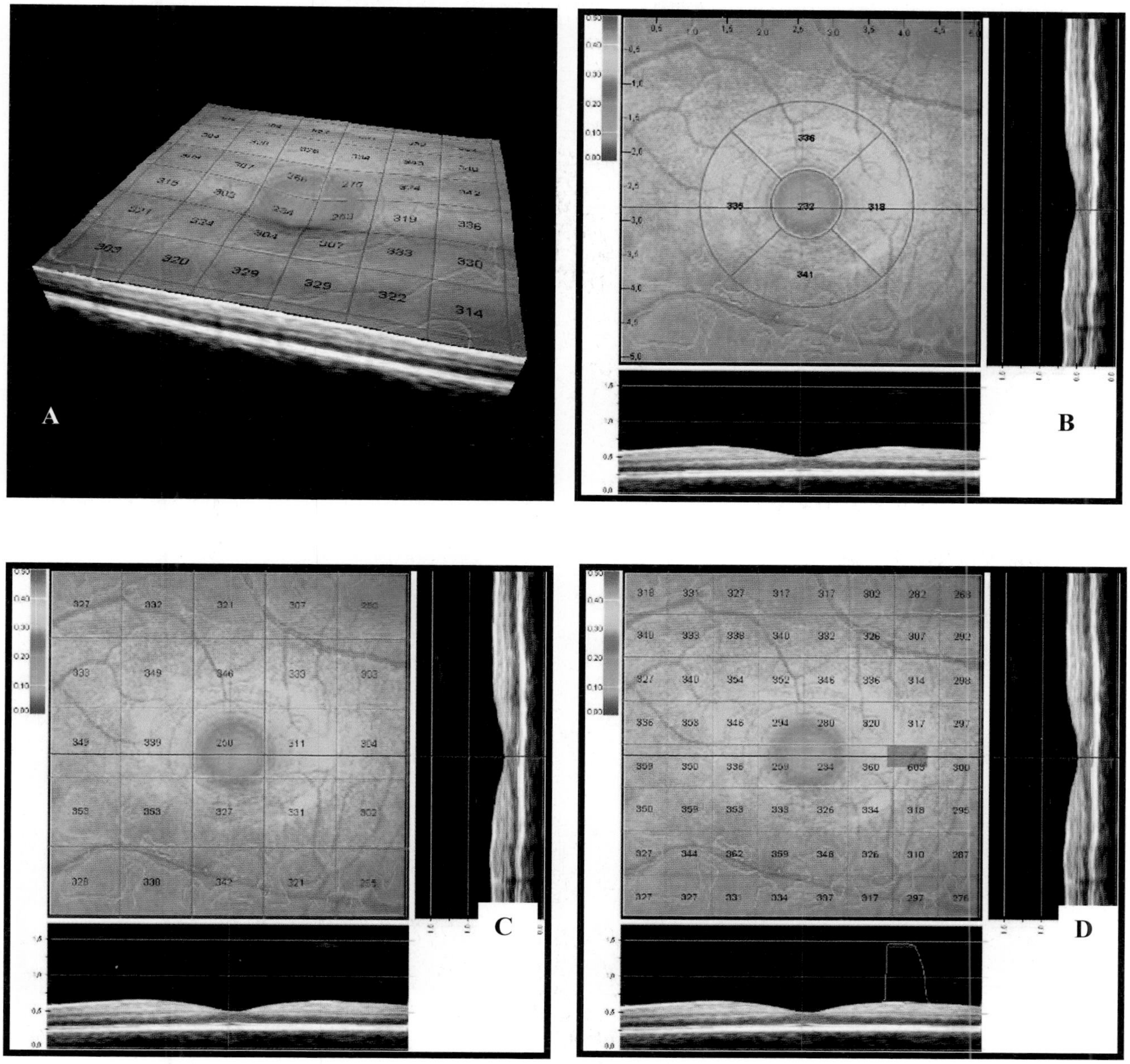

Figure 4. Graphic representation of retinal topography.

A): Prospective vision of retinal topography.

B): Retinal topography.

C): Retinal topography subdividing the retina into sectors for analysis of the macular area.

D): Example of manual correction of an erroneous line.

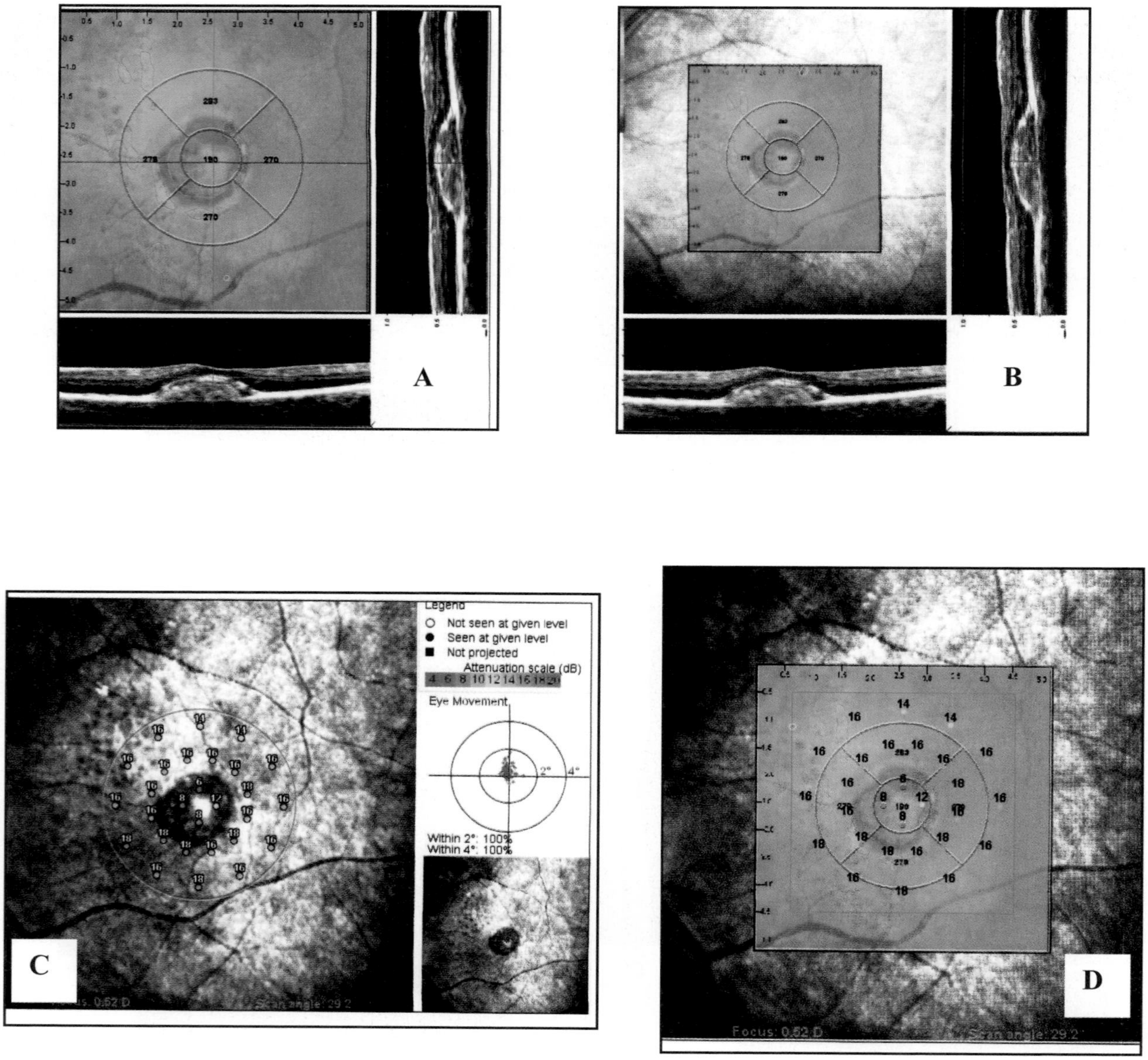

Figure 5.

A): **Retinal thickness mapping** in a case of pseudo-vitelliform macular degeneration. The numbers on the map correspond to the mean retinal thickness of the zone. The retinal thickness scale is situated on the left.

B): **Overlay of retinal mapping** onto an SLO fundus photograph.

C): **SLO microperimetry** in a case of pseudo-vitelliform macular degeneration. Retinal sensitivity is indicated in decibels. Values below 14 decibels are pathological.

D): **SLO microperimetry overlaid** onto retinal thickness mapping. The *OTI** instrumentation allows automatic alignment of the two images by superimposing the capillaries. Retinal thickness and retinal sensitivity are therefore displayed simultaneously on the map.

References

1. **Menke MN, Sato E, Van De Velde FJ, Feke GT.** Combined use of SLO microperimetry and OCT for retinal functional and structural testing. *Graefes Arch Clin Exp Ophthalmol. 2006 May;244(5):634-8*
2. **Carpineto P, Ciancaglini M, Di Antonio L, Gavalas C, Mastropasqua L.** Fundus microperimetry patterns of fixation in type 2 diabetic patients with diffuse macular edema. *Retina. 2007 Jan;27(1):21-9.*
3. **Vujosevic S, Midena E, Pilotto E, Radin PP, Chiesa L, Cavarzeran F.** Diabetic macular edema: correlation between microperimetry and optical coherence tomography findings. *Invest Ophthalmol Vis Sci. 2006 Jul;47(7):3044-51.*
4. **Okada K, Yamamoto S, Mizunoya S, Hoshino A, Arai M, Takatsuna Y.** Correlation of retinal sensitivity measured with fundus-related microperimetry to visual acuity and retinal thickness in eyes with diabetic macular edema. *Eye. 2006 Jul;20(7):805-9.*
5. **Carpineto P, Ciancaglini M, Aharrh-Gnama A, Agnifili L, Cerulli AM, Cirone D, Mastropasqua L.** Optical coherence tomography and fundus microperimetry imaging of spontaneous closure of traumatic macular hole: a case report. *Eur J Ophthalmol. 2005 Jan-Feb;15(1):165-9.*
6. **Ojima Y, Tsujikawa A, Hangai M, Nakanishi H, Inoue R, Sakamoto A, Yoshimura N.** Retinal sensitivity measured with the micro perimeter 1 after resolution of central serous chorioretinopathy. *Am J Ophthalmol. 2008 Jul;146(1):77-84*
7. **Charbel Issa P, Helb HM, Holz FG, Scholl HP; MacTel Study Group.** Correlation of macular function with retinal thickness in nonproliferative type 2 idiopathic macular telangiectasia. *Am J Ophthalmol. 2008 Jan;145(1):169-175*

OCT INTERPRETATION

Clinical Analysis and Interpretation of OCT Characteristics in AMD Comparison with Angiography

Gabriel COSCAS
Florence COSCAS, Sabrina VISMARA,
Alain ZOURDANI, C.I. Li CALZI

(Créteil and Paris)

Introduction

Optical coherence tomography (OCT) imaging has been widely accepted by ophthalmologists as an attractive imaging modality. It not only provides a wealth of information, but it is also non-invasive and easy to perform.

In particular, OCT can provide an overview of the neurosensory retina, retinal pigment epithelium (RPE), Bruch's membrane, and choroid in age-related macular degeneration (AMD)

For example, the presence of **intraretinal fluid, subretinal fluid,** or fluid underneath the RPE may indicate *abnormal leakage* derived from choroidal neovascularization.

The evaluation of the leakage can be precisely quantified, which is useful for monitoring progression of disease or response to treatment.

Although retinal thickness is a precise and informative measurement, OCT can provide much more additional insight.

Detailed examination of changes observed on cross-sectional images of the macular region allows:

- *Analysis* of each layer of the neurosensory retina, retinal pigment epithelium (RPE), Bruch's membrane, and choroid to establish a **definitive diagnosis**.

- *The interpretation of OCT signs* is based on recognizing patterns of abnormalities induced by various lesions and their complications.

For each OCT image, the following should be considered:

- **Alterations of normal structures:**
  - There can be changes in the different tissue layers: the choroid, Bruch's membrane, RPE, neurosensory retina, or in the potential **spaces** between these layers.

- **Additional structures**:
  Pathologic lesions have characteristic variations of reflectivity, which allow their identification. For example, drusen, choroidal neovascularization, hemorrhage, fluid accumulation, pigment deposits, and exudates all appear distinct on OCT.

- **Grouping of the various signs** induced by the combination of these different alterations allows a **more precise diagnosis** of the *type and stage of AMD*, and particularly, the etiology for vision loss, such as choroidal neovascularization or progression to atrophy.

- The **polymorphic natural history** and response to treatment accounts for the different and numerous clinical forms of AMD that should be identified in order to guide treatment.

Besides OCT, *traditional angiography* is still essential to identify choroidal neovascularization and localize it in relation to the fovea.

Fluorescein angiography (FA) is the gold standard for detecting classic choroidal neovascularization (CNV), while **indocyanine green angiography (ICG)** helps visualize occult CNV, and the almost always associated pigment epithelial detachments (PED).

Although OCT cannot directly illustrate choroidal neovascularization like angiography does, it can show highly suggestive **indirect signs**.

An advantage of OCT examination over angiography for the patient is that it does not require an intravenous injection of dye.

Recent developments in imaging systems allow simultaneous display of FA, ICG, and OCT.

This remarkable progress allows exact spatial correlation of angiography with OCT, which helps draw more effective conclusions.

Interpretation of an OCT Image

Interpretation of OCT images must therefore avoid assumptions based on a global, intuitive approach. The examiner should proceed systematically in each case as if completing a reading chart or grid.

*

* *

- **First step:**

The first step is to identify and follow the ***RPE* band,** looking for:

- Irregularities, thickening, fragmentation, effraction, disruption, or shadowing.

The RPE must also be examined for:

- Potential separation of the RPE from Bruch's membrane, which then becomes visible and distinct from the RPE.

*

* *

Posterior to the RPE band:

The analysis continues by studying variations behind the RPE, essentially looking for:

- The presence of **hyper-reflectivity** extending posteriorly throughout the choroid, suggesting atrophy, or on the other hand,
- **Hypo-reflectivity, which** suggests shadowing derived from overlying structures.

Anterior to the RPE band:

Retinal thickness, anterior to the RPE, must then be analyzed for:

- The presence of *cavities* or *deposits*, and
- Analysis of *the neurosensory retinal layers*, membranes, and vitreous.

*

* *

Spectral-Domain OCT

Spectral-Domain OCT (SD-OCT) has transformed analysis of the **external layers of the retina.**

This new technology allows:

- High-resolution visualization of *retinal layers*, and
- Easy distinction of the *interfaces* between the various structures.

This can be obtained as a result of noise reduction and enhanced contrast.

*

* *

This **separate analysis** of the structures and their various abnormalities observed on an OCT section is clearly *schematic and somewhat arbitrary.*

There are virtually no cases in which a pathological lesion affects only one layer or only one tissue.

Therefore, interpretation of localized lesions must also take changes in adjacent structures into account.

I. Retinal Pigment Epithelium

In the Normal Eye

Time-Domain OCT

In Time-Domain OCT, the RPE appears to be clearly visible, as it is a distinct and hyper-reflective structure compared to adjacent structures.

However, this structure actually corresponds to the RPE-Bruch's membrane-choriocapillaris *complex* that is difficult to dissociate, except in pathological conditions.

Spectral-Domain OCT

This technology allows much more detailed analysis, but paradoxically, leaves a larger number of unknowns.

- **The retinal pigment epithelium (RPE)** appears to present (according to some authors) not one, but two, distinct hyper-reflective bands separated by a thin hypo-reflective band (**Figures 1 and 2**).

This feature was first observed with ultrahigh-resolution OCT systems.

The *outer hyper-reflective band* appears to correspond to the pigment epithelium cell bodies, but the origin of the *inner band* has not been clearly elucidated.

Some authors consider this inner band to correspond to *Verhoeff's membrane*, composed of tight junctions between pigment epithelial cells.

According to another hypothesis, this inner band corresponds to basal infoldings and apical processes that enclose photoreceptor outer segments.

This feature is only visible with ultrahigh-resolution systems (or systems associated with adaptive optics) and in normal eyes.

These two bands are *more difficult to distinguish* in the presence of pathological changes, which could have a prognostic value.

- **Bruch's membrane (BM)** is usually not visible on OCT in a normal eye.

It is only really visible and distinct when there is a loss of localized adhesion and it is separated from the RPE with a more or less marked elevation of the RPE band, like in a retinal pigment epithelial detachment.

- The **choriocapillaris** remains poorly visualized and its alterations are almost impossible to analyze.

In the future, the use of longer wavelengths in the infrared spectrum will probably allow better visualization of the choroid.

- The **thickness of the RPE** cannot be measured by Time-Domain OCT but can be measured manually by Spectral-Domain OCT.

Different structures **anterior to the RPE** can now be analyzed:

- The **external limiting membrane** (ELM), which is a fused structure corresponding to the alignment of structures between photoreceptors and Müller cells.
- The **interface** (or **junction**) between photoreceptor inner segments and outer segments (**IS/OS**).

Photoreceptor **inner segments** and **outer segments** can therefore be more precisely evaluated by visualization of these hyper-reflective lines and the hypo-reflective zones on either side.

The **distance** between the RPE and the IS/OS interface increases in the foveal region, corresponding to the longer outer segments of cones in this region (**Figures 1 and 2**).

These normal findings can be used to methodically follow the RPE band from the perimacular zone (usually normal) to the central lesion.

NORMAL RETINAL PIGMENT EPITHELIUM AND RETINAL LAYERS RETINIENNES NORMALES

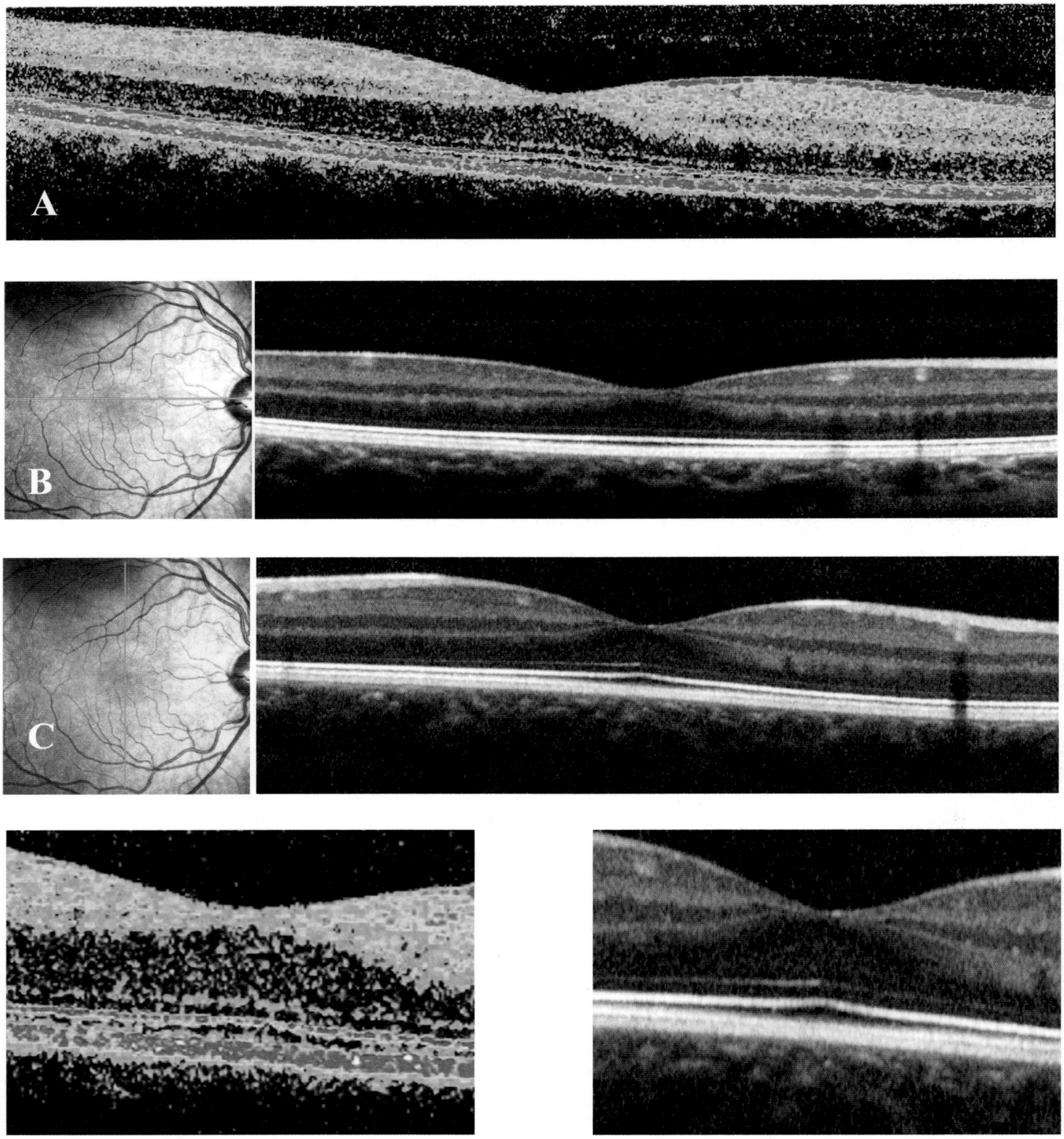

Figure 1: Normal SD-OCT (*Spectralis) section.**
A): Color image. **B** and **C**): Black and white images at different magnifications.
This section delineates the external limiting membrane, the inner segment/outer segment interface, the retinal pigment epithelium, and the choroid. Two distinct layers in the RPE can be seen.
These images are shown with reference red-free images with a horizontal OCT section (B) and an OCT vertical section (C). Fluorescein angiography and SLO-ICG angiography images can also be selected.

NORMAL RETINAL PIGMENT EPITHELIUM AND RETINAL LAYERS

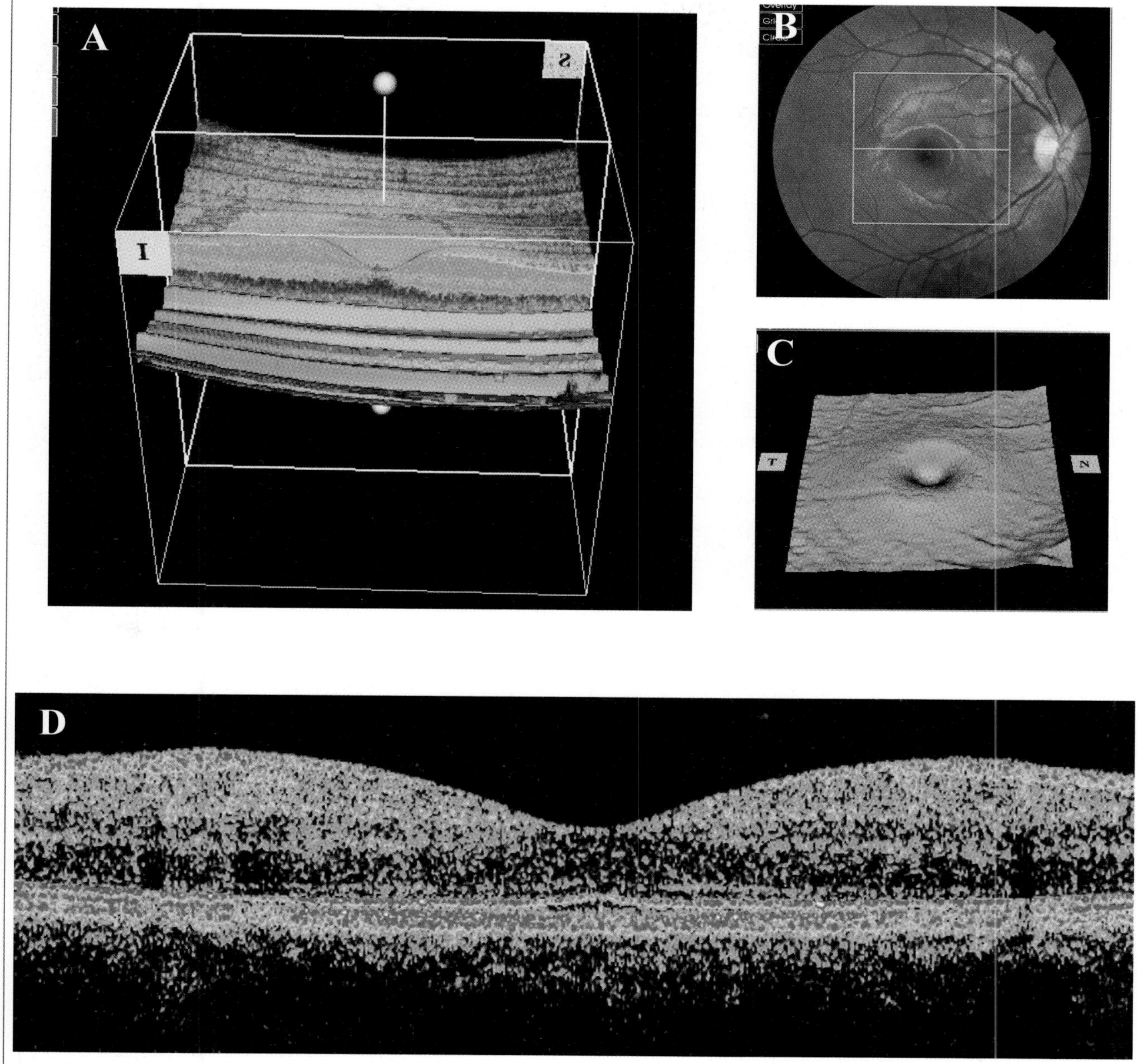

Figure 2: Normal SD-OCT (*Topcon) section.**

A): Volume image with partial segmentation, allowing analysis of the axial cross section (through the center of the fovea) and of the different surfaces.

B): Color reference images showing the zone of examination.

C): False-color image of the retinal surface.

D): Axial section showing the external limiting membrane, the inner segment/outer segment interface, the retinal pigment epithelium, and the choroid.

In Clinical Practice

SD-OCT can be used to detect and evaluate:

- Variations of *thickness*, *contour*, *irregularities*, and *fragmentation*, which must be distinguished from shadowing artifacts.
- *Detachment* of Bruch's membrane.
- The presence of *abnormal structures* located **anterior** or **posterior** to the RPE.

Each of these abnormalities are usually visible on Time-Domain OCT, but they are demonstrated much better on SD-OCT.

The use of SD-OCT is often able to distinguish more subtle abnormalities, which may not be detectable by other modalities.

Enlarged OCT images are useful to precisely analyze these minute structures, whose physiological role and pathological alterations are so important.

In macular diseases and AMD, lesions are rarely larger than a **20° field**, and SD-OCT magnified images provide satisfactory demonstration of pathological details.

Bruch's Membrane

Bruch's membrane (BM) becomes visible when there is a loss of adhesion between itself and the RPE.

This loss of adhesion is usually due to abnormal exudation from choroidal neovascularization underneath the RPE.

In this context, Bruch's membrane is seen as a very regular, homogeneous, slightly hyper-reflective, and relatively thin line.

This line should be used as the outer limit for retinal thickness measurements (**Figure 3**).

Inner Segment/Outer Segment Interface

The inner segment/outer segment interface (IS/OS) is visible as a hyper-reflective line anterior to the RPE.

There is a dark, hypo-reflective space delineated by the RPE on one side and the IS/OS interface on the other side. This space corresponds to *photoreceptor outer segments.*

Another hypo-reflective space is bordered by the IS/OS interface and the external limiting membrane and corresponds to *photoreceptor inner segments.*

These three boundaries (BM, IS/OS interface, and external limiting membrane) constitute essential landmarks during assessment of AMD (**Figure 4**).

RETINAL PIGMENT EPITHELIUM AND OUTER RETINAL LAYERS

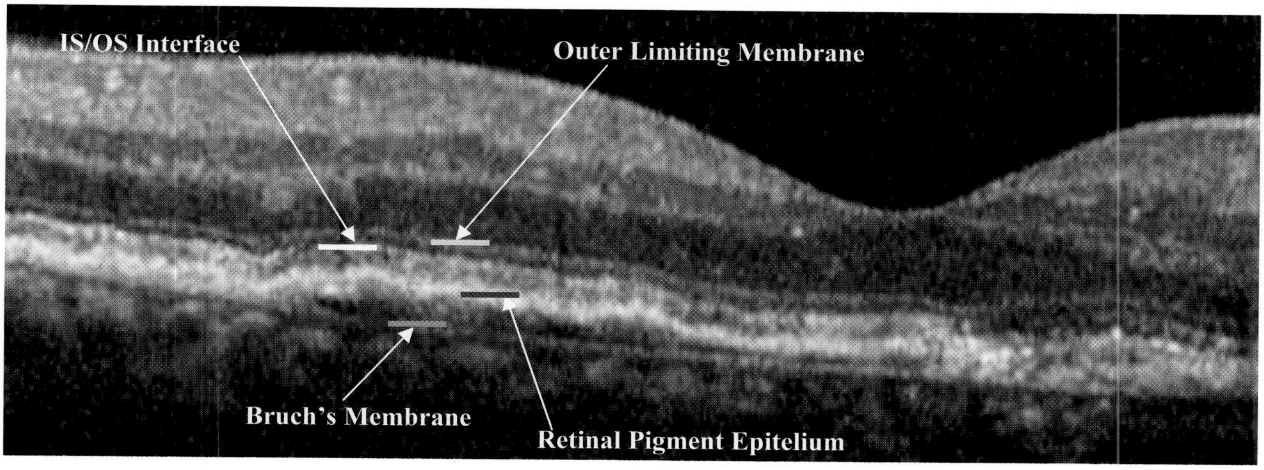

Figure 3: SD-OCT section showing a very limited PED, allowing distinction between the inner segment/outer segment interface, the external limiting membrane, the RPE band, Bruch's membrane, and the choroid (*Spectralis**).

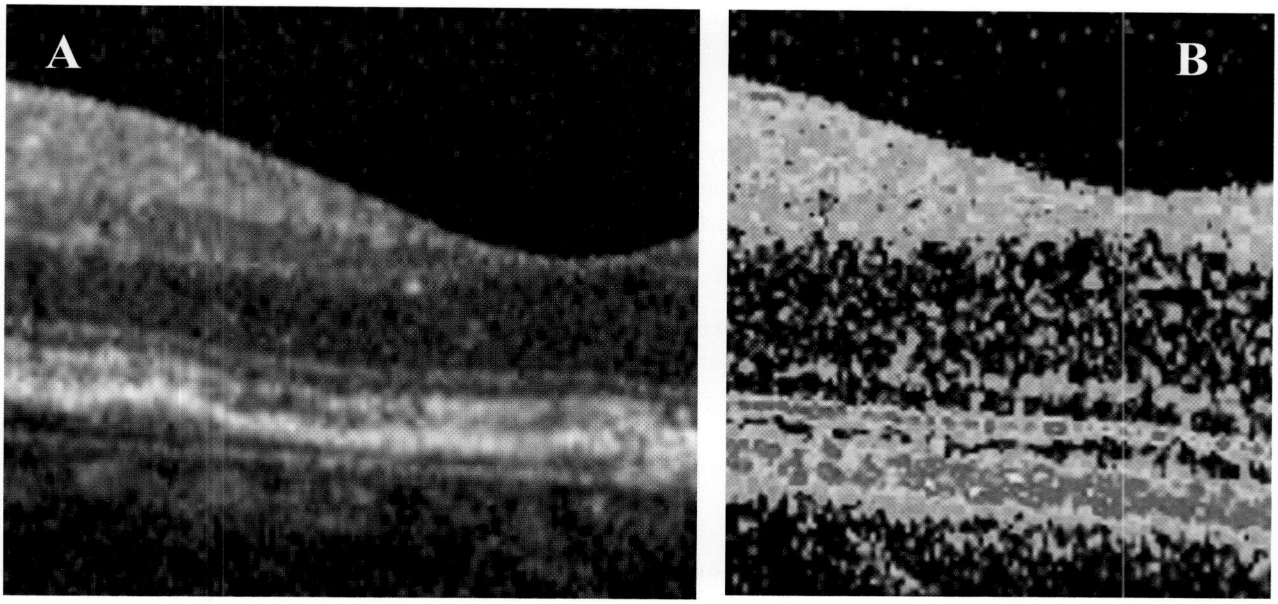

Figure 4: SD-OCT section (same case as in Figure 2).

A): The enlarged image clearly reveals 4 hyper-reflective lines (Bruch's membrane, RPE, IS/OS interface, external limiting membrane), and the hypo-reflective bands that separate these structures, particularly the outer and inner segments and limited PED.

B): The reference cross-section in a normal patient (false-color) reveals the IS/OS interface and the external limiting membrane but with lower resolution. Note the increased thickness of the outer segments in the center of the fovea.

Main Abnormalities of the RPE Band

Variations of RPE thickness are usually relatively mild and difficult to measure precisely because the limits of the RPE are poorly-demarcated, at least on Time-Domain OCT.

However, these variations can be assessed by observing more or less localized enhancement or attenuation of reflectivity.

Evaluation of these changes is more difficult on Time-Domain OCT due to the presence of relatively frequent undulations, which are artifacts due to eye movements.

RPE analysis is more precise with Spectral-Domain OCT, although changes related to the presence of drusen must be taken into account (**Figures 5 and 6**).

RPE Band Thickening

RPE band thickening could possibly be due to proliferation of the RPE, as observed on histological sections. RPE proliferations are barely perceptible on Time-Domain OCT.

Certain features on Spectral-Domain OCT are suggestive of localized proliferation of the RPE and are fairly frequently associated with occult choroidal neovascularization underneath the RPE, which itself may not be directly visible on OCT (**Figures 7 and 8**).

However, OCT correlation with pathology specimens of normal and AMD affected eyes are not available at the present time.

Marked thinning of the RPE can be observed, particularly in case of **RPE atrophy**.

The band corresponding to the RPE appears to be markedly thinned, usually linear, associated with hyper-reflectivity extending posteriorly into the zone of atrophy and enhancing this area.

Thinning of the entire neurosensory retina may also be observed over an RPE atrophy area, especially when it is extensive.

Spectral-Domain OCT can confirm this thinning, essentially corresponding to **alterations of outer layers**, as the external limiting membrane and IS/OS interface are interrupted and absent over atrophic RPE (**Figure 9**).

In more severe atrophy, the outer nuclear layer is altered or no longer detectable and the RPE appears to be in direct contact with the outer plexiform layer (**Figure 10**).

In extreme cases, such as after an RPE tear, the choroid (more or less atrophic) and the residual Bruch's membrane are exposed by the rolled up retracted RPE and are in contact with the inner layers of the retina (**Figure 11**).

Interruptions of the RPE

In some cases, discontinuity of the RPE is due to effraction or break of the RPE, which allows subretinal or intraretinal protrusion of choroidal structures.

The most typical example is that of chorioretinal anastomoses between choroidal neovascularization and juxtafoveal retinal vessels.

This type of lesion is rarely well-visualized on Time-Domain OCT but is better demonstrated on Spectral-Domain OCT.

The appearance of a chorioretinal anastomoses is even more marked with simultaneous angiography, which provides point by point overlay (**Figure 12**).

The **features of attenuated** RPE are usually due to shadowing or accentuated masking.

Masking is related to the presence of highly reflective structures (eg, pigment, hard exudates, and CNV) in the inner retinal layers. Masking is partial and progressive and corresponds to the density of overlying structures.

Masking may be due to retinal hemorrhage or accumulation of melanin pigment or lipofuscin.

Shadowing due to a hyper-reflective structure, such as the presence of classic CNV, must be recognized for early treatment (**Figure 1**).

IRREGULARITIES OF THE RPE

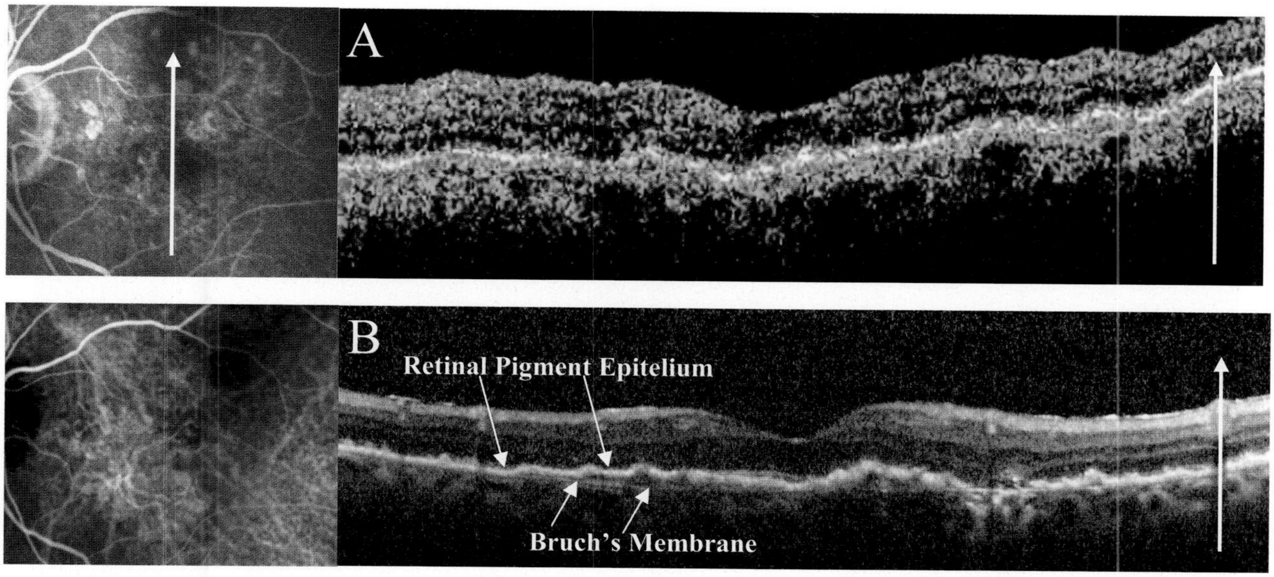

Figure 5: Thickness variations and irregularities of the RPE.

A): *Stratus vertical section shown with fluorescein angiography** (*abnormal choroidal network*):
Undulations from motion artifact limit the visibility of retinal structures.

B): *Spectralis vertical section correlated with ICG angiography** (*same patient*):
Multiple, more or less marked thickness irregularities over the entire length of the section.
Note the presence of several drusen and ability to visualize Bruch's membrane (short arrows), indicating an early PED.

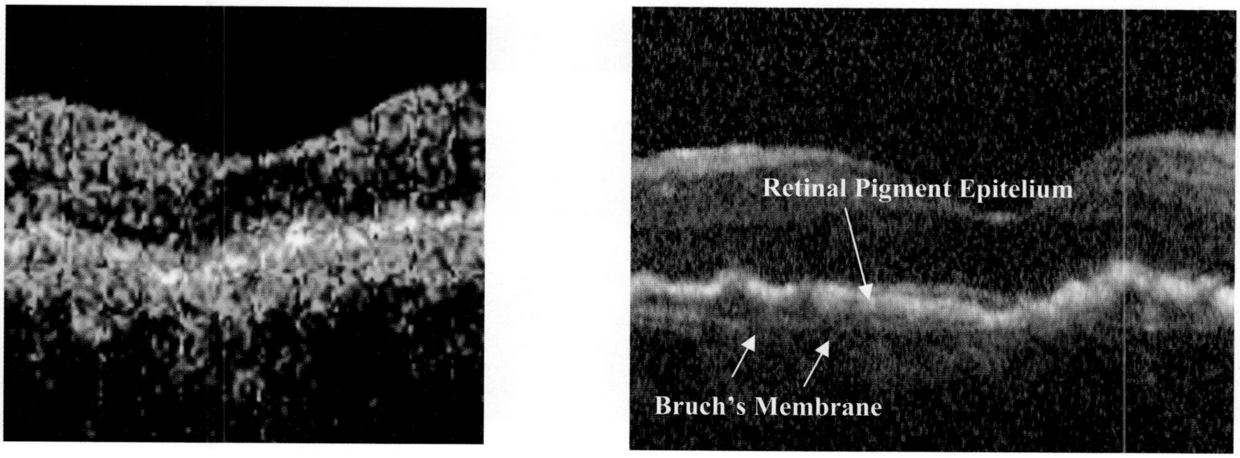

Figure 6: Thickness variations and irregularities of the RPE (same case as in Figure 7).

These enlarged views facilitate analysis of minimal changes in the thickness and reflectivity of the RPE and various alterations in adjacent layers.

RPE THICKENING AND PROLIFERATION

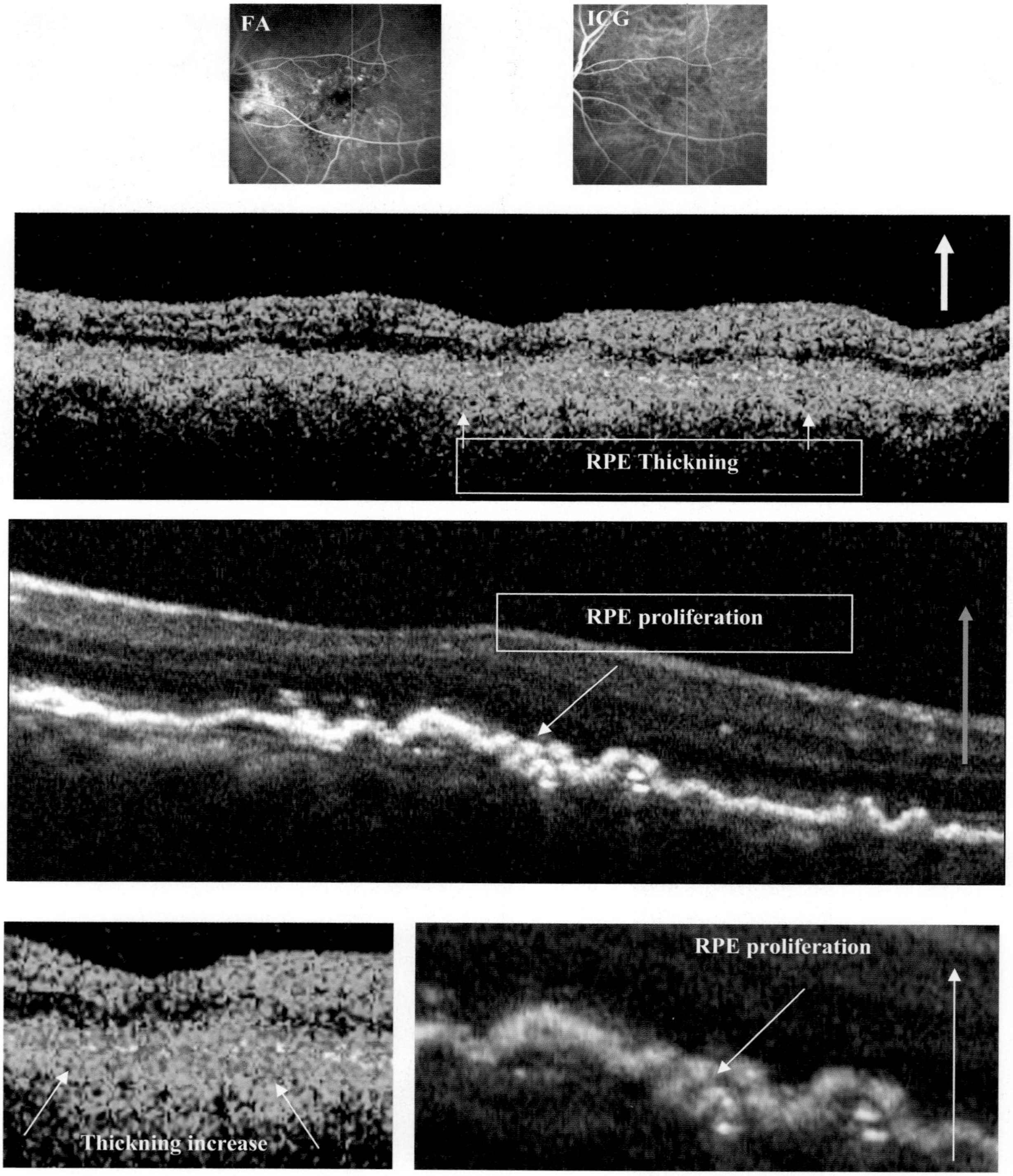

Figure 7: Increased thickness and proliferation of the RPE with limited detachment of the RPE.
A): *Stratus vertical section shown with fluorescein angiography** (*early occult CNV*): increased thickness only (arrows).
B): *Spectralis vertical section correlated with ICG angiography** (*same patient*): fairly marked irregularities of thickness with proliferation of the RPE (arrow) in the area of the CNV.
C): Increased thickness and proliferation of the RPE: Magnified view.

RPE PROLIFERATION

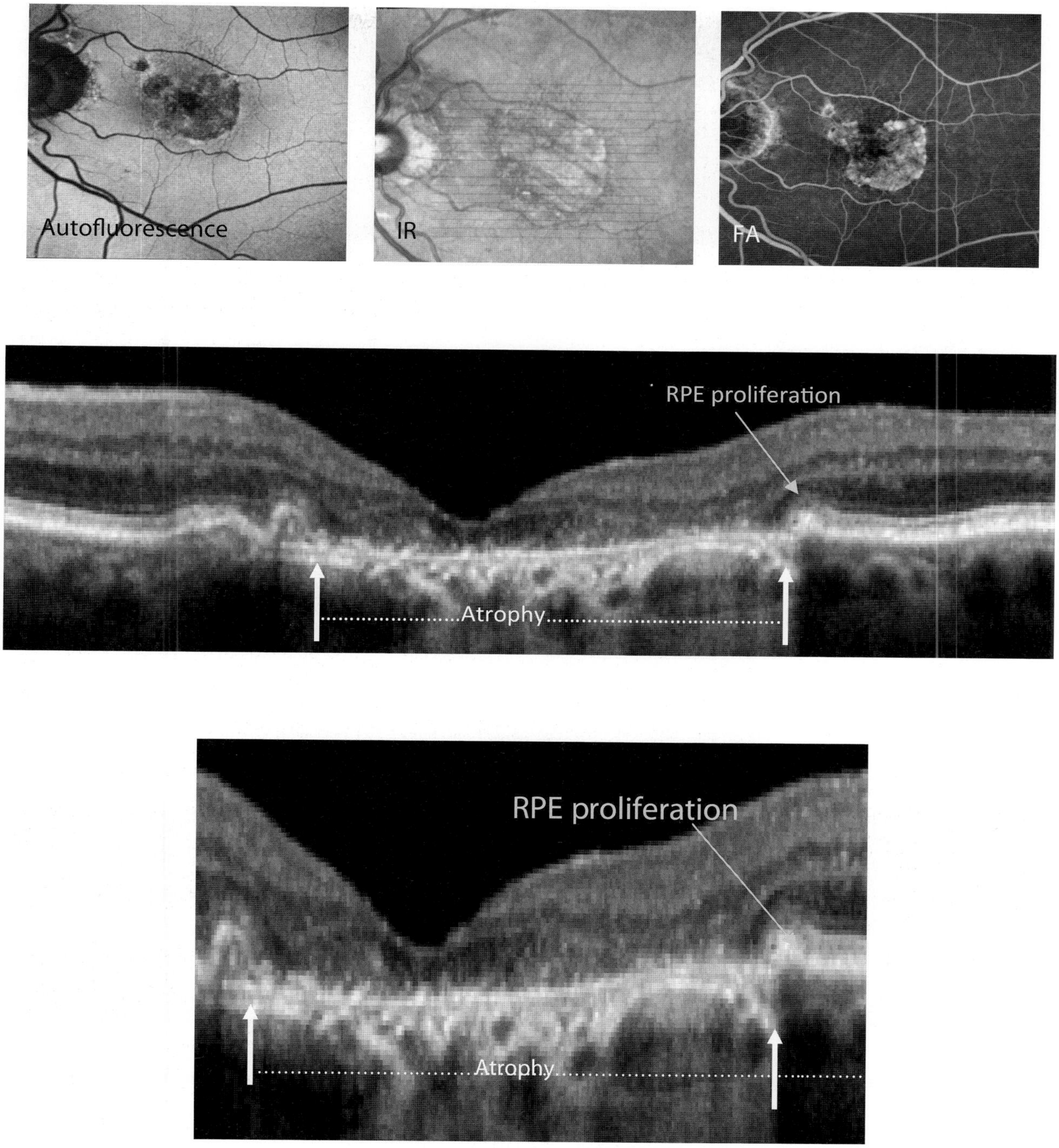

Figure 8: Proliferation of the RPE (adjacent to an area of laser-induced atrophy):

***Spectralis** section correlated with fluorescein angiography:**
Presence of a prominence on the RPE band, due to hypertrophy and underlying fibrosis, adjacent to the inferior para central laser scar (clearly visible with thinning of the retina, atrophy of the RPE, and hyper-reflectivity extending well posteriorly).

RPE THINNING AND ATROPHY

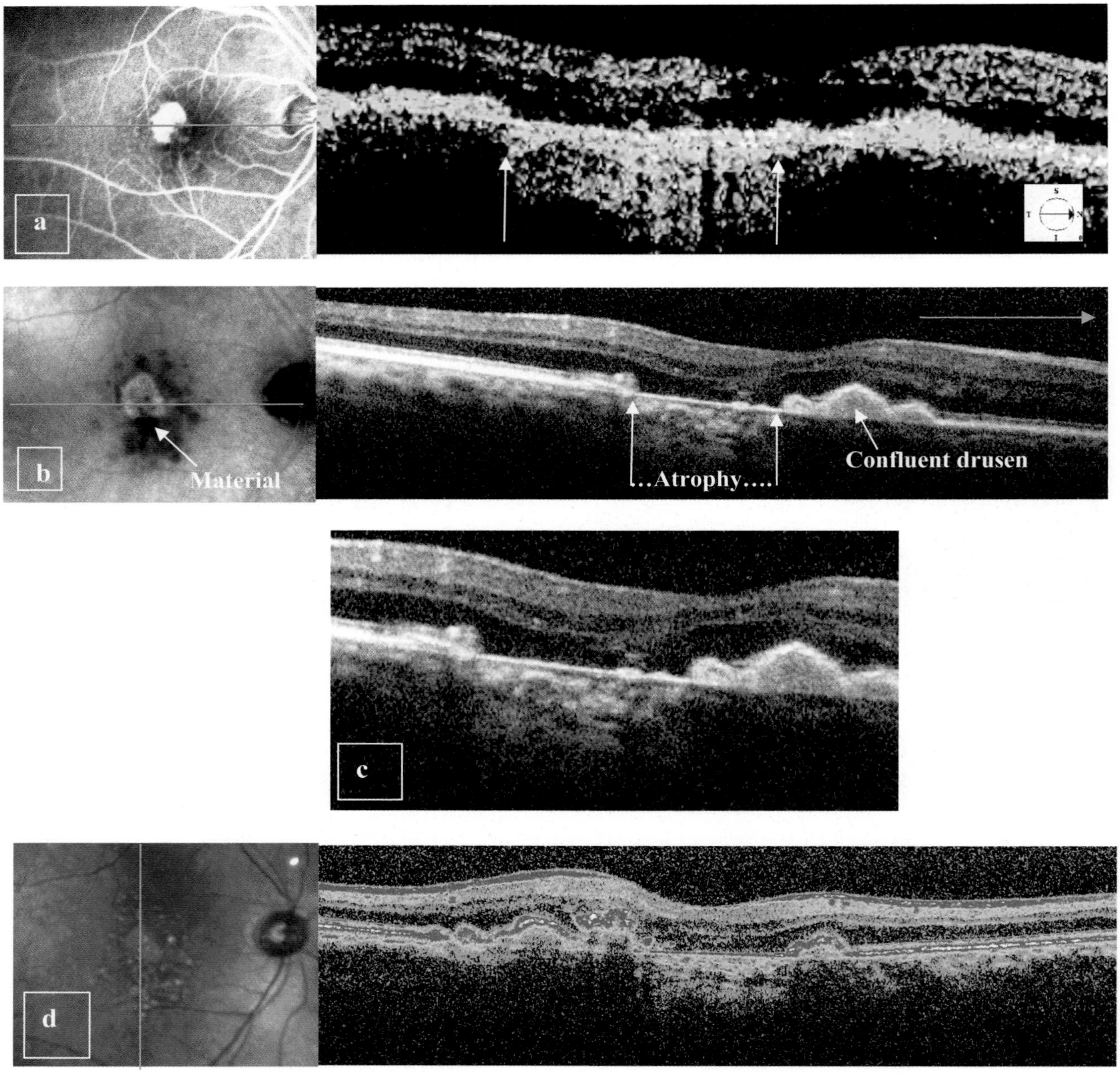

Figure 9: Area of RPE atrophy related to spontaneous resorption of deposits and associated with confluent soft drusen:

a): *Stratus horizontal section shown with fluorescein angiography** (*hyper-fluorescence related to atrophic resorption of deposits*). **On OCT**, the area of RPE atrophy is seen as thinning of the RPE and posterior hyper-reflectivity.

b): *Spectralis horizontal section correlated with ICG angiography** (*black residual material; localized RPE atrophy [same patient]*). **On SD-OCT**, the IS/OS interface and external limiting membrane are no longer visible in this atrophic zone. Note the prominent confluent soft drusen on either side of the atrophic zone.

c): *Spectralis horizontal section**: enlargement of image (**b**).

d): *Spectralis vertical section correlated with an autofluorescence image** (*the residual material is autofluorescent*). **On SD-OCT**, the false-color image also clearly demonstrates the localized atrophy of the RPE and the outer layers of the retina.

RPE THINNING AND ATROPHY AND LOSS OF PHOTORECEPTORS

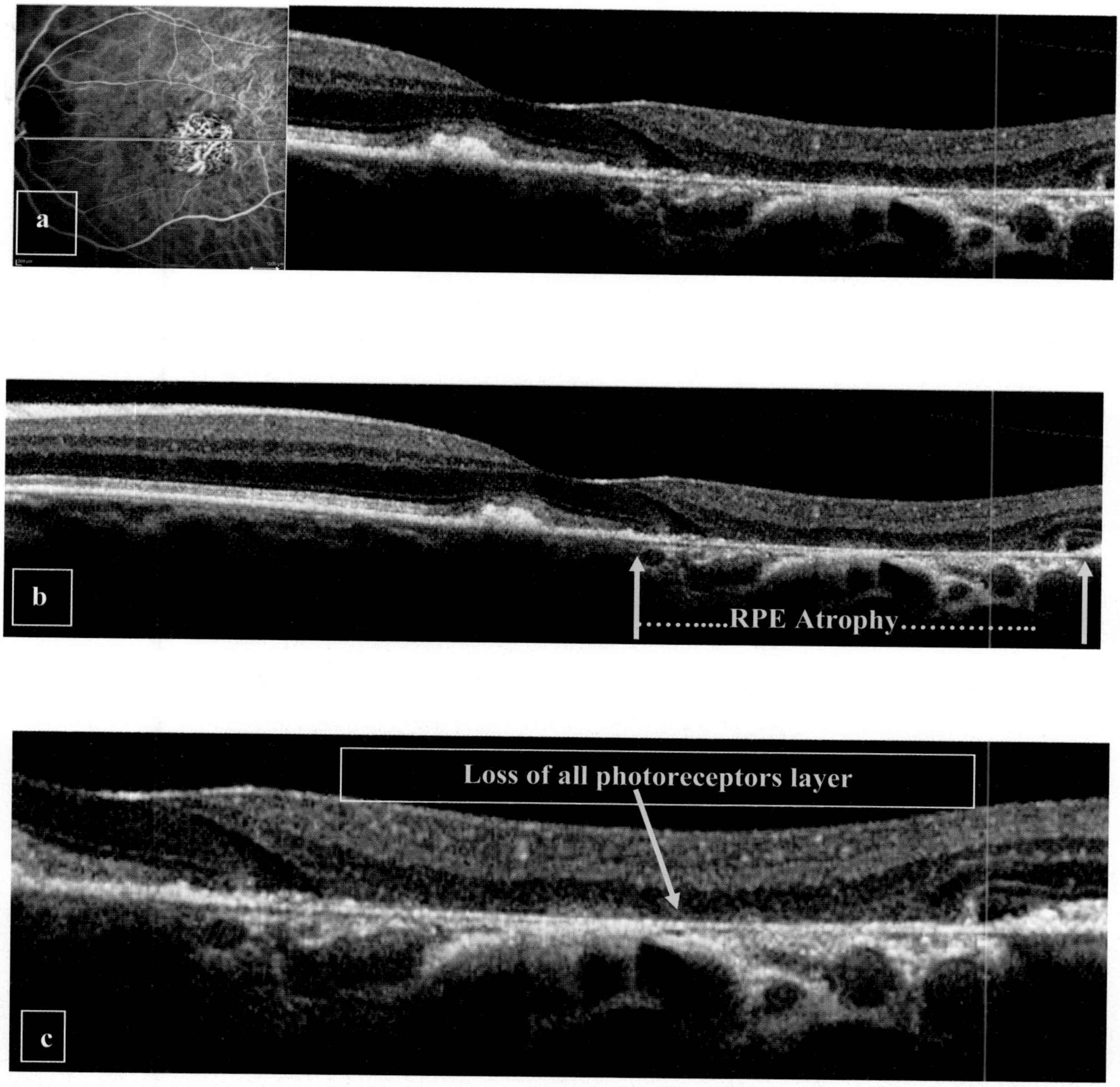

Figure 10: Area of thinning and RPE atrophy (related to resorption of deposits).

a): ICG angiography: *only a few large choroidal vessels are visible in the atrophic RPE area and choriocapillaris.*

b): *Spectralis horizontal section correlated with ICG angiography:** the localized RPE atrophy (yellow arrows) is associated with loss of the IS/OS interface, external limiting membrane, and even the outer nuclear layer, which is the result of the photoreceptor layer loss.

c): Enlarged view: Only the inner plexiform layer and retinal layers are still visible.

LOCALIZED LOSS OF THE RPE

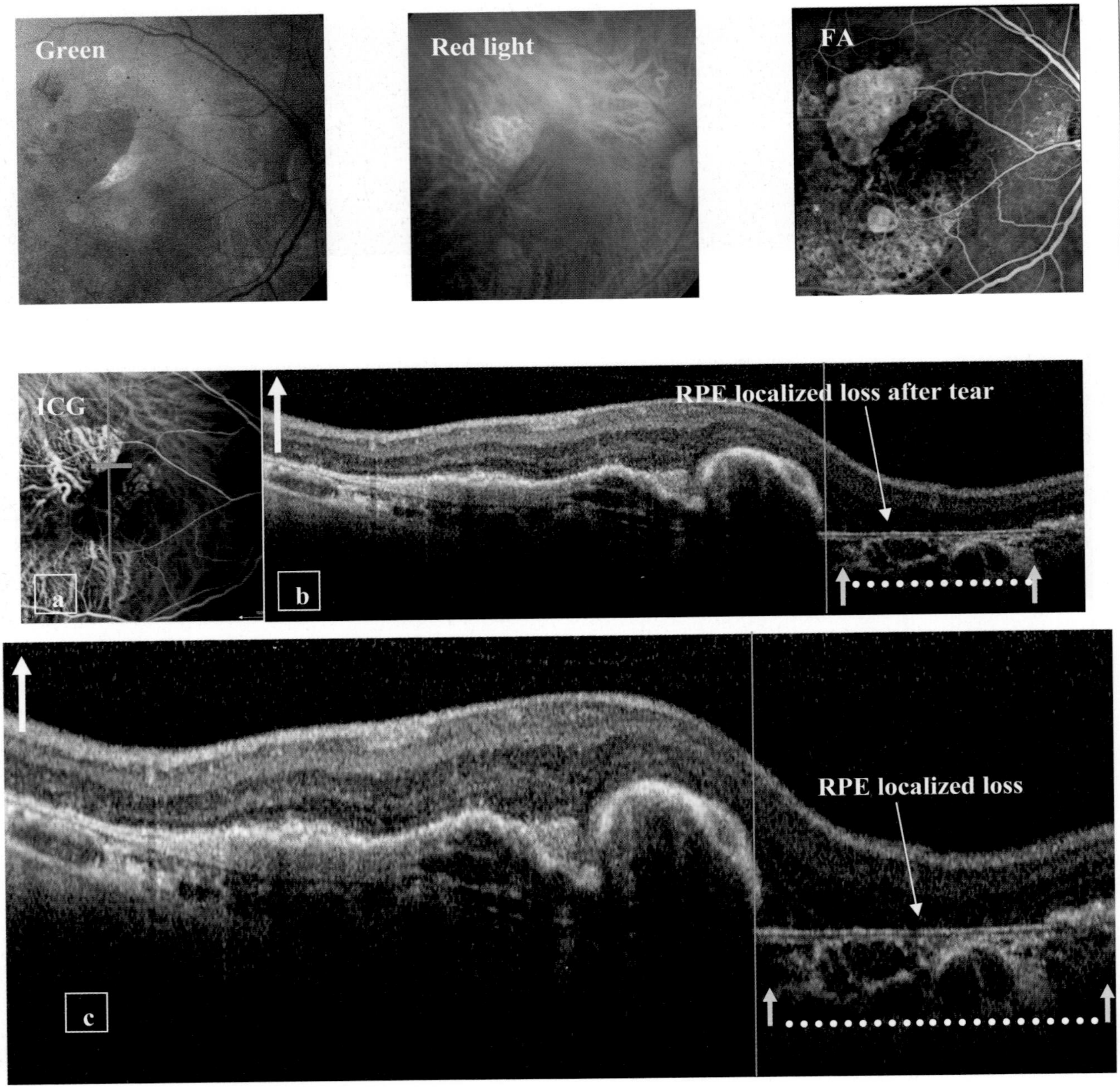

Figure 11: Localized absence of the RPE due to retraction after a tear.

a): ICG angiography: *in the superior region, a choroidal area is exposed by by the rolled-up retracted RPE that appears very dark and hypofluorescent. The inferior part corresponds to the residual PED.*

b): *Spectralis vertical section correlated with ICG angiography**: the residual PED is clearly visible, delineated by the retracted RPE. The RPE is no longer visible in the exposed zone. The atrophic choroid and Bruch's membrane are in contact with the inner retinal layers. The green line and calliper are located at the edge of the tear.

c): Enlarged view.

LOCALIZED DISRUPTION OF THE RPE

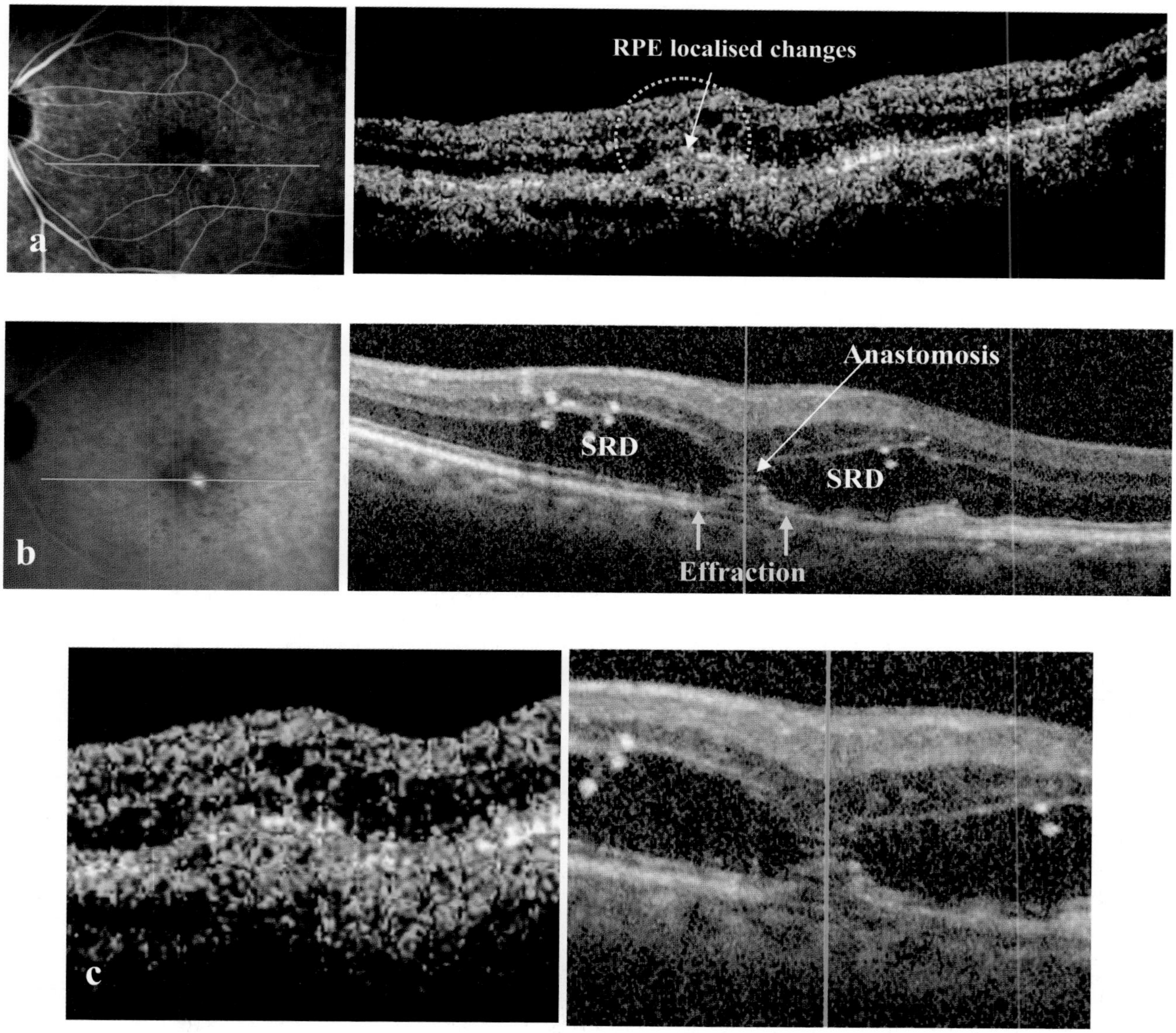

Figure 12: Break of the RPE (chorioretinal anastomosis).

a): *Stratus horizontal section shown with fluorescein angiography** (*juxtafoveal hot-spot*): the RPE band presents an isolated, limited, and localized abnormality: this juxtafoveal irregularity is accompanied by a small PED.

b): *Spectralis horizontal section correlated with ICG angiography (*same patient*)**: the RPE band is clearly visible almost throughout this image, accompanied by the parallel line of the the IS/OS interface. These two lines are suddenly interrupted over a limited juxta-foveal zone.

This break or effraction of the RPE exposes a moderately reflective structure, which appears to penetrate into the neurosensory retina, suggesting the presence of a chorioretinal anastomosis. It is demonstrated on angiographies and confirmed by other associated signs (small PED, accentuated exudation, SRF, intraretinal cysts).

c): Enlargement of previous images.

This zone of RPE rupture is not simply due to back-shadowing and should be clearly identified.

II. Posterior to the RPE Band

Many changes or signs located posterior to the RPE band are observed in the course of AMD.

Analysis of these signs provides a wealth of information. These changes are observed on both sides of **Bruch's membrane** (BM).

Bruch's membrane is adherent to the RPE and is not visible in normal eyes.

Visualization of the BM as a *distinct entity from the RPE* indicates localized loss of adhesion and ***detachment of the RPE***. This detachment may be minimal, moderate, or extensive.

The following signs may be observed between BM and RPE:

- *Accumulation of material* of variable density (drusen, deposits, fibrovascular tissue), or
- *Accumulation of fluid.*

This fluid may be:

- Either **serous** and optically empty, or
- **Fibrinous** and moderately reflective, or
- **Hemorrhagic** and blocking light.

1. Accumulation of Material Posterior to the RPE: Drusen

Drusen

Drusen, frequently present in AMD, cause **elevation of the RPE**.

Drusen can be detected as soon as they are larger than the classical definition of soft drusen (greater than 63 μm). They may be isolated or multiple.

They induce very little loss of visual acuity when they are small but can have a more dramatic impact when larger.

TD-OCT

Drusen are *not optically empty*, but their cross-section appears to be **moderately hyper-reflective**, which distinguishes them from serous detachments.

This is a particularly important characteristic sign.

This moderate hyper-reflectivity (false green color with the *Stratus**) nevertheless allows visualization of the regular line of Bruch's membrane (**Figures 13 and 14**).

SD-OCT

Analysis of the IS/OS interface and **outer nuclear layer** over the drusen is very useful to assess their **effects**.

These structures remain clearly visible, continuous, and only slightly modified over *small or medium-sized drusen*.

However, **large confluent drusen** protrude into and alter adjacent retinal layers:

- The outer nuclear layer may appear thinned, sometimes with a jagged appearance.
- The external limiting membrane and IS/OS interface present localized disruptions over the apex of the drusen (**Figures 15-17**).

However, this disruption and alteration of these lines are sometimes more extensive, especially when adjacent to small areas of RPE atrophy (**Figure 18**).

Examination of these layers on sufficiently enlarged images provides direct signs of photoreceptor inner and outer segment damage, which may have a major prognostic value for follow-up of high-risk drusen.

ELEVATION OF THE RPE BY DRUSEN

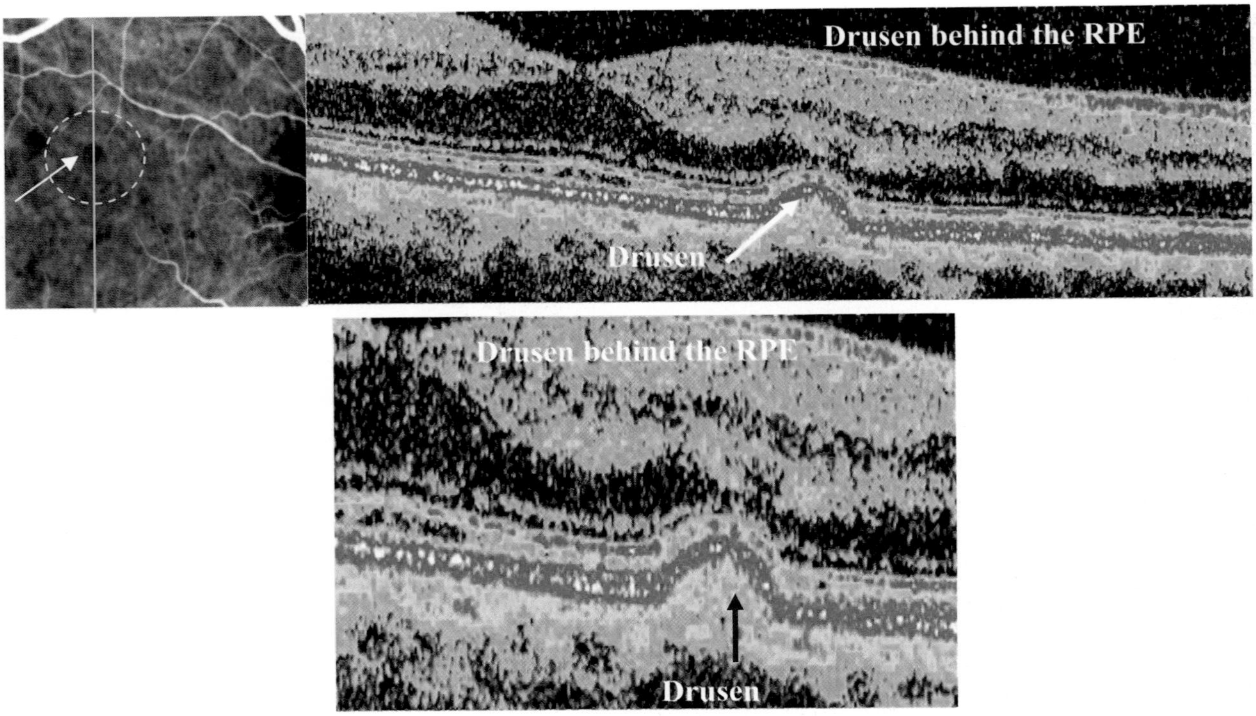

Figure 12: Localized elevation of the RPE related to the presence of a large soft drusen.
Spectralis *** vertical section combined with ICG angiography** (*persistent hypo-fluorescence of a large drusen*).
The drusen (arrow) induces moderately hyper-reflective elevation of the RPE without posterior shadowing. Bruch's membrane remains clearly visible. Note that the IS/OS interface and external limiting membrane are not disrupted but slightly altered with relative thinning of the outer nuclear layer.

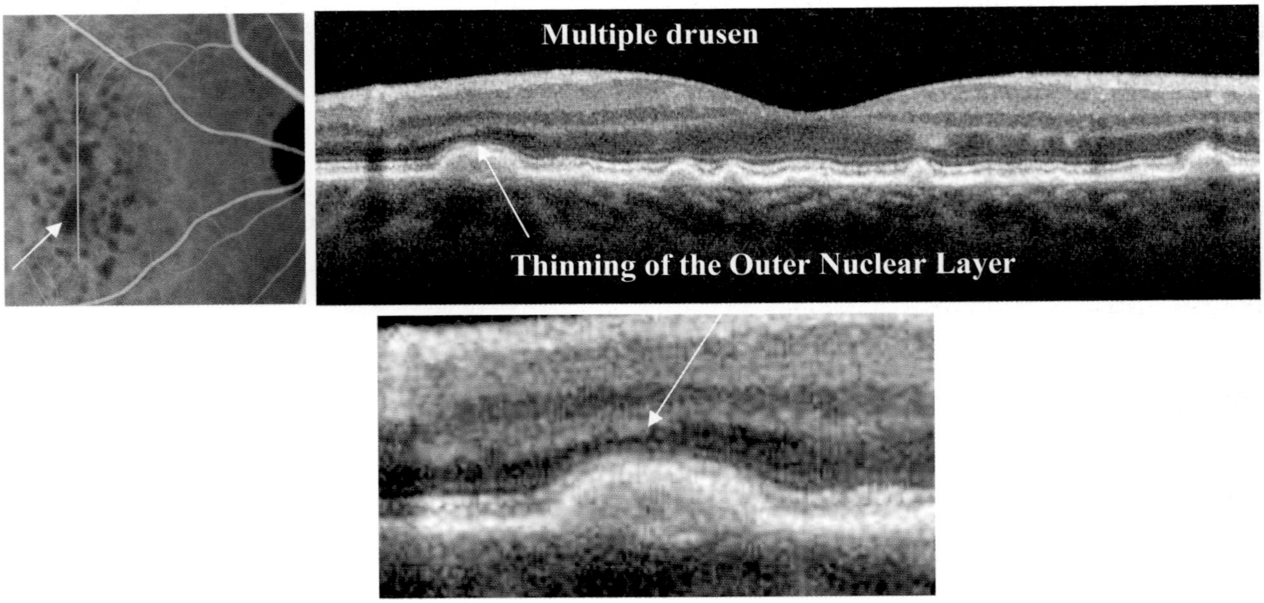

Figure 13: Multiple elevations of the RPE related to the presence of many soft drusen.
Spectralis *** vertical section combined with ICG angiography** (*persistent hypo-fluorescence of the drusen*).
The large drusen (enlarged view) induces marked elevation of the RPE, but the IS/OS interface and external limiting membrane are not disrupted and remain visible. However, the outer nuclear layer is considerably thinned.

MULTIPLE ELEVATIONS OF THE RPE BY DRUSEN

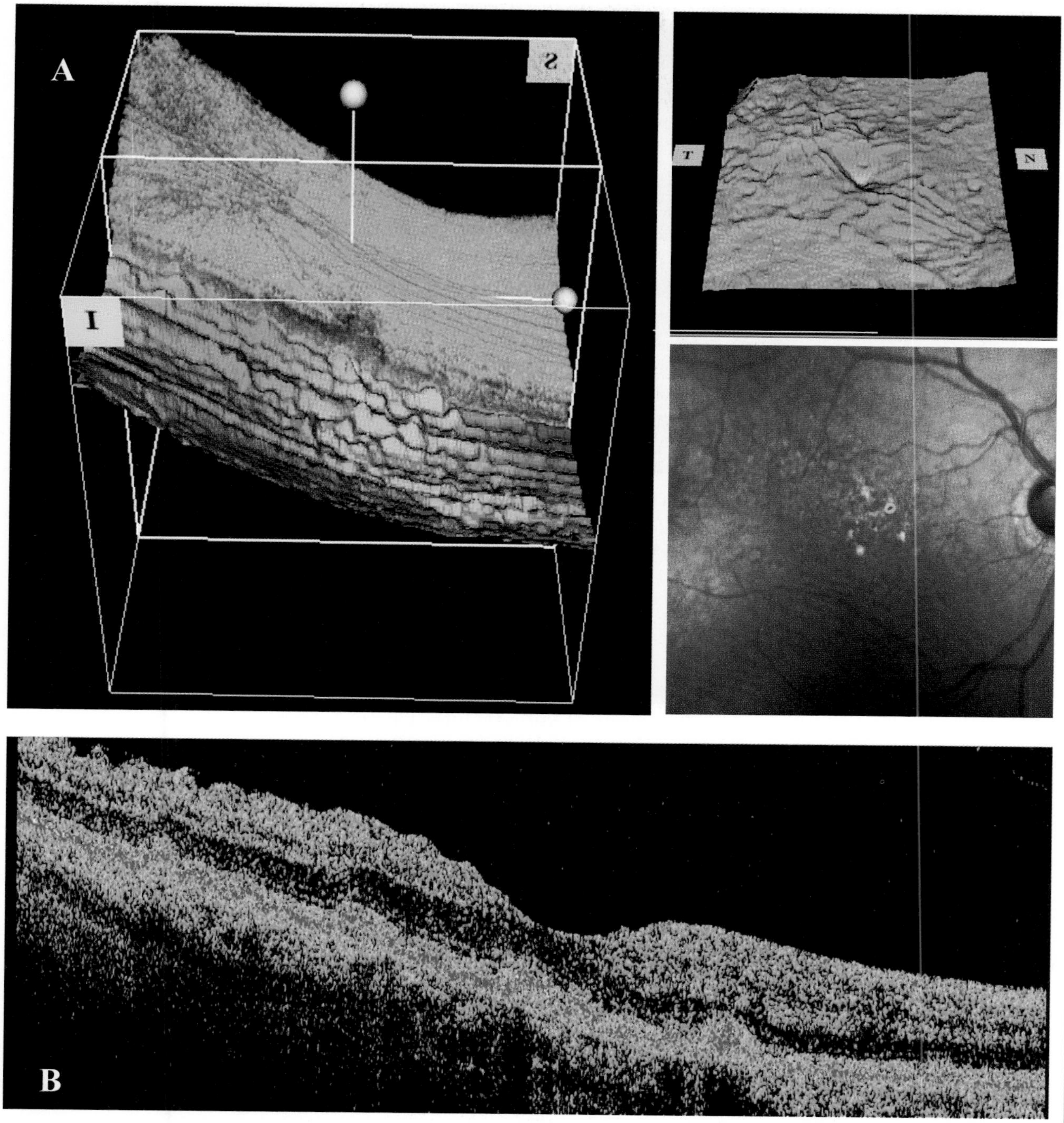

Figure 14: Multiple localized elevations of the RPE related to the presence of drusen.

Topcon*: **3D image associated with surface images immediately posterior to the RPE.**

A): Section through the inferior part of the fovea, demonstrating multiple drusen immediately posterior to the RPE.

B): High-definition horizontal section demonstrating numerous drusen displacing the RPE.

MULTIPLE ELEVATIONS OF THE RPE BY DRUSEN

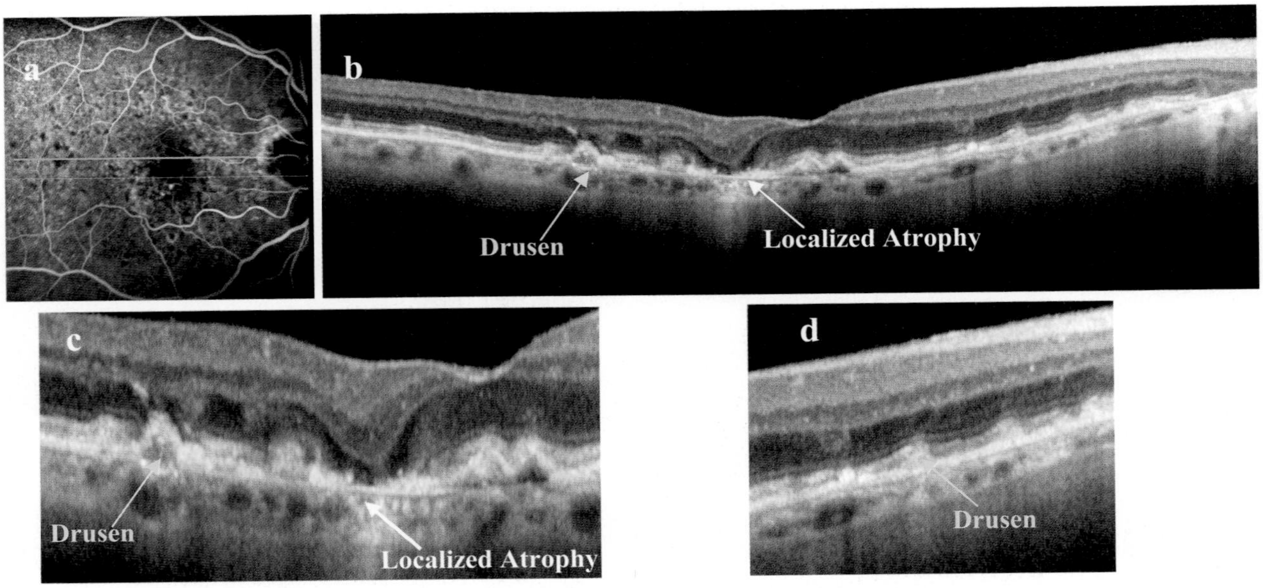

Figure 15: Multiple localized elevations of the RPE related to the presence of drusen.
a and b): *Spectralis horizontal section** *correlated with fluorescein angiography: slow staining of multiple drusen.*
On SD-OCT, drusen (*yellow arrow*) are moderately hyper-reflective with no posterior shadowing. Bruch's membrane is clearly visible.
c and d): Enlarged images: the prominent drusen modify and alter the continuity and thickness of the hypo-reflective outer nuclear layer, which appears thinned over the drusen. Note a small area of juxtafoveal atrophy (*white arrow*).
d): the external limiting membrane and IS/OS interface over the small drusen are not modified.

MULTIPLE ELEVATIONS OF THE RPE BY DRUSEN
Alterations of Retinal Outer Layers

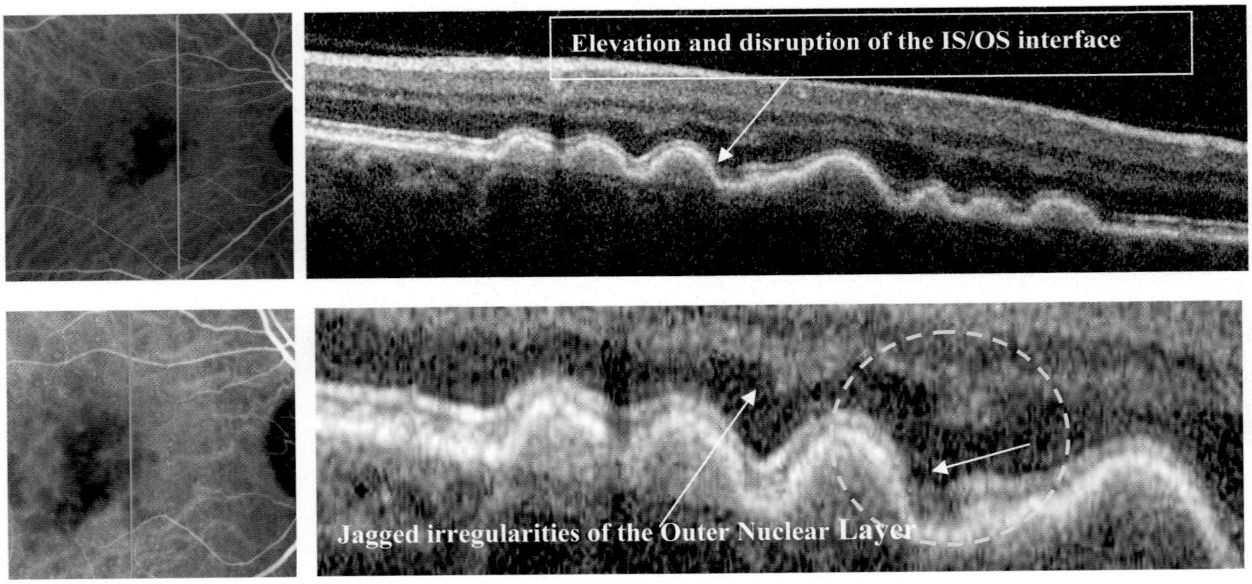

Figure 16: Multiple elevations of the RPE related to the presence of large soft drusen.
***Spectralis** vertical section correlated with ICG angiography** (*hypo-fluorescence of confluent drusen*).
The drusen have a homogeneous, slightly reflective content, which is well-delineated posteriorly by Bruch's membrane and causes moderate shadowing due to their volume.
The IS/OS interface and external limiting membrane remain visible, almost continuous, and only slightly modified with a localized disruption. The outer nuclear layer has several irregularities with a jagged appearance.

ELEVATION OF THE RPE BY LARGE DRUSEN

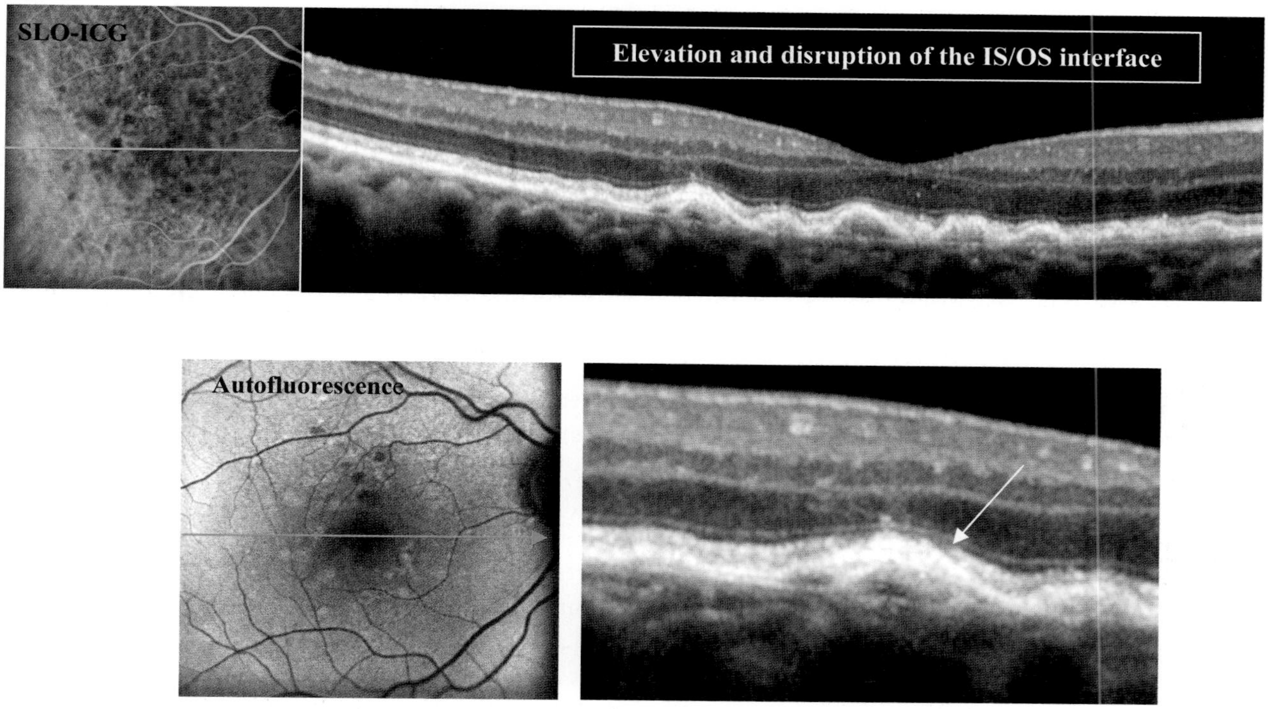

Figure 17: Elevation of the RPE, over a large soft drusen.

***Spectralis** horizontal section correlated with ICG angiography** (*hypo-fluorescence of drusen*).

Multiple drusen of various sizes are clearly delineated posterior to Bruch's membrane. The external limiting membrane remains clearly visible, but the IS/OS interface is disrupted at the apex of the drusen with slight alteration of the outer nuclear layer.
Note on the autofluorescence image, several dark areas of RPE atrophy over drusen.

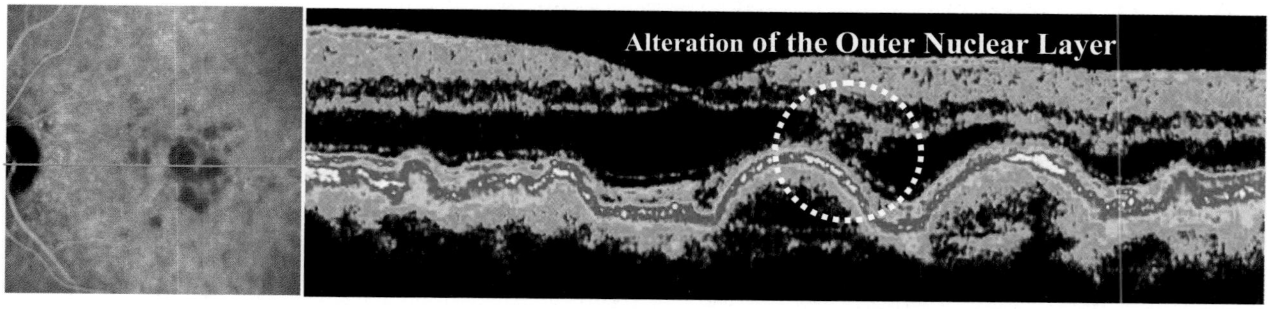

Figure 18: Multiple elevations of the RPE over very large drusen.

***Spectralis** horizontal section correlated with ICG angiography** (*hypo-fluorescence of drusen*).

The cavity of the drusen presents a moderate but variable reflectivity. The BM is visible.
The outer nuclear layer is displaced and thinned over the apex of the drusen with increased density in some areas (*circle*).
The IS/OS interface is irregular and sometimes disrupted.

2. Accumulation of Material Posterior to the RPE: Drusenoid PED

Confluent soft drusen can cause more pronounced and more irregular elevation of the RPE.

Confluent drusen are sometimes sufficiently large to cause **drusenoid pigment epithelium detachments (PED)**.

A drusenoid PED, characterized by its irregular shape, is slowly but noticeably filled with dye and enhanced on *fluorescein angiography*.

Pigment migrations are often present in drusenoid PEDs, forming geometric or star shapes, and lipofuscin pigment accumulation may sometimes be observed.

On ICG angiography, drusenoid PED remains markedly hypo-fluorescent until the very late phase of the angiogram.

TD-OCT

The RPE remains regular and homogeneous but can also be thickened and have irregularities. Many drusen are visible adjacent to the RPE.

The cavity of a drusenoid PED is not optically empty but moderately hyper-reflective, similar to that of soft drusen, leaving the straight line of Bruch's membrane clearly visible. Partial or minor shadowing may be observed.

SD-OCT

Modifications of the IS/OS interface and external limiting membrane may be minor or moderate, with simple displacement of these structures by the drusenoid PED.

However, most cases present marked alterations at the apex of the PED, similar to those observed with large drusen.

Alterations of the IS/OS interface (thickened or undetectable), and disruptions of the external limiting membrane may be observed.

Alterations of the outer nuclear layer are even more important for prognosis. The outer nuclear layer may be thinned, more highly reflective, and irregular with a jagged appearance in drusenoid PEDs.

When the lesion is mainly central, all of this area may be displaced with loss of the foveal depression (**Figures 19 and 20**).

Patients presenting these alterations must be carefully examined to detect the presence of *intraretinal fluid*, suggestive of neovascular complications that should be identified as early as possible.

3. Accumulation of Material Posterior to the RPE

Posterior to the RPE (and sometimes also in contact with and/or anterior to the RPE), lipofuscin deposits can raise a number of problems.

Clinically, these deposits are **polymorphous** and vary in dimension, location, or in their association with extensive lesions. They may sometimes be reorganized as a result of complications.

On OCT sections, this **vitelliform** material may be situated anterior to or fused with the RPE, causing regular and moderate elevation of the RPE, but without an *exudative reaction*.

Accumulation of material induces posterior **masking** of the choroid (**Figure 21**).

These features are sometimes difficult to distinguish from choroidal neovascularization. The diagnosis is based on the presence or absence of associated exudative signs.

This material may be responsible for posterior hyper-reflectivity, simulating fibrosis and sometimes optically empty zones, suggesting a neovascular process. This material can also spread and proliferate anterior to the RPE and even extend into the neurosenory retinal layers (**Figures 22-26**).

ELEVATION OF THE RPE BY DRUSENOID PED VOLUMINEUX

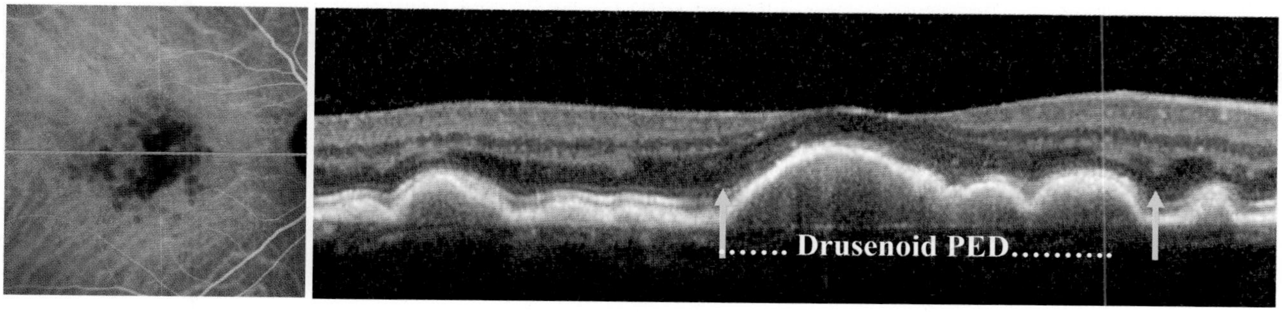

Figure 19: Elevation of the RPE–confluent soft drusen with a central drusenoid PED.

***Spectralis** horizontal section correlated with ICG angiography** (*drusen and drusenoid PED appear black*).

The **SD-OCT** section demonstrates several drusen of different sizes that have become confluent in the central zone measuring half a disc diameter. Retinal layers are displaced but their normal architecture is preserved.
However, the external limiting membrane and the IS/OS interface are relatively poorly-defined. There are no signs of abnormal fluid accumulation.

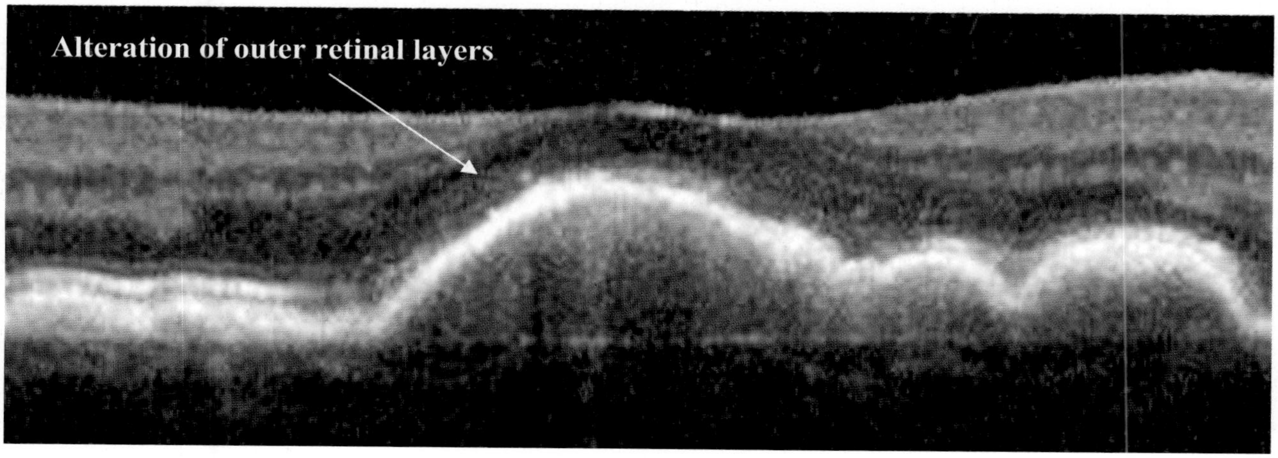

Figure 20: Elevation of the RPE–confluent soft drusen with a central drusenoid PED.

***Spectralis** horizontal section (enlargement of the previous image).**

The line of the IS/OS interface and the thinner line of the external limiting membrane are less clearly visible over the dome of the drusenoid PED.
The IS/OS interface appears to be replaced by a more dense signal, extending into the outer nuclear layer.
These features are suggestive of localized photoreceptor damage.

Note displacement of all of the retina and loss of the foveal depression. However, the normal architecture of all retinal layers appears to be not significantly altered.

ELEVATION OF THE RPE–ACCUMULATION OF VITELLIFORM MATERIAL

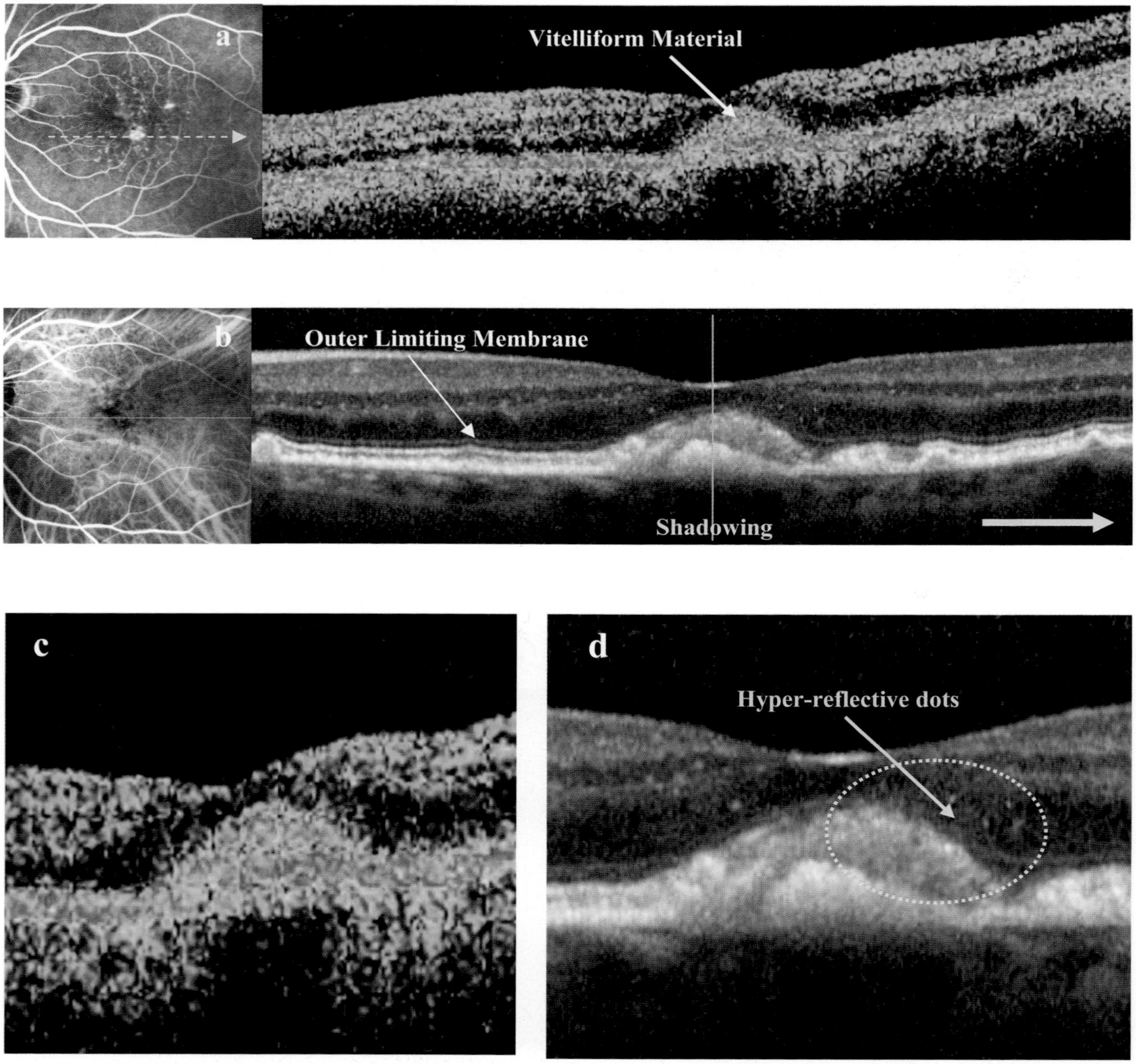

▫ Figure 21: Elevation of the RPE–Accumulation of material posterior and anterior to the RPE (VA: 20/50).

a): *Stratus horizontal section correlated with fluorescein angiography** *(late staining of the material).*
On **TD-OCT**, this material seems to bulge or thicken the RPE with a pronounced posterior shadowing.
This lesion could also be suggestive of classic CNV, but there is no fluid or fluorescein leakage.

b): *Spectralis horizontal section combined with ICG angiography** *(material still hypo-fluorescent on late phase).*
On **SD-OCT**, the material forms a heterogeneous, protruding area, which merges with the RPE and displaces the IS/OS interface making it less clearly visible. The external limiting membrane remains clearly visible. Note the presence of intraretinal hyper-reflective bright spots.

c and d): enlargements of **(a)** and **(b).**

ELEVATION OF THE RPE - ACCUMULATION OF VITELLIFORM MATERIAL

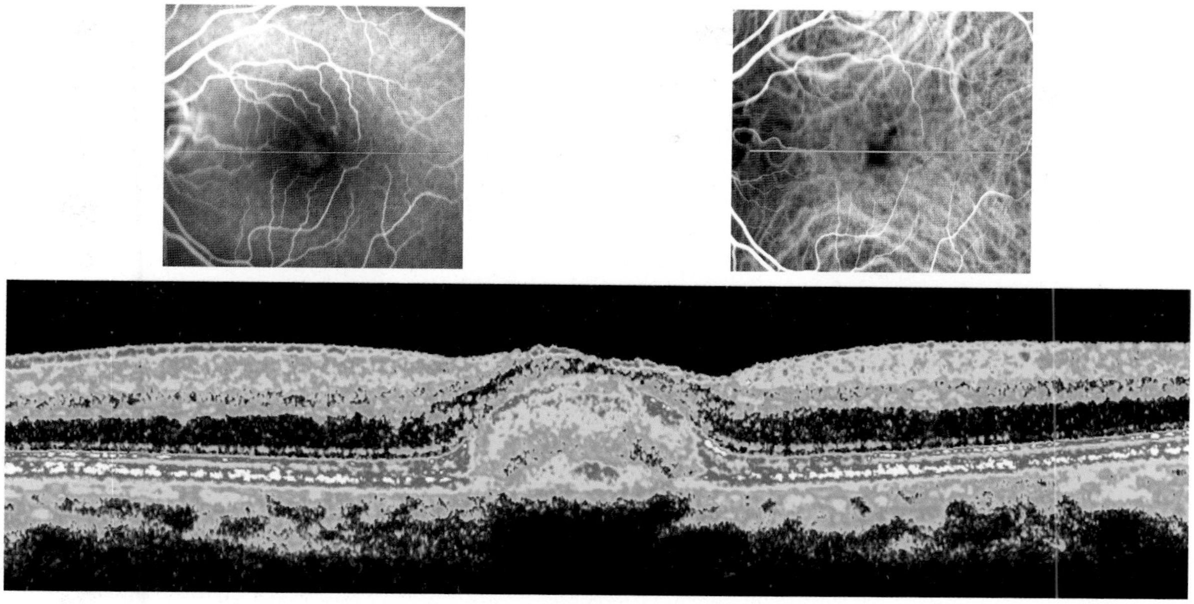

Figure 22: Elevation of the RPE–Accumulation of material posterior to the RPE, suggesting pseudo-vitelliform dystrophy (VA: 20/40).

***Spectralis** horizontal section combined with fluorescein angiography** (*progressive hyper-fluorescence, while ICG angiography shows persistent hypo-fluorescence).*

On OCT, the material is bulging or thickening the RPE with marked posterior shadowing. This lesion could also be suggestive of occult CNV, but ICG angiography and the absence of fluid exclude this diagnosis.

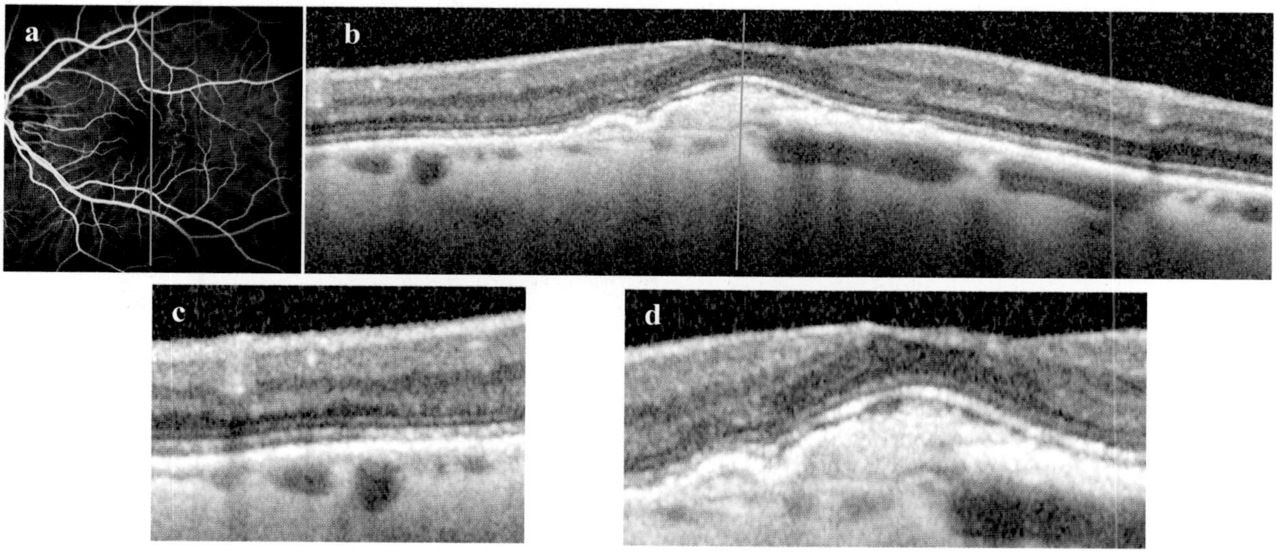

Figure 23: Elevation of the RPE–Accumulation of material posterior to the RPE (VA: 20/32).

a and b): *Spectralis vertical section combined with ICG angiography** (*partial late staining of the material*).

On OCT, the heterogeneous material lifts the RPE, displacing the IS/OS interface, which appears thicker and denser. Both the IS/OS interface and the external limiting membrane appear fragmented.

c and d): Enlarged images: compare the outer layers in the normal zone to the area of material accumulation, which shows marked irregularities and thinning of the outer nuclear layer. The foveolar zone is only slightly modified, accounting for the good visual acuity.

ELEVATION OF THE RPE–ACCUMULATION OF MATERIAL

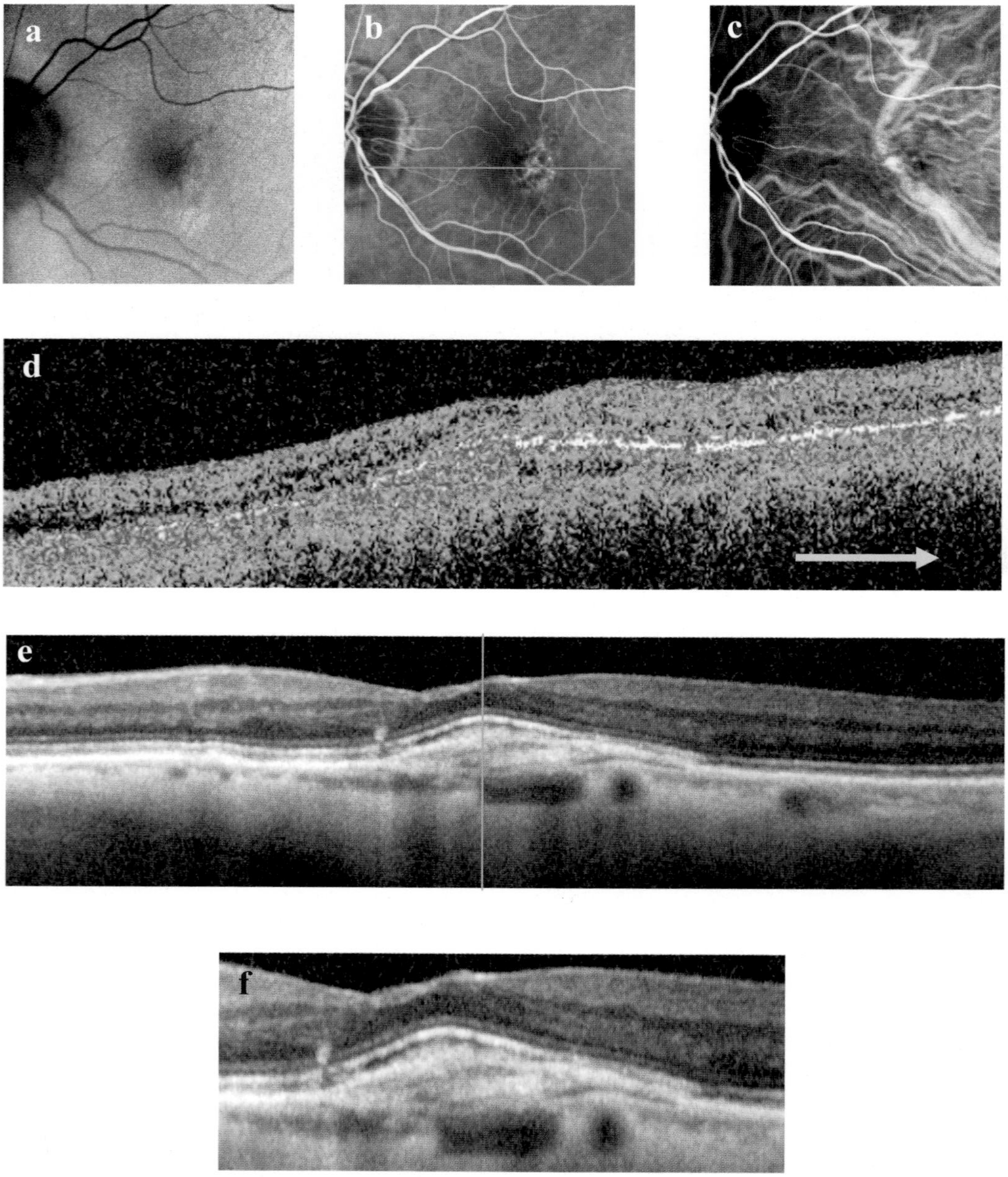

Figure 24: Elevation of the RPE–Accumulation of material posterior to the RPE (VA: 20/40).

a, b, and c): Autofluorescence, fluorescein angiography, and ICG angiography: *Juxtafoveal and subfoveal deposit of heterogeneous material with late hyper-fluorescence but without leakage.*

d): *Stratus horizontal section: On TD-OCT**, the material is heterogeneous, dense in the nasal part and, on the contrary, hypo-reflective in the temporal part, which could suggest an exudative reaction. However, the absence of fluorescein leakage argues against a neovascular complication.

e): *Spectralis horizontal section: On SD-OCT**, the material raises the band of RPE with a heterogeneous structure adherent to the RPE. The IS/OS interface (which remains clearly visible) is displaced with the external limiting membrane. Note the outer nuclear layer thinning.

f): Enlargement of image (e).

ELEVATION OF THE RPE–ACCUMULATION OF MATERIAL

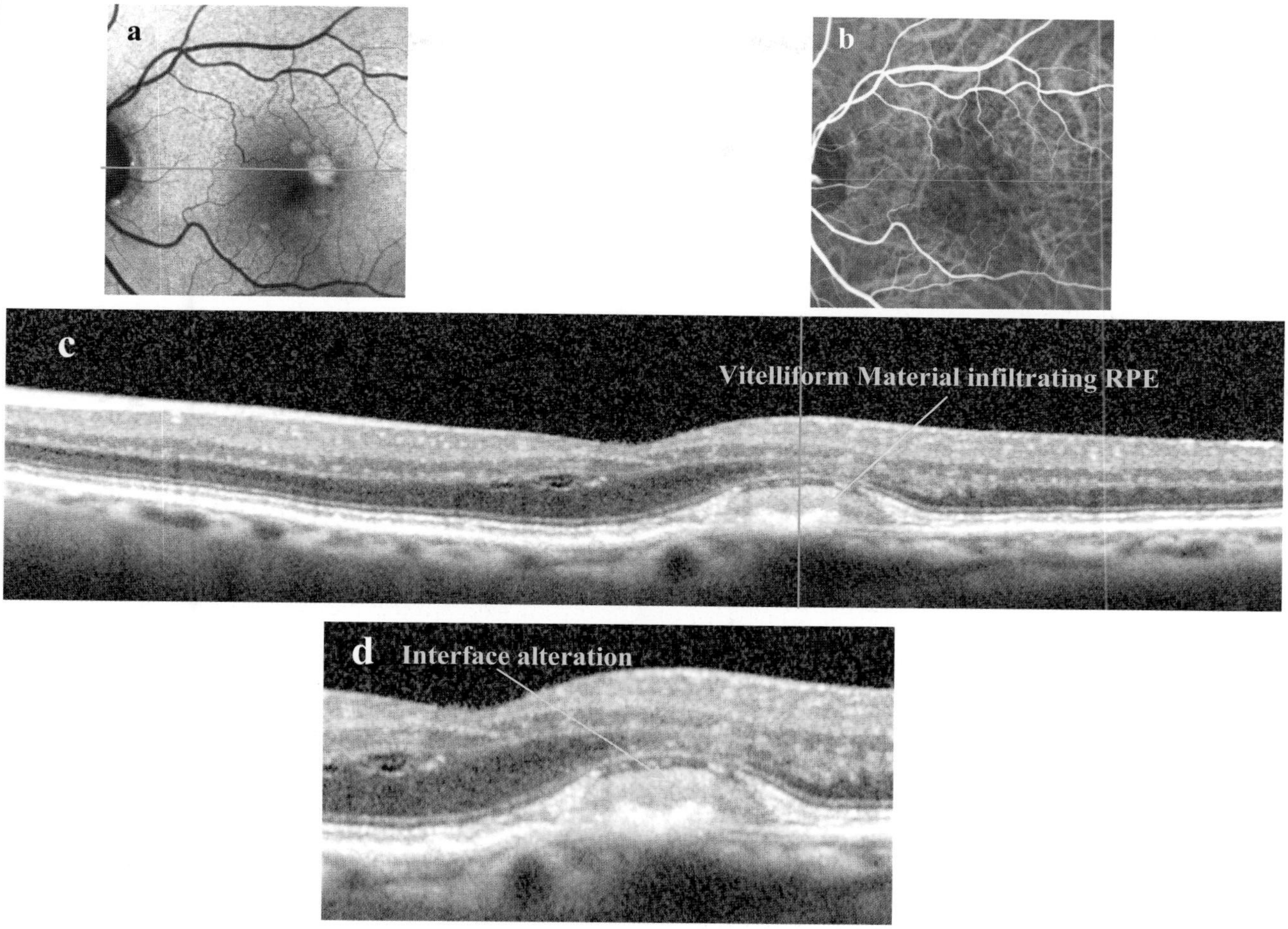

Figure 26: Elevation of the RPE–Accumulation of material posterior and anterior to the RPE.
a and b): Autofluorescence and ICG angiography: *presence of a dark temporo-foveal area of autofluorescent material with delayed ICG staining.*
c): *Spectralis vertical section.**
d): Enlarged image of (c): On SD-OCT thickening and hyper-reflectivity of the RPE in the center of the lesion induces relative masking. The material also accumulates anterior to the RPE, lifting and deforming the IS/OS interface and nuclear layer.

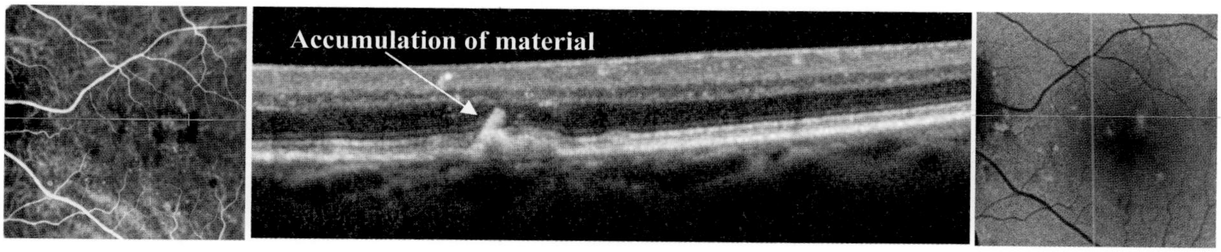

Figure 26: Elevation of the RPE–Accumulation of material posterior and anterior to the RPE (VA: 20/63).
***Spectralis** horizontal section combined with ICG angiography** *(hypo-fluorescent material).* The material is hyper-fluorescent on the autofluorescence image.
On OCT, the material lifts the RPE, but also appears to extend within the retina.

4. Posterior to the RPE: Serous and Fibrovascular PED

Proliferation of choroidal neovascularization underneath the RPE (occult CNV) directly induces detachment of the RPE, which separates from BM.

The pigment epithelium detachment (PED), initially minimal then moderate, may, depending on the volume of exudation and the extent of the choroidal neovascularization (CNV), become very large.

a) Predominantly Serous PED

Accumulation of fluid in the space between the RPE and BM may be predominant or may even **appear to be isolated** depending on the location of the cross-section.

- *The PED* is then **essentially serous** and appears optically empty. The RPE band outlines the detachment. The elevation is regular, **dome-shaped**, of variable prominence and gently sloping (at least in the early stages) (**Figure 27**).

- *Choroidal occult neovascularization* is barely visible on OCT.

- During natural history or after treatment, the PED may take on a **multi-lobed** appearance with a wavy surface and variable size (**Figure 28**).

Successive OCT scans and the various **graphic representations** demonstrate either persistence, flattening, or scarring, as well as other retinal inflammatory response.

This sub-RPE exudative reaction appears to be much **less sensitive to treatment** than subretinal fluid accumulation or intraretinal infiltration.

The PED thickness should be frequently assessed in retinal thickness measurements after treatment to distinguish thickness related to leakage from that related to the presence of fibrous tissue.

b) Fibrovascular PED

- Exudation from CNV and fibrovascular tissues is less pronounced, and the PED cavity is **moderately hyper-reflective and heterogeneous**.

Only part of the cavity appears to be optically empty and filled by fluid.

Moderately reflective zones (false-green color on TD-OCT) are also observed.

The hyper-reflectivity is often limited to a **small band underneath the RPE**, but can fill almost the entire cavity (**Figure 29**).

- **Typical fibrovascular PEDs** are probably the most frequent form of ***occult sub-RPE choroidal neovascularization in AMD***.

Choroidal neovascularization in fibrovascular PEDs is rarely visible on OCT but usually seen on ICG angiography (**Figure 30**).

Various signs of progression on OCT (*hyper-reflective bright spots, dense zones, alterations of outer layers*) may be associated.

c) Two types of vascularized PED

- Predominantly bullous and serous or,
- Predominantly fibrovascular (slightly leaking).

These two forms can also coexist in varying degrees during the course of the disease.

This is especially the case for chronic forms that gradually become *organized*. All these lesions induce little or no posterior shadowing and Bruch's membrane remains visible.

- During the course and usually in response to treatment, the PED detachment gradually collapses. The vascularized PED often becomes **multi-lobed with a wavy** appearance and an extensive but relatively flat profile.

At the same time, its cavity becomes organized and increasingly reflective, suggesting the development of fibrosis (**Figures 31-34**). This is confirmed by fluid resorption and progressive reattachment of the retina.

However, on SD-OCT, changes, organization, or even loss of the outer retinal layers persist or may be accentuated over the fibrosis and are associated with gradual and **irreversible functional impairment**.

POSTERIOR TO THE RPE: SEROUS PED

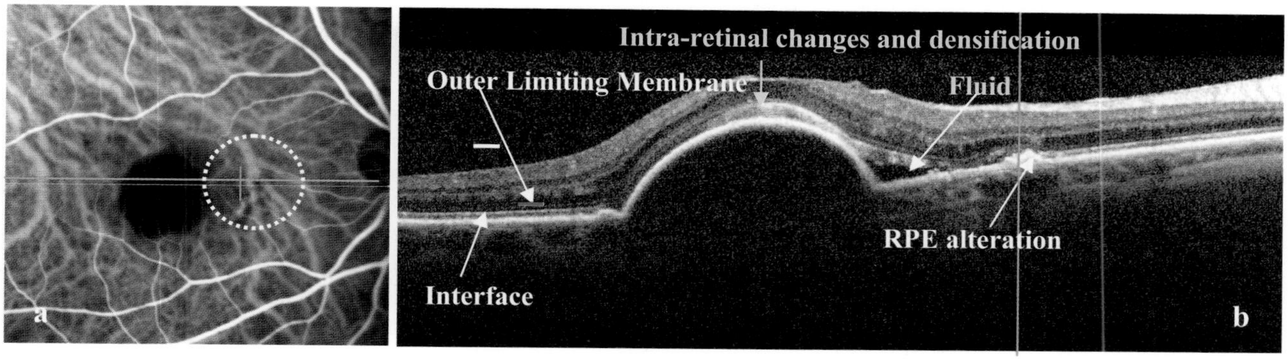

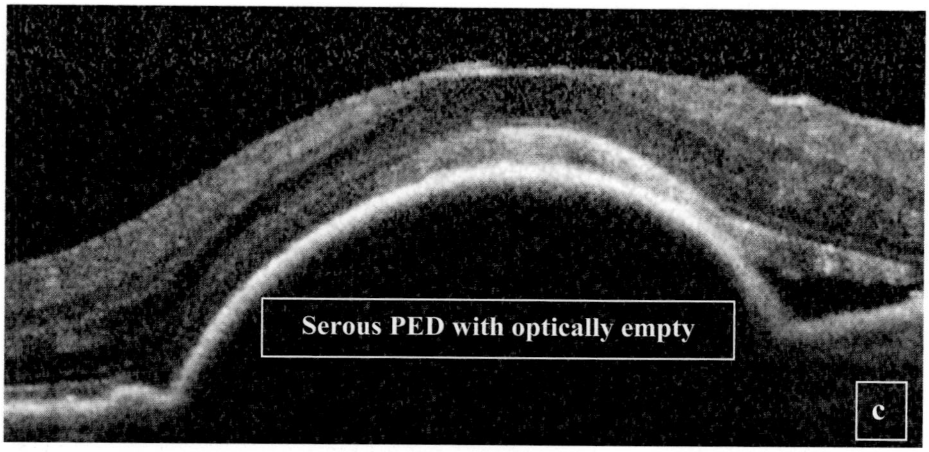

Figure 27: RPE detachment: Large serous detachment posterior to the RPE and occult CNV.

a): ICG angiography: *serous PED adjacent to occult CNV. The PED is rounded and markedly hypo-fluorescent. It is well-delineated with a nasal notch which corresponds to the CNV.*

b): Spectralis* horizontal section.

On SD-OCT, the RPE band is abruptly detached from Bruch's membrane and forms a regular, fairly prominent, rounded, gently sloping dome. The cavity appears to be optically empty with slight shadowing; the BM is just visible.

The external limiting membrane and IS/OS interface are clearly visible away from the lesion. They are less clearly visible over the PED but remain continuous.

A hyper-reflective zone over the apex of the PED appears to displace retinal layers. A small zone of subretinal fluid is seen in the nasal sector.

c): Enlargement of image (a): the BM is partially attenuated in the zone of the PED. It can nevertheless be identified below the regular and homogeneous RPE band, forming a dome over an optically empty cavity. This serous PED is related to the presence of occult CNV at its nasal margin (*circle*). It is associated with *inflammatory response signs,* mainly anterior to the RPE and at the level of the outer retinal layers.

POSTERIOR TO THE RPE: SEROUS PED, FOLLOW-UP

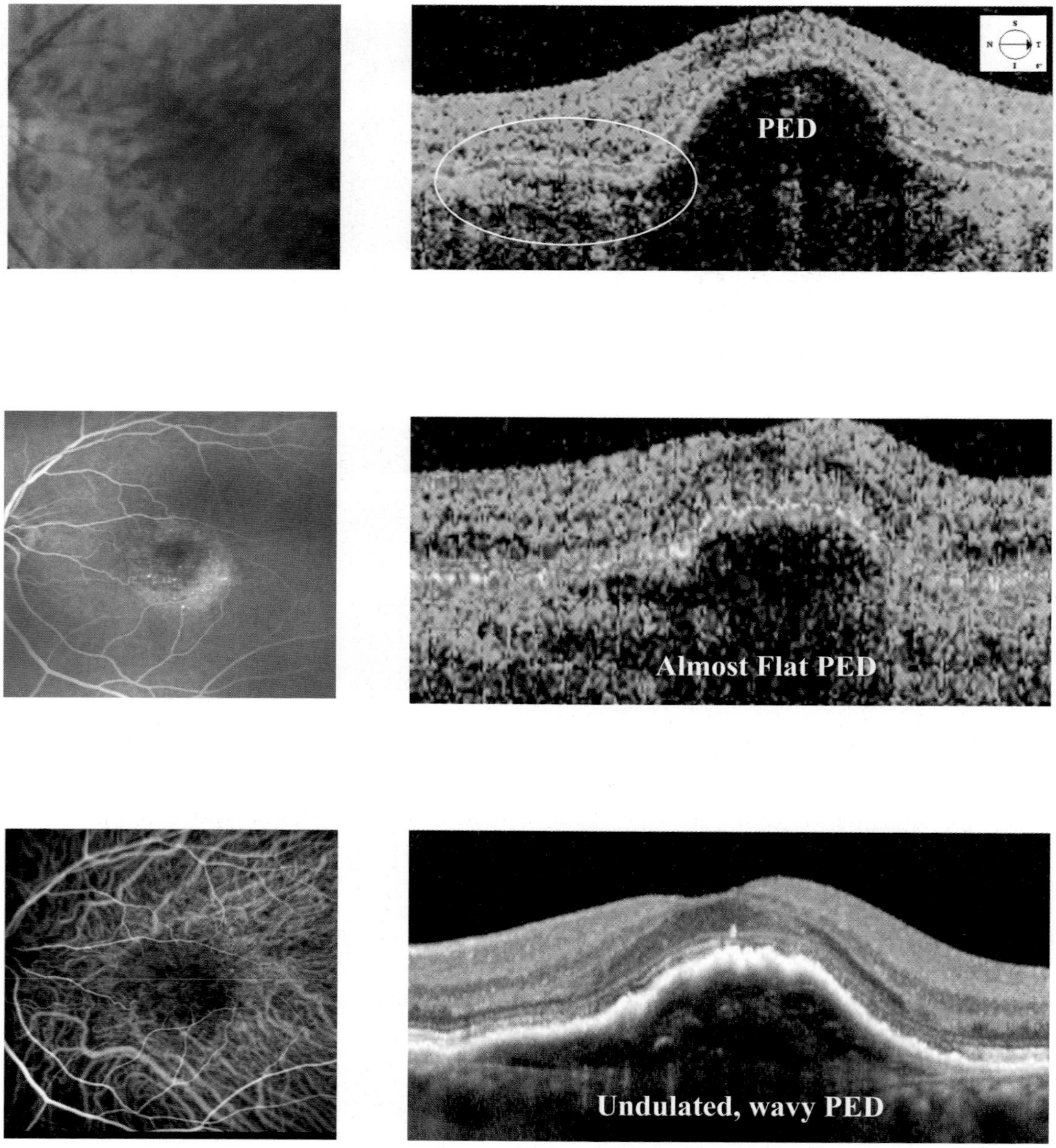

■ Figure 28: Elevation of the RPE: Very large serous PED associated with occult CNV–Good response to anti-VEGF therapy over a period of 10 months (VA 20/80 → 20/32).

***Stratus** and *Spectralis** horizontal sections associated with monochromatic or angiographic images.**

On **TD-OCT**, rounded, regular, fairly prominent gently sloping dome-shaped PED. The cavity appears to be optically empty with slight shadowing leaving the BM visible.

Various features may be observed during the course of a PED: the PED can gradually collapse and become less regular with wavy margins. The cavity might become slightly reflective, probably reflecting fibrous organization.

POSTERIOR TO THE RPE: FIBROVASCULAR PED

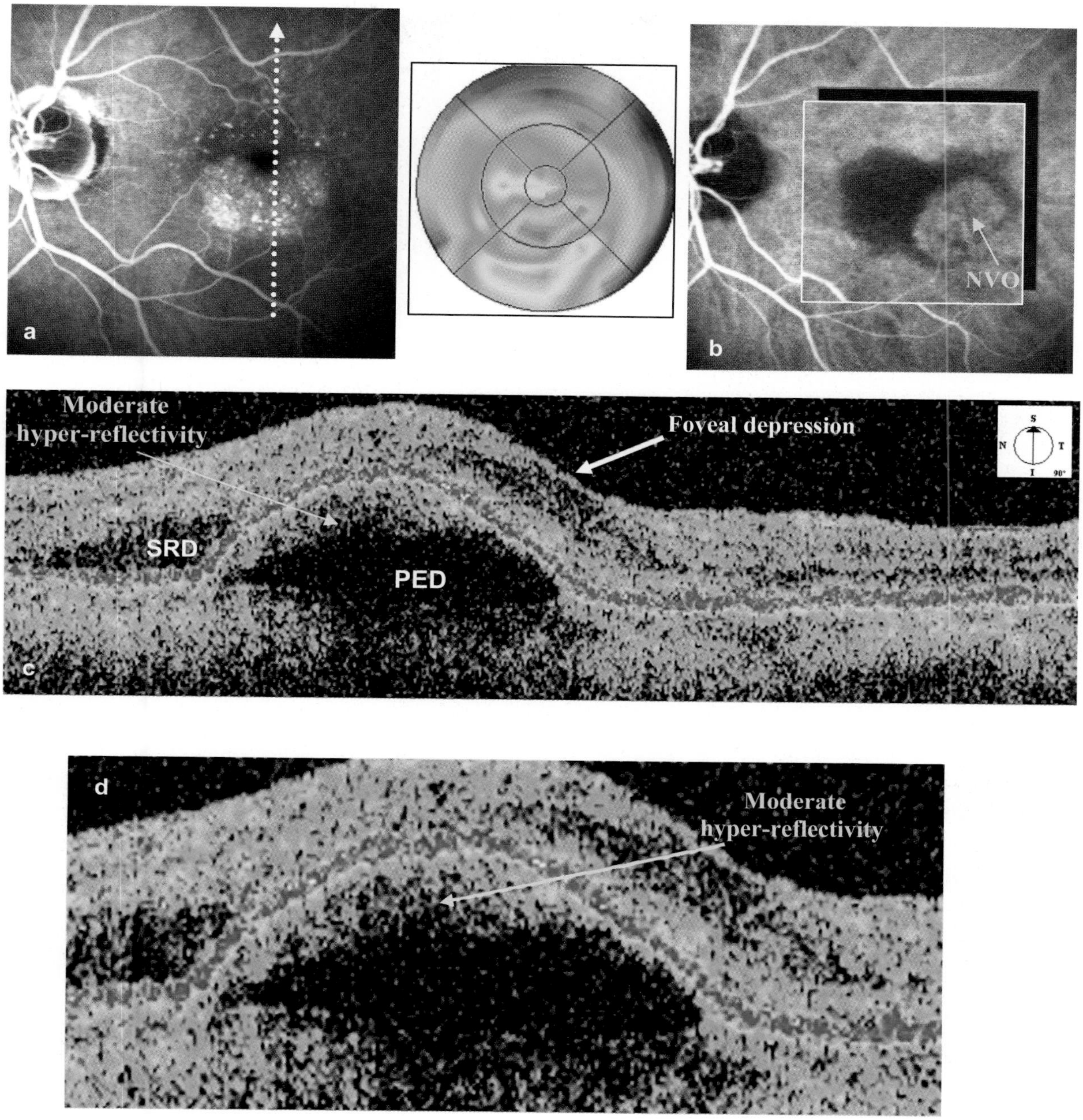

Figure 29: Elevation of the RPE: Vascularized PED partially invaded by occult CNV.

a and b): Fluorescein angiography and ICG angiography: *CNV clearly visible in the serous PED.*

c and d): ***Stratus**** **horizontal section.**

On **TD-OCT**, the RPE is hyper-reflective and clearly visible, raised in a very regular dome shape pattern with a mostly optically empty cavity.
The cavity is actually occupied by a moderately reflective band (*yellow arrow*) just posterior to the RPE, corresponding to the inferior part of the PED with CNV.

POSTERIOR TO THE RPE: FIBROVASCULAR PED

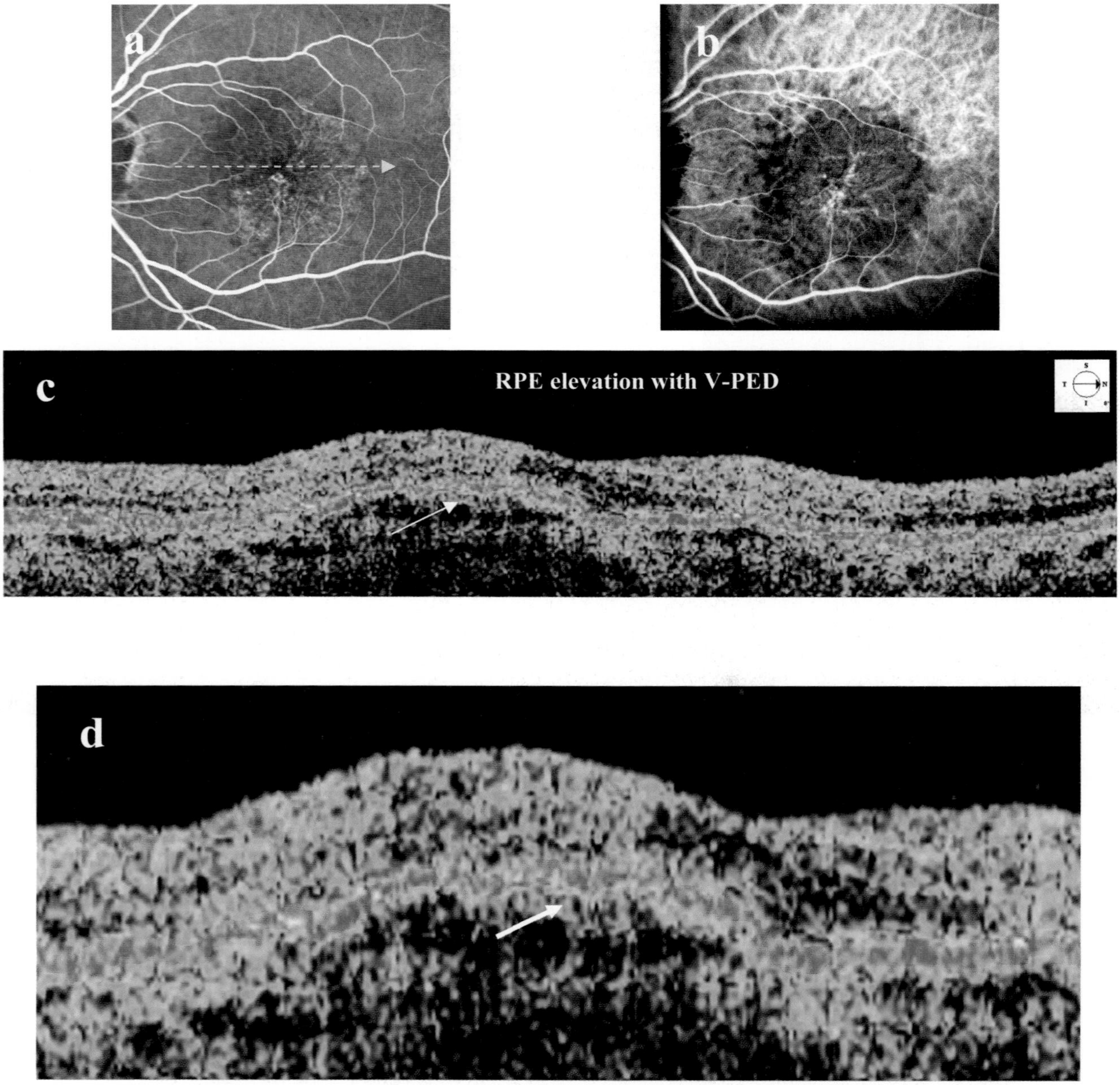

Figure 30: Elevation of the RPE: Fibrovascular PED associated with occult CNV (VA 20/80).

a and b): Fluorescein angiography and ICG angiography: *neovascular network invading all of the vascularized PED cavity.*

c and d): *Stratus horizontal section.**

On **TD-OCT**, the RPE is separated from the plane of Bruch's membrane (*arrow*) with a slight, heterogeneous elevation and partial shadowing. The cavity appears to be moderately reflective, suggesting partial organization.

d): Enlarged image (c): irregular thickness of the RPE and progressive fibrosis of the vascularized PED and intraretinal changes (infiltration and disorganization) reflecting the retinal reaction to choroidal neovascularization.

POSTERIOR TO THE RPE: FIBROVASCULAR PED

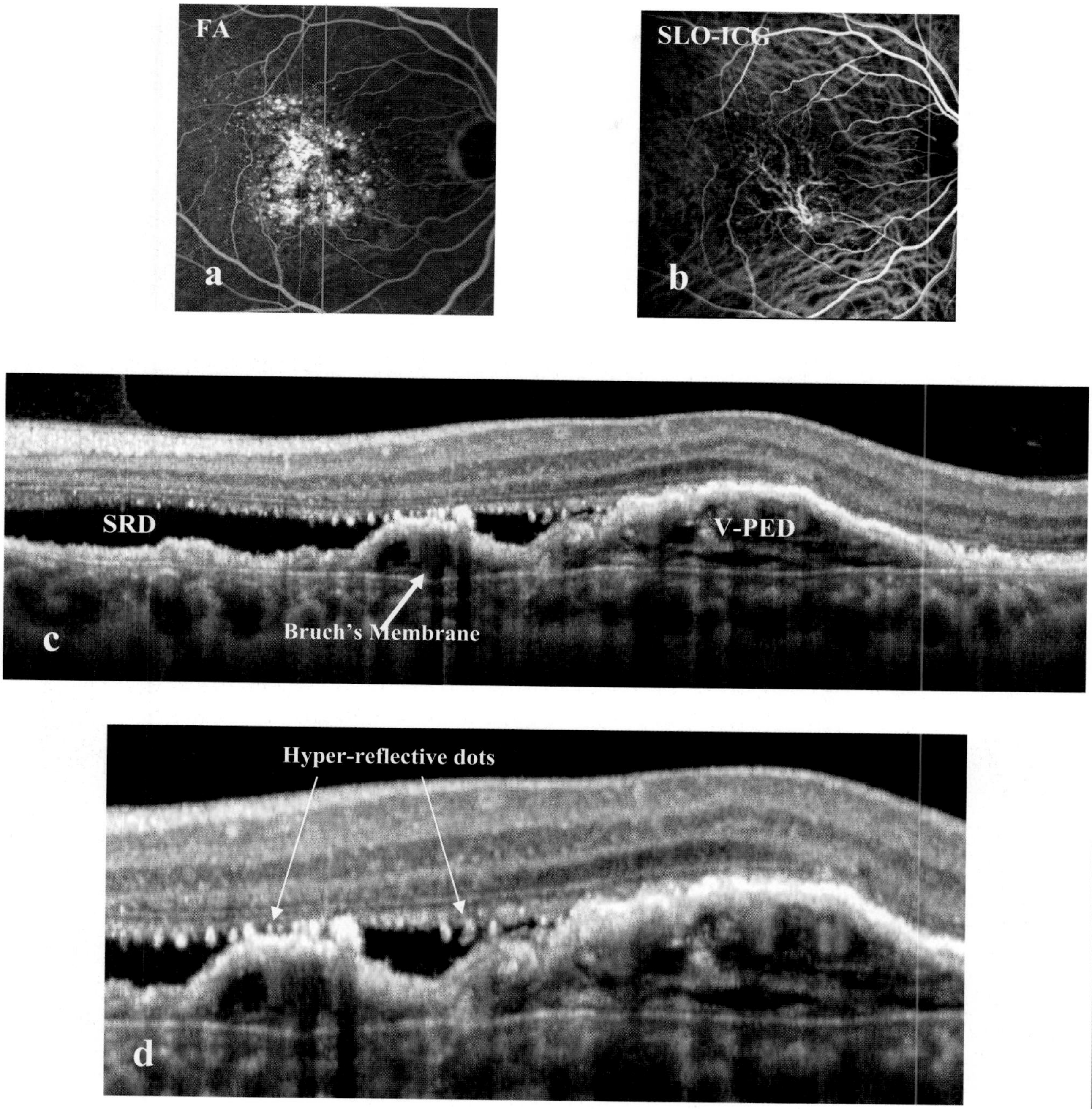

Figure 31: Elevation of the RPE: Fibrovascular PED associated with occult CNV.

a and b): Fluorescein angiography and ICG angiography: *CNV is clearly visualized on ICG angiography, invading all of the vascularized PED.*

c): *Spectralis vertical section:**

On SD-OCT, the RPE (irregular and thickened) is separated from Bruch's membrane (*arrow*) with a small heterogeneous elevation, corresponding to fibrovascular tissue and partial organization.
Spectral-Domain OCT demonstrates, not only persistence of subretinal fluid, but with hyper-reflective bright spots, which are a sign of activity (*double white arrows*). The preserved organization of inner and outer retinal layers is indicative of a favorable prognosis.

POSTERIOR TO THE RPE: ADVANCED FIBROVASCULAR PED

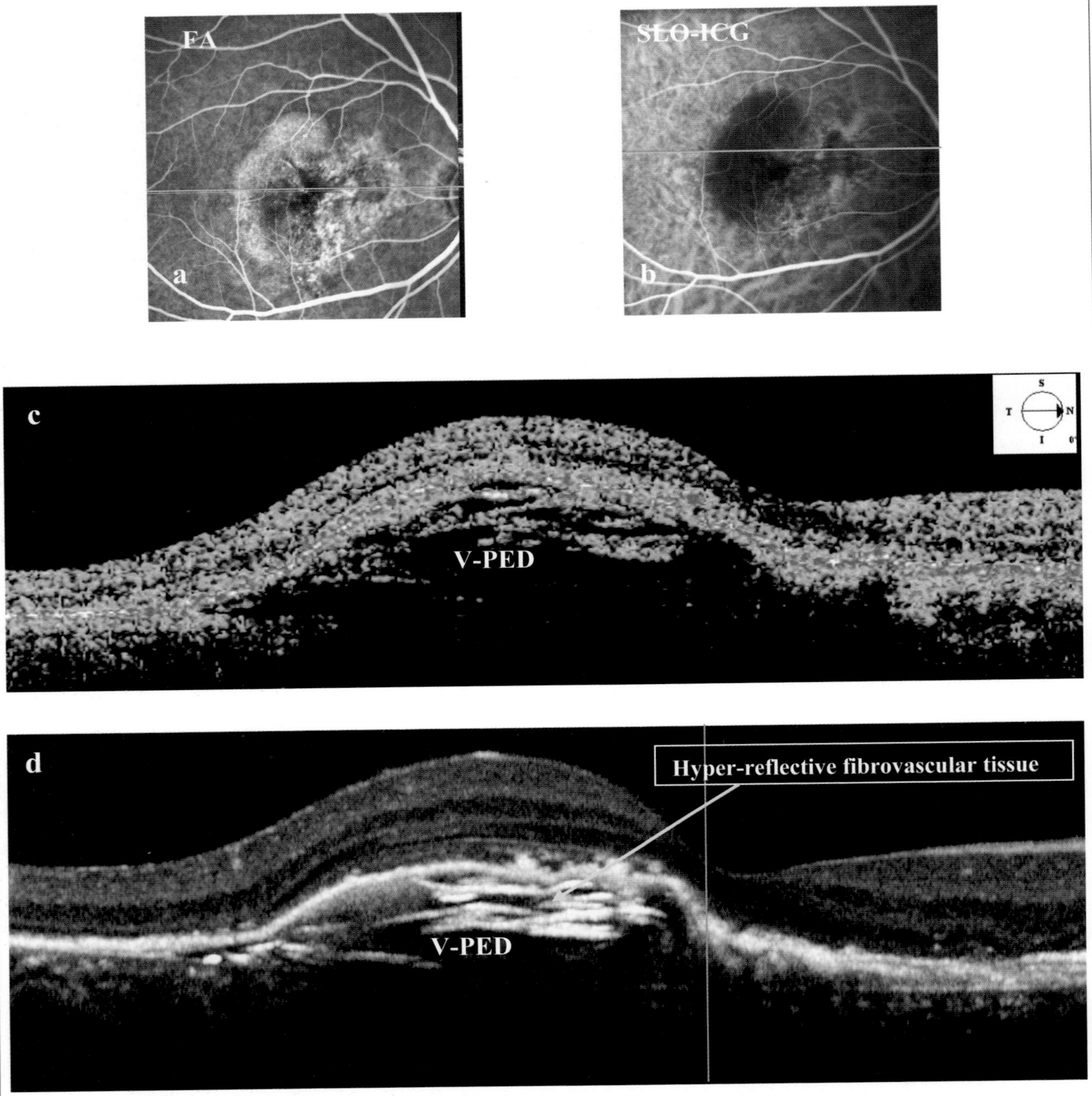

Figure 32: Elevation of the RPE: Advanced fibrovascular PED with extension of occult CNV and progressive fibrosis.

a and b): Fluorescein angiography and ICG angiography: *CNV is clearly visualized on ICG angiography, invading all of the vascularized PED.*

c): *Stratus horizontal section:** On TD-OCT, the elevated and bulging RPE delineates a cavity containing a large number of fibrous or fibrovascular elements with apparently little activity, inducing only moderate leakage, but more pronounced posterior shadowing.

d): *Spectralis horizontal section:** On SD-OCT, the hyper-reflective fibrovascular tissue is clearly visible with posterior shadowing. Note the irregularities of the RPE and slight alterations of the outer layers over the apex of the vascularized PED.

POSTERIOR TO THE RPE: PROGRESSIVE FIBROSIS

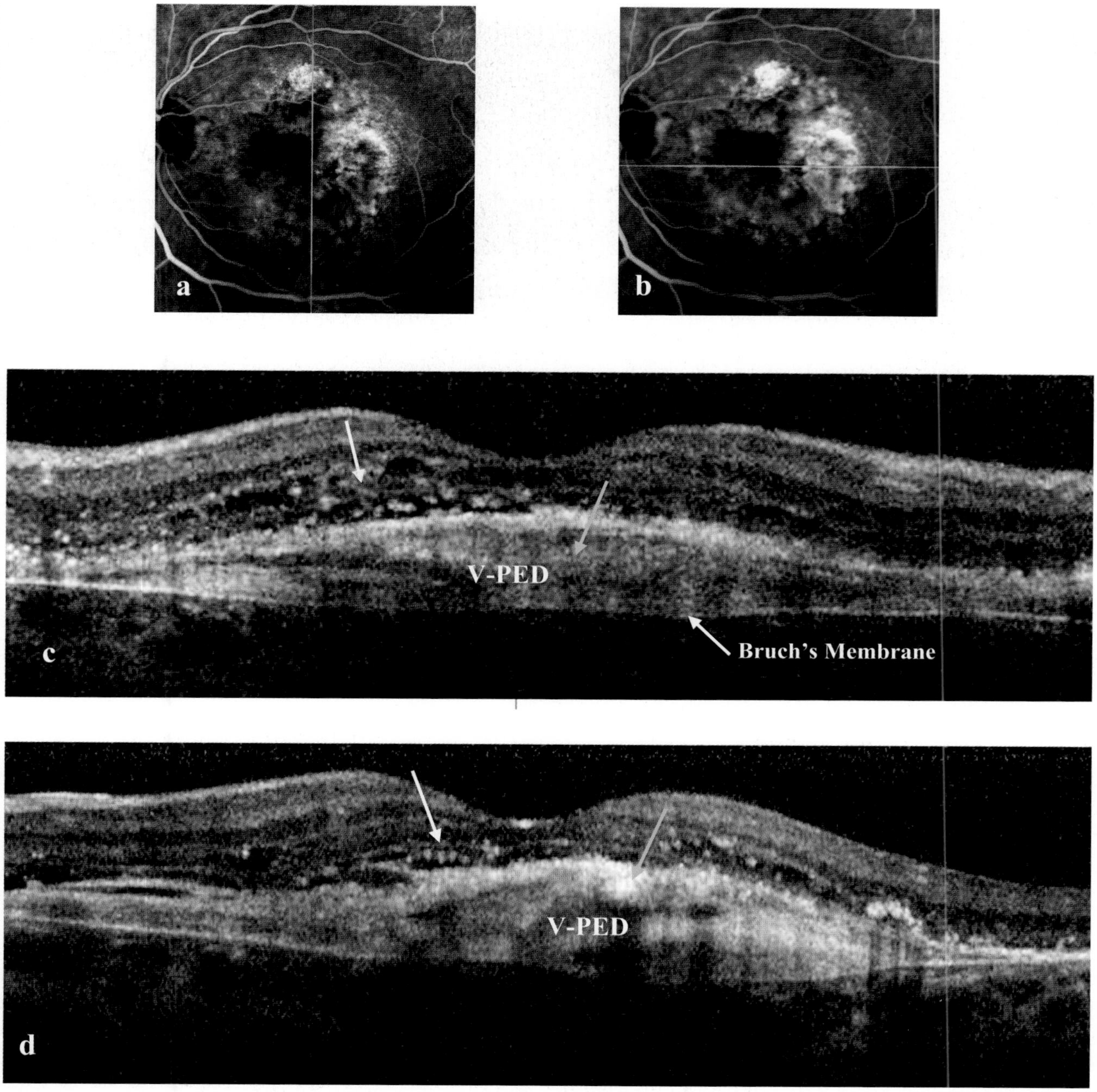

Figure 33: Elevation of the RPE: Progressive fibrosis posterior to the RPE.
a and b): Fluorescein angiography: *complex, extensive lesion, still active after 3 intravitreous injections.*
c): *Spectralis vertical section.**
On **SD-OCT**, the PED is flat but has a heterogeneous hyper-reflective cavity until Bruch's membrane, which remains visible. Despite this early fibrosis, the lesion is still active with fluid infiltration and numerous hyper-reflective bright spots (white arrow). Early signs of organization and probable fibrosis are seen.
d): *Spectralis horizontal section (same patient, after further treatment).**
The hyper-reflectivity posterior to the RPE (probable fibrosis) has increased. This progressive fibrosis is accompanied by resolution of the anterior reactive signs: decreased retinal thickness and hyper-reflective bright spots. The outer nuclear layer is barely visible, but organization of the other retinal layers is almost normal.

POSTERIOR TO THE RPE: FIBROTIC SCAR

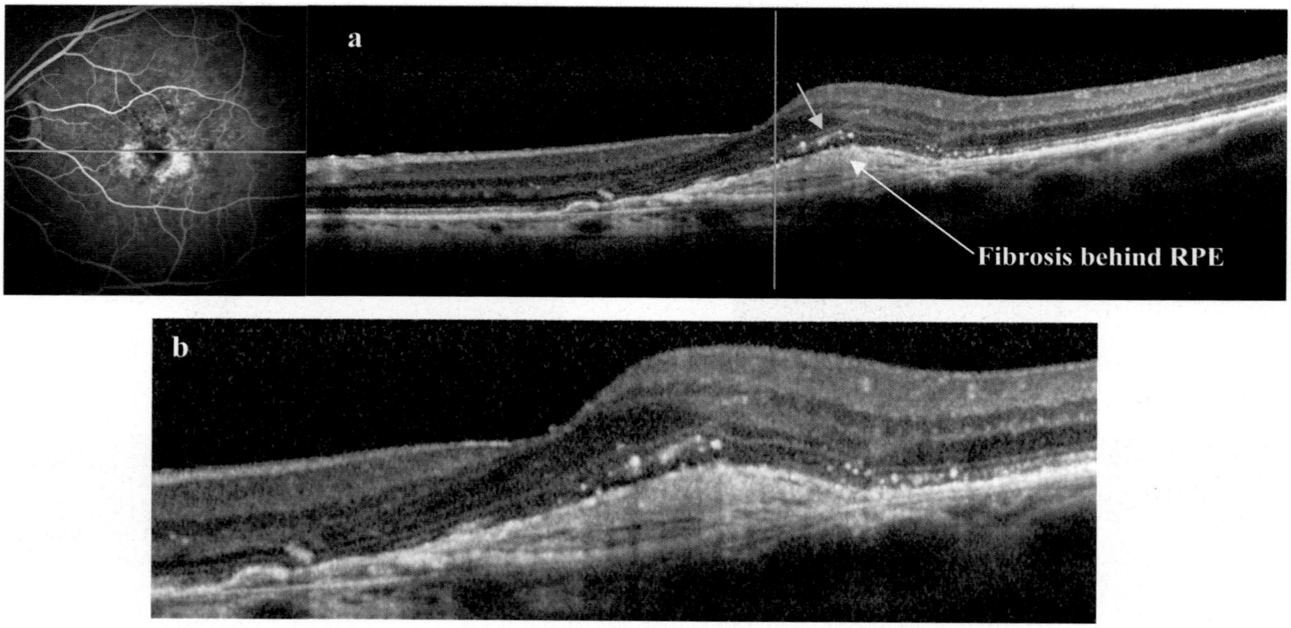

Figure 34: Elevation of the RPE: Fibrovascular PED, at the scarring stage, with fibrosis posterior to the RPE.
a): *Spectralis, horizontal section combined with fluorescein angiography** (*staining of the fibrotic lesion).*
On SD-OCT, the PED is relatively flat with a hyper-reflective, homogeneous cavity. Bruch's membrane remains slightly visible.
After repeated intravitreous injections, the fibrovascular PED has become organized with probable fibrosis. There is no more fluid accumulation and the organization of the retinal layers has almost returned to normal.
b): Enlargement of the *Spectralis section (a):** The external limiting membrane is continuous but the IS/OS interface is altered with a few persistent bright hyper-reflective bright spots (*yellow arrow*); the outer nuclear layer is barely visible.

7

5. Posterior to the RPE: Shadowing or Hyper-Reflectivity

Pronounced hyper-reflectivity may be observed with *atrophy of the retinal layers* (or *post-laser atrophic scars*).

- This **atrophy** allows abnormal passage of light into the choroid. This hyper-reflectivity may immediately draw the examiner's attention.
- Atrophy of retinal layers in the central part of the fovea is mainly observed in advanced forms, either spontaneously or after treatment. In these cases, pronounced thinning of the neurosensory retina allows increased passage of light (**Figure 35**).
- Atrophy of the RPE may also be associated with resorption of lipofuscin deposits (**Figure 8**), a previous RPE tear (**Figure 9**), or laser treatment (**Figure 36**).

Inversely, the presence of various *hyper-reflective structures in the inner retinal layers* can also cause changes on OCT.

- These alterations can induce **back-shadowing**, which may extend posteriorly to the choroid, when no light penetrates into this layer.

This is the case with retinal hemorrhage, accumulation of material, or classic CNV (**Figures 37-40**).

Similarly, lipid exudates (**Figure 41**), large retinal vessels, or dense clumps of pigment can induce back shadowing, even until the level of the choroid (**Figures 42 and 43**).

POSTERIOR TO THE RPE: HYPER-REFLECTIVITY AND SHADOWING

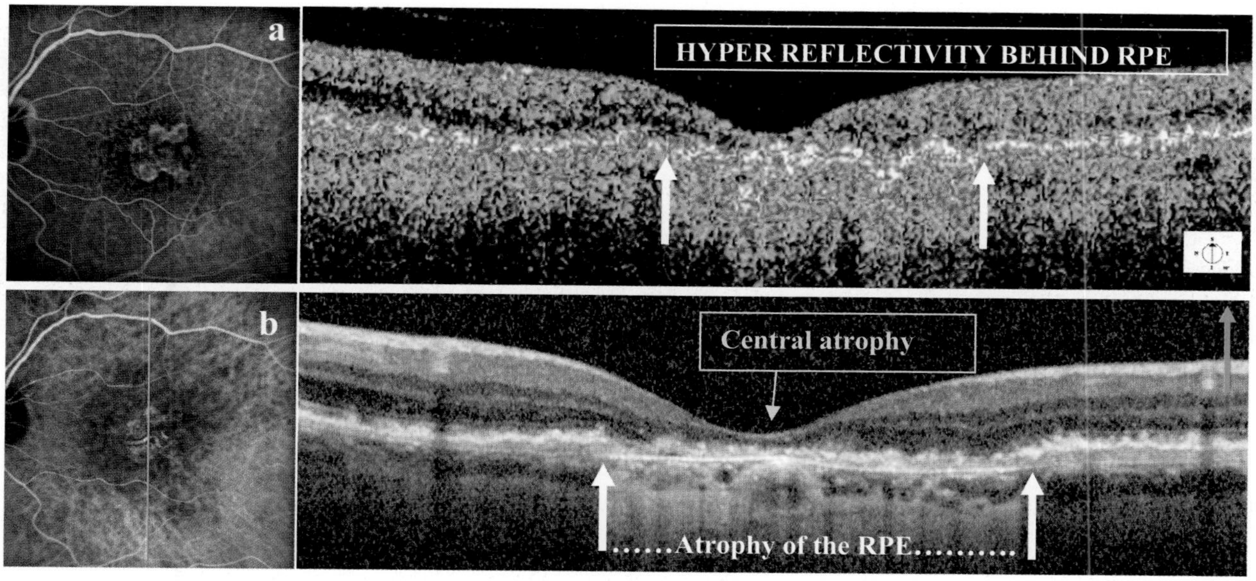

Figure 35: Posterior hyper-reflectivity due to atrophy of the neurosensory retina.

a): *Stratus vertical section correlated with fluorescein angiography** (*geographic atrophy due to resorption of drusen).*

b): *Spectralis vertical section combined with ICG angiography** (*same patient*). Thinning of the central neurosensory retina is associated with atrophy of the RPE and pronounced hyper-reflectivity towards the choroid. Note the loss of the outer retinal layers in the atrophic area.

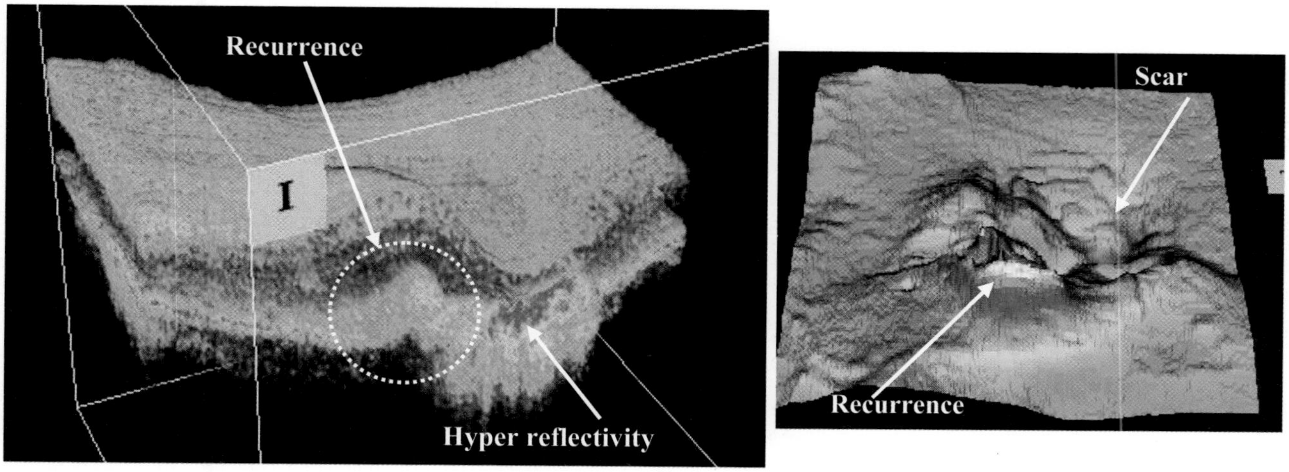

Figure 36: Posterior hyper-reflectivity due to post-laser atrophy.

***Topcon** 3D volume and surface mapping section**: post-laser atrophy and adjacent subfoveal recurrence.

The laser scar causes posterior hyper-reflectivity and thinning on retinal mapping, reflected by a blue color.
The hyper-reflectivity in choroidal layers is clearly visible and is associated with an atrophy, not only of the RPE, but also of the neurosensory retina. The can be seen particularly in the central foveal zone, which accounts for the irreversible loss of VA (20/100).

POSTERIOR TO THE RPE: MASKING BY HEMORRHAGE

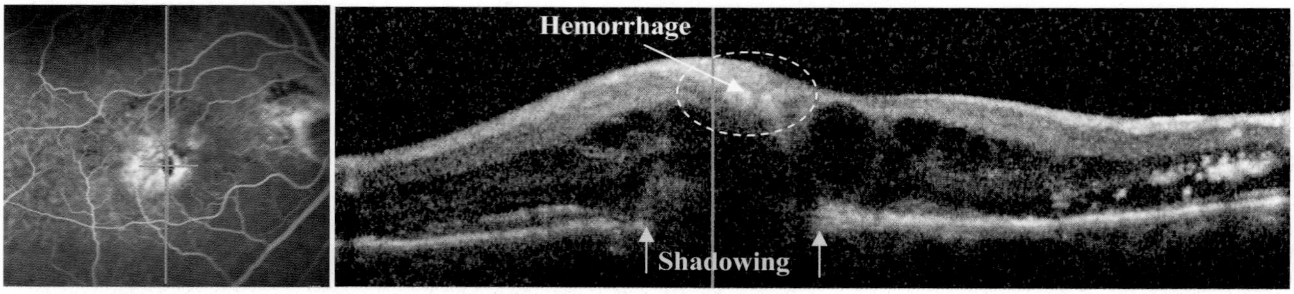

Figure 37: Localized masking of the RPE due to the presence of retinal hemorrhage.

***Spectralis** vertical section combined with fluorescein angiography**: *localized hyper-fluorescence partially masked by dense and superficial retinal hemorrhage.*

Hemorrhage causes posterior shadowing which masks not only the RPE, but also all intraretinal structures and features posteriorly, such as the choroid.

POSTERIOR TO RPE: MASKING BY DEEP HEMORRHAGE

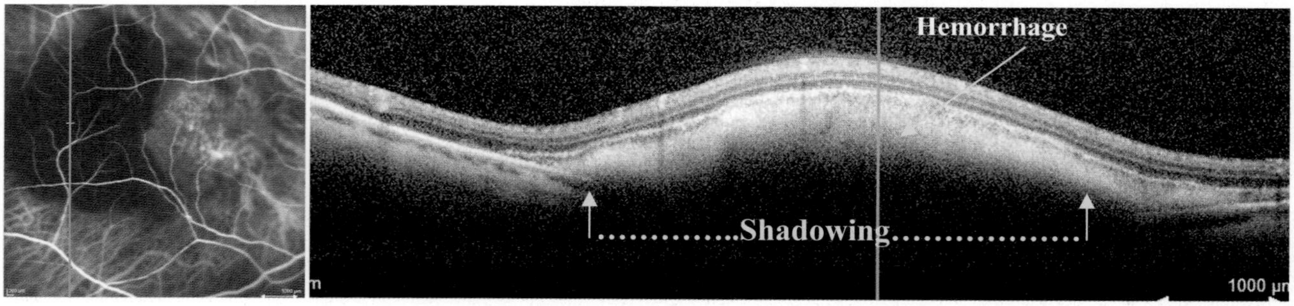

Figure 38: Localized masking of the RPE due to the presence of a large hemorrhagic detachment of the RPE.

***Spectralis** vertical section combined with ICG angiography**: *marked hypo-fluorescence corresponding to the hemorrhage adjacent to a deep neovascular network visible in the PED.*

Hemorrhage induces pronounced hyper-reflectivity with major shadowing, as the light does not penetrate through the layers of blood. This induces posterior masking not only of Bruch's membrane but of all posterior structures including the choroid.

POSTERIOR TO THE RPE: SHADOWING BY MATERIAL

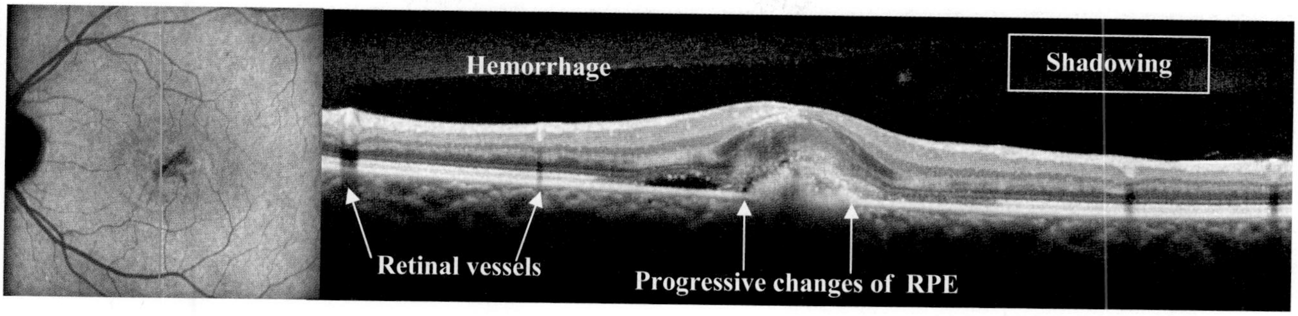

Figure 39: Partial masking of the RPE related to the presence of lipofuscin deposits.

***Spectralis** vertical section combined with ICG angiography, late phase**: *the material remains markedly hypo-fluorescent.*

On **SD-OCT**, the material accumulated in front of the RPE is cone-shaped with maximum thickness in the center, corresponding to maximum masking of the RPE. The RPE remains visible, although attenuated on either side.

Note that the large vessels of the superior and inferior temporal arcades causes clearly visible and well-defined shadowing from peripheral layers (the site of the vessels) towards the choroid.

POSTERIOR TO THE RPE: LOCALIZED MASKING BY NEOVASCULARIZATION

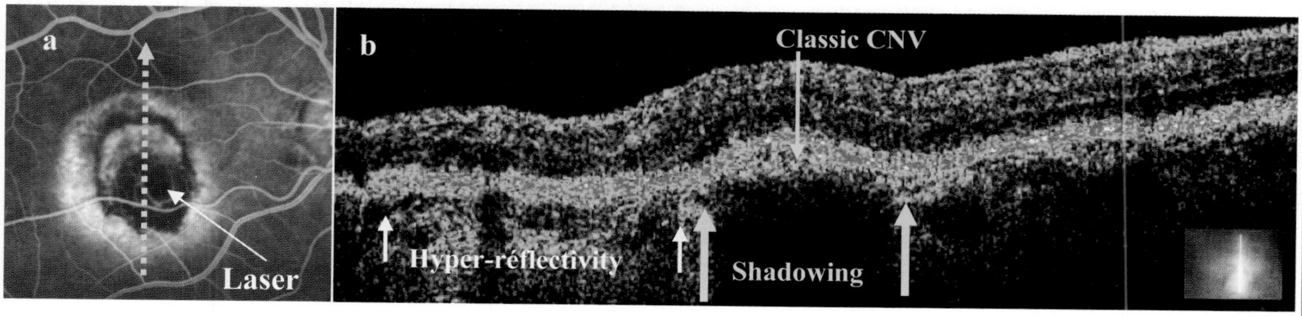

Figure 40: Shadowing with masking of the RPE, related to the presence of classic CNV.

a): Fluorescein angiography: *inferior parafoveal laser scar and recurrence of classic CNV on its superior edge.*

b): *Stratus vertical section.**

The **TD-OCT** section initially passes through the inferior scar, causing marked posterior hyper-reflectivity. The section then passes through the recurrent CNV on the superior edge of the scar: CNV induces a bulging cone-shaped zone of hyper-reflectivity accompanied by posterior shadowing.

POSTERIOR TO THE RPE: LOCALIZED MASKING BY LIPID EXUDATES

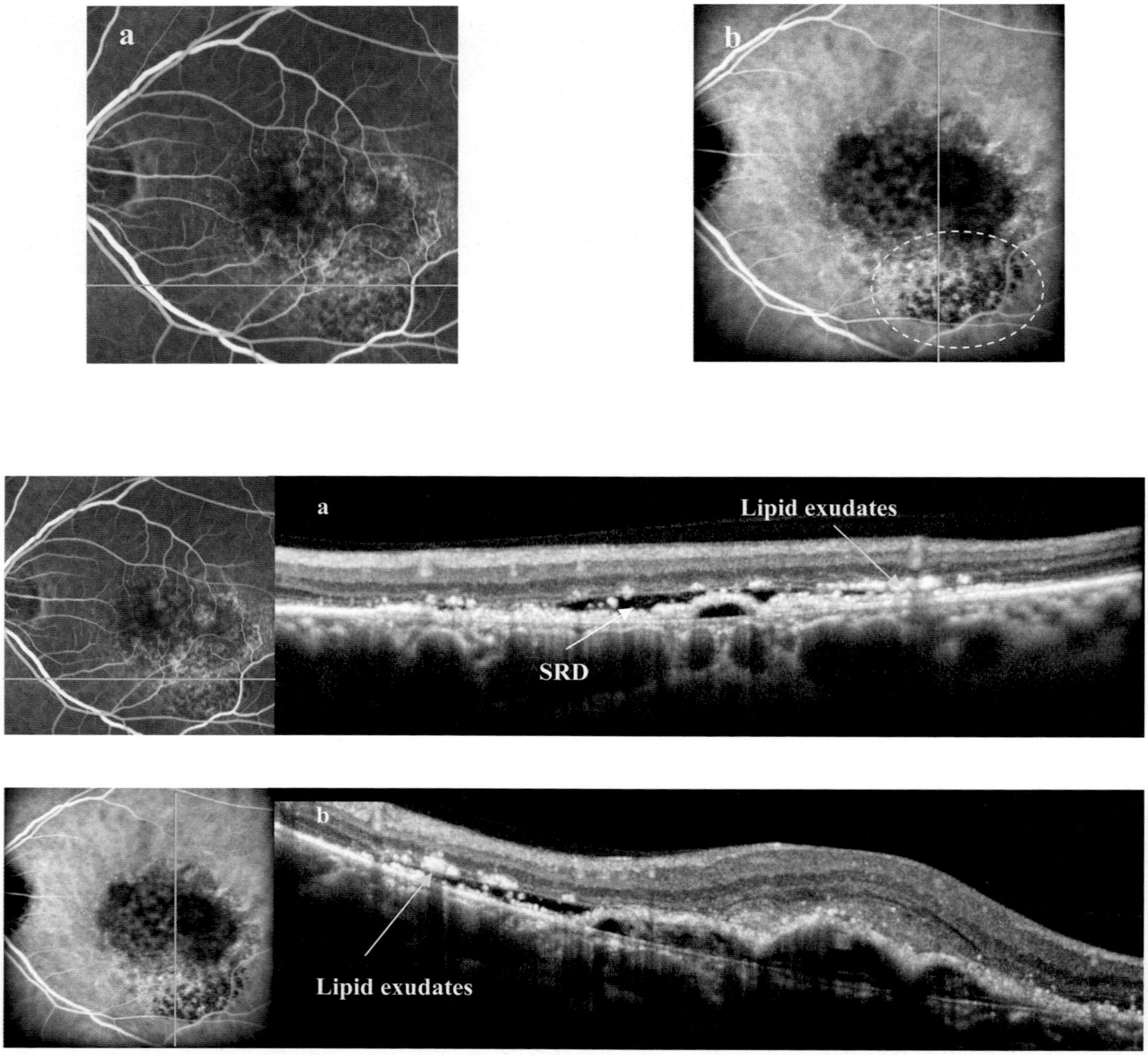

▫ Figure 41: Shadowing related to the presence of lipid exudates at the periphery of CNV.

a): *Spectralis horizontal section combined with fluorescein angiography** (*extensive occult CNV with serous retinal detachment and accumulation of exudates at its inferior edge).*

On **SD-OCT**, exudates are seen as tightly packed hyper-reflective clumps in the outermost layers of the retina.

This is similar to the hyper-reflective bright spots usually associated with active CNV (as in the more temporal zone of the section).

b): *Spectralis vertical section combined with ICG angiography** (*same patient*): Similar appearance of lipid exudates in the outer layers of the retina.

POSTERIOR TO THE RPE: LOCALIZED MASKING BY NORMAL RETINAL VESSELS

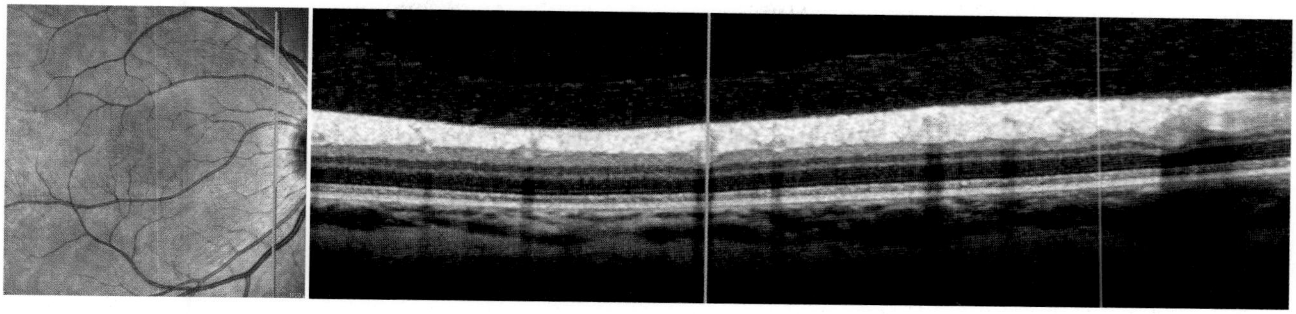

Figure 42: Shadowing by retinal vessels.

***Spectralis** vertical section combined with a reference red-free image.**

The **SD-OCT** section passes adjacent to the optic disc and shows the large retinal vessels.

These vessels are clearly visible and induce a small zone of hyper-reflectivity followed by masking over a narrow zone, which corresponds to the diameter of the vessel. The effect crosses all layers of the retina even until the RPE and choroid. The vessel's walls are usually highly reflective.

In some cases, it is even possible to distinguish the vessel lumen and its associated backward-masking in the outer layers.
This type of masking is easily recognized and is often used as a landmark for comparison with angiography.

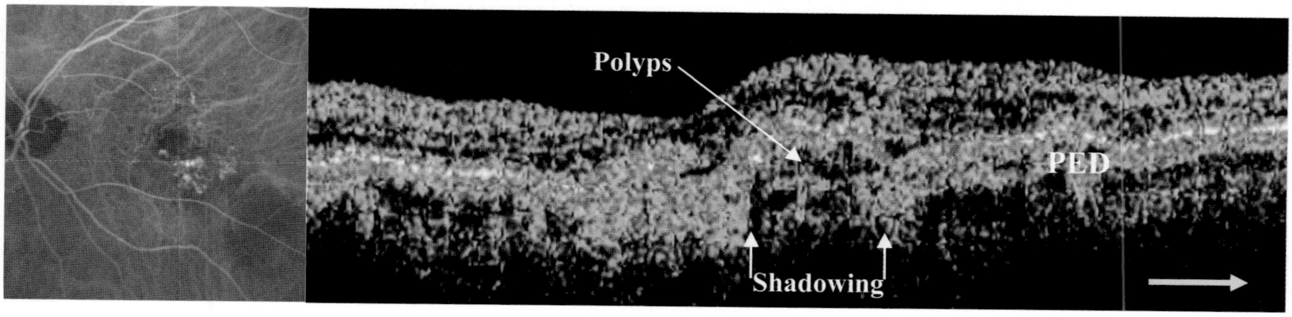

Figure 43: Shadowing induced by the presence of polypoidal formations.

***Stratus** horizontal section shown with ICG angiography** (*clearly demonstrating very dense polyps, the normal choroidal network, and the inferior macular PED).*

On **TD-OCT**, this is immediately suggestive with the steeply sloped multi-lobed prominence, which lifts the RPE and induces relative posterior masking.
The superior pole of the PED is visible and continues temporally.
Also note the subfoveal fibrosis inducing posterior hyper-reflectivity.

III. Anterior to the RPE Band

TD-OCT

Reactive signs related to the presence of different features of AMD, either *precursors* or *complications* (atrophic or neovascular), can gradually accumulate.

- **Fluid accumulation** is the most easily detectable and quantifiable sign in exudative AMD and is therefore routinely evaluated. It essentially corresponds to *intraretinal* or *subretinal* fluid infiltration and accumulation.

These intraretinal fluid collections can be *diffuse* or associated with *cystoid spaces*. Cystoid spaces can progress to become more numerous, larger, and eventually confluent, especially in the central foveolar zone.

The **inner layers** of the retina are only slightly modified in the early stages, but subsequently become disorganized due to fluid infiltration and an inflammatory response.

The various stages of AMD along with the indications for and results of treatment are often assessed based on the amount of leakage.

This leakage appears *easy to evaluate and quantify* on OCT, at least in terms of fluid accumulation and retinal thickness, which are measureable.

- **Central retinal thickness** (CRT) is certainly an easy criterion to use, but it is not sufficient to fully describe the polymorphous clinical forms of AMD and their course.

- Hyper-reflective **pre-retinal vascular proliferations** can be fairly easy to identify and localize, but they must be clearly distinguished from accumulation of non-vascular material or fibrin deposits, which appear as part of the healing process.

More extensive imaging and particularly angiography is essential in these situations.

SD-OCT

- **Other reactive signs** can now be appreciated on OCT with the advent of Spectral-Domain technology.

These advantages are most apparent when evaluating the outer retinal layers (*outer nuclear layer, external limiting membrane, photoreceptor cell bodies, and inner segment/outer segment interface*).

- Additional signs appear to reflect the presence of active CNV, their abnormal permeability, and the inflammatory response they elicit. These signs include:
  - *Bright hyper-reflective* spots adjacent to fluid and outer layers but sometimes disseminated as far as the inner layers.
  - *Dense zones with enhanced reflectivity*, displacing or spreading inside the outer nuclear layer and sometimes extending as far as the inner layers.

1. Fluid Accumulation Anterior to the RPE: Sub-Retinal Detachments (SRD)

The presence of serous fluid is visualized as a homogeneous optically empty space, and therefore is hyporeflective and dark on OCT images. The space situated between the neurosensory retina and the RPE is an **easily detachable potential space**. Any abnormal exudation can accumulate in this space and create a serous detachment of the neurosensory retina (SRD).
During the course of disease, the size of the SRD can progressively change. The SRD is sometimes minimal and limited to a barely visible thin layer of fluid, which is usually associated with a highly suggestive localized intraretinal infiltration. (**Figure 44**).

Active CNV causes more marked leakage, creating a more elevated SRD, which is usually also associated with intraretinal cysts (**Figure 45**).
When the retina is already raised by a serous detachment of the RPE, fluid accumulation anterior to the RPE appears to be limited to or localized around the PED and therefore has a fairly characteristic triangular shape on OCT cross-sections (**Figure 46**).
Diverse changes in the relative degree of fluid accumulation under the neurosensory retina (ie, SRD), RPE (ie, PED), or intraretinal cysts may be observed during the subsequent course of disease.

MINIMAL SRD

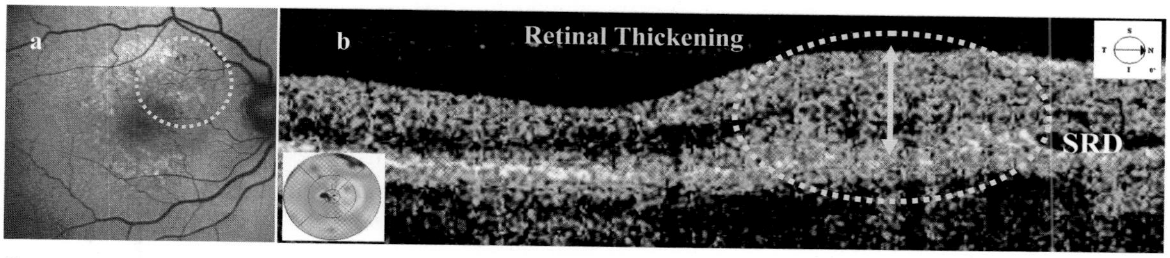

Figure 44: Fluid accumulation anterior to the RPE with minimal SRD.

a) Autofluorescence: multiple perifoveal hyperfluorescent areas.

b) *Stratus TD-OCT horizontal section**: early lesion in the nasal and superior sectors of the fovea with intraretinal fluid accumulation and increased retinal thickness (*circle*) associated with a limited adjacent SRD.

MODERATE SRD

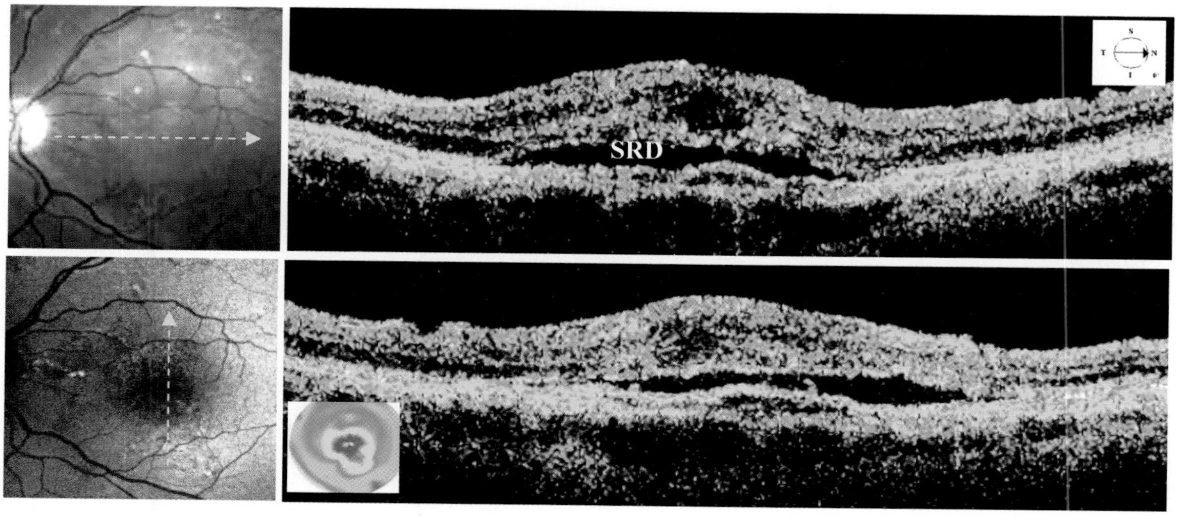

Figure 45: Fluid accumulation anterior to the RPE.

***Stratus** horizontal and vertical sections correlated to red-free and autofluorescence images.**

This OCT section demonstrates elevation of the macular region with loss of the foveal depression.

The SRD is an optically empty, black spindle-shaped zone between the RPE and neurosensory retina.

Anteriorly, the retina is thickened and infiltrated with a large central cyst, but retains an almost normal configuration.

Posteriorly, a PED can be seen, suggesting the presence of an occult CNV.

SRD ASSOCIATED WITH A PED

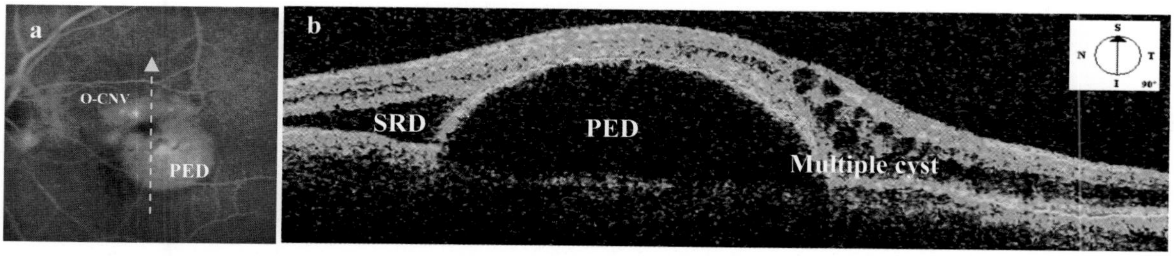

Figure 46: Fluid accumulation anterior to the RPE associated with a serous PED.

a): Fluorescein angiography: serous PED with a small area of occult CNV at its superior edge.

b): *Stratus OCT vertical section**: dome-shaped elevation of the RPE related to the serous PED.

In the inferior part, localized, triangular SRD with fluid accumulation anterior to the RPE. In the superior part, multiple cysts and intraretinal fluid. At the summit of the dome of the PED, the retina is in contact with the RPE and has a normal thickness.

2. Fluid Accumulation Anterior to the RPE

Features of SRD and its Evolution

Active choroidal neovascularization is accompanied by enlargement of the serous retinal detachment (SRD), with frequent shifting of subretinal fluid.

The presence and size of serous retinal detachment must therefore be studied completely on serial sections of the macula (**Figure 47**).

Regression of the SRD

Rapid regression of the SRD, particularly after the first injections of anti-VEGF, suggests treatment efficacy and is also generally accompanied by a rapid and marked functional improvement.

This regression then becomes slower, decreasing intraretinal fluid and cysts but leaving a limited yet persistent band of SRD.

The subretinal detachment may even paradoxically increase, followed later by gradual regression (**Figures 48-50**).

Persistent Fluid

The fluid layer of the SRD sometimes *chronically* persists. This occurs especially when treatment is delayed and fibrosis has already begun (**Figures 51 and 52**).

Persistent fluid is sometimes compatible with a relatively stable and fair visual acuity if subretinal fibrosis remains moderate. In this situation, the presence of subretinal fluid is not an absolute indication for retreatment (**Figure 53**).

Complications

Some complications are often associated with (recurrent) exudative lesions. The presence of a limited SRD, detectable only on OCT sections, may explain the occurrence of symptoms such as metamorphopsias and decreased visual acuity.

This could detect early recurrences of CNV for example at the edge of a known laser scar (**Figures 54 and 55**).

Extensive leakage may also be observed in cases of RPE tears, mainly from the exposed choriocapillaris (**Figure 56**) or in cases of active occult CNV (**Figure 57**).

The incidence of SRD is lower than that usually reported.

SRD is not a constant feature in early forms of AMD or during a stable course, but it is often a sign of active disease.

The thickness of the SRD usually remains moderate or limited, and the SRD is often only discovered on vertical sections or sections of the inferior part of the macula.

In a study of 150 consecutive cases of wet AMD, SRD was present in only 28% of eyes.

The SRD was more clearly visible or more accentuated in the prone position and on vertical sections in two-thirds of cases.

The SRD was associated with cystoid spaces in one-half of cases.

The SRD was minimal (defined as an increase of less than 100 μm) in one-third of cases (30%); moderate (increase of 100 to 200 μm) in about one half of cases (45%); and marked (increase greater than 200 μm) in only a quarter of cases (25%).

The SRD regressed in response to treatment, but persisted to a lesser extent in 80% of cases after three intravitreous injections of anti-VEGF, (minimal in 25% of cases, moderate in 44% of cases, and marked in 31% of cases of persistent SRD).

Conversely, diffuse intraretinal fluid or intraretinal cysts (with variable shape and volume) appear to be much more frequent and are more often responsible for the increased central retinal thickness.

PREDOMINANTLY SHIFTING SRD

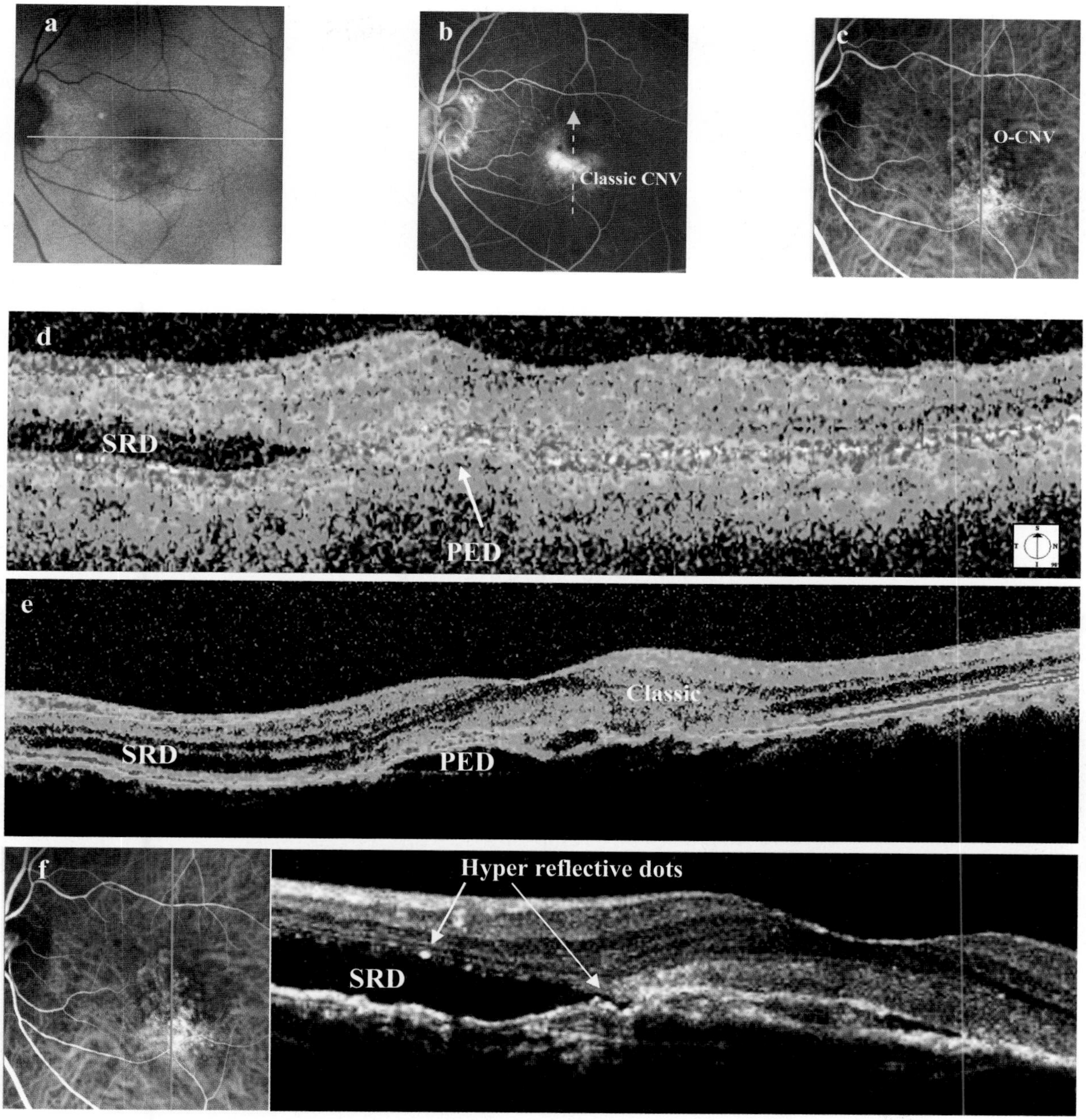

Figure 47: Fluid accumulation anterior to the RPE associated with advanced occult CNV.
a, b, and c): Autofluorescence, fluorescein angiography, and ICG angiography *(mixed, occult, and classic CNV).*
d): *Stratus OCT vertical section**: relatively marked SRD but limited to the inferior foveal region. The central retina appears slightly thickened but with no cysts. The hyper-reflective zone anterior to the RPE is suggestive of the presence of classic CNV. Note the flat PED with thickening of the RPE.
e): *Spectralis 110° vertical section** demonstrating the profile of the lesion with subfoveal mixed CNV and an inferior SRD.
f): Enlarged image associated with ICG angiography *(showing the real extent of the lesion).*
On SD-OCT, the SRD is even more clearly visible. Note the bright hyper-reflective spots on the internal limits of the SRD. They are probably reflecting active inflammatory response and damage to outer segments.
The external limiting membrane is still visible on all cross-sections. Note many irregularities on the RPE band. Bruch's membrane is clearly visible delimitating a partially organized PED.
In the subfoveal area, between the external limiting membrane and the RPE, there is a relatively dense and thick material which appears to occupy or surround the IS/OS interface, which is probably an inflammatory response around classic CNV.

PARTIAL REABSORPTION OF SRD

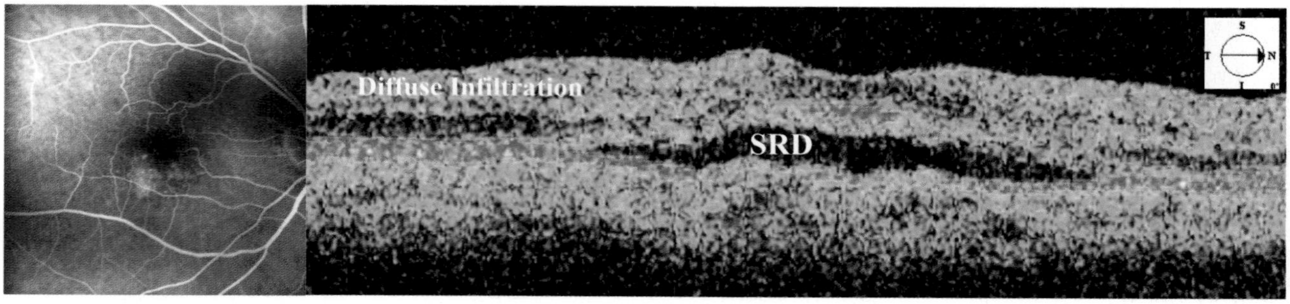

Figure 48: Fluid accumulation anterior to the RPE, resolving after treatment.

***Stratus** horizontal section associated with fluorescein angiography** *(showing resolution of occult CNV).*

The TD-OCT horizontal section shows a clearly visible subfoveal SRD. The central retina is still slightly thickened, with a visible but flattened foveal depression without any cystoid edema.
The SRD is not completely optically empty, but presents minimal hyper-reflectivity, possibly related to the presence of proteins.

PARTIALLY RESOLVED SRD

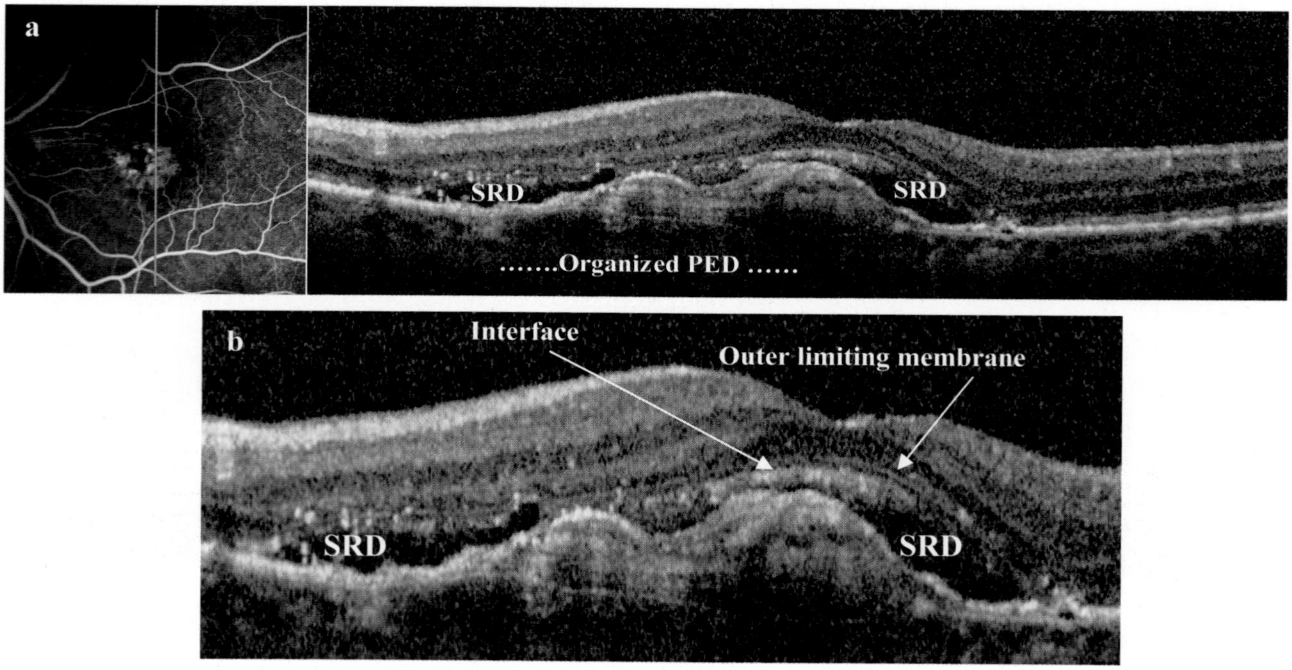

Figure 49: Fluid accumulation anterior to the RPE, partially resolved after treatment.

a): *Spectralis vertical section associated with fluorescein angiography** *(persistence of an area of occult CNV with moderate leakage).*
The OCT section shows persistence of the SRD anterior to a wavy and partially organized vascularized PED.

b): Enlarged view: despite improvement in response to treatment, the SRD and its limits are still marked by many bright hyper-reflective spots. The IS/OS interface is discontinuous but thickened in the subfoveal zone. The outer nuclear layer remains thinned and irregular, except in the subfoveal zone. The external limiting membrane is clearly visible and continuous, and the other retinal layers appear to be well-organized.

RESIDUAL SRD IN THE INFERIOR ZONE

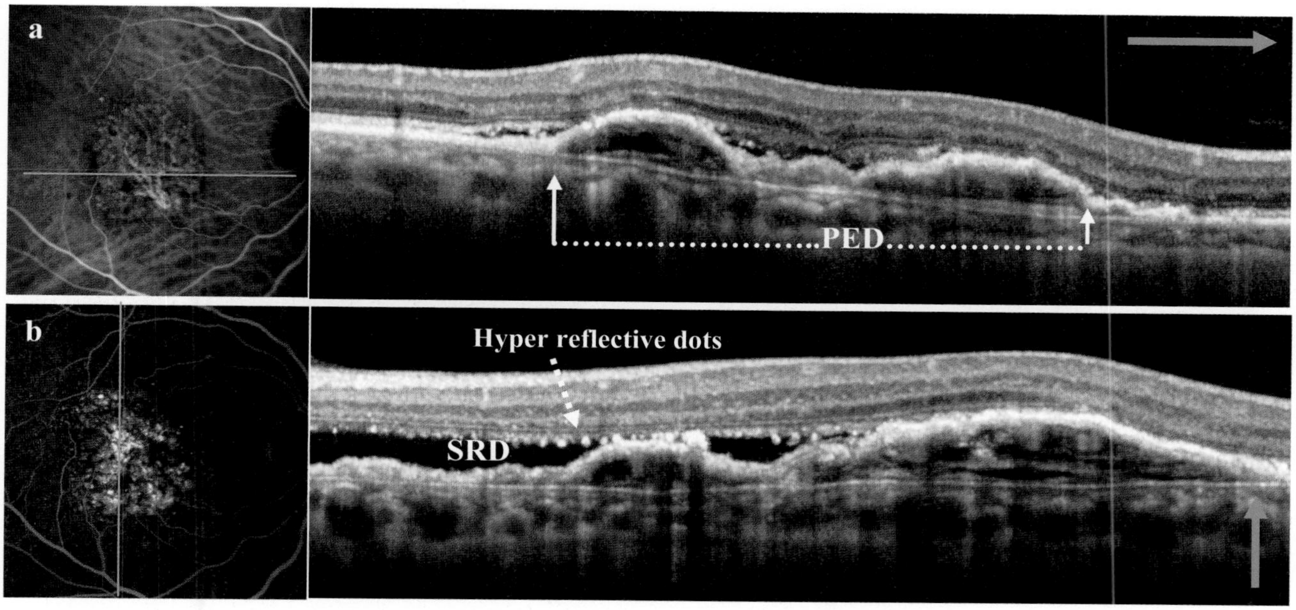

Figure 50: Fluid accumulation anterior to the RPE, partially resolved after treatment.

a): Spectralis* horizontal section, associated with ICG angiography *(persistence of the neovascular network).*
On SD-OCT, the SRD has almost completely resolved but persists at the edges and between the different domes of the vascularized PED.

b): ***Spectralis**** **vertical section, associated with fluorescein angiography.**
SD-OCT also shows persistence of shifting intraretinal fluid, and then, only visible on the vertical section. Note the multiple bright hyper-reflective spots at the edges of the SRD.

LONG DURATION SRD

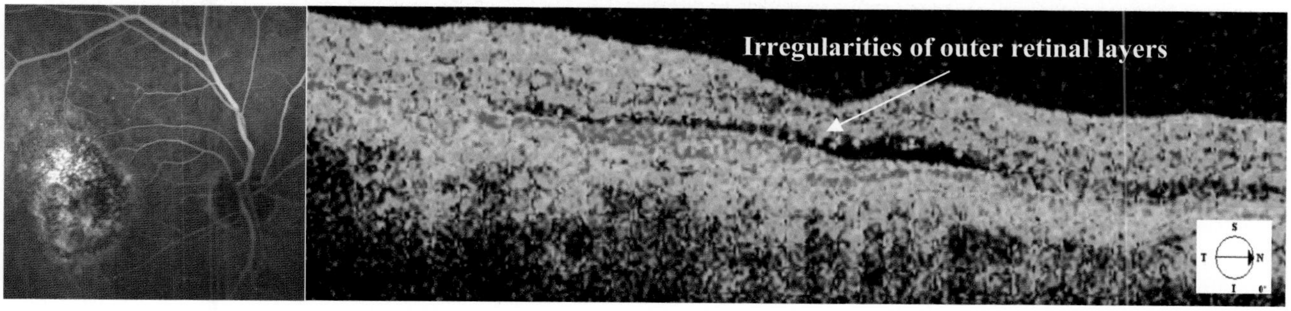

Figure 51: Fluid accumulation anterior to the RPE, partially resolved after multiple treatments.

Stratus* **horizontal section correlated with fluorescein angiography**: some leakage is still visible.

On TD-OCT, ongoing fibrosis (hyper-reflective band) associated with a thin layer of fluid anterior to this fibrosis.
Note the multiple irregularities of the photoreceptors often observed in chronic SRD.

LONG DURATION SRD WITH FIBROSIS

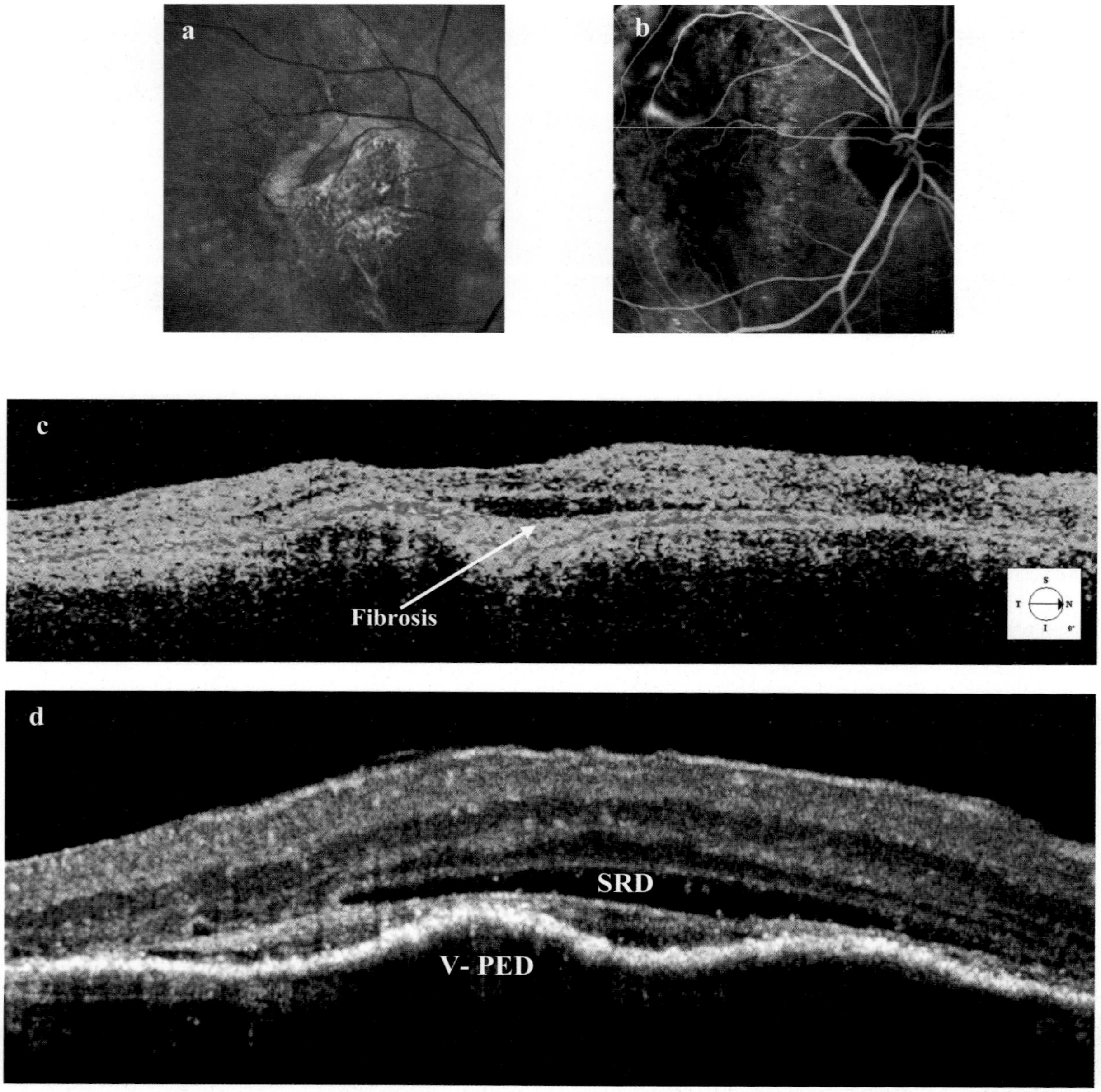

Figure 52: Fluid accumulation anterior to the RPE, persistent and chronic after treatment.

a and b): Red-free photography and fluorescein angiography: old vascularized PED in the process of healing with retraction towards the central fibrosis. The lesion is still thick and raised.

c): *Stratus horizontal section.**
On TD-OCT, a layer of moderately reflective fibrosis has formed anterior to the residual PED. A moderately thick SRD persists over this fibrosis, despite the absence of intraretinal fluid.

d): *Spectralis horizontal section.**
On SD-OCT, a small persistent pseudo-cystic space is visible between the IS/OS interface (persistent fluid) and the fibrous tissue that has proliferated anterior to the RPE band. The vascularized PED has become almost completely flattened.
The different outer retinal layers are disorganized and poorly distinguishable.

MINIMAL PERSISTENT SRD

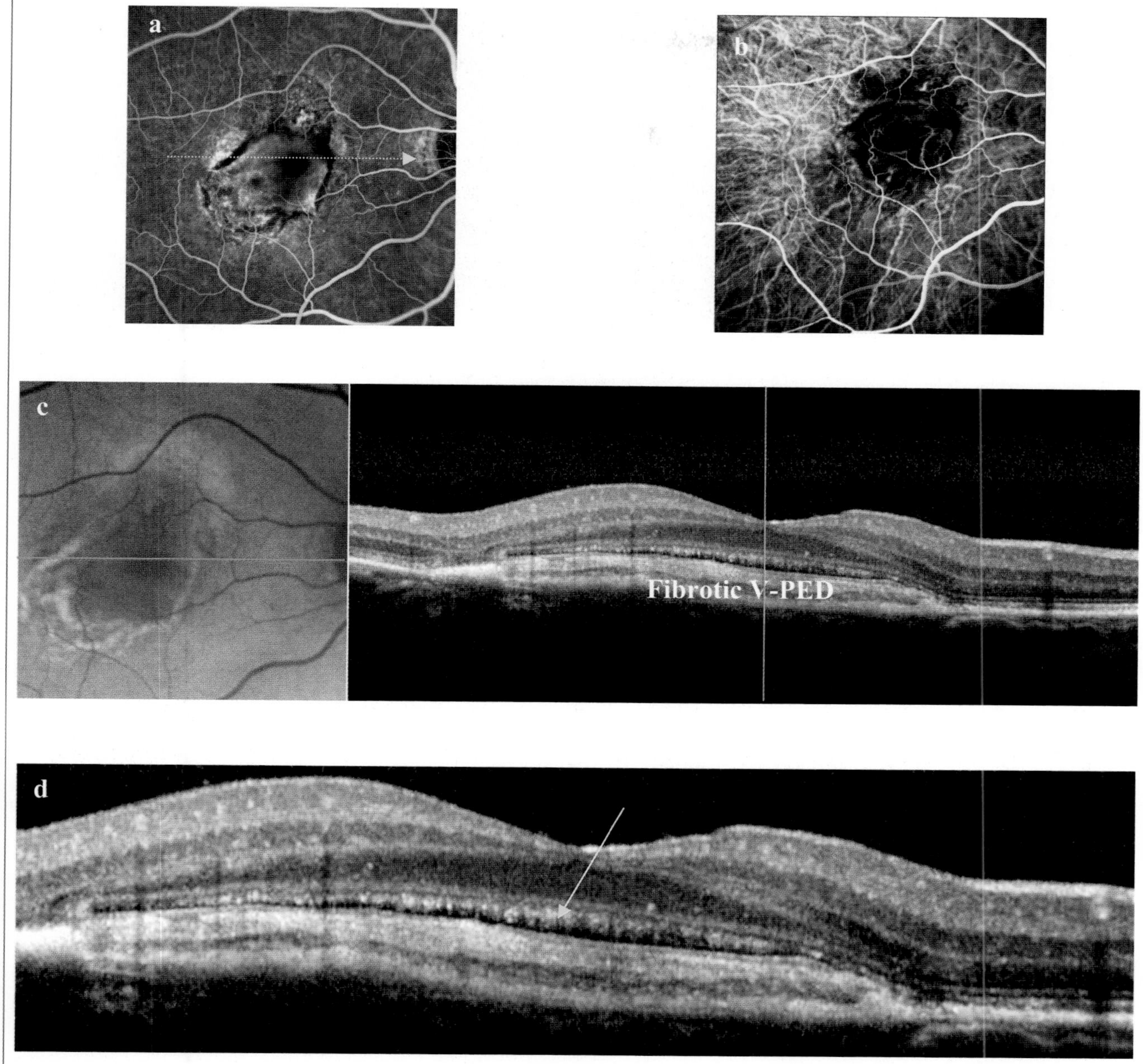

Figure 53: Chronic fluid accumulation anterior to the RPE persisting after treatment.

a and b): Fluorescein and ICG angiography: retracted and fibrotic classic CNV membrane.

c): *Spectralis horizontal section, associated with autofluorescence image.**
On SD-OCT, anterior to the residual organized and hyper-reflective PED, there is a limited but persistent layer of fluid. Many bright hyper-reflective spots (*arrow*) are visible at the outer limit of the retina and also a few disseminated in all of the layers.

d): Enlarged view: the IS/OS interface and external limiting membrane remain visible and continuous. The other nuclear layer, the plexiform layers and the foveal depression remain well organized. This is well correlated with the fair visual acuity (20/32).

RECURRENCE AND SRD

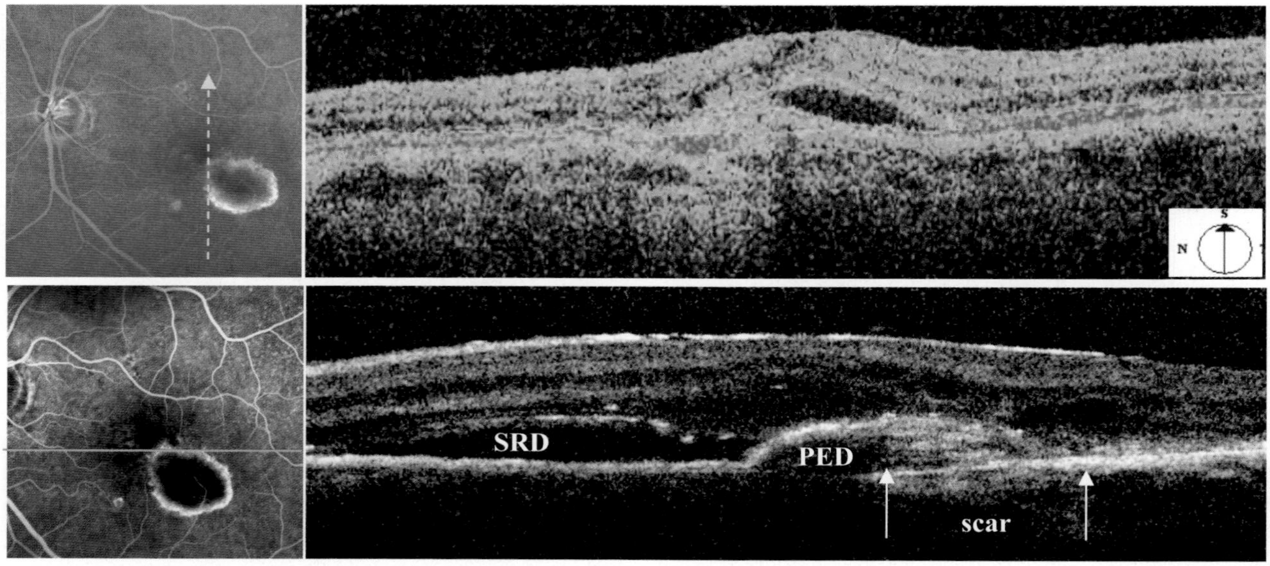

Figure 54: Recent fluid accumulation anterior to the RPE suggesting a juxtafoveal recurrence.

***Stratus** vertical section, associated with fluorescein angiography** *(minimal changes on the foveal edge of the scar).*
On TD-OCT, the scar is hyper-reflective. Note at the foveal edge of the scar, a minimal elevation of the RPE due to recurrence, combined with an adjacent SRD.

***Spectralis** horizontal section, associated with fluorescein angiography.**
SD-OCT shows a dense hyper-reflective scar with back-shadowing. The recurrence and the PED are adjacent to the scar, with an accentuation of the SRD. Note the bright hyper-reflective spots and the moderate intraretinal fluid accumulation.

RECURRENCE AND SRD

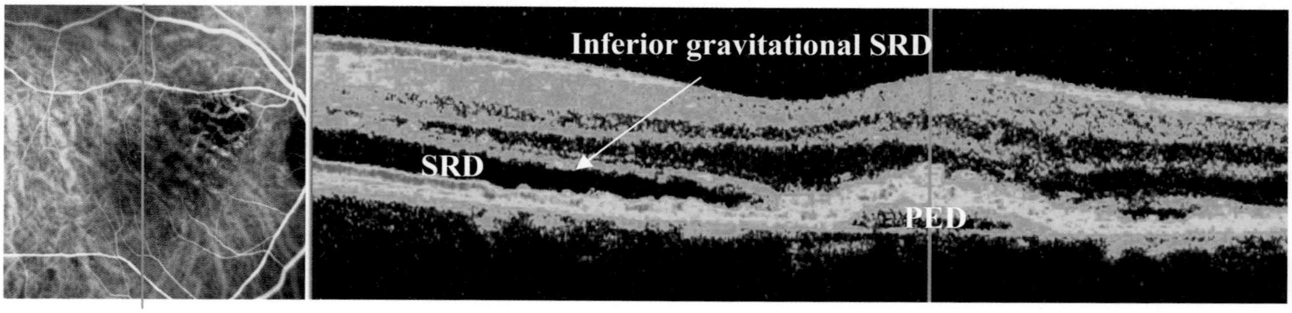

Figure 55: Fluid accumulation, anterior to the RPE and predominantly downward shifting.

***Spectralis** horizontal section, associated with ICG angiography** *(supero- nasal post-laser scar associated with an occult subfoveal recurrence with PED and shifting SRD).*

On SD-OCT, the inferior SRD is accentuated and visible in the inferior part of the vascularized PED.
Note several bright spots and intraretinal fluid but still good organization of the retinal layers. VA: 20/40.

SRD and RPE TEAR

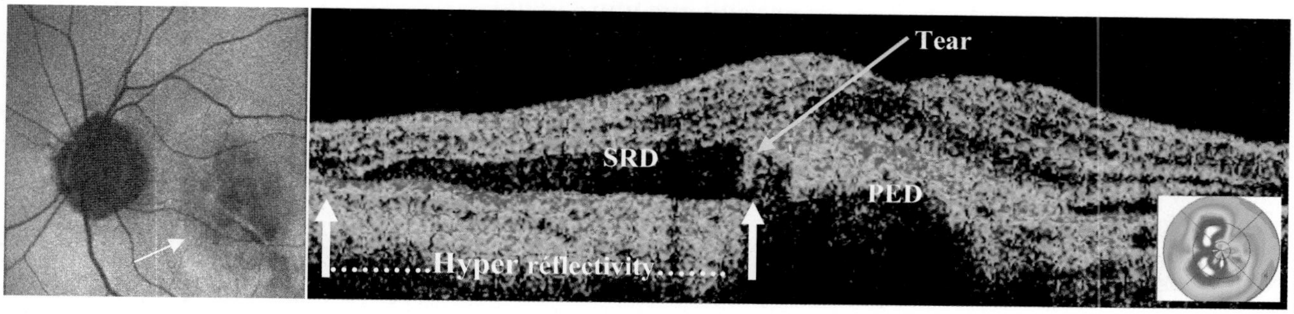

Figure 56: Fluid accumulation, anterior to the RPE, over a recent tear of the RPE.

a): **Autofluorescence:** Note the inferonasal RPE-tear and adjacent exudative reaction (*arrow*).

b): *Stratus horizontal section.**
On **TD-OCT**, extensive SRD over all of the choroidal zone exposed by the RPE tear and retraction.

Note the hyper-reflectivity in this zone, which extends far posteriorly towards the choroid.
In the superior half of the lesion, the PED persists with partial organization of the retracted fibrovascular tissue.

SRD and RETINAL HEMORRHAGE

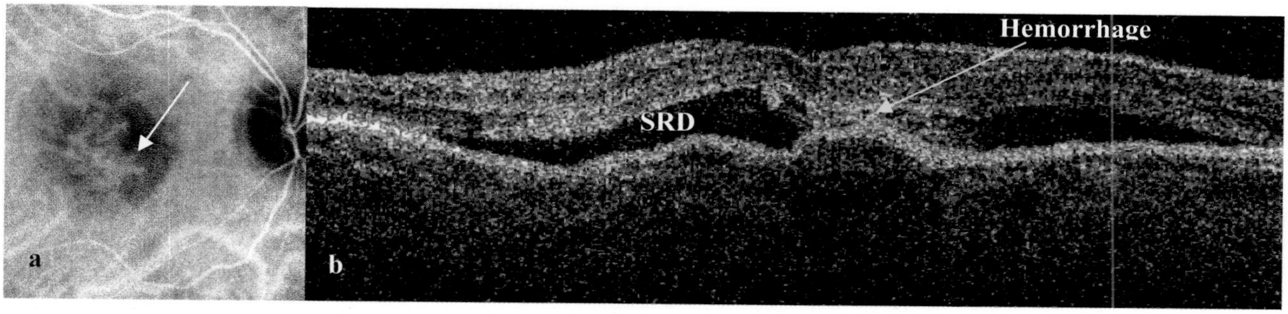

Figure 57: Fluid accumulation, anterior to the RPE, indicating an active phase of occult choroidal neovascularization with retinal hemorrhage.

a): **ICG angiography**: demonstration of the CNV network and hemorrhage (*arrow*).

b): *Stratus horizontal section.**
On **TD-OCT**, the SRD involves the entire surface of the vascularized PED and extends slightly beyond.

Note the zone of hyper-reflectivity corresponding to deep retinal hemorrhage, very close to the center.

3. Fluid Accumulation Anterior to the RPE

Cystoid Macular Edema

Cystoid macular edema, the second type of retinal alteration related to abnormal leakage, is accumulation of serous (or predominantly serous) fluid within the neurosensory retina. It may consist of:

- Diffuse intraretinal fluid, or
- Intraretinal cysts.

Simple intraretinal fluid **infiltration** is a common feature and is easy to measure, as it causes increased retinal thickness, which is particularly important in the central foveal or foveolar region.

This increased central retinal thickness (CRT) in the central 1000 µm of the fovea can be **measured automatically** and rapidly by OCT software. It can also be corrected manually to avoid well known sources of error (**Figure 58**).

All OCT systems are equipped with more or less similar complex **measuring devices**. With SD-OCT, retinal thickness measurements are displayed on numerical representations, false-color scales, and/or map representations (**Figure 60**).

Different images and/or measurements or graph **overlay processes** can be used to follow and analyze the response to treatment. This has been further improved by precise ***eye-tracking*** systems, allowing measurements to be automatically repeated in exactly the same place.

3D images can also be used to easily detect and study the different areas of the macula and to avoid overlooking a slightly eccentric or small lesion.

Intraretinal cystic spaces, suggesting the histological appearance of cystoid macular edema, may be observed at different stages of the disease:

- **Isolated** or **associated** with diffuse intraretinal fluid and/or SRD (**Figures 58-60**),
- **Small** or **large** and/or sometimes very extensive (**Figures 61-63**),
- **Single** or **multiple** (**Figure 64**).

Intraretinal cysts are usually situated in the central macula and the foveal avascular zone, where they often become confluent; they are always larger than more peripheral cysts (**Figures 65 and 66**).

These cystoid spaces can be tightly packed or scattered. They may be organized in one or two layers, with a predilection for the plexiform layers (**Figures 67-69**).

Intraretinal cystoid spaces almost always reflect marked exudation from choroidal neovascularization. They can resolve in response to treatment, often more rapidly than the SRD.

They can also be associated with more chronic, older lesions with marked fibrosis (**Figures 70-72**).

Later in the course, intraretinal cysts can be a sign of **irreversible degeneration** of the neurosensory retina and persist even after resolution of leakage. In these cases, the diagnosis is based on the hyper-reflective zone of fibrosis and the absence of SRD (as well as marked loss of visual acuity).

Intraretinal cysts and diffuse intraretinal fluid are therefore easy to recognize on OCT images and constitute a major sign to be detected and quantified in wet AMD.

These cystoid spaces are rarely isolated. Indirect signs of CNV proliferation are always present, either as a preretinal zone of hyper-reflectivity corresponding to classic CNV or as a vascularized PED, which is always associated with occult CNV.

SD-OCT more precisely visualizes and allows follow-up of associated signs such as bright hyper-reflective spots and intraretinal dense zones, which are probably signs of associated inflammatory response and worsening of the lesions.

DIFFUSE INTRARETINAL FLUID

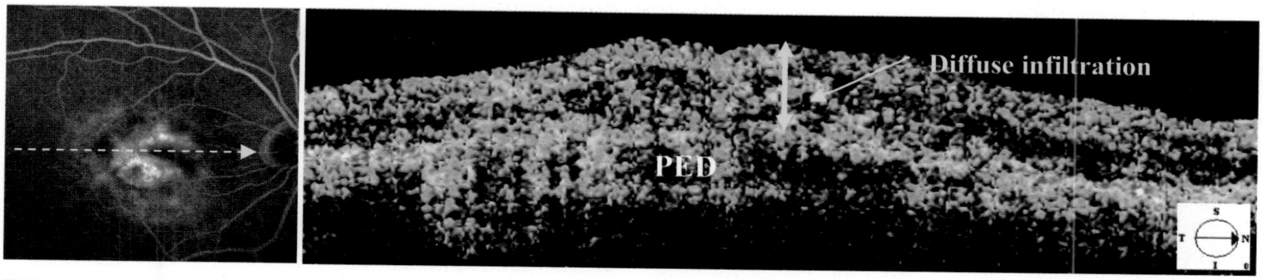

◘ Figure 58: Diffuse intraretinal fluid and thickening of the macular neurosensory retina.
***Stratus** horizontal section, associated with fluorescein angiography** (*leakage and edema*).
On **TD-OCT**, diffuse intraretinal fluid accumulation induces thickening with flattening of the foveal depression. Retinal layers are disorganized anterior to the RPE. The RPE band is poorly visible. Presence of an old PED.

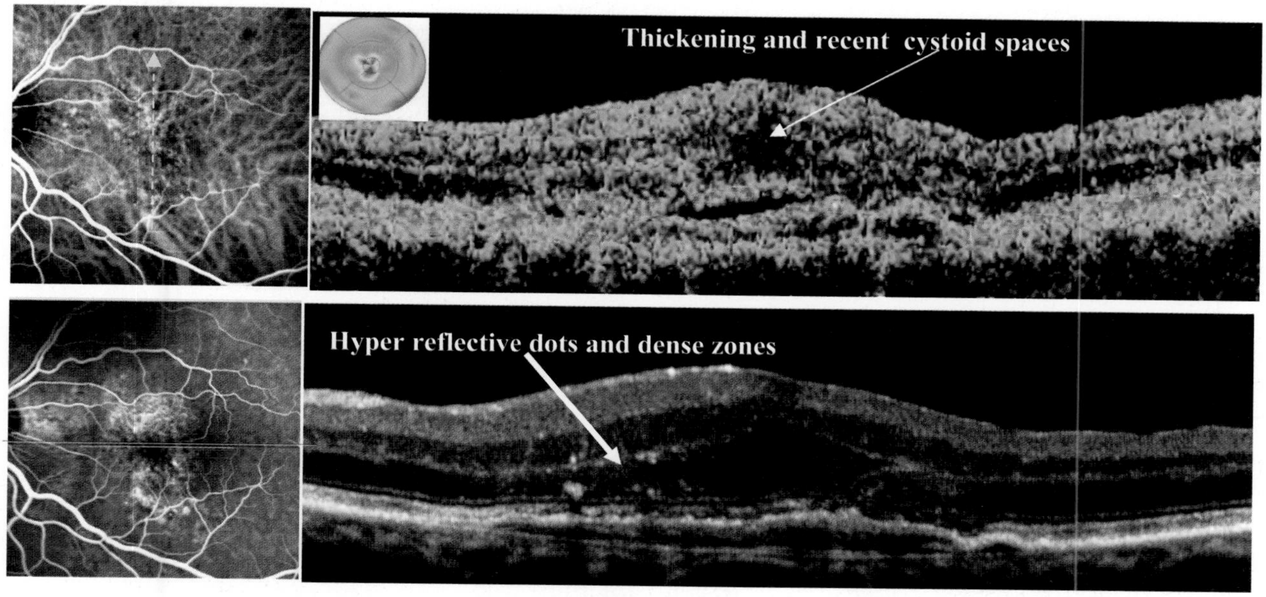

◘ Figure 59: Fluid accumulation anterior to the RPE: diffuse intraretinal fluid, thickening of the macular neurosensory retina and intraretinal cyst.
***Stratus** vertical section associated with ICG angiography demonstrating the occult CNV network.**
On TD-OCT, the retina is thickened with flattening of the foveal depression. Retinal layers are disorganized in the center and replaced by a poorly-delineated cystoid space.
***Spectralis** horizontal section associated with fluorescein angiography.**
The retinal structure is more precisely visualized on SD-OCT: alterations of the outer layers and bright hyper-reflective spots around the cystoid spaces in the outer nuclear layer. Note the dense zones anterior to the external limiting membrane.

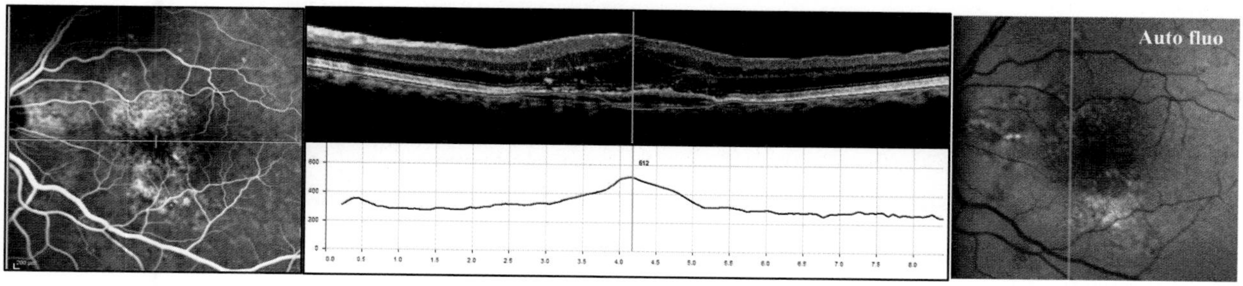

◘ Figure 60: Fluid accumulation anterior to the RPE. Graphic representation of retinal thickness measurements (between the 2 red lines) as far as Bruch's membrane.

CYSTOID SPACES

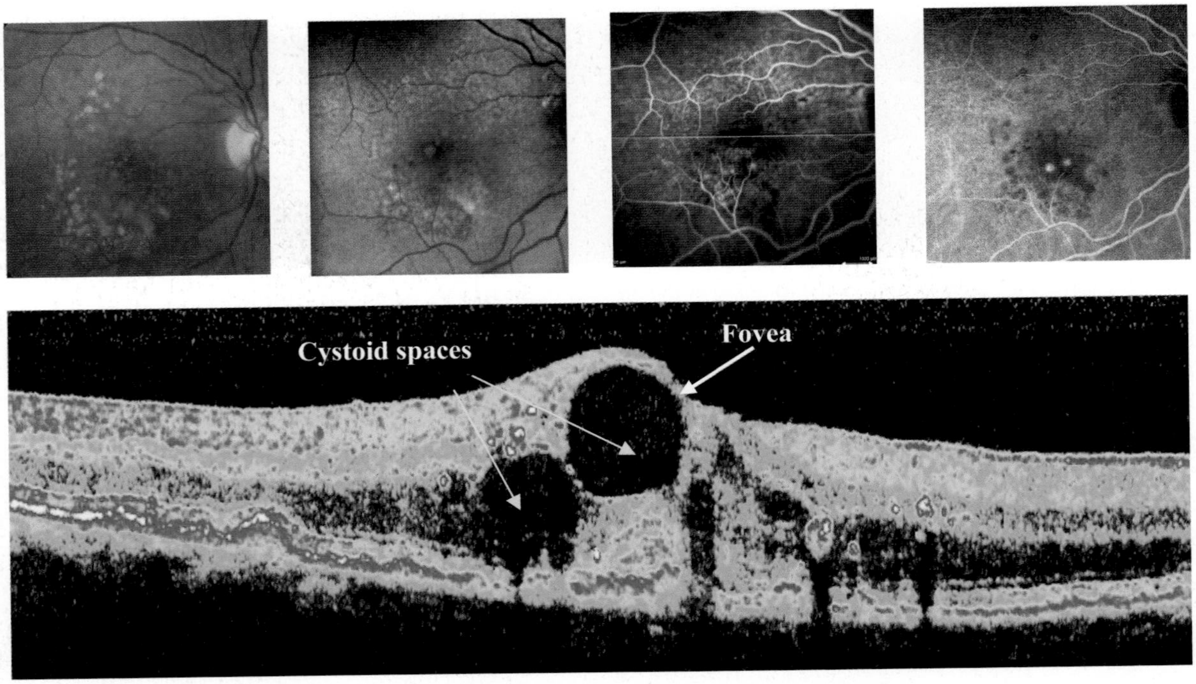

Figure 61: Fluid accumulation anterior to the RPE: two predominant cystoid spaces **in the central area.**
Spectralis * **horizontal section, associated with fluorescein angiography** *(juxtafoveal leakage).*
On SD-OCT, the retina is raised by a large, almost central well-delineated cyst. Note a second, deeper paracentral cyst.
VA: 20/100.

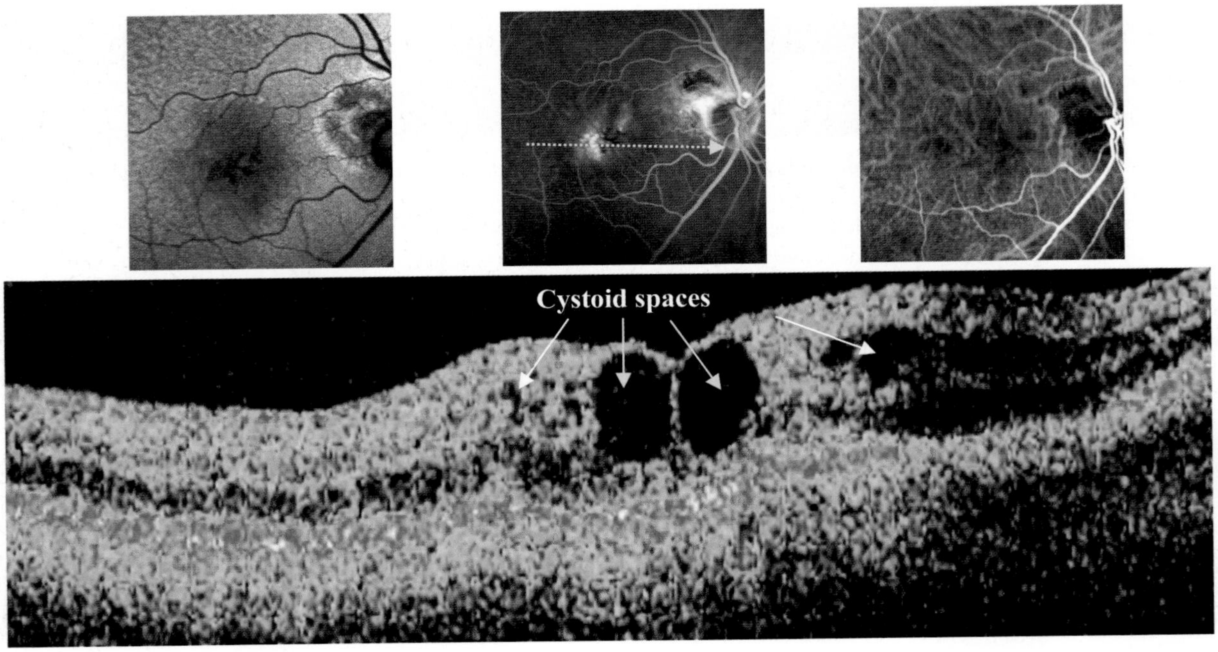

Figure 62: Fluid accumulation anterior to the RPE: two predominant cysts in the central area.
Stratus * **horizontal section shown with fluorescein angiography**: foveal leakage.
On TD-OCT, the retina shows thickening, the foveal depression is raised by two large and very well-delineated central cysts just underneath the inner limiting membrane. Note the presence of several adjacent cysts, much smaller and closely packed. VA: 20/50.

CYSTOID SPACES

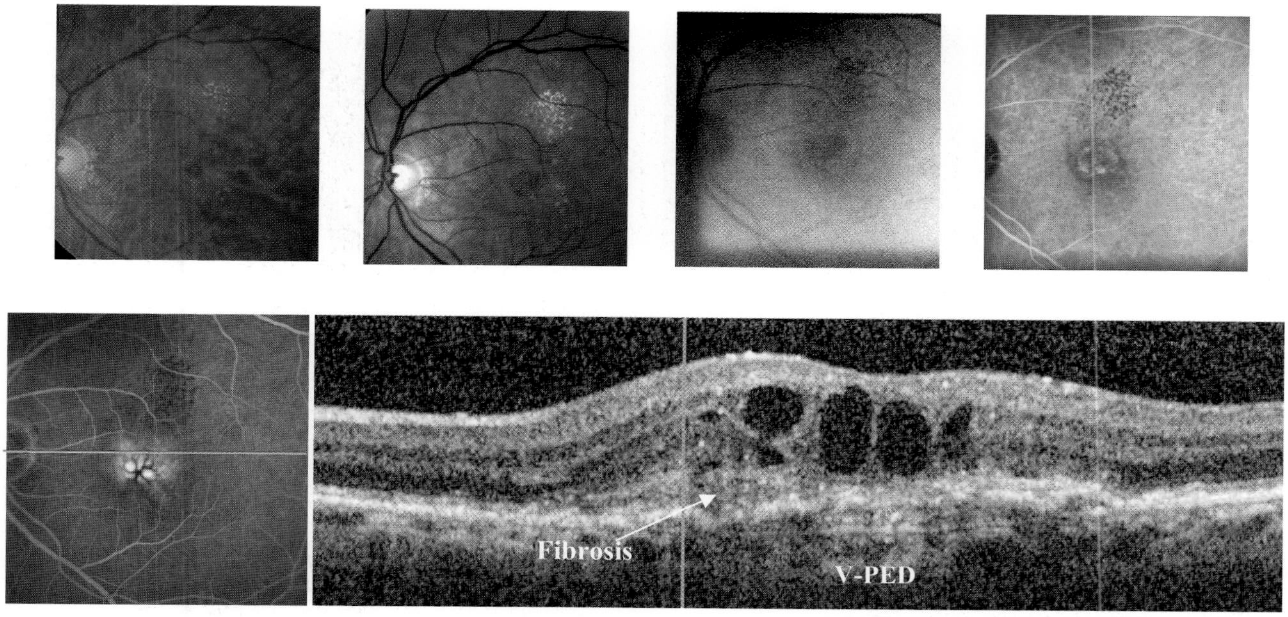

Figure 63: Fluid accumulation anterior to the RPE: old isolated cysts.
***Spectralis** horizontal section associated with fluorescein angiography** (*cystoid macular edema*).
On SD-OCT, the central retina is thickened by large, well-delineated cystoid spaces underneath the inner limiting membrane. Note the absence of SRD. Early signs of fibrosis anterior to the organized vascularized PED are suggestive of an old lesion. VA: 20/80.

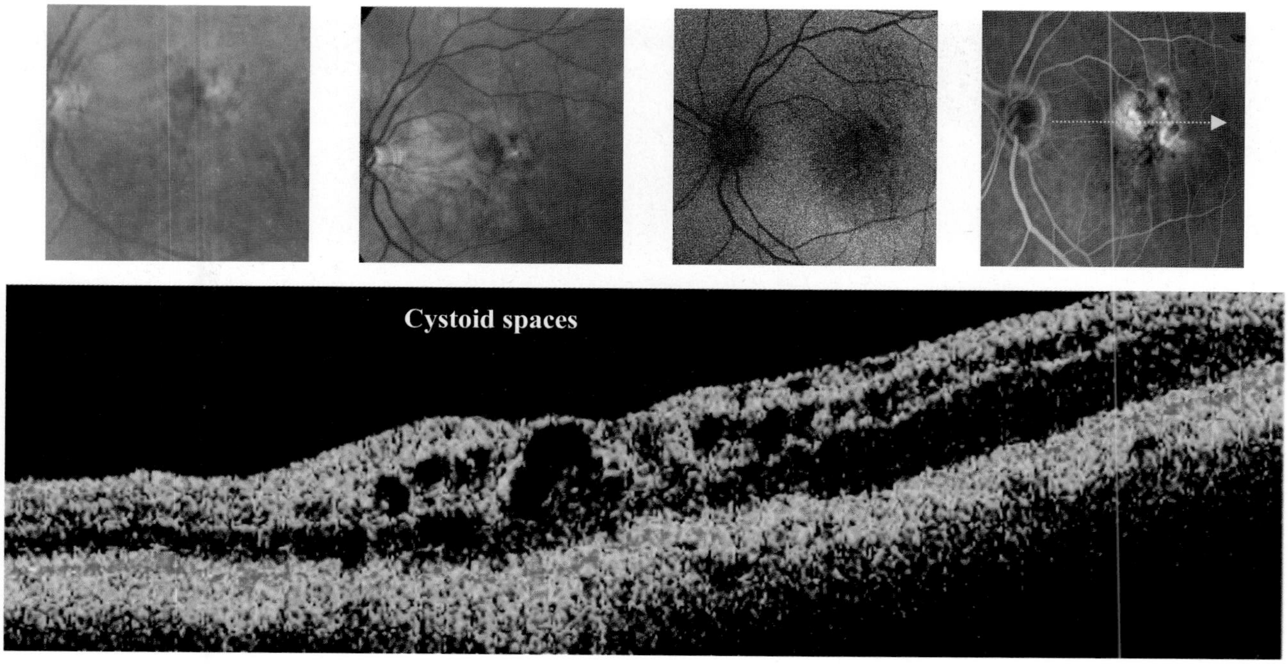

Figure 64: Fluid accumulation anterior to the RPE: large number of multiple cysts. VA: 20/63.
***Stratus** horizontal section associated with fluorescein angiography** *(advanced chorioretinal anastomosis)*.
On TD-OCT, the central retina is thickened by many well-delineated cysts, confluent in the center and associated with diffuse intraretinal fluid accumulation (anterior to a vascularized PED, which is flat on this section).

CYSTOID SPACES

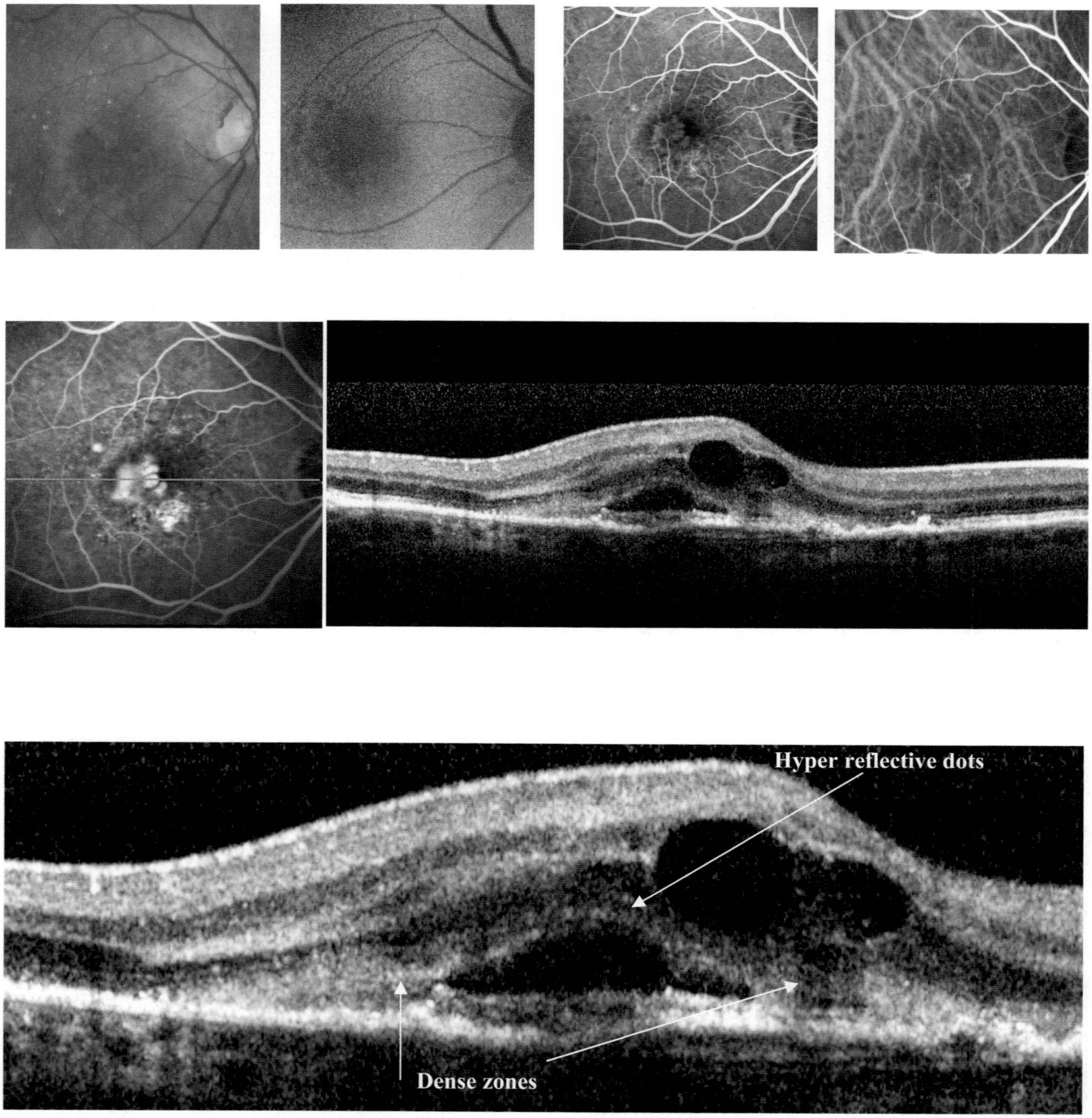

Figure 65: Fluid accumulation anterior to the RPE: large central cysts.

Spectralis ***horizontal section associated with fluorescein angiography** (*mixed CNV*).

On SD-OCT, the enlarged view shows the various tissue changes.

Note the scattered bright hyper-reflective spots predominantly in outer layers and around the cysts. Zones of intraretinal densification are visible at the level of the outer nuclear layer and the external limiting membrane. These layers remain visible in all regions, while the IS/OS interface is severely altered. VA: 20/50.

CYSTOID SPACES

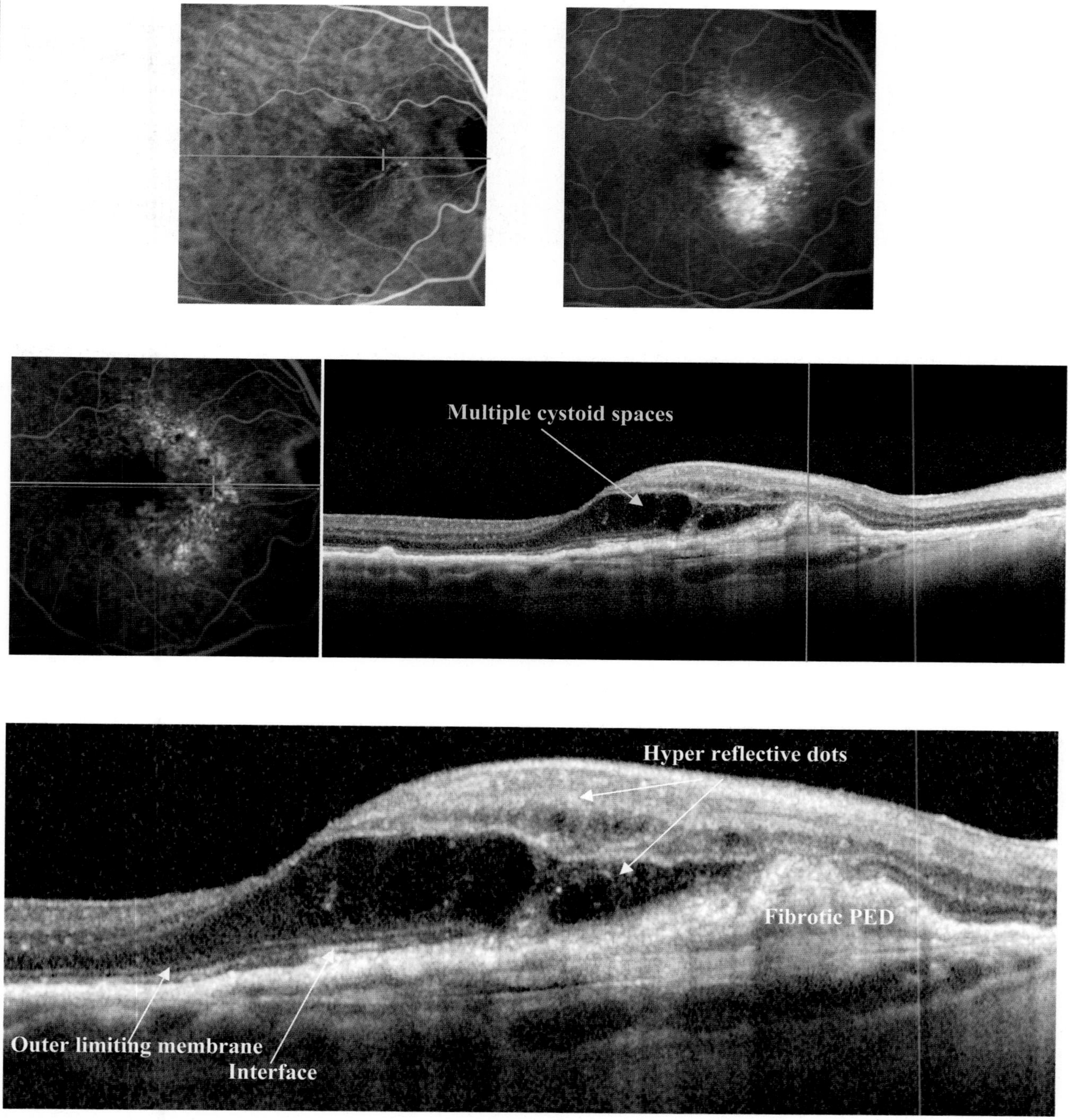

Figure 66 Fluid accumulation anterior to the RPE: large central cysts.

***Spectralis** horizontal section associated with angiography** *(advanced occult CNV).*

On SD-OCT, the enlarged view shows the limits of the cysts delineated by bright hyper-reflective spots, predominantly in the outer layers. Note that the outer nuclear layer, external limiting membrane, and IS/OS interface remain visible, except over the area of occult CNV (indicated by the calliper on the green line). The PED is fibrotic and hyper-reflective. VA: 20/50.

MULTIPLE CYSTS IN SEVERAL LAYERS

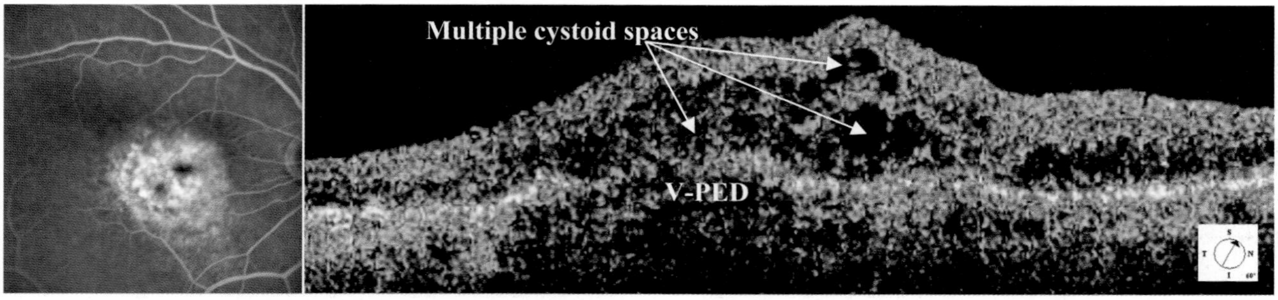

Figure 67: Fluid accumulation anterior to the RPE: multiple central cysts in several layers.
***Stratus** horizontal section associated with angiography** (*occult CNV and advanced multiple anastomosis*).
On TD-OCT, the retina is considerably thickened and infiltrated with multiple large cysts, often confluent and sometimes involving several layers.
Note the old, partially-organized, vascularized PED with a break or disruption of the RPE band.

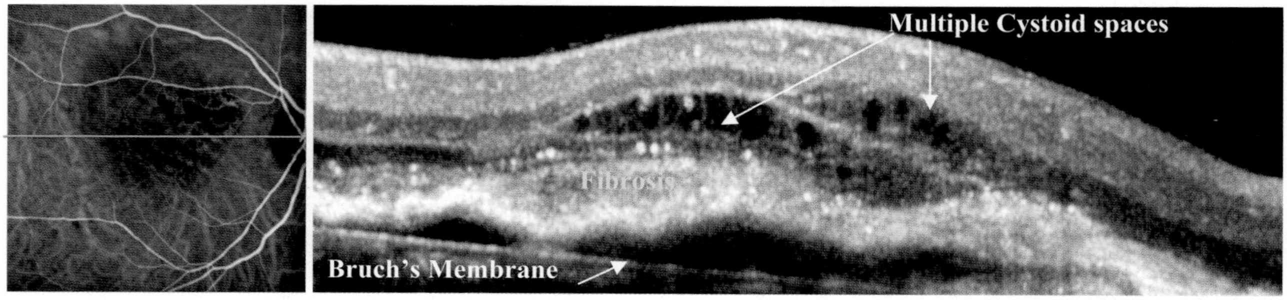

Figure 68: Fluid accumulation anterior to the RPE: multiple central cysts in several layers.
***Spectralis** horizontal section associated with ICG angiography** *(dark persistent PED but poorly perfused, barely visible network).*
On SD-OCT, persistence of multiple, small cysts in the outer layers, despite treatment. These cysts are associated with the persistence of many bright spots and the development of dense, hyper-reflective material anterior to the RPE. The wavy, multilobed, vascularized PED is still visible but is fairly flat.

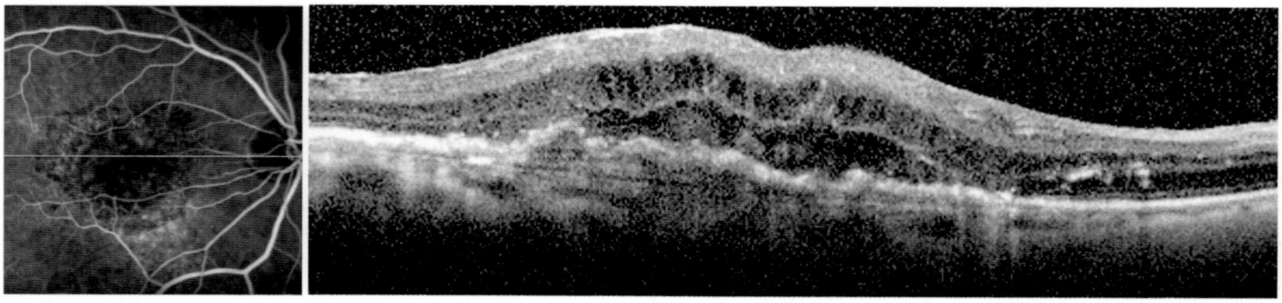

Figure 69: Fluid accumulation anterior to the RPE: large number of small cysts.
***Spectralis** horizontal section associated with fluorescein angiography** *(partial regression of CNV)*.
On SD-OCT, persistence of marked intraretinal fluid accumulation with a large number of cysts in the outer plexiform layer. The outer nuclear layer is modified with a number of bright hyper-reflective spots and partial densification, which persists even after many treatment sessions.
These alterations and cysts are situated anterior to a persistent PED, which has become partially organized despite treatment.
No improvement of visual acuity. VA: 20/800.

RESIDUAL CYSTS AFTER TREATMENT

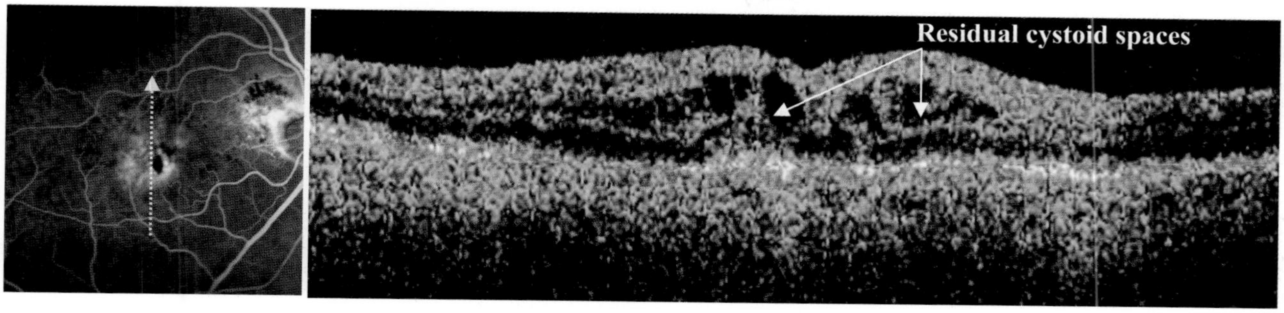

Figure 70: Fluid accumulation anterior to the RPE: large number of small cysts.
***Stratus** vertical section associated with fluorescein angiography** *(partial regression of CNV)*. VA: 20/50.
On TD-OCT, the intraretinal cysts, particularly marked in this case of chorioretinal anastomosis, have only partially regressed and persist with diffuse intraretinal fluid and moderately increased retinal thickness.

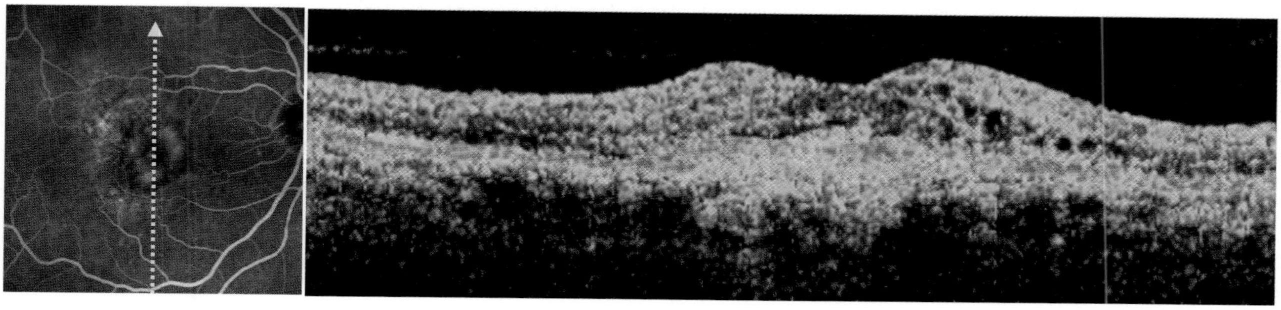

Figure 71: Fluid accumulation anterior to the RPE: multiple small persistent cysts.
***Stratus** vertical section associated with fluorescein angiography** *(partial regression of CNV)*. VA: 20/63.
On TD-OCT, the foveal depression is normalized, suggestive of a good visual prognosis. A moderate thickening of the retina persists with a series of small cysts in the outer plexiform layer, especially in the superior macular region but sparing the center.
Progressive healing of the neovascular membrane with moderate fibrosis.

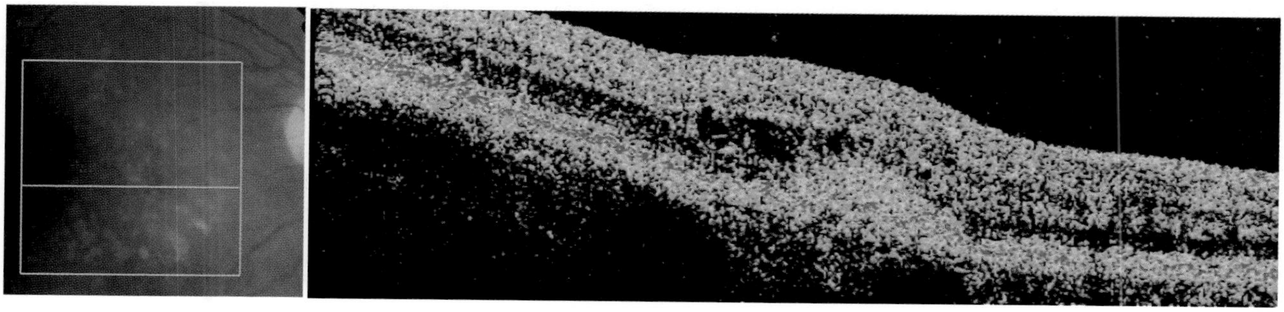

Figure 72: Fluid accumulation anterior to the RPE: persistence of several cysts in front of a moderate fibrosis.
***Topcon** horizontal section associated with a color photograph.** Morphological and functional stabilization.
On SD-OCT, regression of exudative signs is accompanied by reapplication of the retina, which remains moderately thickened. Several cysts are still visible adjacent to the small fibrotic scar. VA: 20/160.

Study on the Characteristics of Intraretinal Cysts in AMD

A consecutive series of 150 patients with wet AMD was analyzed in an independent and blinded study to compare fluorescein angiography, SLO-ICG angiography, and OCT.

This study was designed to objectively determine the value of these various imaging modalities (fluorescein angiography, SLO-ICG angiography, and OCT), alone or in combination, for diagnosis, and to guide treatment.

In this context, OCT examinations demonstrated the presence of intraretinal cysts in almost one half of patients (62 patients, 41%).

In this group of 62 patients, cysts were almost always multiple (97%) and were isolated or central in only 2 patients (3%).

Cysts were associated with the presence of diffuse intraretinal fluid with a significant increase of retinal thickness (more than 50 µm or more than 25%) in 36 patients (58%).

The **presence of subretinal fluid** with serous retinal detachment (SRD) was detected in more than one-third of patients (24 patients, 39%).

The **dimensions** of intraretinal cysts varied according to the stage and history of the lesions.

- Small cysts in 70% of cases,
- Large or confluent cysts in 30% of cases.

The **extent** of the cysts also varied according to the history of the lesions:

- Visible in only one layer in 42% of cases,
- Visible in two layers in 58% of cases.

In longstanding, advanced forms associated with varying degrees of **fibrosis**, cysts remained visible in 20 patients (30%), which corresponded to irreversible degenerative lesions with severe loss of visual acuity.

Cysts were usually accompanied by probable **inflammatory response** (bright hyper-reflective spots and dense zones) that showed a similar response to treatment (regression or recurrence).

These reactive signs were accompanied by **disorganization** of the retinal layers.

Bright hyper-reflective spots were clearly visible in most cases (70%).

During treatment, after 3 intravitreous injections of anti-VEGF, cysts were still present in 22 of the 62 patients (35%).

Resolution of cysts appeared to be delayed compared to functional improvement.

Conclusion

The course of intraretinal cysts and intraretinal fluid may follow that of the other signs of AMD, or may be delayed, or they may persist despite resolution of other signs.

The most difficult problem is to distinguish a *residual lesion* that is likely to resolve from persistent cysts reflecting irreversible alteration of the retina.

Other functional studies and imaging modalities are particularly valuable in this setting.

IV. Anterior to the RPE Band: Bright Hyper-reflective Spots and Dense Zones

The combined presence of these signs (bright hyper-reflective spots and intraretinal dense zones) is detected only rarely on TD-OCT.

They are clearly visible and more easily analyzed on Spectral-Domain OCT, especially with the *Spectralis**.

- The presence and integrity of the **external limiting membrane** and **IS/OS interface** must be confirmed.

These relatively dense lines can be altered, disrupted, or on the contrary, thickened over AMD lesions (**Figure 73**).

The external limiting membrane and IS/OS interface constitute landmarks to evaluate the inner and outer segments, which corresponds to hypo-reflective bands situated between these two lines.

- Modifications of the IS/OS interface are particularly marked over active CNV, either classic or occult.

These changes usually resolve in response to treatment, especially when treatment is started early in the course of the disease (**Figures 74 and 75**).

These signs therefore have a prognostic value and should be analyzed and compared on follow-up examinations, in the same way as intraretinal fluid and cysts.

Bright Hyper-reflective Spots

Bright hyper-reflective spots often appear to accumulate on the inner and outer limits of the SRF or cysts (**Figure 76**).

They can also be more disseminated, involving even the innermost layers.

They usually resolve gradually in response to treatment (**Figures 77 and 78**) and can therefore constitute markers of neovascular lesion activity.

Hyper-reflective Material

This relatively dense material probably reflects an inflammatory reaction. It appears to accumulate in the space situated between the external limiting membrane and the IS/OS interface. It also appears to be an important marker related to deterioration of the lesions (**Figure 79**).

Response to Treatment

In most cases, the efficacy of treatment is largely evaluated in terms of regression of intraretinal fluid and reattachment of the retina.

In parallel, bright hyper-reflective spots and dense material appear to be reliable markers of the activity of the lesions. Their resolution usually indicates a good response to treatment (**Figures 79 and 80**). In contrast, these signs persist and deteriorate in the case of progressive fibrosis (**Figure 81**).

In a series of 30 patients with active occult CNV initially examined by SD-OCT and then reassessed monthly, all patients presented bright hyper-reflective spots and major alterations of the outer nuclear layer and IS/OS interface.

After 3 IVT sessions, bright hyper-reflective spots resolved in parallel with improvement of VA in 20 patients (66%).

In another 8 patients, bright hyper-reflective spots decreased but in the context of progressive fibrosis with loss of visual acuity, and 2 patients had persistent cystoid degeneration.

These alterations of the external limiting membrane, IS/OS interface, and RPE, and the presence and course of bright hyper-reflective spots and dense zones in the outer nuclear layer can provide useful information to evaluate the presence and degree of photoreceptor damage.

EXTERNAL LIMITING MEMBRANE, IS/OS INTERFACE, RPE

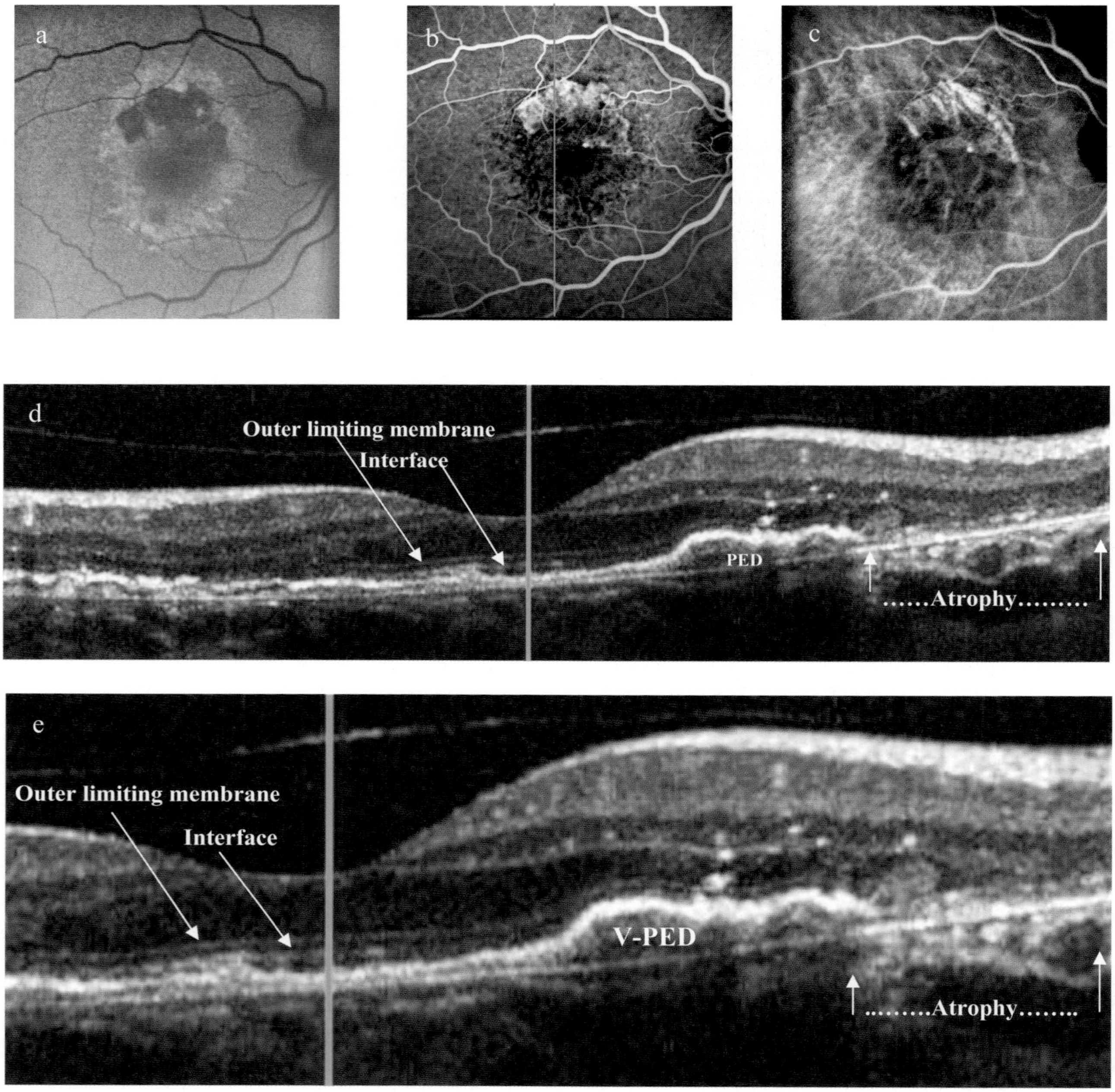

Figure 73: External limiting membrane and IS/OS interface.

a, b, and c): Autofluorescence, fluorescein angiography, and ICG angiography: complex lesion with occult CNV and atrophic areas in the superior part of the macula.

d): *Spectralis SD-OCT horizontal section.**

In the inferior macular region: flat PED; Bruch's membrane is visible, distinct from the irregular and thickened RPE, the IS/OS interface is intermittent, and the external limiting membrane is poorly visible.

In the central foveal zone, the three bands are clearly visible and only slightly altered: visual acuity is maintained at 20/32.

e): Enlarged view: in the superior macular region, over the vascularized PED: the external limiting membrane and IS/OS interface are no longer visible and numerous *bright hyper-reflective spots* can be seen.

In the superior atrophic zone, the RPE, IS/OS interface, external limiting membrane, and even the outer nuclear layer have disappeared.

EXTERNAL LIMITING MEMBRANE, IS/OS INTERFACE, RPE

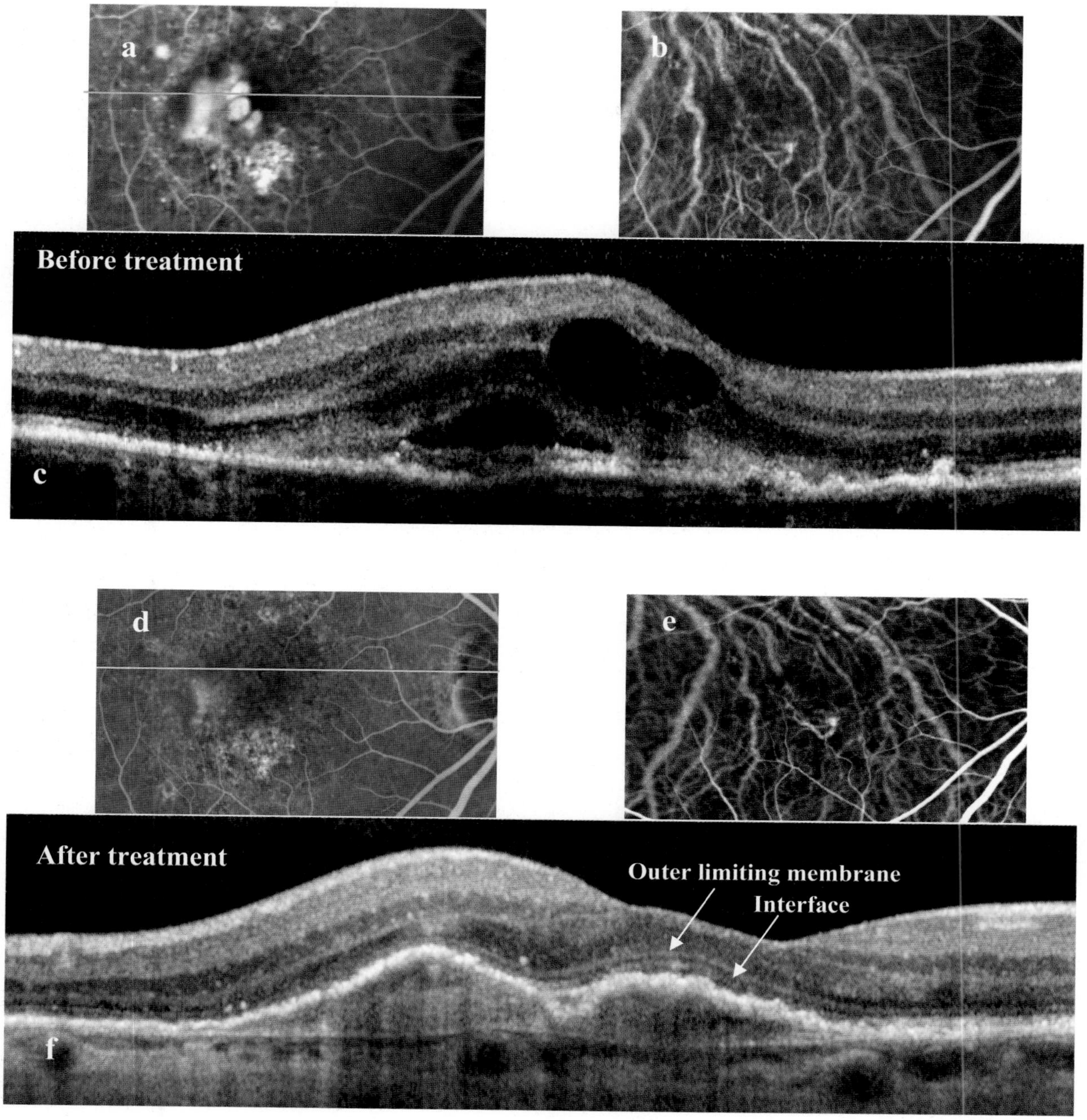

Figure 74: External limiting membrane and IS/OS interface.
a, b, and c): Before treatment:
***Spectralis** horizontal section correlated with fluorescein angiography and ICG angiography** *(mixed lesion with occult and classic CNV and marked cystoid spaces).*
SD-OCT: in the foveal zone, very large cysts with major changes of the three bands and outer nuclear layer invaded by a dense zone and bright hyper-reflective spots. VA: 20/50.
d, e, and f): After treatment:
***Spectralis** horizontal section**: reattachment and decreased thickness of the retina and almost normal appearance of the external limiting membrane, IS/OS interface, and outer nuclear layer. VA: 20/32.

EXTERNAL LIMITING MEMBRANE, IS/OS INTERFACE, RPE

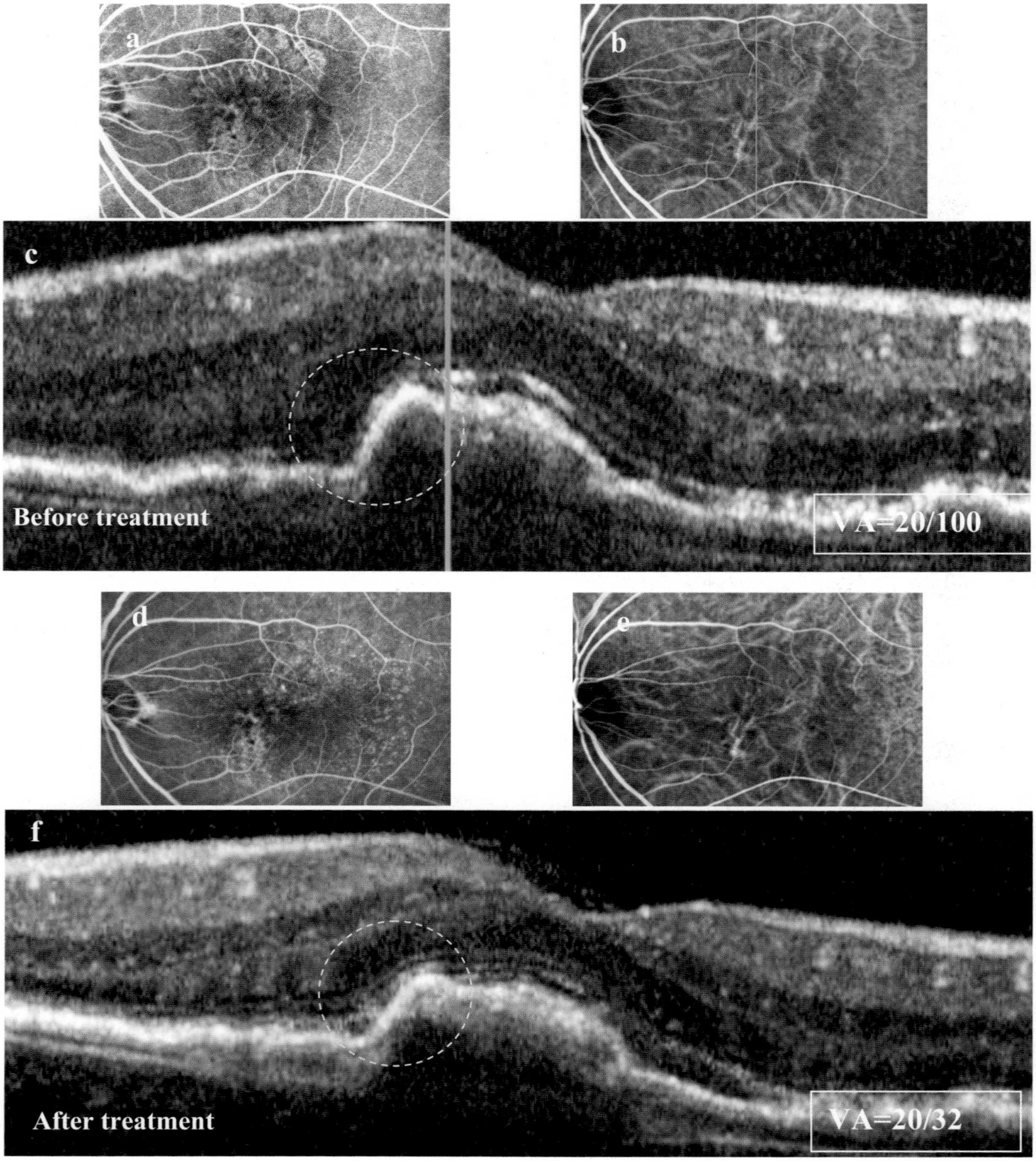

Figure 75: External limiting membrane and IS/OS interface.

a, b, and c): Before treatment. VA: 20/100.
***Spectralis** horizontal sections**: occult CNV and vascularized PED.
SD-OCT: in the foveal zone, irregularities and alterations of the three bands and disruption of the IS/OS interface (*circle*).
d, e, and f): After treatment, VA: 20/32.
After an injection of anti-VEGF, decreased thickness and almost normal appearance of the external limiting membrane, IS/OS interface, and outer nuclear layer (*circle*).

EXTERNAL LIMITING MEMBRANE, IS/OS INTERFACE, RPE

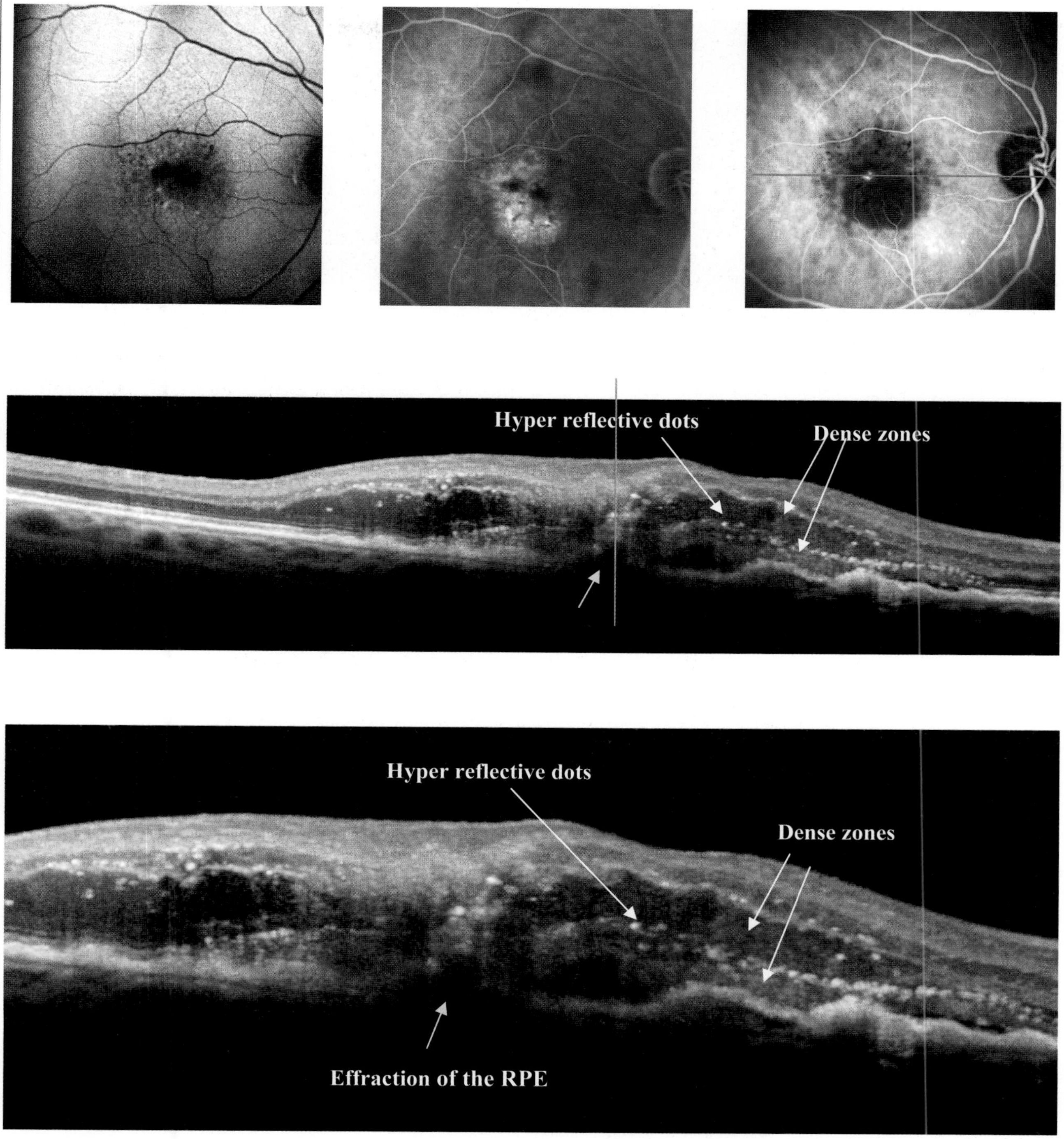

Figure 76: Hyper-reflective spots and dense zones.

Autofluorescence, fluorescein angiography, and ICG angiography: vascularized PED and probable chorioretinal anastomosis.
***Spectralis** horizontal section:**
SD-OCT: retina detached and thickened by numerous cysts in the foveal zone with numerous bright hyper-reflective spots highlighting the limits of the cysts, the IS/OS interface, and external limiting membrane (which are poorly visible). Large dense zone in the outer nuclear layer.
Note the break of the RPE at the site of the anastomosis (*yellow arrow*). VA: 20/80.

BRIGHT HYPER-REFLECTIVE SPOTS AND DENSE ZONES

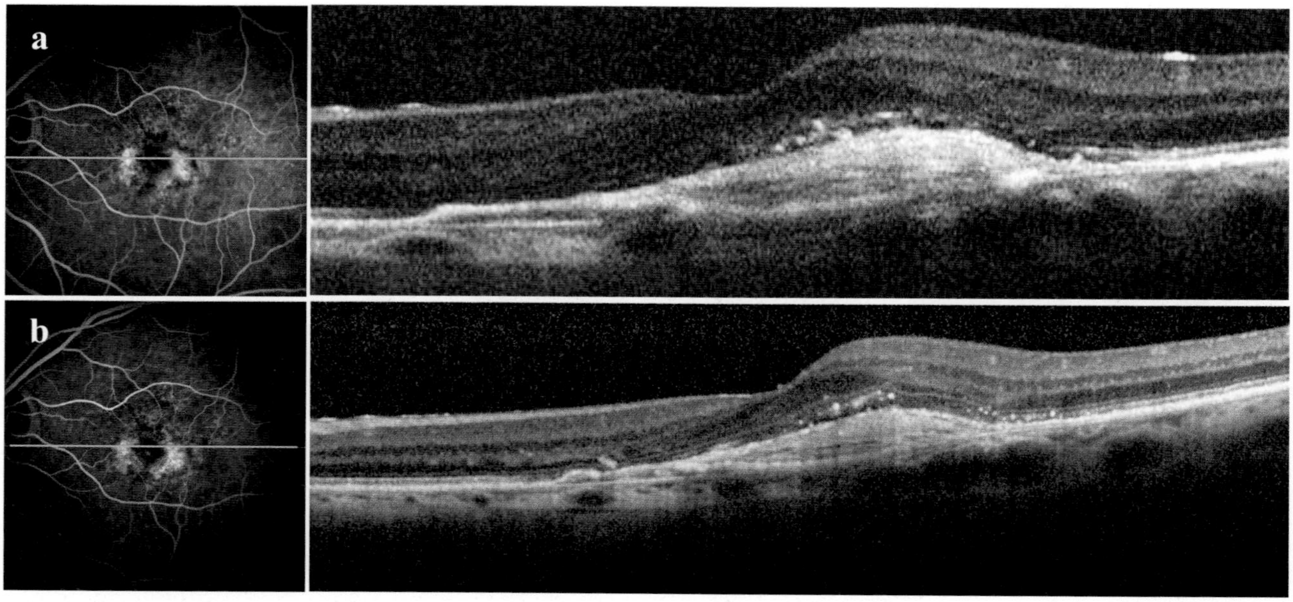

Figure 77: Bright hyper-reflective spots and dense zones.
***Spectralis** horizontal sections correlated with fluorescein angiography and ICG angiography** *(occult CNV during treatment).*
SD-OCT: **a):** Before treatment, in the foveal zone, numerous bright hyper-reflective spots masking the IS/OS interface and external limiting membrane. These are located anterior to the vascularized PED, which is in the process of re-organizing. The outer nuclear layer is poorly visible. VA: 20/80.
b): After treatment, re-attachment and decreased thickness of the retina; reduction of bright hyper-reflective spots and restoration of the external limiting membrane and IS/OS interface. The outer nuclear layer is almost normal. VA: 20/40.

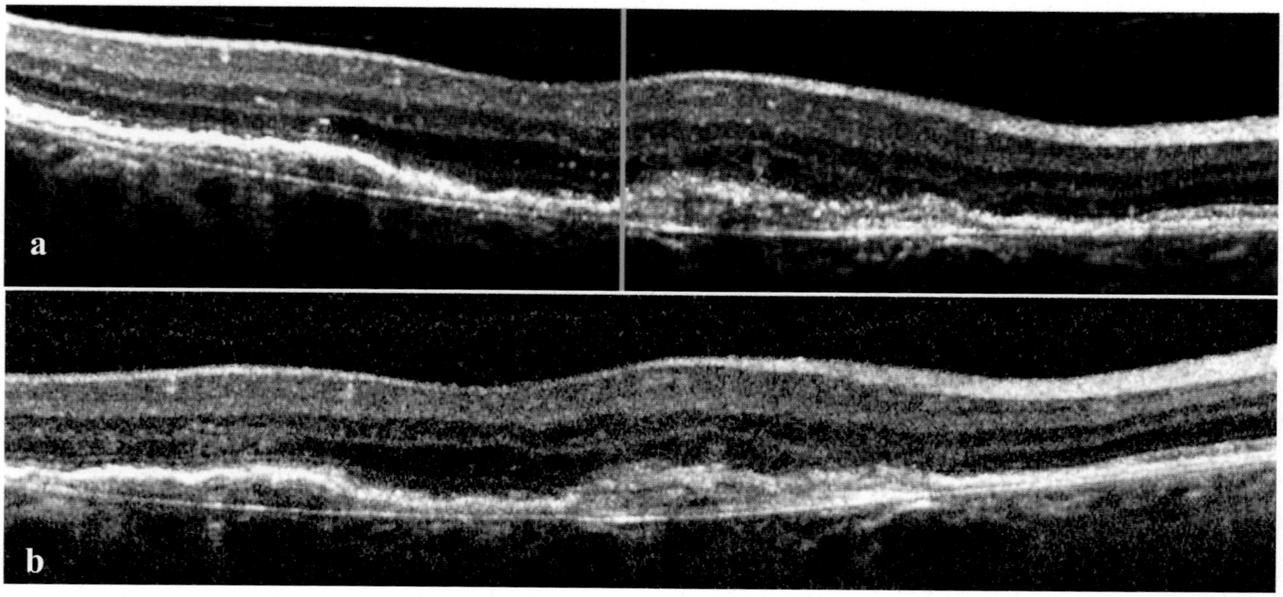

Figure 78: Bright hyper-reflective spots and dense zones.
***Spectralis** horizontal sections**: occult CNV with slightly raised but very extensive PED during anti-VEGF therapy.
SD-OCT: a): at the beginning of treatment, moderate diffuse intraretinal fluid with accumulation of bright hyper-reflective spots at the limits of this cystic space contiguous with the raised RPE. VA = 20/63.
b): After 3 IVT sessions, relative reduction of retinal thickness and the number of bright hyper-reflective spots. VA = 20/32.

BRIGHT HYPER-REFLECTIVE SPOTS AND DENSE ZONES

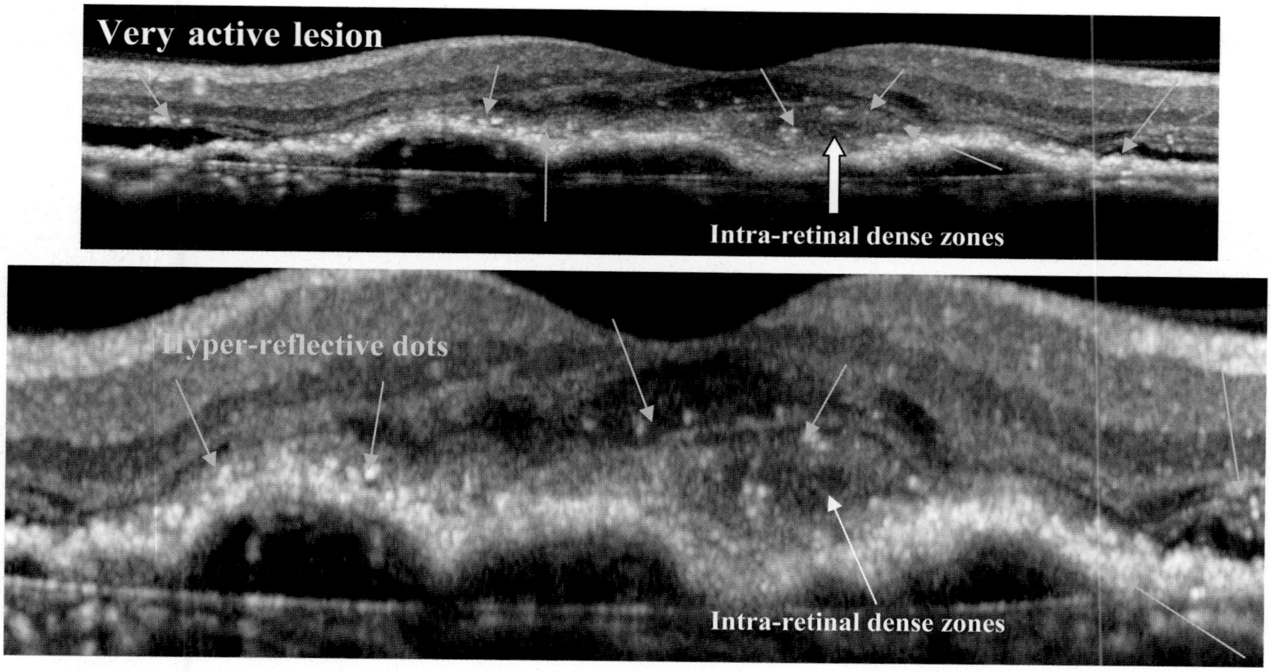

Figure 79: Bright hyper-reflective spots and dense zones.
Spectralis* **horizontal section**: advanced, extensive, irregular, wavy vascularized PED.
SD-OCT: thickened retina, raised by the vascularized PED. Numerous bright hyper-reflective spots, (yellow arrows), disseminated in the retinal tissue, predominantly in the outer layers, highlighting the limits of the IS/OS interface and external limiting membrane (which are poorly visualized).
Large zone of moderately reflective increased intraretinal density (white arrow) in the outer nuclear layer contiguous to the RPE. VA: 20/80.

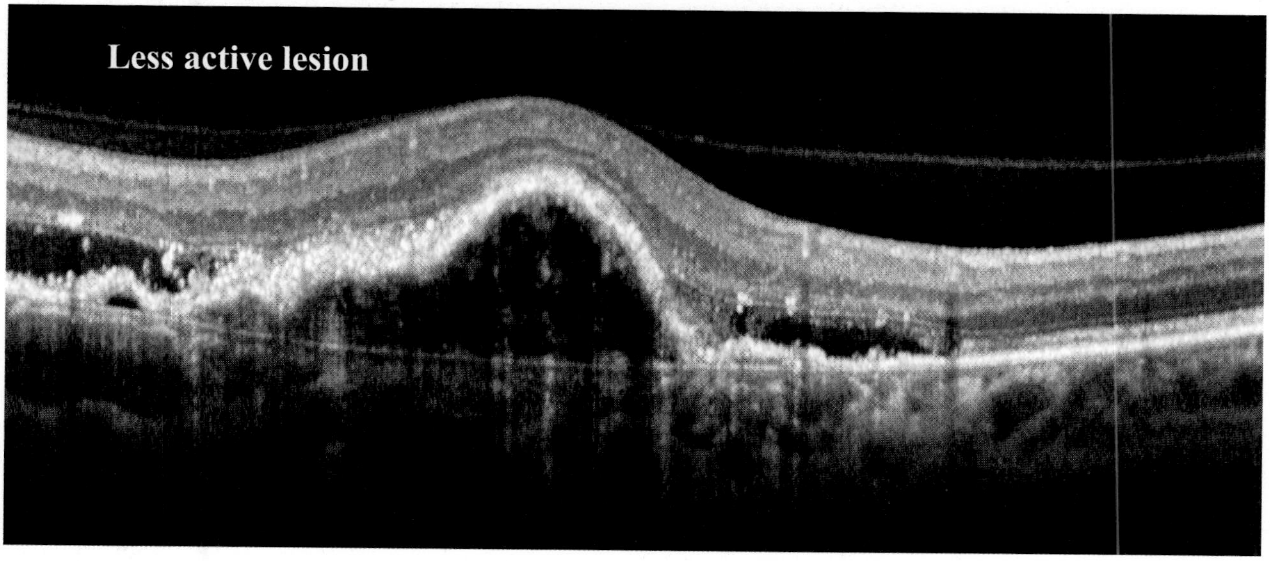

Figure 80: Bright hyper-reflective spots and dense zones.
Spectralis* **horizontal section**: advanced vascularized PED during anti-VEGF therapy.
SD-OCT: Progressive re-attachment of the retina which has resumed an almost normal configuration.
A large number of bright hyper-reflective spots persist, predominantly in the outer layers, highlighting the limits of the persistent SRD. The IS/OS interface and external limiting membrane are now visible and almost continuous. The outer nuclear layer remains poorly visible over the vascularized PED. VA: 20/40.

BRIGHT HYPER-REFLECTIVE SPOTS AND DENSE ZONES

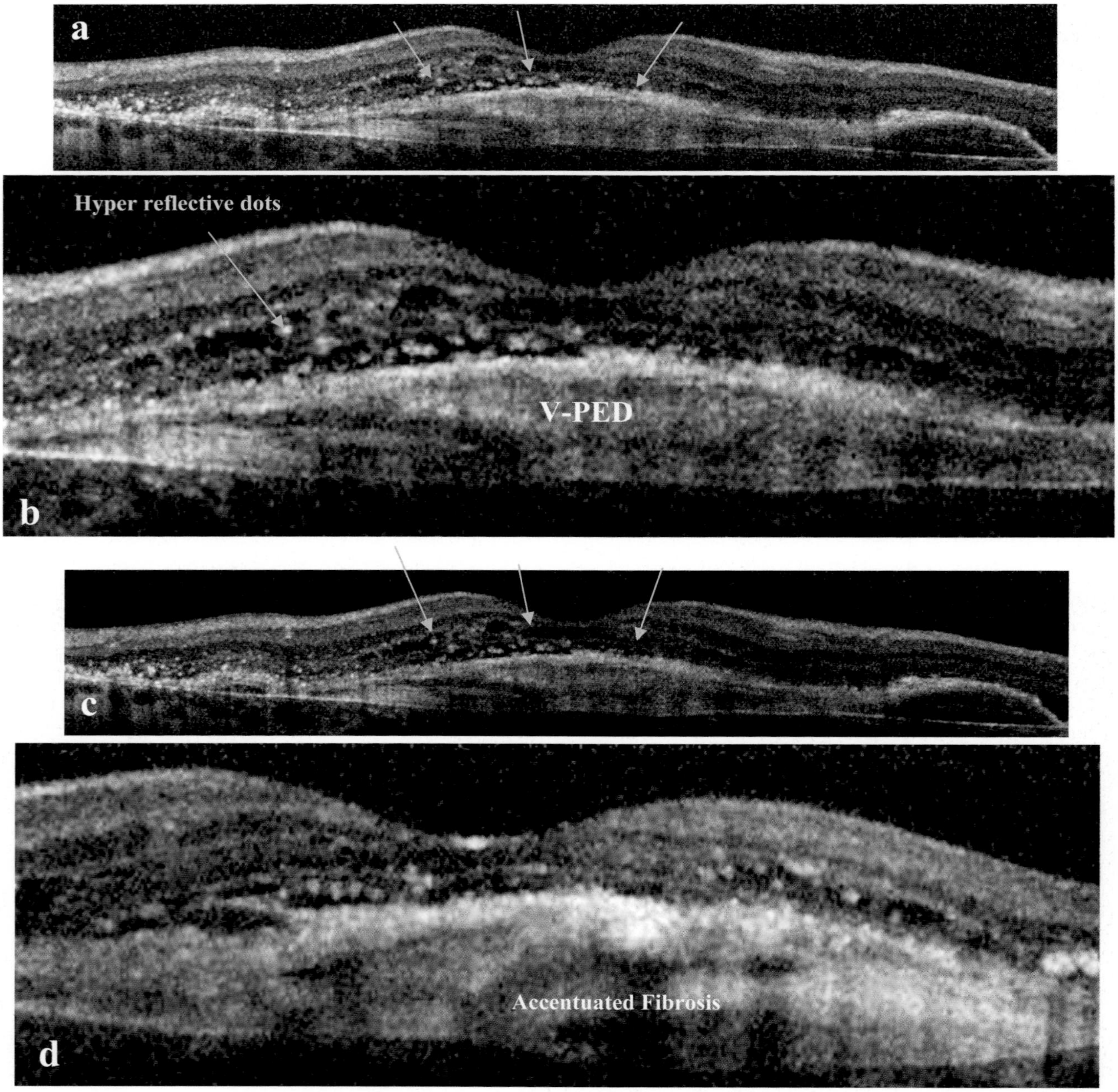

Figure 81: Bright hyper-reflective spots and dense zones: progression to fibrosis.

a and b): Before treatment: persistent vascularized PED progressing to fibrosis despite anti-VEGF therapy.

***Spectralis** SD-OCT horizontal sections**: advanced lesion with a very active appearance consisting of intraretinal fluid and numerous bright hyper-reflective spots. VA: 20/100.

c and d): After treatment: after 4 IVT sessions, persistence of the intraretinal fluid and bright hyper-reflective spots and accentuated hyper-reflectivity of the vascularized PED, suggesting progressive fibrosis and lack of response to treatment. VA: 20/200.

V. Anterior to the RPE: Retinal Hemorrhage

Choroidal neovascularization is frequently accompanied by retinal hemorrhage, responsible for characteristic signs and constituting one of the major elements of biomicroscopic examination. Retinal hemorrhages have a polymorphous appearance.

Large hemorrhages mask the neovascularization responsible for the bleeding and are difficult to interpret on angiography and sometimes even on indocyanine green angiography.

The exact site of the hemorrhage cannot always be easily determined, although some signs are very characteristic such as the hemorrhagic margin around classic CNV or the localized juxtafoveal retinal hemorrhage of chorioretinal anastomosis.

Spectral-Domain OCT is able to specify the site and extent of these hemorrhages and their relationship with CNV and can provide additional signs.

Four types of hemorrhages can be distinguished (**Figures 82-84**):

- **Group I**: hemorrhages accompanying occult choroidal neovascularization,
- **Group II**: hemorrhages accompanying chorioretinal anastomosis,
- **Group III**: hemorrhages associated with classic choroidal neovascularization,
- **Group IV**: hemorrhages complicating polypoidal choroidal vasculopathy.

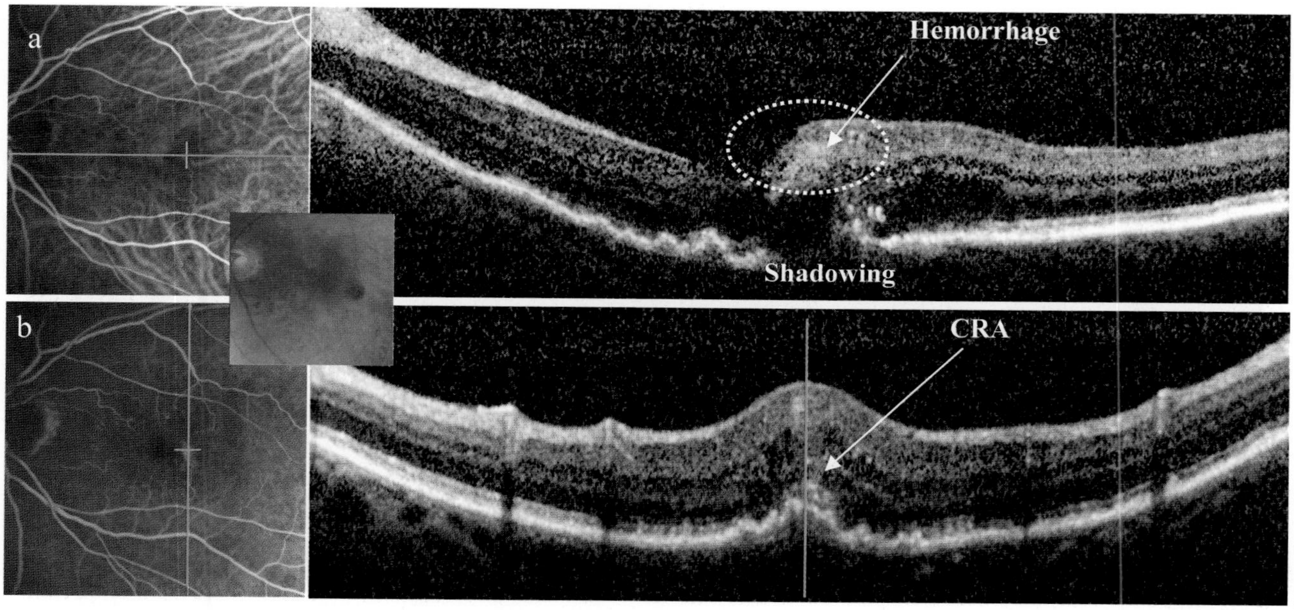

Figure 82: Retinal hemorrhage associated with chorioretinal anastomosis.

a): *Spectralis horizontal section correlated with ICG angiography.**
On SD-OCT, hemorrhage induces a denser and more hyper-reflective zone in the inner layers of the juxtafoveolar retina and is accompanied by back-shadowing with masking of all layers, including the RPE.

b): *Spectralis vertical section correlated with fluorescein angiography**: the green calliper is placed on fluorescein leakage partially masked by the hemorrhage.
The **SD-OCT** section passes adjacent to a hemorrhage and demonstrates a localized PED, the chorioretinal anastomosis, and intraretinal cysts.

7

RETINAL HEMORRHAGE

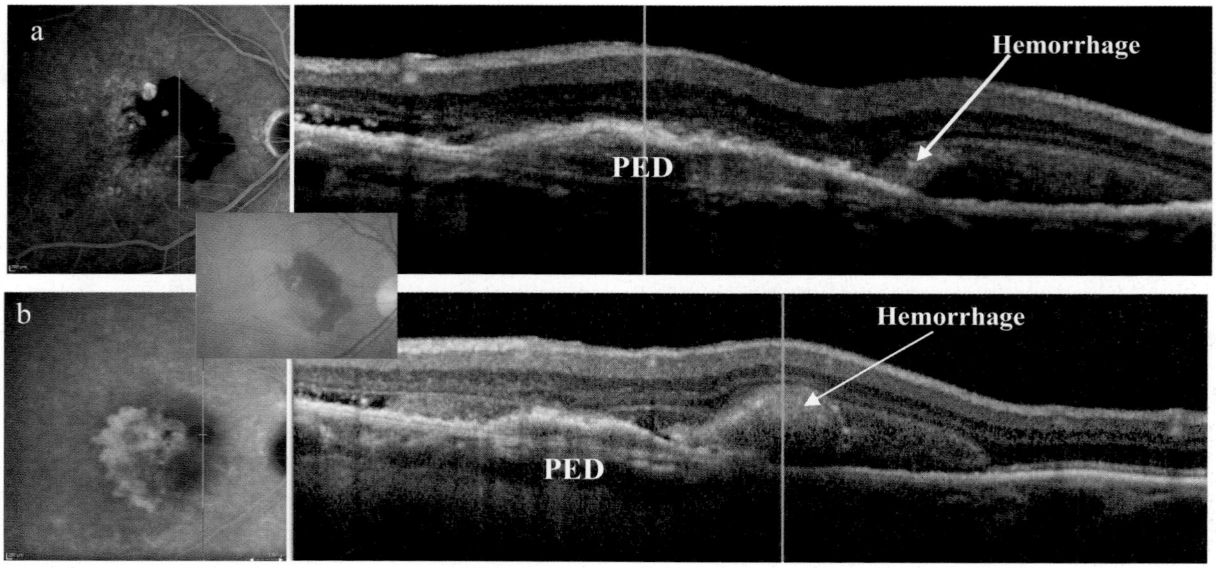

Figure 83: Retinal hemorrhage associated with an area of occult CNV.
a): *Spectralis vertical section correlated with fluorescein angiography**: nasal and superior arcuate hemorrhage partially masking the occult CNV.
On SD-OCT, clearly visible and well-delineated vascularized PED with fluid accumulation and bright hyper-reflective spots. In the superior half, the hemorrhage presents as a fairly dense, hyper-reflective zone between the outer layers of the retina and the RPE, causing partial back-shadowing.
b): *Spectralis vertical section correlated with ICG angiography revealing partially occult CNV.**
On SD-OCT, the section shows the inferior part of the PED, and a deep, fairly dense, hyper-reflective zone of hemorrhage between the outer layers and the RPE.
In the most dense zone, the light is blocked by the hemorrhage with a back-shadowing effect.

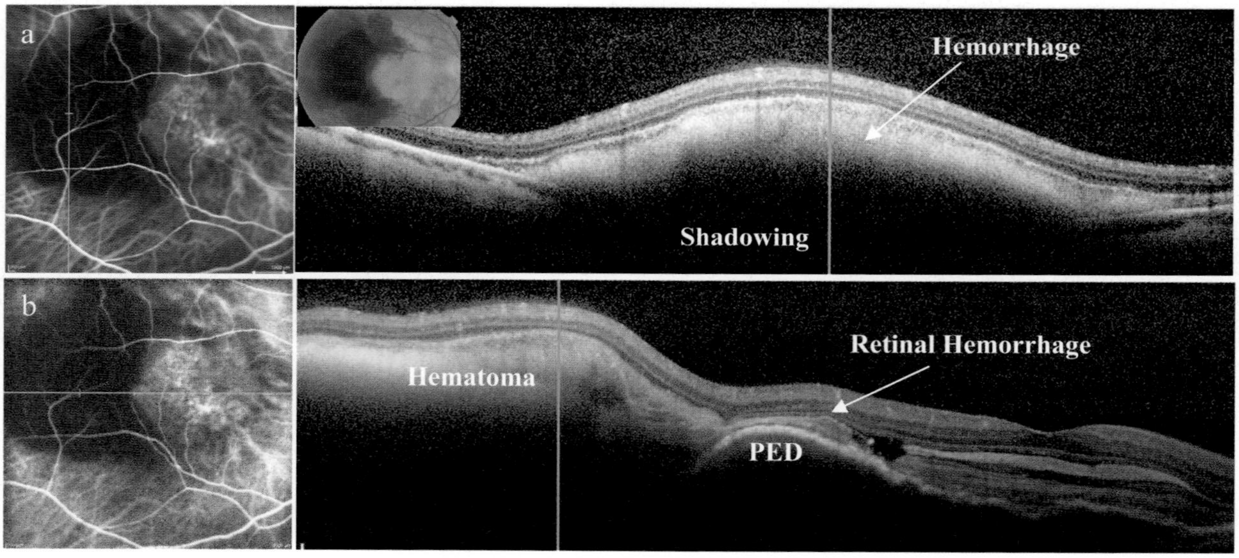

Figure 84: Macular hemorrhage associated with an area of occult CNV.
a): *Spectralis vertical section correlated with ICG angiography**: adjacent massive hemorrhage.
On SD-OCT, the hemorrhage infiltrates the outer retinal layers and completely masks the RPE and choroid.
b): *Spectralis horizontal section correlated with ICG angiography.**
On SD-OCT, the hemorrhage completely blocks the light causing back-shadowing. Note the changes in the outer retina layers anterior to the vascularized PED.

RETINAL HEMORRHAGE

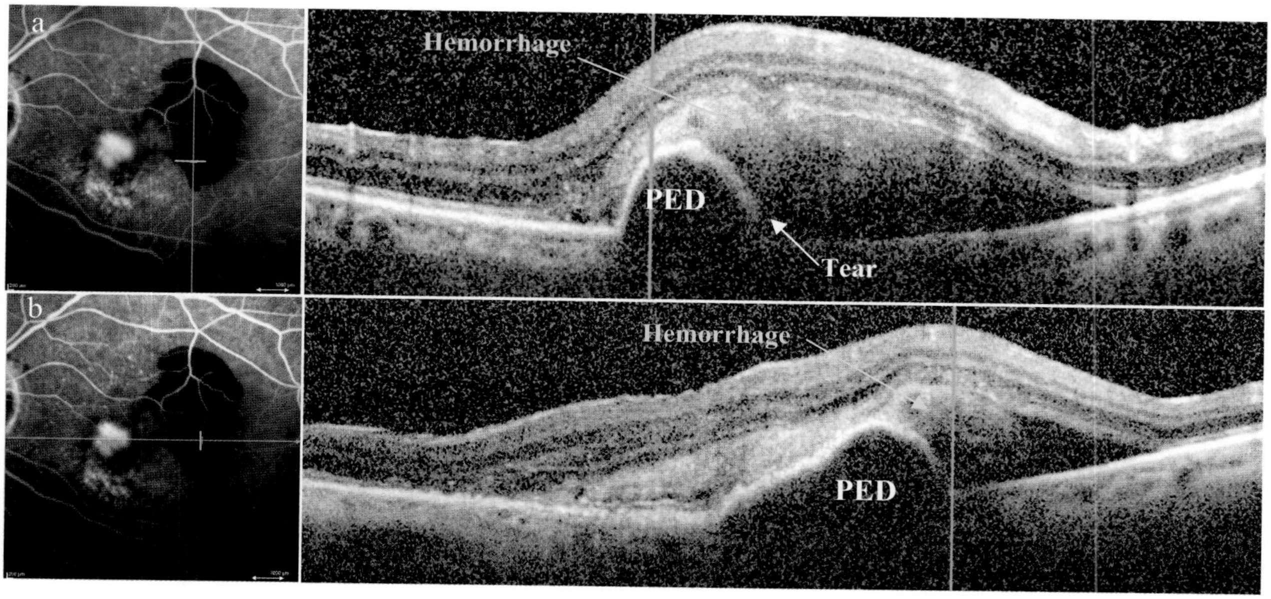

Figure 85: Arcuate hemorrhage associated with an RPE tear.

a): ***Spectralis**** **vertical section correlated with fluorescein angiography**: hemorrhage masking the tear.
SD-OCT: extensive hemorrhage anterior to the PED and anterior to the choroidal zone exposed by the tear.
b): ***Spectralis**** **horizontal section correlated with fluorescein angiography.**
On SD-OCT, the hemorrhage is visible as a white, hyper-reflective zone, partially blocking the light and causing back-shadowing.

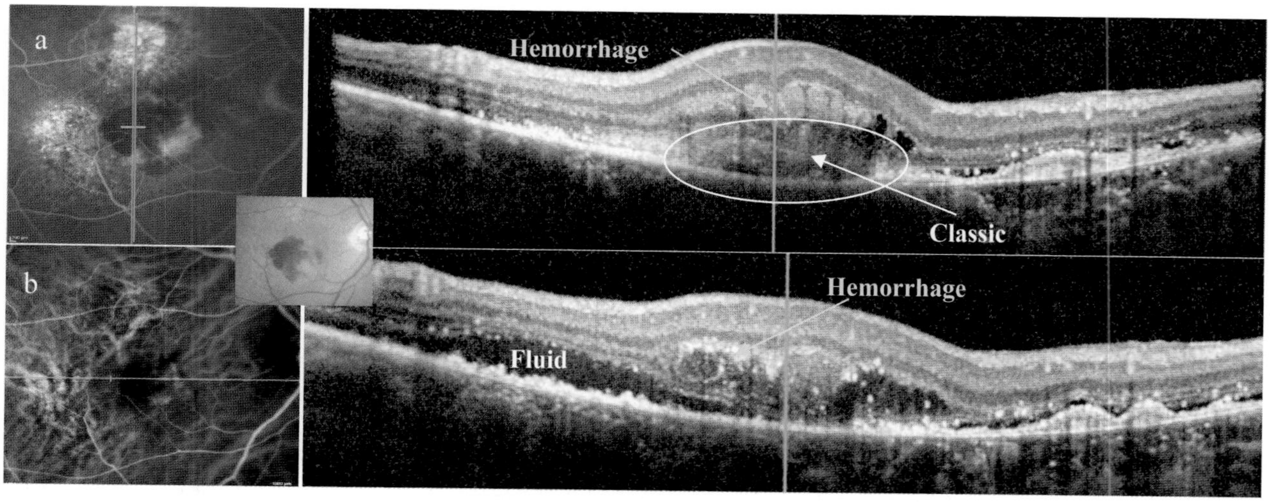

Figure 86: Retinal hemorrhage associated with classic CNV.

a): ***Spectralis**** **vertical section correlated with fluorescein angiography**: hemorrhage partially masking classic CNV.
SD-OCT: the hemorrhage is visualized as a dense, homogeneous, spindle-shaped zone in the outer retinal layers that lifts the retina. The hemorrhage is just anterior to and in contact with a classic CNV membrane proliferating anterior to the RPE. It induces changes of the IS/OS interface and outer nuclear layer with bright hyper-reflective spots and cysts.
b): ***Spectralis**** **horizontal section correlated with fluorescein angiography**. Same hyper-reflective appearance between the outer retinal layers and the altered IS/OS interface.

Clinical Features and Natural History of AMD

1. Age-Related Maculopathy

Gabriel COSCAS
Florence COSCAS, Sabrina VISMARA,
Alain ZOURDANI, C.I. Li CALZI

(Créteil and Paris)

1. Age-Related Maculopathy

Introduction

Over recent years, OCT has become an essential part of the examination in routine follow-up for AMD to guide clinical practice and analyze the response to treatment. OCT examinations can clearly demonstrate the efficacy of treatment by showing regression or persistence of leakage. Moreover, alterations of the outer retinal layers can also be analyzed.

Therefore, OCT has rapidly acquired an indispensable place in diagnosing, treating, and following patients with AMD.

New OCT Techniques

New Spectral-Domain OCT techniques now provide more than mere quantification of macular thickness and intraretinal or subretinal fluid accumulation by allowing clear visualization of the effect on photoreceptors of CNV proliferation.

CNV can occur posterior to the RPE (occult CNV), or more rarely, anterior to the RPE (classic CNV).

The outer layers of the retina comprise the photoreceptors as well as structures on either side of the photoreceptors (external limiting membrane and the IS/OS interface). Better analysis of the outer retinal layers will allow more accurate prognosis and will help identify either reversible or fibrotic late lesions.

All these data are important to guide patient care and specifically to decide whether to stop or continue treatment.

Imaging Modalities

Despite its apparent simplicity and its noninvasive nature, OCT cannot replace all other ophthalmological investigations.

In fact, OCT cannot directly visualize choroidal neovascularization, its degree of perfusion, or its exact location, but OCT does provide valuable and suggestive indirect signs.

Fluorescein angiography (for classic CNV) and SLO-ICG angiography (for the more frequent occult CNV) remain the "gold-standard" to diagnose the various clinical forms of CNV as precisely as possible.

A combination of these various imaging modalities probably remains the best way to assess how choroidal neovascularization responds to treatment, to identify good and poor responders, and to define indications for combined treatment modalities.

Correlations

Functional and *morphological* correlations are essential to guide the treatment strategy, taking into account not only measurements of central visual acuity, but also microperimetry to evaluate macular function.

Comprehensive evaluation of these different signs by the ophthalmologist guides not only the initial indication for treatment but also the imaging modalities during follow-up for AMD and the frequency and duration of intravitreal injections.

These imaging methods and treatment strategies mainly concerns *wet AMD*. They must also be applied in *age-related maculopathy*, for the early detection of choroidal neovascularization.

Clinical Practice

This chapter covers the detailed analysis of OCT images by describing the *natural history* and the *response to treatment* of each of the main clinical forms of AMD.

Clinical cases will be used to illustrate the contribution of OCT compared to that of angiographies and functional investigations in order to guide first-line treatment (currently consisting of intravitreal anti-VEGF injections).

The modalities and duration of post-treatment follow-up and the decision to repeat injections are also based on the investigations discussed above.

In many cases, treatment must be continued for several months or even longer. This is a delicate treatment strategy that should be tailored to the individual patient.

Age-Related Maculopathy

Current classifications group all of the **precursor** signs of age-related macular degeneration under the term "**age-related maculopathy**" (ARM) comprising:

- The various clinical forms of drusen,
- Alterations of the RPE, either hypo-pigmentation or hyper-pigmentation,
- Deposits of autofluorescent lipofuscin material, which are possibly related to the above findings.

8

These lesions are frequently observed in populations over the age of 50, and their frequency increases considerably with age. They can evolve over many years and sometimes throughout the subject's lifetime without causing any complications.

In the majority of cases, the disease remains stable for many years, with no progression to the advanced or complicated stages of true AMD.

I. Different Types of Drusen

Diffuse Deposits

Diffuse deposits or *basal laminar drusen* are mainly composed of lipoproteins located between the RPE basement membrane and plasma membrane. These deposits are early markers of ARM.

However, even with SLO-ICG angiography or OCT examination, they cannot be identified on clinical examination.

Detection of the first drusen on *biomicroscopy* therefore constitutes the initial clinical stage of the disease.

Hard Drusen

Small, well-defined hard drusen are easily detected on biomicroscopy or angiography but are barely visible on OCT (**Figures 1a and 2**).

Hard drusen are usually stable and complications are relatively rare. They only occur fairly late in the course of the disease.

This distinguishes them from soft drusen, which are associated with an increasing risk of neovascular or atrophic complications over time (after 5 or 10 years).

Hard drusen could change gradually, starting with *clusters* then sero-granular drusen and can even give rise to complications (**Figures 1b and 2**).

Hard drusen can be transformed into typical soft drusen after many years. A few hard drusen frequently persist around the central part of the fovea where large, soft drusen accumulate (**Figure 1b, c, and Figure 2**).

Soft Drusen

Soft drusen are often still only characterized by their dimensions. They are considered to be a part of AMD. (**Figure 1c and d; Figures 3, 4, and 5**). They are fairly common, observed in 10% of patients between the ages of 50-60 years and 25-30% by the age of 80 years.

Typical, soft drusen are pale yellow, with irregular and poorly-demarcated contours.

On **fluorescein angiography**, they stain late and progressively but without leakage.

SLO-ICG angiography better visualizes soft drusen, which are dark and hypo-fluorescent throughout the angiographic sequence and well-defined in the late phase. The hypo-fluorescence of even small soft drusen on SLO-ICG angiography is a diagnostic characteristic (**Figures 3, 4, and 5**).

OCT

On **OCT**, soft drusen are clearly visible as an elevation of the RPE with a moderately reflective cavity, which partially reveals Bruch's membrane with little or no posterior shadowing.

They have variable dimensions and are generally larger towards the center of the fovea. The most important contribution of SD-OCT in this scenario is to demonstrate associated alterations of the outer retinal layers (**Figure 2**).

The various stages of the natural history of drusen have been precisely classified to define *risk factors* for the appearance of complications of AMD. These **risk factors** are based on drusen number, size, confluence, and associated pigment migration.

HARD, SOFT AND MIXED DRUSEN

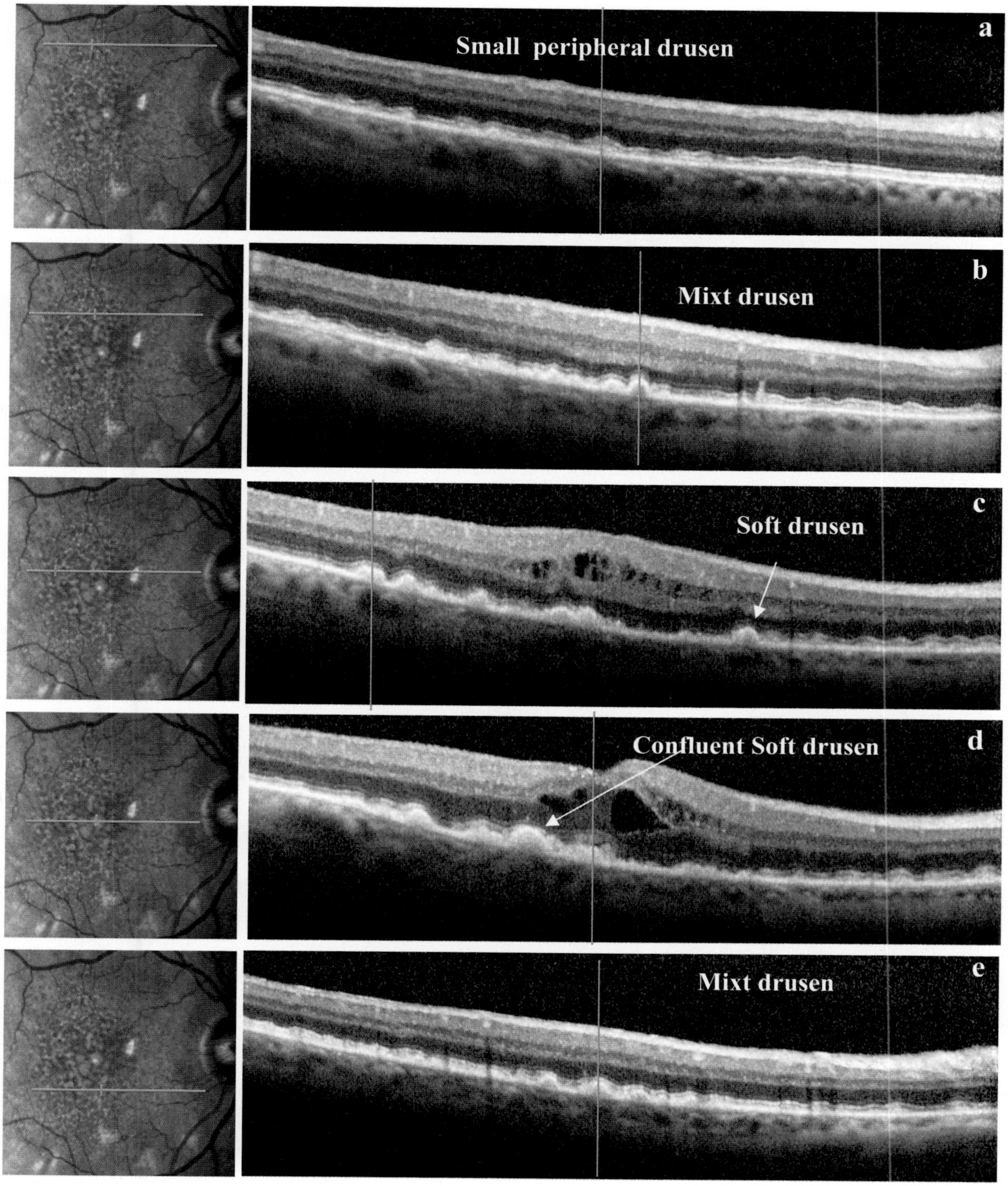

Figure 1. Presence of large soft drusen in the center of the fovea. Smaller hard drusen are mainly in the periphery.

a and b): in the periphery, the drusen are smaller, more numerous, and barely visible even with *Spectralis** SD-OCT. Several hard drusen are grouped in clusters with rare soft drusen.
c and d): in the central region, numerous, tightly packed, medium-sized soft drusen that are sometimes confluent.
e): in the inferior periphery, small soft drusen and many small, barely visible drusen.

8

HARD, SOFT AND MIXED DRUSEN

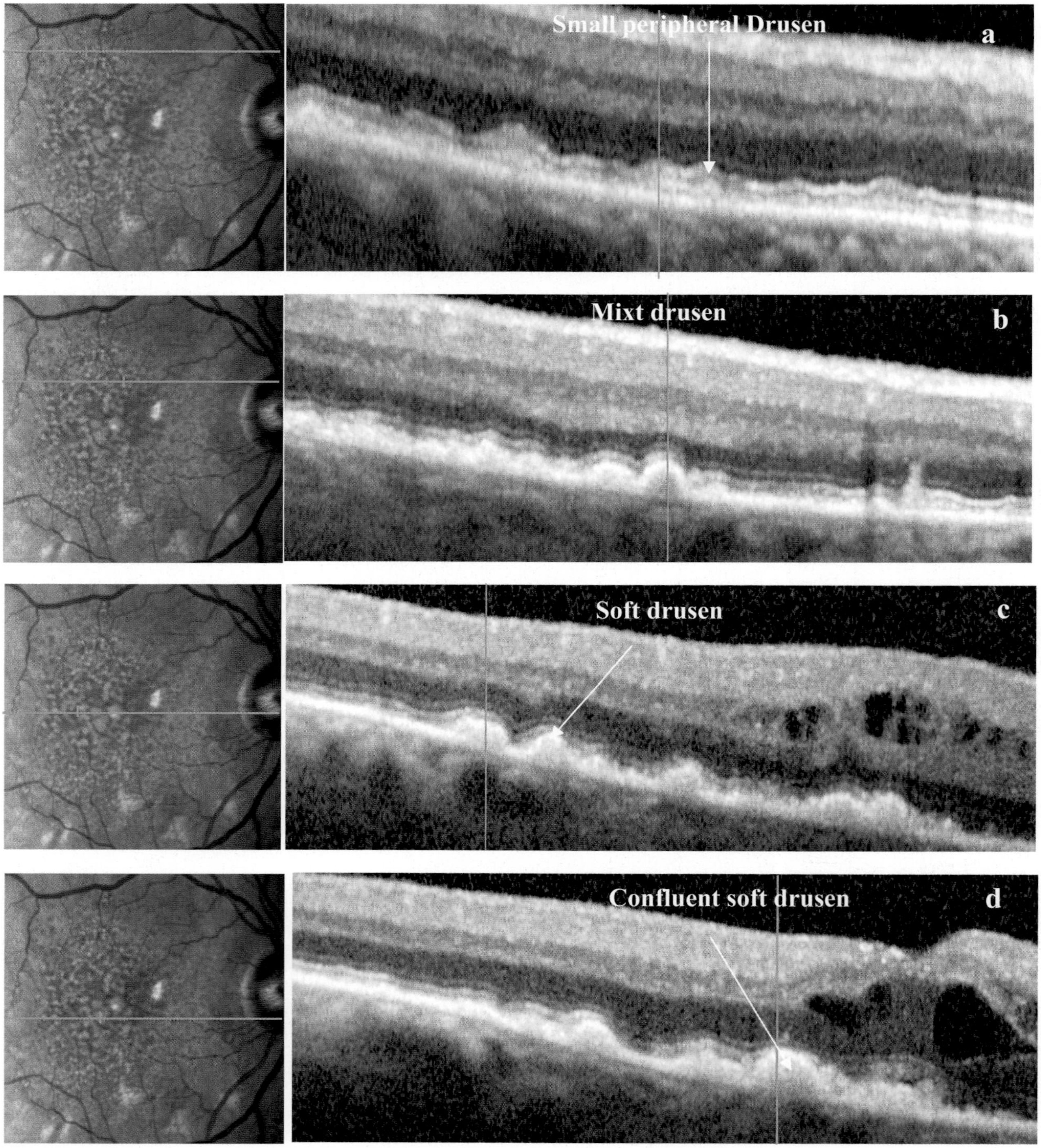

Figure 2. Mixed drusen. Enlarged images of Figure 1. *Spectralis horizontal sections.**

The enlarged images clearly visualize changes of the outer retinal layers.
a and b): In the periphery, the outer nuclear layer and external limiting membrane are slightly modified except over the larger drusen. The IS/OS interface shows several minor alterations of reflectivity.
c and d): in the central zone, the modifications are more accentuated over the dome of the larger drusen with irregularities, disruptions, and thickening of the IS/OS interface, especially over confluent drusen.

SMALL AND MEDIUM-SIZED SOFT DRUSEN

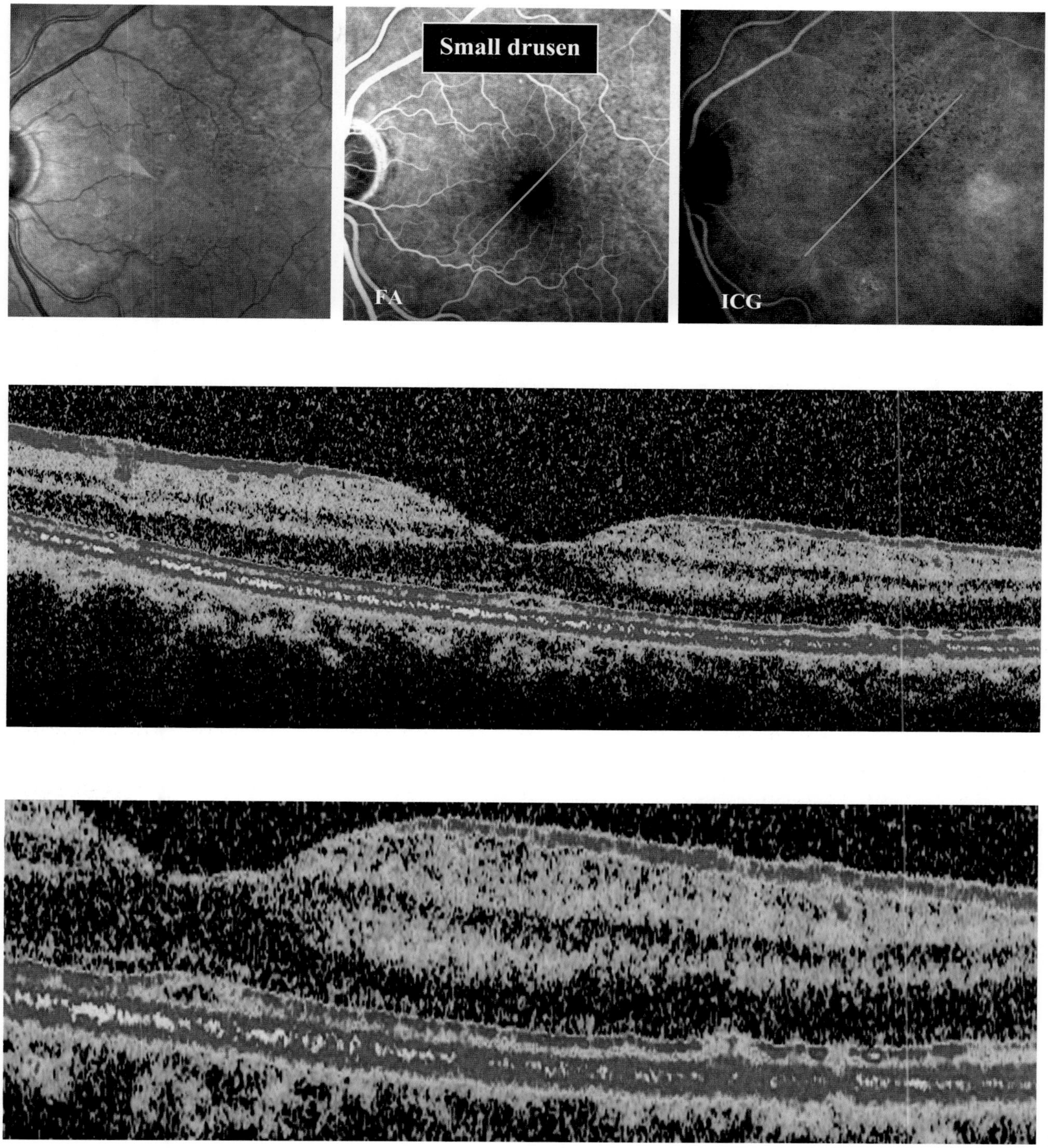

Figure 3: Numerous perifoveal hard drusen.

***Spectralis** color-coded oblique section correlated with fluorescein angiography and ICG angiography** *(the numerous small drusen, all the same size, are visible as hyper-fluorescent spots on fluorescein angiography and hypo-fluorescent spots on SLO-ICG angiography).*
On SD-OCT sections, the RPE is only slightly modified with a few small irregularities in thickness. Some of these irregularities are more marked and probably correspond to drusen, inducing relatively moderate elevation of the IS/OS interface with no other retinal effect at this stage.

SMALL AND MEDIUM-SIZED SOFT DRUSEN

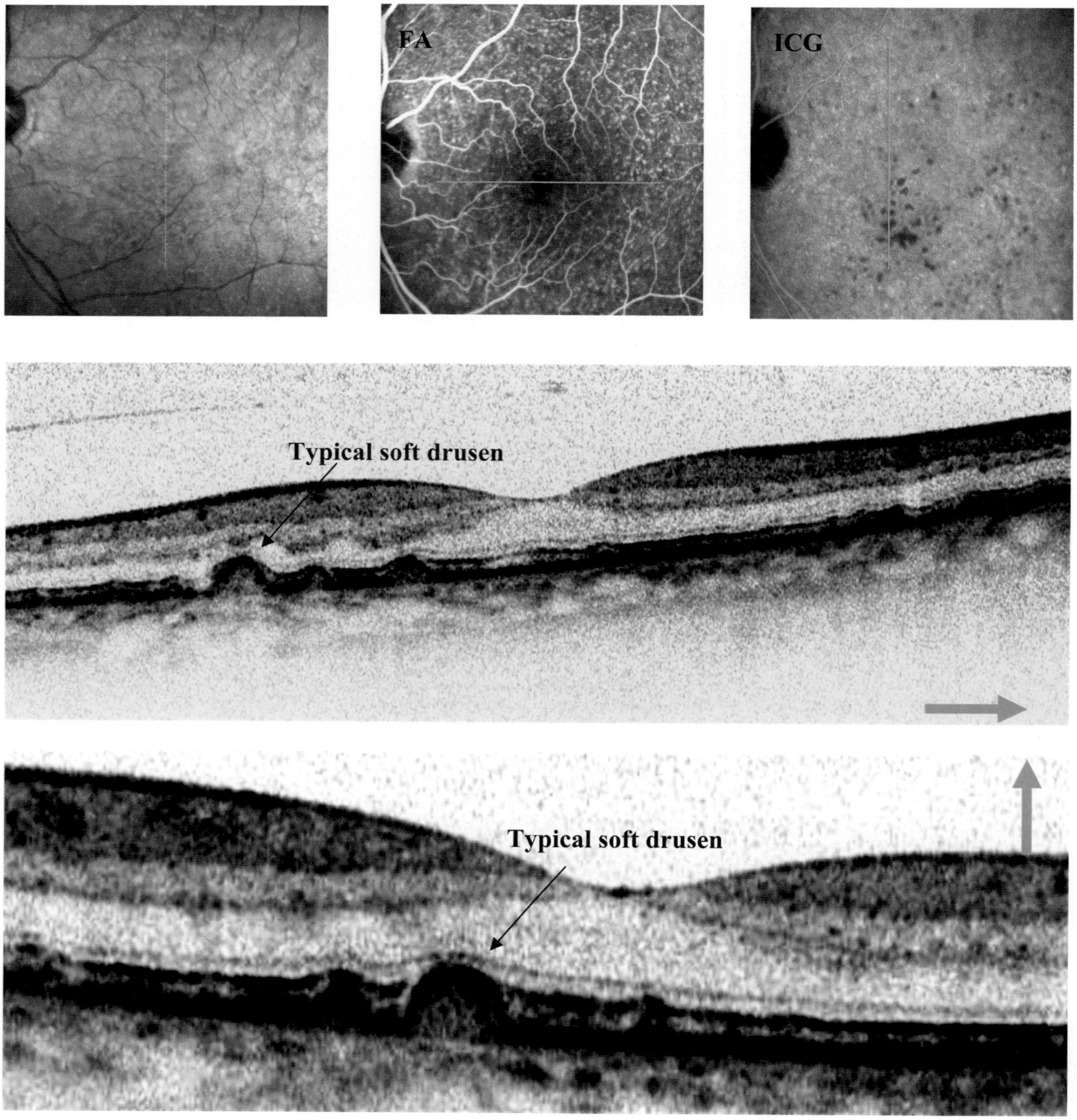

Figure 4: Several medium-sized soft drusen (VA: 10/10).

***Spectralis** black and white horizontal section correlated with fluorescein angiography** *(numerous small drusen with a few soft drusen and several hard drusen in the periphery).*

On SD-OCT, the retina is only slightly abnormal. Hard drusen are barely detectable. Occasional soft drusen are visible (*arrow*), raising the RPE and outer nuclear layer, with few reactive lesions. Note the heterogeneous appearance of the soft drusen.

***Spectralis** vertical section: correlated with** ICG angiography *(the drusen are hypo-fluorescent until the late phases).*

The SD-OCT section through the largest soft drusen demonstrates their typical appearance at this early stage (elevation, partial shadowing, clearly visible Bruch's membrane) and the absence of any reactive lesions.

MULTIPLE SOFT DRUSEN

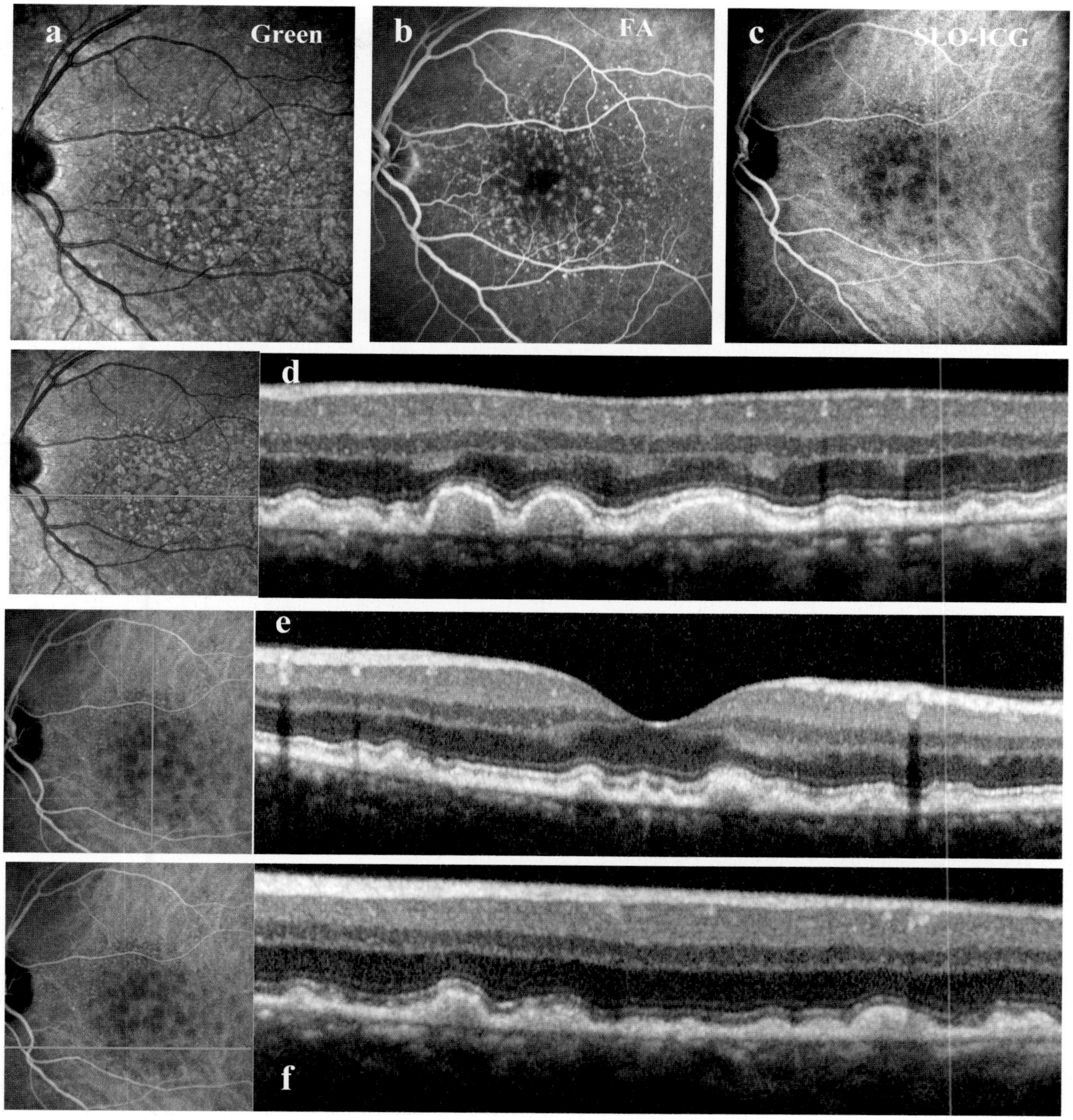

Figure 5: Numerous, large and confluent soft drusen (VA: 20/32).
a, b, and c): Red-free fluorescein angiography and SLO-ICG images: numerous drusen occupying all of the posterior pole, large in size in the central region and much smaller in the periphery. Soft drusen stain only in the late phases of fluorescein angiography. Only soft drusen are visible on SLO-ICG as hypo-fluorescent and black spots.
d): *Spectralis horizontal section**: numerous typical regular dome-shaped soft drusen. The material underneath the RPE is moderately hyper-reflective, leaving Bruch's membrane visible without shadowing.
Note the zone of flatter and wider confluent drusen. The IS/OS interface and external limiting membrane are visible, continuous, and only slightly modified, but the outer nuclear layer appears to be displaced and thinned over the drusen with a characteristic jagged appearance.
e): *Spectralis vertical section**: the central zone is spared with only two small drusen and a normal appearance of Henle fibers, compatible with the good visual acuity.
f): *Spectralis eccentric horizontal section**: the SD-OCT section demonstrates early changes of the IS/OS interface and outer nuclear layer just over the dome of the larger drusen.

The presence of **reticular drusen** (especially visible in blue light) adjacent to the temporal arcades is an additional *risk factor for wet AMD*. They are hardly seen on TD-OCT sections of perimacular zones.

These reticular drusen are much more clearly visible on SD-OCT and enlarged views, which show a thickening band and undulations of the RPE but with no alteration of the outer nuclear layer (**Figure 6**).

Drusen and Outer Retinal Layers

Moreover, **one of the major advantages of SD-OCT** is to visualize reactions in the outer retinal layers when present.

8

As drusen increase in size, they raise the RPE band, IS/OS interface, and external limiting membrane, which then can appear irregular, thinned, and disrupted. The *outer nuclear layer* can also be modified, thinned, and invaded by a homogeneous or jagged moderately reflective zone (**Figure 6**).

These alterations reflect damage to inner and outer segments and photoreceptors as a whole over the largest drusen. They therefore constitute valuable signs of the impact of drusen and possible *photoreceptor damage*.

Analysis of drusen is based not only on anteroposterior scans, but also on 3D scans. Future clinical trials of **drusen volume** measurements will allow even more reliable quantitative assessment of their course (**Figure 7**).

Natural History

Atrophy

Drusen usually progress towards atrophy as the material regresses and is replaced by a zone of atrophy of the RPE (**Figure 8**). Atrophy can be seen on monochromatic images and especially on red-free images.

On **fluorescein angiography**, RPE atrophy causes hyper-fluorescence due to a window defect with late and progressive staining, while atrophy is hypo-fluorescent on ICG angiography.

The **OCT examination** easily confirms the diagnosis of RPE atrophy by showing thinning of the RPE band associated with thinning or even loss of the outer retinal layers.

These areas of atrophy replace perifoveal drusen and then gradually spread to the center of the macula causing loss of vision (**Figure 9**).

Drusenoid PED

Soft drusen usually increase in size and become confluent, resulting in the appearance of a **drusenoid PED** (**Figure 10**). *Biomicroscopic findings* are already suggestive with a wavy, irregular elevation and pigment migration, which can be star-shaped or web-shaped.

On *fluorescein angiography*, hypo-fluorescence due to pigment migration and xanthophyll pigment contrast with the zone of progressive hyper-fluorescence corresponding to the drusenoid PED.

However, on *SLO-ICG angiography*, drusenoid PEDs and the surrounding soft drusen remain hypo-fluorescent even in late images.

On **OCT**, the RPE band is elevated with gently sloping or sometimes wavy edges. The underlying drusenoid material is usually moderately hyper-reflective and Bruch's membrane becomes visible.

Pigment migrations induce zones of fairly intense hyper-reflectivity that alter and sometimes disrupt the IS/OS interface and external limiting membrane. They can also extend into the retina, causing localized disorganization (**Figure 11**).

Neovascular Complications

Drusen may evolve spontaneously to choroidal neovascularization, which can be characterized by fluorescein leakage. The presence or absence of leakage on fluorescein angiography and the presence of subretinal or intraretinal fluid on OCT are the most reliable diagnostic signs.

OCT can also demonstrate slight **intraretinal fluid**, even at a subclinical stage. This would suggest the presence of choroidal neovascularization. *OCT should therefore be considered in all patients with soft, confluent drusen or a drusenoid PED who present with functional changes such as metamorphopsias or vision loss.*

CNV can lead to the formation of a vascularized PED, precisely detectable on OCT, as illustrated by the following example (clinical case No. 1, page 184, **Figures 12, 13, and 14**).

RETICULAR PSEUDO-DRUSEN

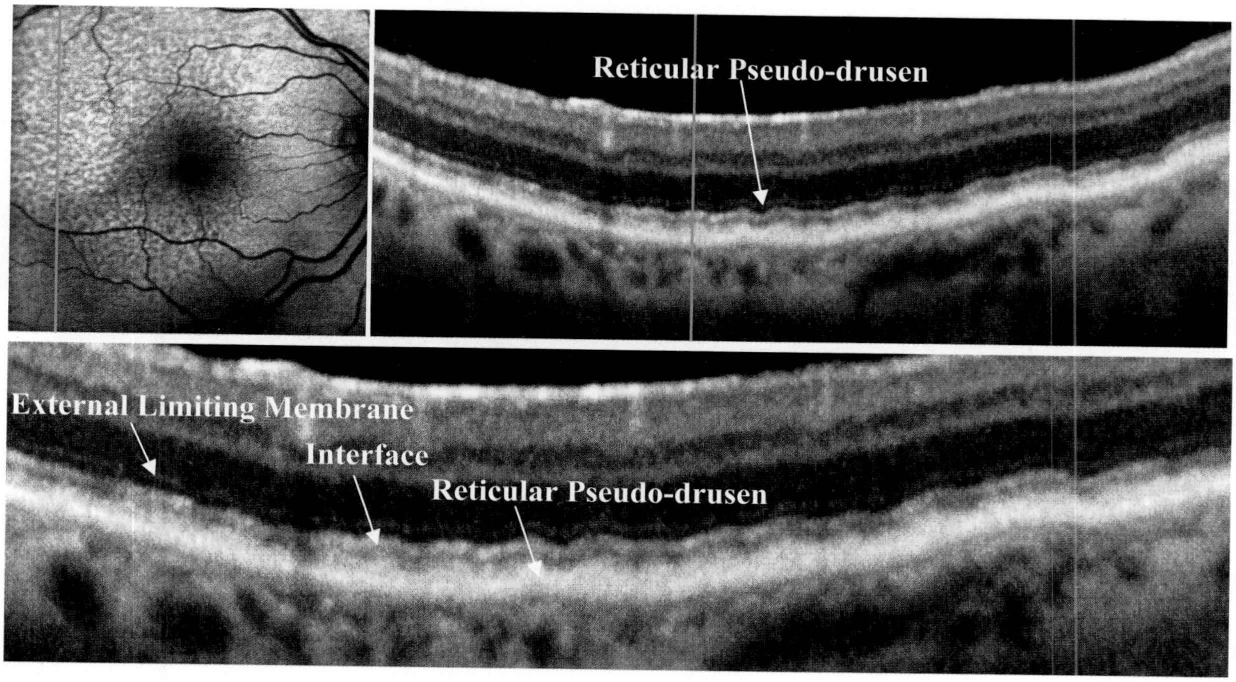

Figure 6: Reticular drusen visible in blue light and on autofluorescence (VA: 20/32).
a): *Spectralis eccentric vertical section correlated with an autofluorescence image** *(numerous reticular pseudo-drusen with a polypoid appearance in the region of the temporal arcades, also visible in blue light).*
On SD-OCT, these lesions are seen as a series of localized thickenings of the RPE, raising the IS/OS interface and external limiting membrane but with no breaks or change in thickness of these lines.
b): Enlarged images of the SD-OCT image confirming the absence of alteration of the outer nuclear layer.

3D IMAGE OF DRUSEN

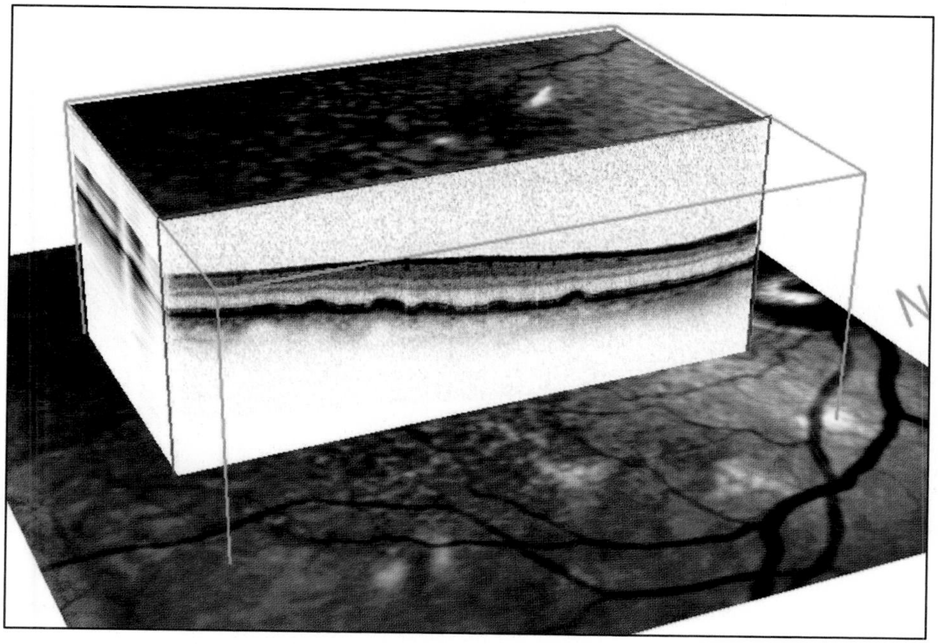

Figure 7: 3D image of drusen (*Topcon).** Each SD-OCT section can be analyzed by comparison with the fundus image and studied frame by frame or as a video sequence.

8

DRUSEN AND ATROPHIC ZONES

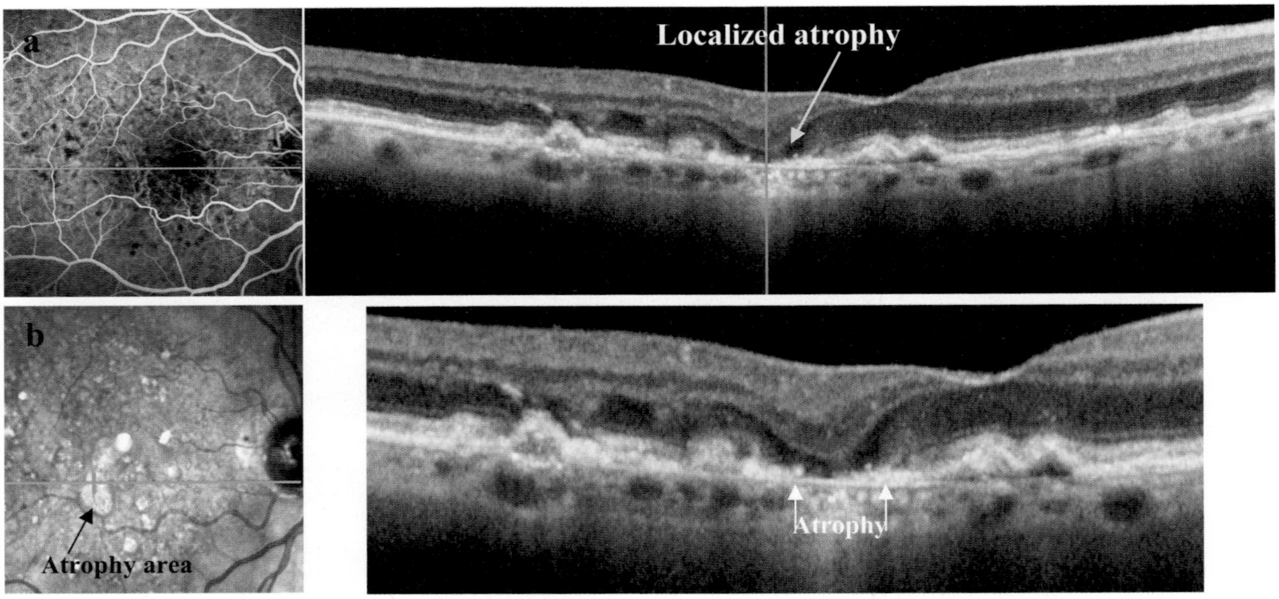

Figure 8: Soft drusen: natural progression to atrophy (VA: 20/50).
a): *Spectralis horizontal section correlated with a monochromatic image and fluorescein angiography**: numerous soft drusen some of which have resulted in atrophy.
On SD-OCT, loss of drusen in the atrophic area, thinning of the RPE, loss of the external limiting membrane and IS/OS interface and alteration of the outer nuclear layer.
The inner layers of the retina remain almost normal.
b): Enlargement of the SD-OCT image confirming changes in the outer retinal layers.

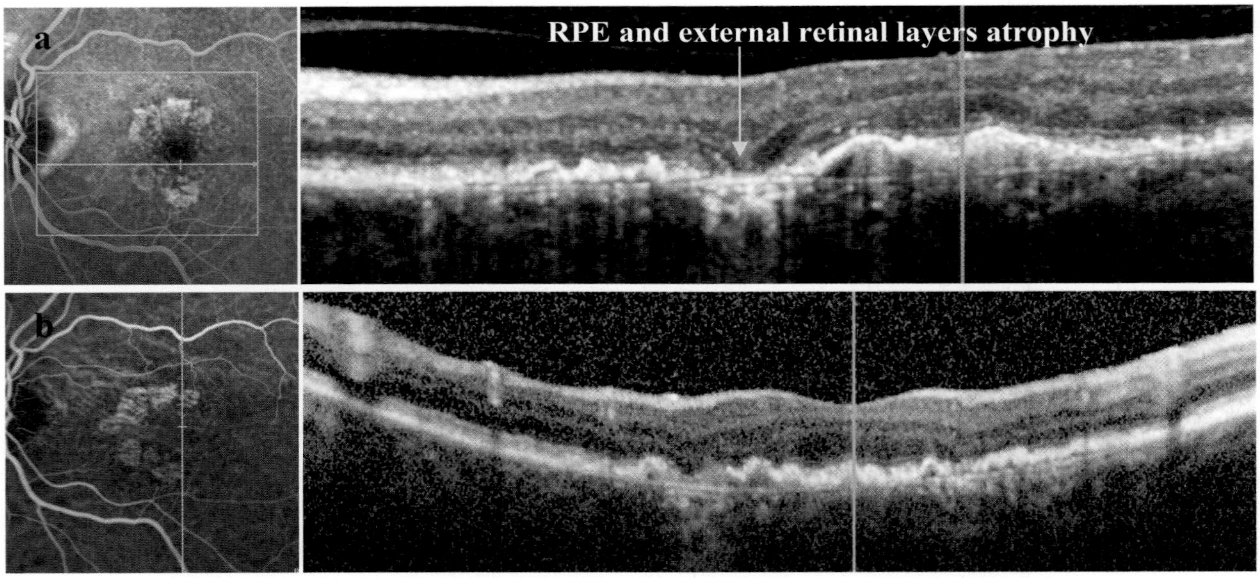

Figure 9: Numerous soft drusen and perifoveal atrophic areas.
a and b): *Spectralis horizontal and vertical sections correlated with fluorescein angiography and ICG angiography** *(most of the soft drusen have been replaced by areas of perifoveal atrophy and atrophy of the outer layers).*
On SD-OCT, numerous soft drusen associated with irregularities of the RPE and areas of atrophy with loss of the RPE and outer retinal layers and marked posterior hyper-reflectivity.

DRUSENOID PED

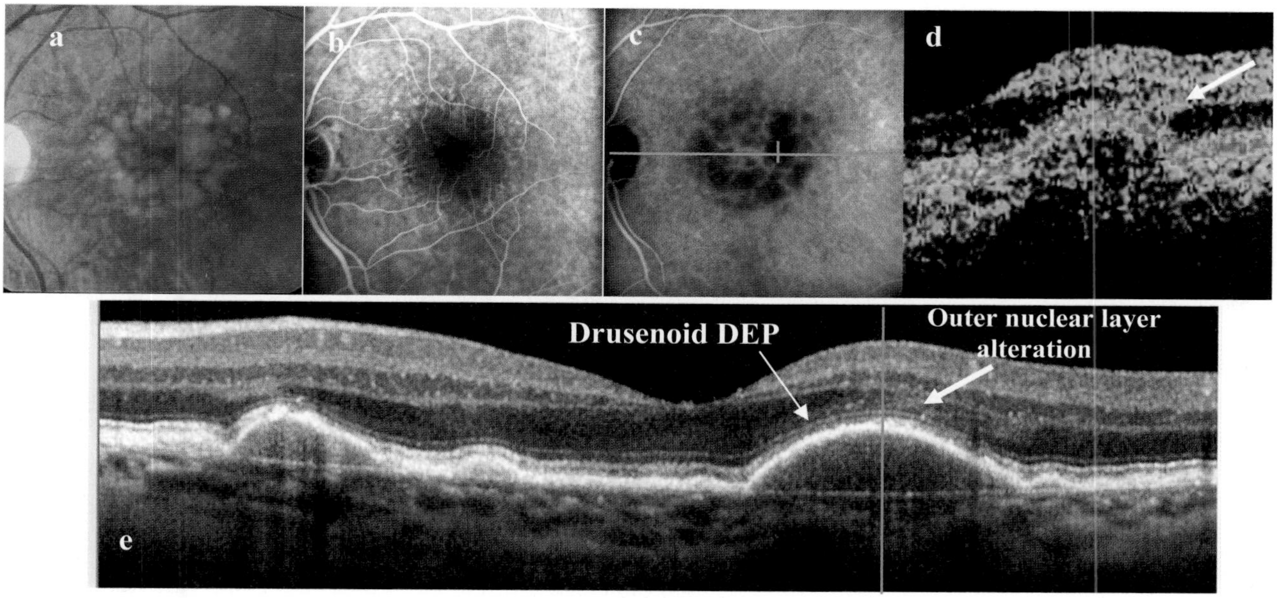

Figure 10: Confluent soft drusen with a small drusenoid PED (VA: 20/25).
a-d): Color photograph, fluorescein angiography, SLO-ICG, and *Stratus OCT.**
e): *Spectralis horizontal section**: this small, regular dome-shaped juxtafoveal drusenoid PED (*thin arrow*) has a less reflective cavity, allowing good visualization of Bruch's membrane.
Note the adjacent alterations of the IS/OS interface and the denser zone that invades the outer nuclear layer. This abnormality can also be seen on *Stratus** OCT (*arrow*).

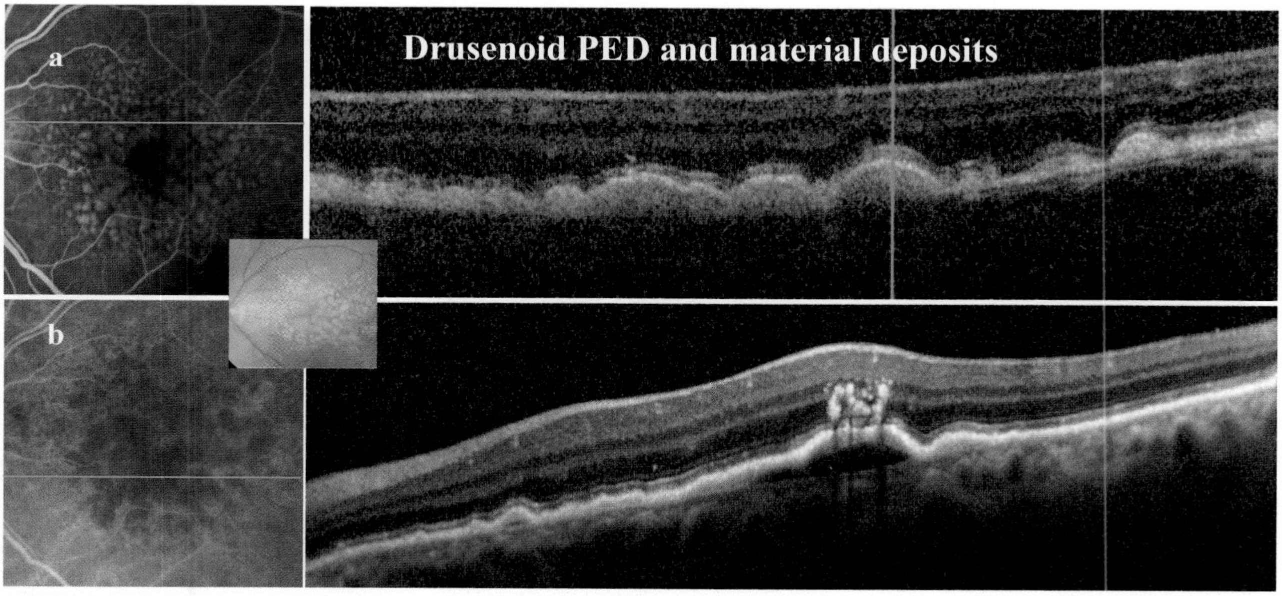

Figure 11: Small drusenoid PED and deposits (VA: 20/63).
a): *Spectralis horizontal section correlated with fluorescein angiography** *(numerous soft drusen with a central hypo-fluorescent area).*
On SD-OCT, numerous tightly packed soft drusen of various sizes, causing changes in the photoreceptor layer and decreased thickness of the outer nuclear layer over the large drusen.
b): *Spectralis horizontal section correlated with ICG angiography** *(numerous large, hypo-fluorescent, confluent soft drusen, especially in the center, forming a small drusenoid PED).*
On SD-OCT, the IS/OS interface appears to be thickened over the dome of the drusenoid PED, the outer nuclear layer is partially displaced or thinned and deposits have invaded the outer retinal layers.

CLINICAL CASE No. 01 MIXED DRUSEN AND CNV

Clinical Signs

A 75-year-old patient followed for decompensation of occult CNV in his first eye, presented with the absence of any symptoms, signs of ARM on routine examination of the fellow eye. This eye had fairly numerous, tightly packed mostly hard drusen of various sizes. The largest drusen are slightly autofluorescent. VA RE: 20/32 - VA LE: 20/20.

Angiography shows rapid and early staining of numerous hard drusen, sometimes in clusters or even confluent and sero-granular. Soft drusen are not stained at this stage. There is no fluorescein leakage.

SLO-ICG shows the presence of a small number of dark, hypo-fluorescent perifoveal soft drusen.

At this stage, these lesions therefore correspond to mixed, predominantly hard drusen without complications (**Figure 12a-d**).

Six Months Later

The patient reported moderate symptoms with minimal metamorphopsias and moderate loss of visual acuity in the left eye (20/32).

Biomicroscopic examination revealed a recently developed, moderately dense macular hemorrhage measuring 1/2 disc diameter with a relatively flat, eccentric SRF which was clearly visible on autofluorescence.

On angiography, an irregular hyper-fluorescent area with pinpoint leakage occupied the nasal half of the fovea, with diffuse fluorescein leakage. This lesion was lined by hemorrhage. **SLO-ICG** showed a dark PED, which was seen as hyper-fluorescence of an occult choroidal neovascularization.

> *Suggested Diagnosis:*
> Recent occult CNV with hemorrhage detected during routine follow-up of mixed drusen (**Figure 13a, b, and c**).

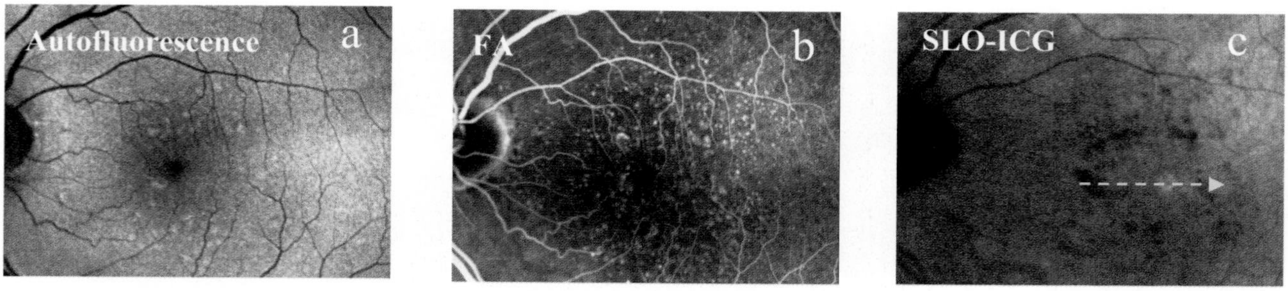

Figure 12a, b, and c): mixed Drusen with no complications during the observation period.

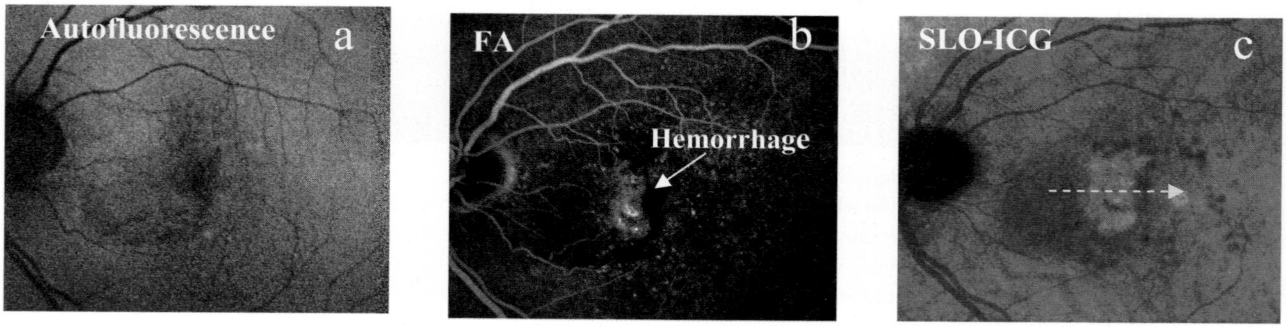

Figure 13a, b, and c): six months later: occult choroidal neovascularization with hemorrhagic complications.

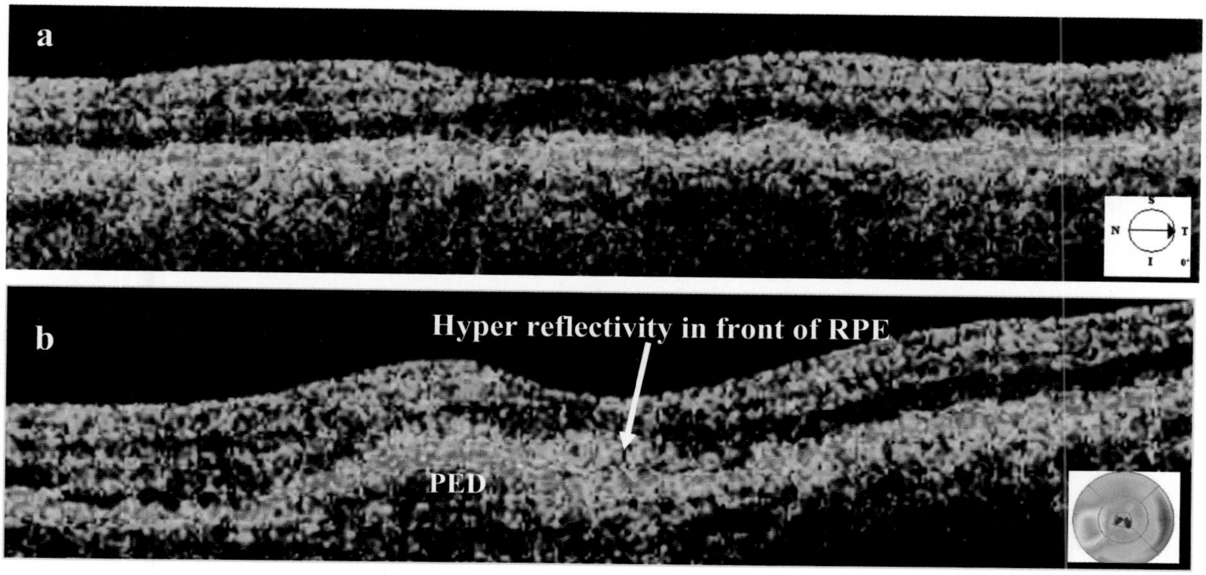

Figure 14a): hard drusen and several soft drusen without complications.
b): six months later, minimal PED with hemorrhagic neovascularization.

Contribution of OCT

During Follow-Up

*Stratus** horizontal section: almost normal appearance (**Figure 14a**).

At the level of the RPE band: several irregularities and limited elevations of the RPE with no posterior shadowing and with poorly reflective material, suggesting small soft drusen. No hard drusen are visible.

Posterior to the RPE: no alteration.

Anterior to the RPE: retinal layers have a normal appearance. Note the slight asymmetry of the hypo-reflective zone corresponding to Henle fibers.

Six Months Later

*Stratus** horizontal section: appearance highly suggestive of CNV (**Figure 14b**).

At the level of the RPE band: moderate but regular elevation of the hyper-reflective band of the RPE.

Posterior to the RPE: the PED cavity is slightly reflective allowing visualization of Bruch's membrane.

Anterior to the RPE: diffuse increase of retinal thickness and presence of subfoveal hyper-reflective material, which probably corresponds to retinal hemorrhage.

Diagnosis

The **OCT examination** demonstrated a *limited PED* (corresponding to the hypo-fluorescent area visible on SLO-ICG angiography).

The PED appears to be relatively flat but is characterized by the visibility of Bruch's membrane, which has become distinct from the RPE.

A small amount of *intraretinal fluid* can be seen anterior to the RPE with increased retinal thickness, which is especially visible in the nasal sector.

In the central zone, the hypo-reflective band of the outer nuclear layer is thinned and partially displaced by a hyper-reflective zone, probably corresponding to retinal hemorrhage.

These signs are suggestive of a small zone of **subfoveal classic CNV**.

Fluorescein angiography confirms the presence of CNV by showing more marked localized hyper-fluorescence in this zone with fluorescein leakage.

On **ICG angiography**, the PED is localized and clearly visible. The sub-RPE fluid accumulation is due to leakage from occult CNV. A small area of classic CNV is also detected (but too small to show the features of a characteristic network).

This **"minimally classic" CNV** shows signs of recent decompensation, confirmed by hemorrhage, fluorescein leakage, the dark PED on ICG angiography, elevation of the RPE band on OCT, and moderate loss of visual acuity.

Anti-VEGF intravitreal injection is indicated, which has to be followed regularly by VA and imaging.

Follow-Up

The proposed treatment of monthly intravitreous injections of anti-VEGF (Lucentis*) was monitored each month by visual acuity, OCT, and fluorescein and ICG angiography with follow-up of one year.

Visual acuity initially declined with recurrence of symptoms during the second month then rapidly improved to become stable at 20/25 by the third month (ie, after the second injection).

A third injection of anti-VEGF was administered to maintain the result.

OCT

- The thickness of the neurosensory retina decreased by the *first month,* but a prominent SRF, (which was confirmed with angiography) was observed after the first injection.

However, symptoms and loss of visual acuity were observed only at the third month.

The presence of a fine layer of subretinal fluid, which increased despite improvement of visual acuity, prompted continuation of treatment (**Figure 15a-d**).

- At the *fourth month*, the situation was greatly improved with resolution of leakage and minimal persistence of a flat, partially organized PED.

- However, *one month later*, recurrence of a marked SRF with signs of photoreceptor damage, justified another IVT injection (**Figure 15e and f**).

- Subsequent follow-up OCT examinations showed a stable appearance with persistence of a small SRF but with no symptoms.

Despite partial normalization of the outer layers, SD-OCT and the enlarged images showed signs of **damage to outer segments,** which had become abnormally visible and irregular at the edge of the SRF (**Figure 15g and h**).

Fluorescein Angiography

The lesion appeared to have paradoxically increased in size after the first injection, extending superiorly and inferiorly.

It then stabilized with almost no change of irregular hyper-fluorescence. No signs of hemorrhage were visible, and the surface area of the lesion did not increase.

ICG Angiography

The neovascular network remained barely visible for the first 6 months. The dark PED can be seen but with poor delineation and poor contrast.

However, at the last 2 follow-up examinations, the neovascular network became more clearly visible and well-defined without an increase in size and appeared to be poorly perfused.

Conclusion

This case of **drusen with a recent hemorrhagic complication** of minimally classic CNV illustrates rapid subjective and objective improvement during the third month, after the second injection. Visual acuity became 20/25 and remained stable on two successive examinations, therefore justifying temporary suspension of IVT injections.

However, a small recurrence was observed 2 months later that resolved immediately after the 4th injection. The situation then remained stable until the 12th month with no further treatment.

This improvement contrasts with the persistent SRF observed on OCT, possibly due to fluid accumulation, with signs of **damage to outer segments,** before complete resorption.

These discordant findings indicated monthly follow-up.

FOLLOW-UP AFTER TREATMENT

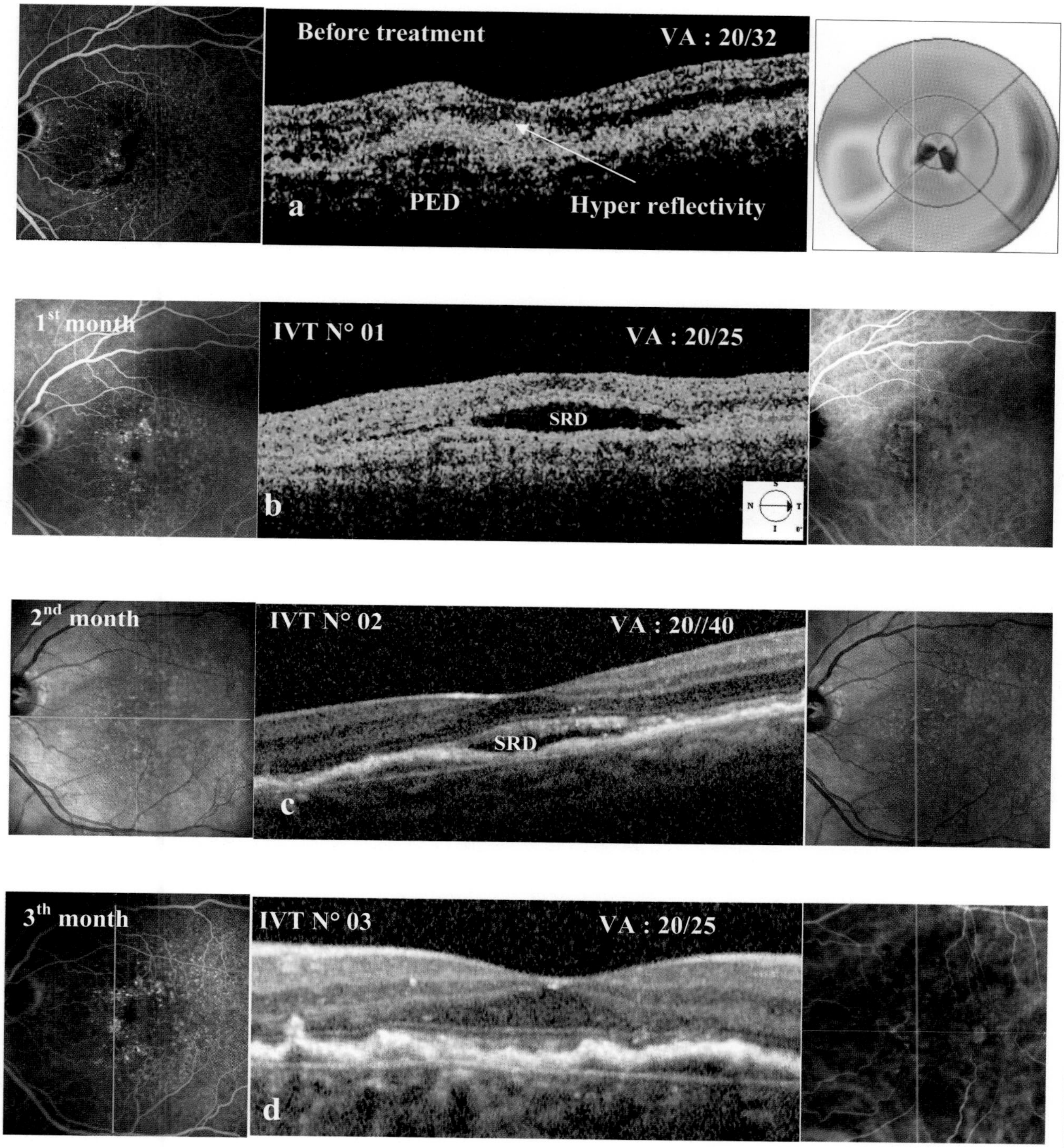

Figure 15: Occult CNV complicating mixed drusen: follow-up after 1 year by VA, fluorescein angiography, ICG angiography, and OCT.

a): Before treatment: elevation of the RPE revealing Bruch's membrane: increased retinal thickness; hyper-reflective subfoveal material, corresponding to the hyper-fluorescent zone with fluorescein leakage on angiography.
b): After the first IVT injection: rapid functional improvement but formation of SRF.
c): 2nd month: loss of visual acuity and persistence of the SRF à 2nd IVT.
d): 3rd month: improvement of visual acuity to 20/25, no signs of SRF and complete re-attachment (vertical section) à 3rd IVT. A third IVT injection was performed to maintain the result.

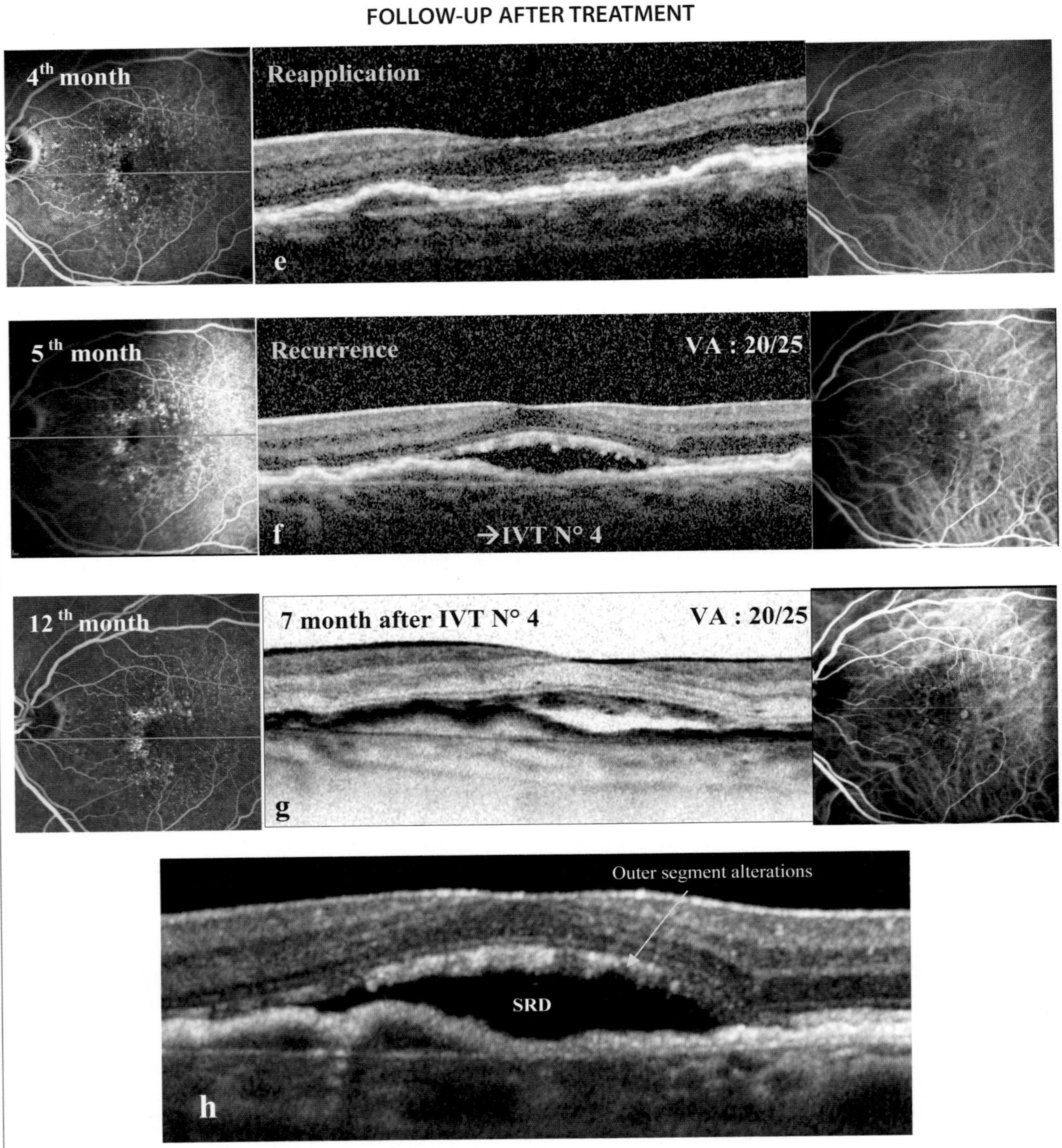

Figure 15 (continued): Occult CNV complicating mixed drusen: follow-up at 1 year by VA, fluorescein angiography, ICG angiography, and OCT.

e): 4th month: no symptoms, VA 20/25 with stable and persistent retinal re-attachment.
f): 5th month: recurrence of leakage with no loss of visual acuity à 4th IVT.
g): 12th month: stable situation: no new symptoms, good visual acuity but with little change in angiographic signs and persistent SRF → no further treatment.
h): Enlarged image (g): the outer layers have returned to normal, but signs of damage to outer segments lining the SRF. Follow-up should be continued for several months.

Conclusion

The various types of drusen remain the best markers of early changes in age-related maculopathy.

The **clinical presentation** of drusen is variable and they are also considerably, but gradually modified during the course of the disease.

Drusen have often been used to analyze the various stages of ARM in order to create a severity index, which would allow ophthalmologists to predict progression to true macular degeneration, either atrophic or especially neovascular.

Biomicroscopic examinations and counting of drusen on color fundus photographs are widely used as they are inexpensive and easy to perform.

However, drusen are more readily visible and much more numerous on red-free photographs and especially fluorescein angiography.

SLO-ICG angiography allows simple and precise visualization of soft drusen, their confluence, and their progression towards drusenoid PED.

OCT is an added advancement, which demonstrates elevation of the RPE band, visibility of Bruch's membrane, and the homogeneous or heterogeneous appearance of drusen deposits.

Spectral-Domain OCT has provided even greater advancement, as it can be used to analyze alterations of the external limiting membrane, IS/OS interface, and the outer nuclear layer, to detect signs of *photoreceptor damage.*

SD-OCT 3D volume reconstruction allows calculation of drusen volume, which would be useful for statistical studies.

Drusen volume is an inexpensive and quantifiable prognostic indicator that can be used to accurately monitor the response to treatment.

SD-OCT analysis of drusen, combined with fluorescein and ICG angiography, is useful for early diagnosis of complications and to differentiate from other diagnoses, which also cause RPE atrophy or lipofuscin deposits.

II. Deposits

Accumulation of **autofluorescent material**, such as lipofuscin, can be observed at various stages of age-related maculopathy or ARM.

Biomicroscopy

This **deposit of material** has a polymorphous appearance on biomicroscopy.

It may present as small clumps of lesions with no reactive phenomena, or larger accumulations resulting in large and much more prominent lesions.

Fluorescein Angiography

On fluorescein angiography, perifoveal deposits often consist of small clumps of hypo-fluorescent yellowish-brown pigment surrounded by a hyper-fluorescent halo.

Perifoveal deposits may also have a highly suggestive, more or less extensive and complex web-like or reticular appearance.

This material is hypo-fluorescent on the early phases of angiography and then slowly and incompletely stains later, starting at its edges.

SLO-ICG Angiography

On SLO-ICG angiography, the material has a fairly characteristic appearance with definite and *persistent hypo-fluorescence* until the late phases.

During its natural course, **progressive atrophy** of this material is associated with atrophy of the RPE.

On OCT

This hyper-reflective material is visualized anterior to the RPE, either in contact with or even fused with the RPE, or it can also be clearly distinct from the RPE.

These deposits displace the IS/OS interface and external limiting membrane and can even protrude into the outer nuclear layer or beyond.

Small deposits induce only minor changes of adjacent structures and usually remain asymptomatic (**Figure 16**). Larger deposits acquire a hyper-reflective cone-shaped appearance in contact and just anterior to the RPE, inducing slight shadowing.

Changes in the Outer Retinal Layers

In contact with these deposits, the IS/OS interface is often thickened and the outer nuclear layer appears thinned and displaced (**Figures 17 and 18**).

Clumps of material are often associated with the presence of soft drusen of various sizes (**Figure 19**).

This material can spread into the central fovea, with or without a surrounding reticular arrangement.

It is clearly visible on ICG angiography as it remains hypo-fluorescent until the late phases. These deposits are also well-visualized by SD-OCT (**Figure 20**).

During the subsequent course, this accumulation may be associated with various features of age-related maculopathy, such as drusen and particularly pigment migration (**Figure 20**).

Complications

It can also be associated with other degenerative complications, such as a lamellar macular hole (**Figure 21**).

These deposits fairly frequently, although slowly, progress to atrophy with irreversible functional loss.

During this process, the zone of hyper-reflectivity related to the substance in contact with and anterior to the RPE may be associated with an optically empty zone suggestive of fluid accumulation.

This fluid accumulation may raise difficult diagnostic problems as it is important to exclude the presence of neovascular complications (**Figure 22**).

The diagnosis can only be clearly established by comparing all imaging modalities.

DEPOSITS

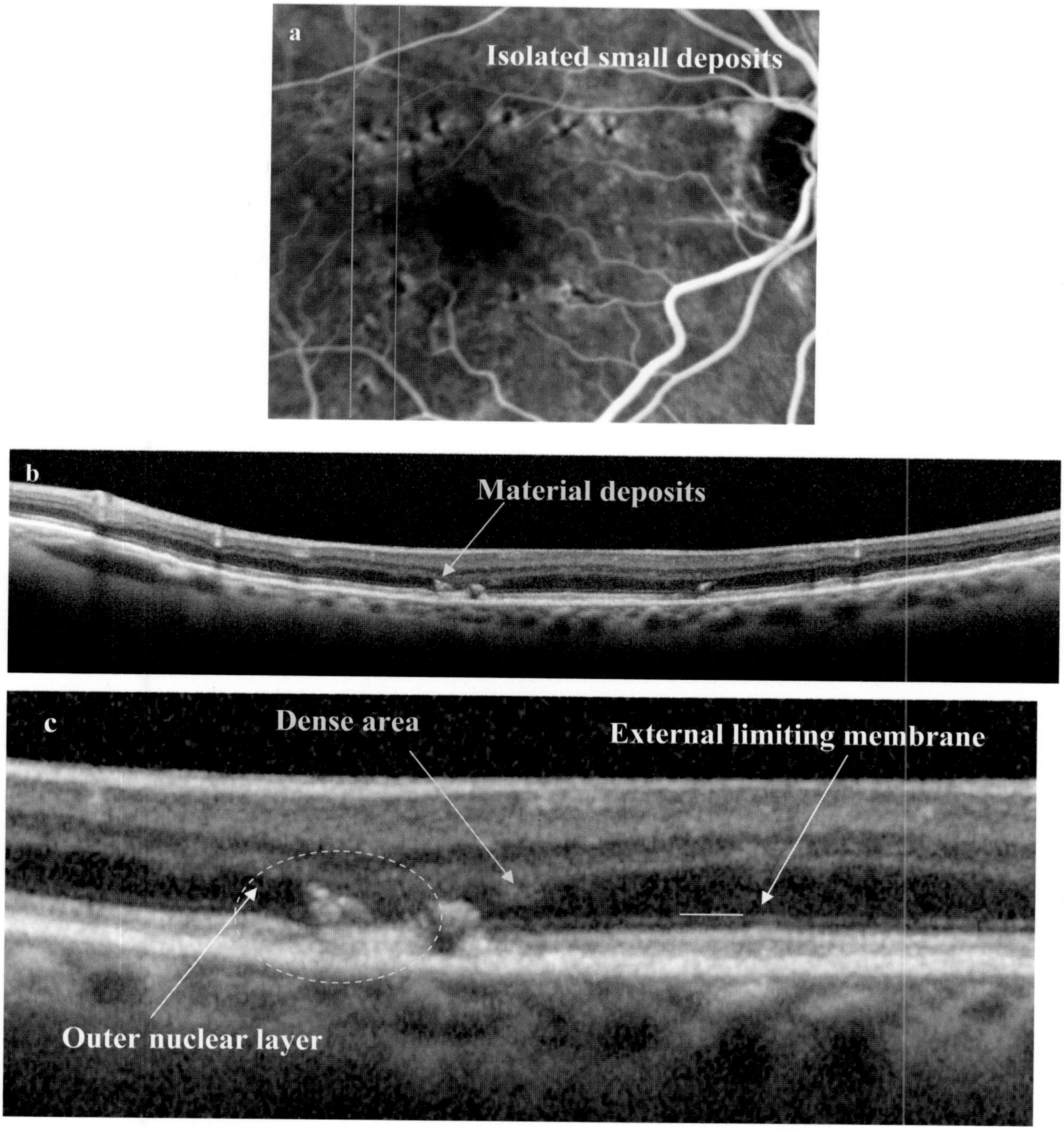

Figure 16: Isolated clumps of small perifoveolar deposits.

a): Fluorescein angiography: material visible in the form of small dark spots surrounded by a hyper-fluorescent halo.
b): *Spectralis supramacular horizontal section.**
On SD-OCT, clumps of hyper-reflective material are clearly visible anterior to the RPE, sometimes inducing posterior shadowing and raising the external limiting membrane, which is disrupted.
c): Enlarged image: the deposits are in the outer nuclear layer, with slightly increased density around the deposits. The other retinal layers remain unchanged without functional repercussions.

DEPOSITS

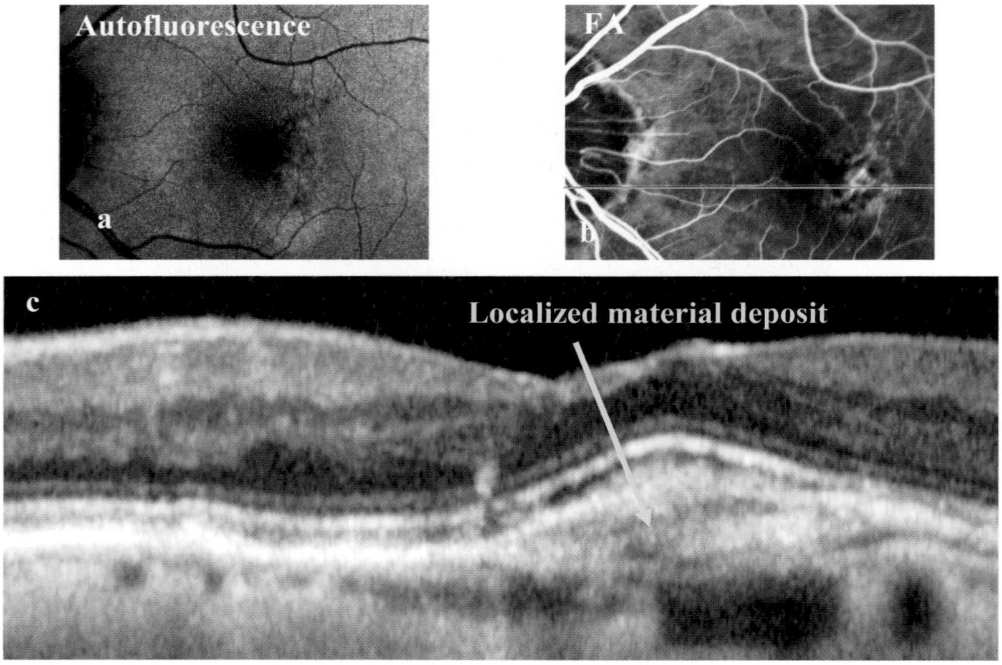

Figure 17: Vast area of temporo-macular deposits. VA: 20/40
a): **Autofluorescence**: the material is clearly visible in the temporo-macular zone.
b): **Fluorescein angiography**: zone of irregular material with late staining but no leakage.
c): ***Spectralis** supramacular horizontal section.**
On SD-OCT, the deposits are juxtafoveal and subfoveal, in contact with and anterior to the RPE, which is partially masked by shadowing. The deposits lift the IS/OS interface, which appears thickened but with no other marked changes. Another clump of deposits can be seen more anteriorly to the IS/OS interface.

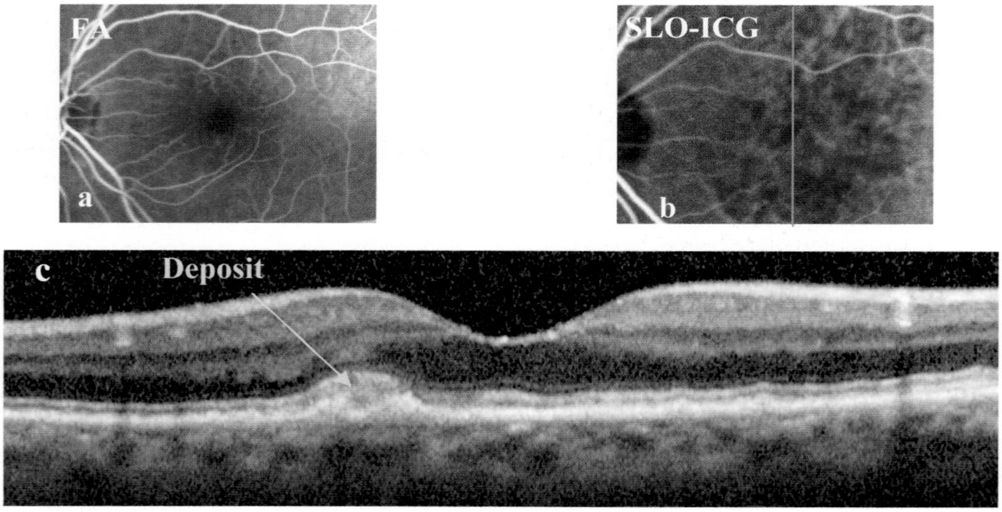

Figure 18: Clump of low-density deposits in the posterior pole.
a): **Fluorescein angiography**: the material is poorly visible.
b): **ICG angiography**: disseminated material seen as hypo-fluorescent spots.
c): ***Spectralis** macular vertical section.**
On SD-OCT, the material is moderately hyper-reflective, prominent, and in contact with the RPE, associated with thickening of the IS/OS interface and displacement or thinning of the outer nuclear layer.

DEPOSITS

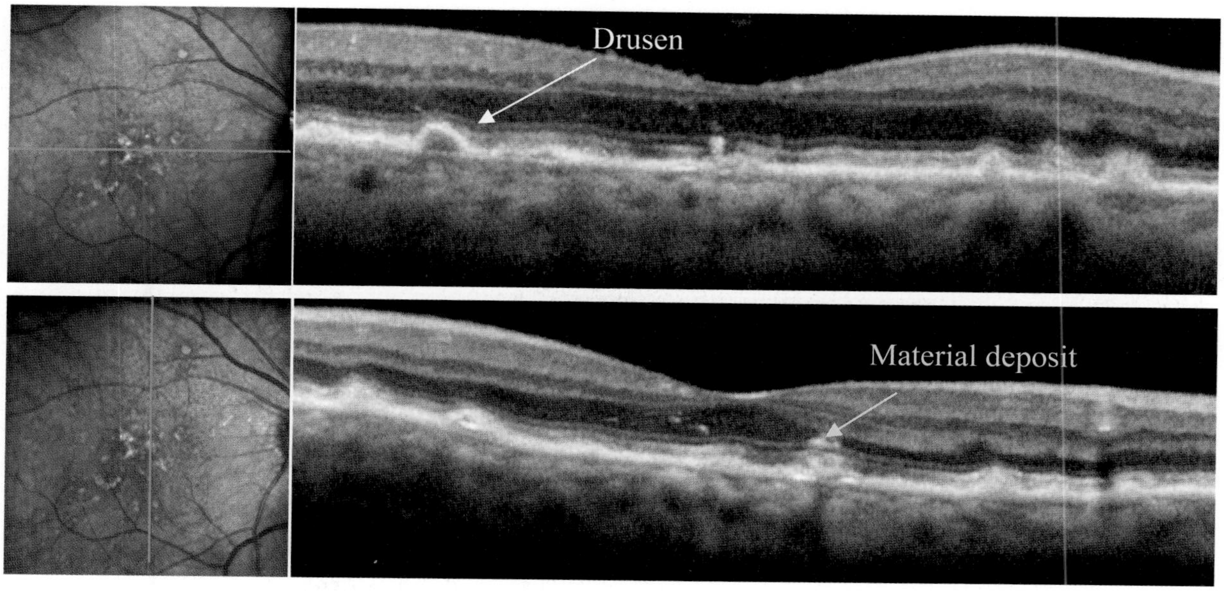

Figure 19: Small clumps of perifoveolar deposits and soft drusen. VA: 20/40.
***Spectralis** macular vertical and horizontal sections correlated with a reference image**: small clumps of pale yellow material in the middle of soft drusen.
On SD-OCT, the clumps of hyper-reflective deposits are clearly visible anterior to the RPE with posterior shadowing. The deposits lift the external limiting membrane and spread into the outer nuclear layer, with slightly increased density around the deposits. The other retinal layers remain unchanged.
Note the presence of several soft drusen with a different appearance and which have limited functional consequences.

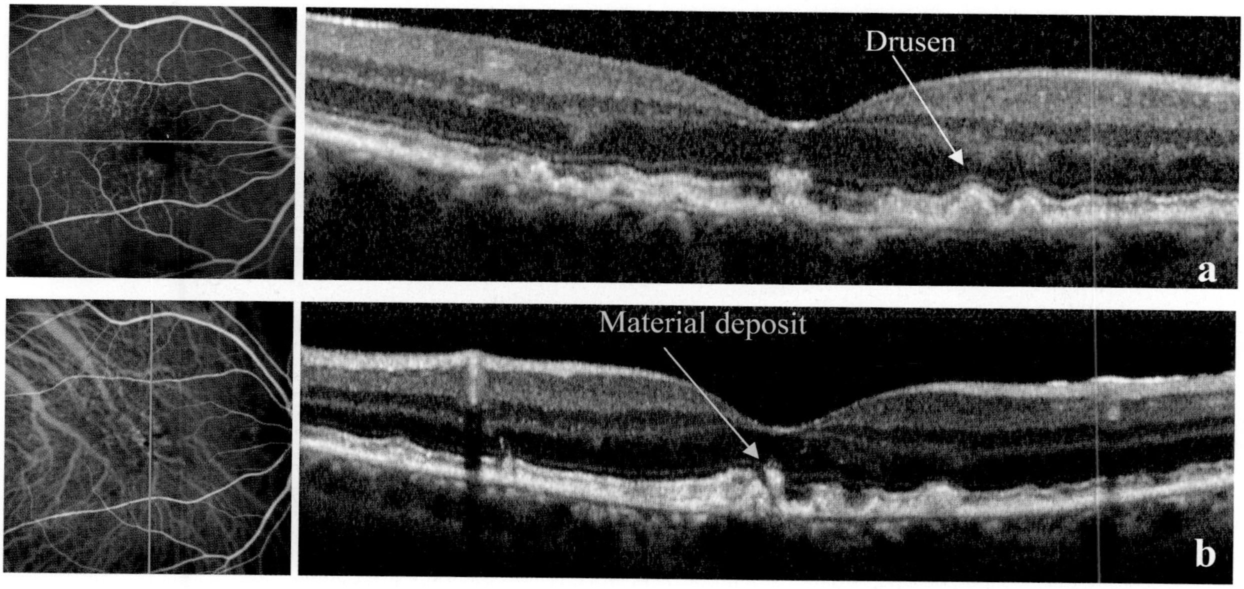

Figure 20: Subfoveal deposits. VA 20/63
a): *Spectralis horizontal macular section correlated with fluorescein angiography** *(dark hypo-fluorescent area).*
SD-OCT shows the presence of clearly visible, subfoveal hyper-reflective material, extending beyond the IS/OS interface and external limiting membrane in the middle of tightly packed drusen (with slight modification of the interface).
b): *Spectralis vertical section correlated with ICG angiography** *(hypo-fluorescent material).*
On SD-OCT, accumulation and proliferation of material, clearly visible anterior to the RPE and under the external limiting membrane.

DEPOSITS

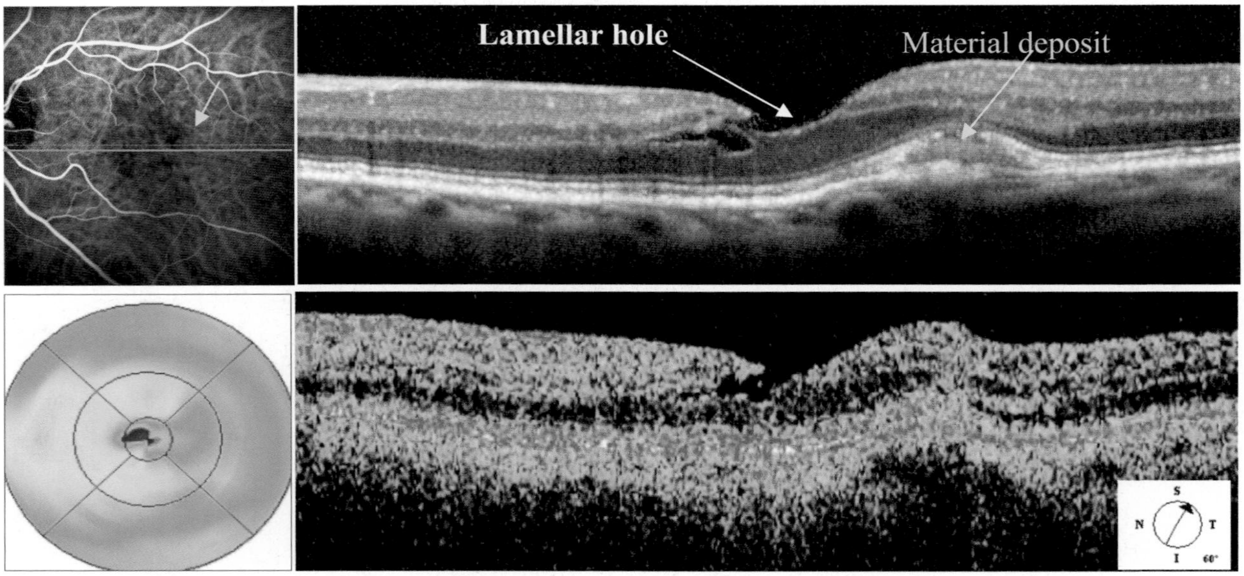

◘ Figure 21: Juxtafoveal deposits associated with a lamellar macular hole. VA: 20/32.
a): *Spectralis horizontal section correlated with ICG angiography** *(hypo-fluorescent juxtafoveal area).*
On SD-OCT, adjacent to the lamellar macular hole, presence of clearly visible, hyper-reflective material, which has accumulated slowly during observation of the fellow eye. Note the alteration of the outer nuclear layer.
b): *Stratus oblique section combined with retinal mapping.**
TD-OCT visualizes the deposits and the alteration of the outer nuclear layer.

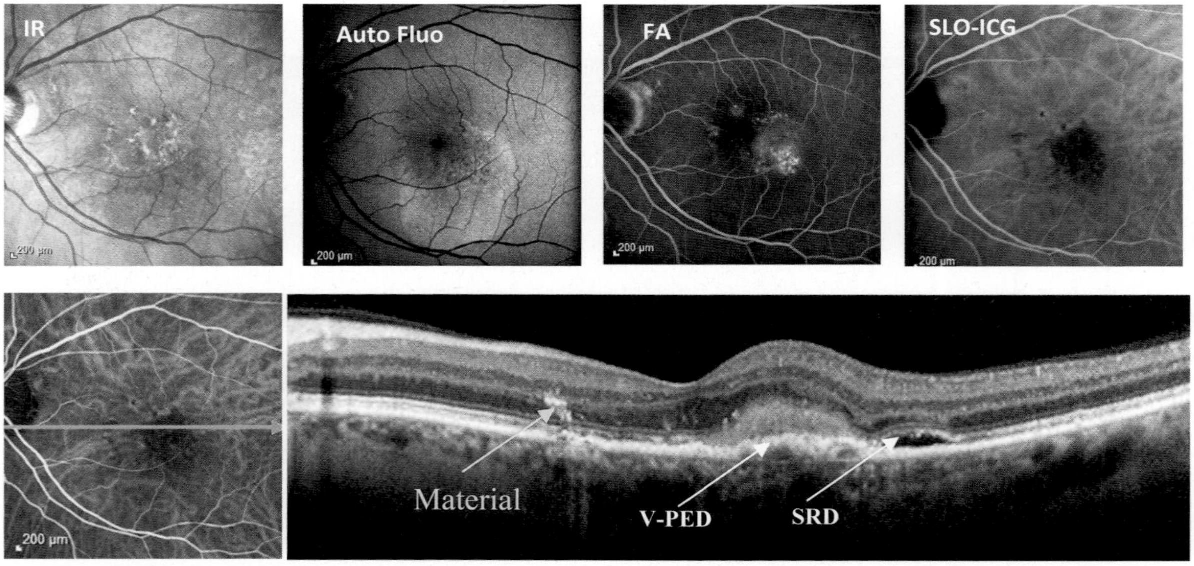

◘ Figure 22: Subfoveal deposits. VA: 20/63.
a): Monochromatic autofluorescence imaging and fluorescein and ICG angiography: vast, slightly raised, autofluorescent and predominantly shifting macular lesion. Fluorescein angiography shows irregular hyper-fluorescence with fluorescein leakage and pinpoint leakage. ICG angiography shows a dark PED and a thin neovascular network. The central black area is suggestive of deposits.
b): *Spectralis horizontal section.**
On SD-OCT, complex lesion comprised of drusen, deposits, a vascularized PED, and occult CNV. SRF and alterations of the outer layers (IS/OS interface, external limiting membrane, and outer nuclear layer) with a dense zone anterior to the PED.

Clinical Features and Natural History of AMD on OCT

2. Age-Related Macular Degeneration

Gabriel COSCAS
Florence COSCAS, Sabrina VISMARA,
Alain ZOURDANI, C.I. Li CALZI

(Créteil and Paris)

2. Age-Related Macular Degeneration

Diagnosis, Observation, and Post Treatment Follow-Up

Introduction

Despite recent progress, age-related macular degeneration (AMD) remains the leading cause of **vision loss** in high-income countries, and its incidence appears to be increasing, probably due to longer life span and improved methods of detection.

The **prevalence** of AMD is higher in women than in men, and most importantly, increases with age, affecting about 3% of the population between the ages of 70 and 80 years and more than 12% after 80 years.

Neovascular AMD

Neovascular AMD represent 50% to 65% of advanced AMD, while the other cases correspond to atrophic forms without neovascularization.

Risk factors influencing the course of wet AMD are similar to those of age-related maculopathy (ARM) and essentially comprise risk factors for arteriosclerosis (hypertension and hyperlipidemia), environmental, and lifestyle factors.

However, recently identified genetic factors also probably play a very important role in the pathogenesis of AMD (*Souïed 2005-2007*).

Wet AMD is usually associated with loss of **central vision and metamorphopsia**.

Classic (pre-retinal) choroidal neovascularization (CNV) generally causes rapid and severe loss of macular vision.

In contrast, occult choroidal neovascularization (subretinal or vascularized pigment epithelium detachment) causes slowly progressive symptoms.

These symptoms may remain undiagnosed for a long time, and all too often, occult CNV is diagnosed at its late stages.

Fundus imaging provides an important contribution to the early and precise detection and diagnosis of AMD.

Monochromatic, color fundus photographs, and autofluorescence images document anatomical landmarks to monitor the progression of signs of ARM along with its exudative (PED, SRF lipid exudates) and hemorrhagic complications.

However, only angiography can directly visualize choroidal neovascularization:

- *Fluorescein angiography* demonstrates classic choroidal neovascularization.
- *Indocyanine green SLO-angiography* demonstrates occult choroidal neovascularization.

Optical Coherence Tomography (OCT) is a noninvasive imaging modality that precisely identifies **indirect signs** related to abnormal exudation (intraretinal fluid and increased retinal thickness).

Modern ***Spectral-Domain OCT*** techniques can also **directly analyze** the impact of choroidal neovascularization on outer retinal layers and evaluate alterations of photoreceptors and inner and outer segments.

Occult Choroidal Neovascularization

Occult choroidal neovascularization is by far the most frequent form of neovascular proliferation during AMD.

This form is described as "occult" because it is poorly-delineated or ill-defined on fluorescein angiography.

First described in 1987 (*Soubrane and Coscas*) as a result of progress in angiographic analysis and subsequently confirmed by indocyanine green angiography, occult CNV appears to represent more than 80% to 85% of all cases of wet AMD. It is often located subfoveally at the time of the diagnosis.

Comparative analysis of OCT and angiography has shown that occult choroidal neovascularization always induces a pigment epithelium detachment from what is now known to be Bruch's membrane (*Coscas F, 2007*).

Clinical Classification of Occult Choroidal Neovascularization

Many **names and classifications** for occult choroidal neovascularization have been successively proposed. These various classifications are essentially designed to guide therapeutic indications.

Clinical Features

Several types of occult CNV can be distinguished according to the type of proliferation, the natural history of the lesion, or its response to available treatments (**Figure 1**).

8

Occult CNV can induce various types of retinal pigment epithelium detachment (PED):

Predominantly Fibrovascular PED

The most frequent from of occult CNV (65%) is a fibrovascular PED, in which the exudative reaction is usually moderate (**Figure 1b and c**).

CNV Accompanied by a Serous PED

This fluid accumulation is due to an intense exudative reaction.

This form (12% to 15% of cases) consists of formation of a bullous PED adjacent to an occult CNV, which is often located in a notch of the PED (**Figure 1d**).

Occult CNV can subsequently invade the entire PED cavity.

Hot Spot Appearance

Occult CNV is juxtafoveal, located inside the PED (**Figure 1e**).

The RPE elevation is essentially serous, rounded, and extends to various degrees.

CNV is associated with chorioretinal anastomosis (12% to 15% of cases).

Polypoidal Choroidal Vasculopathy

Polypoidal choroidal vasculopathy (PCV) is often considered to resemble occult CNV.

PCV does not have all of the features of AMD, but it can be complicated by macular choroidal neovascularization.

Treatment

Direct **thermal laser** photocoagulation of occult CNV is effective in only a limited number of cases.

Photodynamic therapy usually only allows stabilization rather than improvement of the lesions.

Current treatments based on **intravitreal injections of anti-VEGF** appear to have changed the prognosis of occult CNV.

Intravitreal injections of anti-VEGF allow stabilization in almost every case and also improvement of visual acuity in more than one-third of patients, especially when treatment is initiated early.

Combination therapies are currently under evaluation.

MAIN TYPES OF CHOROIDAL NEOVASCULARIZATION

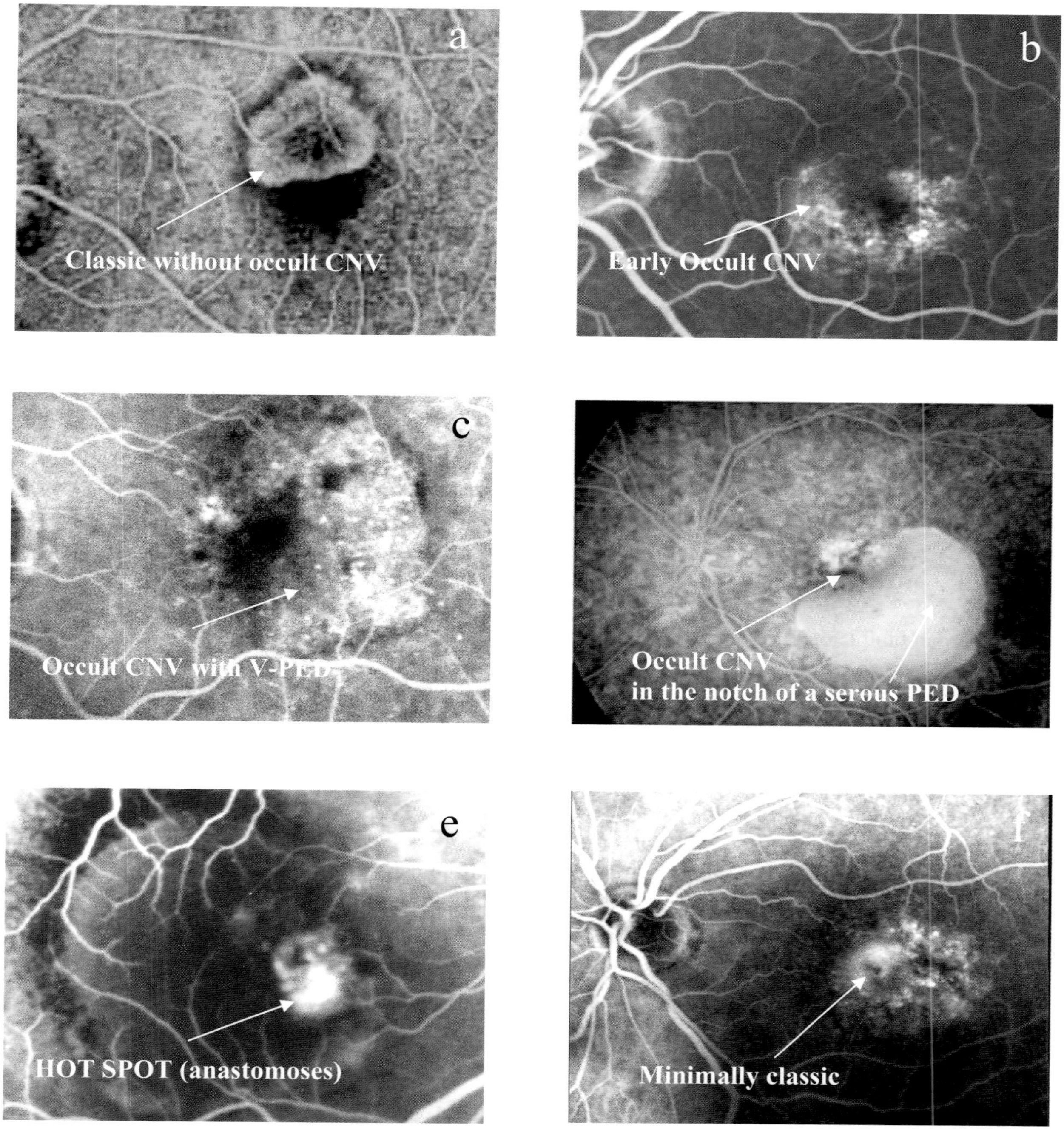

Figure 1: Main types of choroidal neovascularization on fluorescein angiography.

a): Pure classic CNV with no occult CNV.
b): Small-size occult CNV.
c): Extensive occult CNV and fibrovascular PED detachment.
d): Occult CNV in a notch of a bullous serous PED.
e): Hot spot in a serous PED: chorioretinal anastomosis.
f): Mixed CNV with a small area of classic CNV in a zone of occult CNV (*minimally classic*).

CLINICAL CASES

CLINICAL CASE No. 01: OCCULT CNV – INITIAL STAGE, ASYMPTOMATIC
Initial, dormant lesion, discovered on clinical examination of the fellow eye .... Page 206

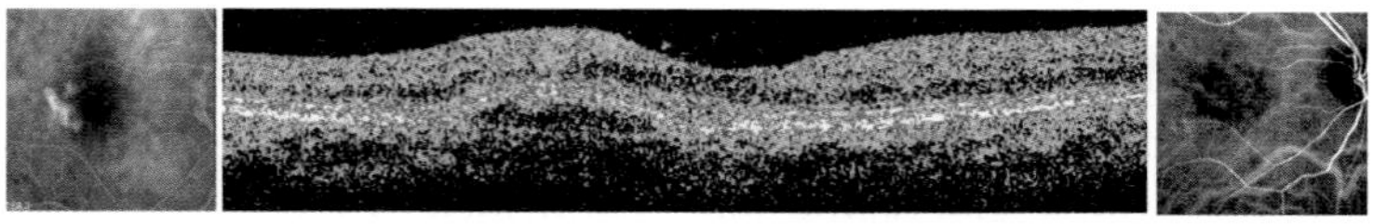

CLINICAL CASE No. 02: OCCULT CNV – INITIAL STAGE, SYMPTOMATIC
Lesion at the initial clinical stage, after onset of the first symptoms .... Page 210

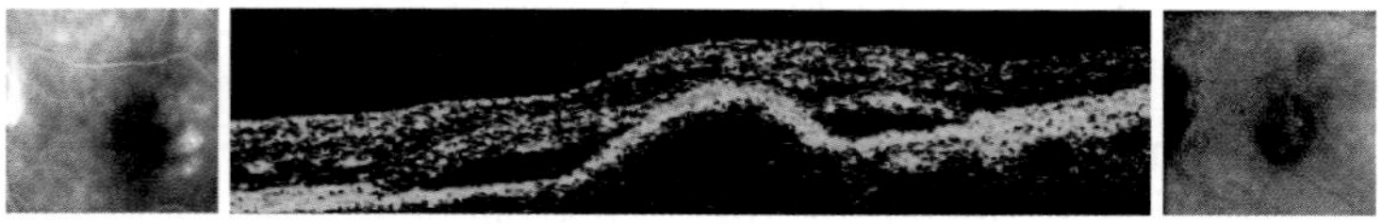

CLINICAL CASE No. 03: OCCULT CNV – EARLY, SMALL
Typical early form, present for several months .... Page 212

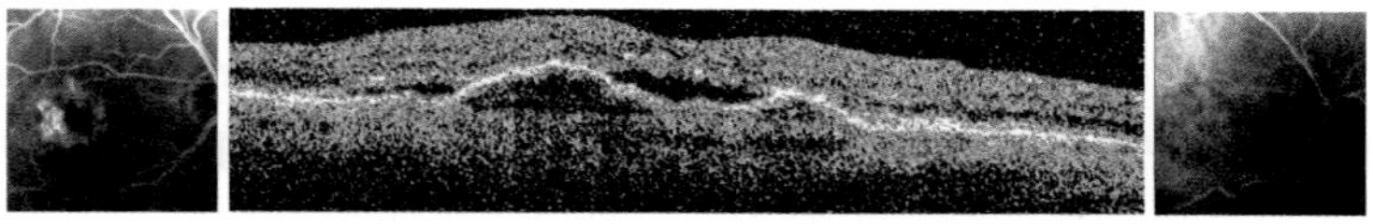

CLINICAL CASE No. 04: OCCULT CNV – MODERATELY LARGE
Occult CNV, with symptoms present for more than 6 months ....Page 216

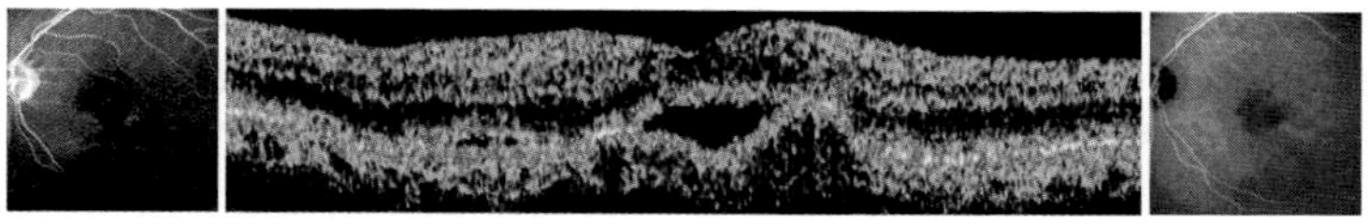

CLINICAL CASE No. 05: OCCULT CNV – MINIMALLY CLASSIC
Occult CNV associated with a small area of *minimally classic* CNV .... Page 222

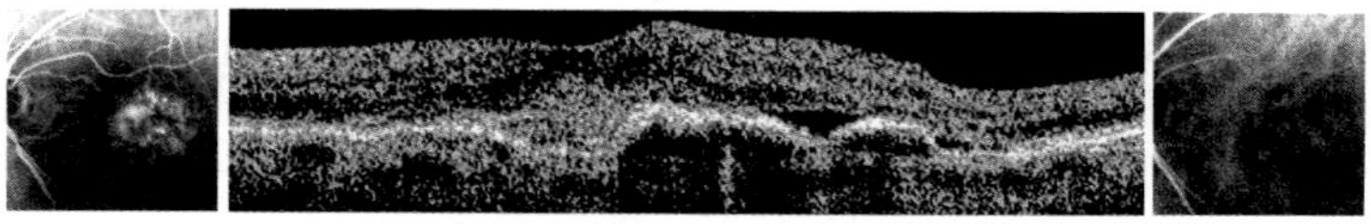

CLINICAL CASE No. 06: OCCULT CNV – MINIMALLY CLASSIC
Occult CNV, recently deteriorated, with symptoms related to minimally classic CNV .... Page 226

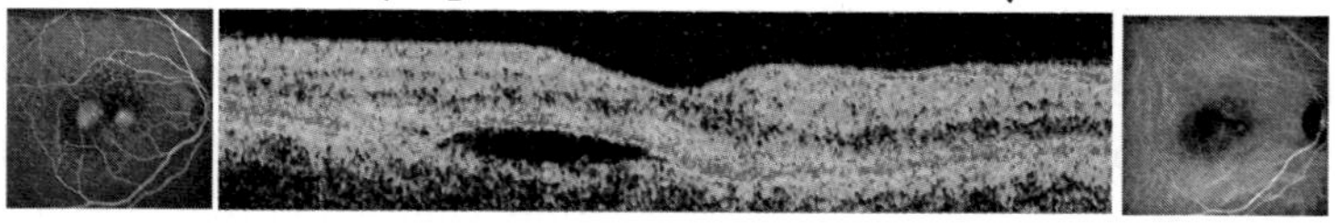

CLINICAL CASE No. 07: OCCULT CNV – LARGE
Occult CNV, progressing over many months, with moderate symptoms .... Page 232

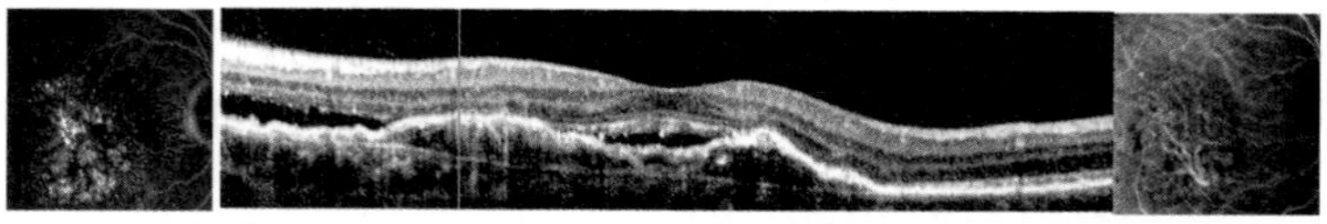

CLINICAL CASE No. 08: MIXED (CLASSIC AND OCCULT) CNV OF EQUAL DIMENSIONS
Mixed CNV, **progressing over many months**, with moderate symptoms .... Page 240

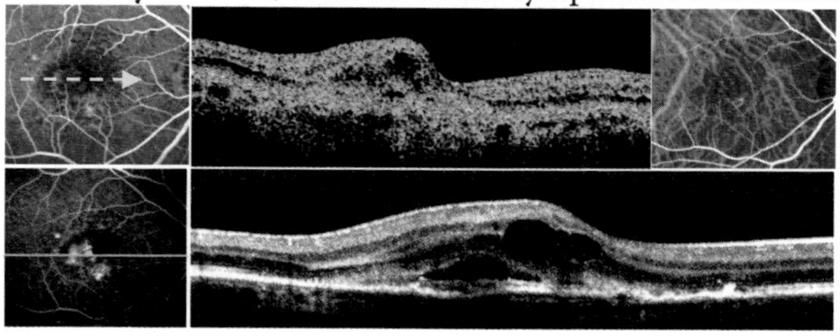

CLINICAL CASE No. 09: PROGRESSIVE PROLIFERATION OF OCCULT CNV
Occult CNV, *gradually deteriorating and recurring on an old laser scar* .... Page 246

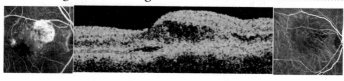

CLINICAL CASE No. 10: OCCULT CNV WITH SEROUS PED
Typical occult CNV, *moderately large with exudation and a dome-shaped PED* .... Page 252

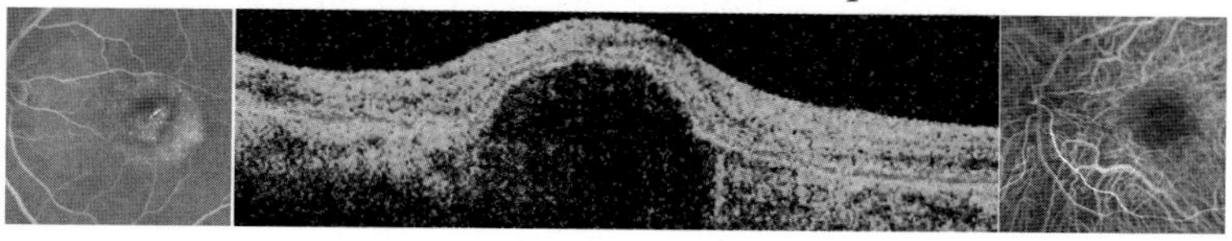

CLINICAL CASE No. 11: OCCULT CNV AT THE EDGE OF SEROUS PED
Bullous and serous PED, *arising at the edge of typical occult CNV* .... Page 256

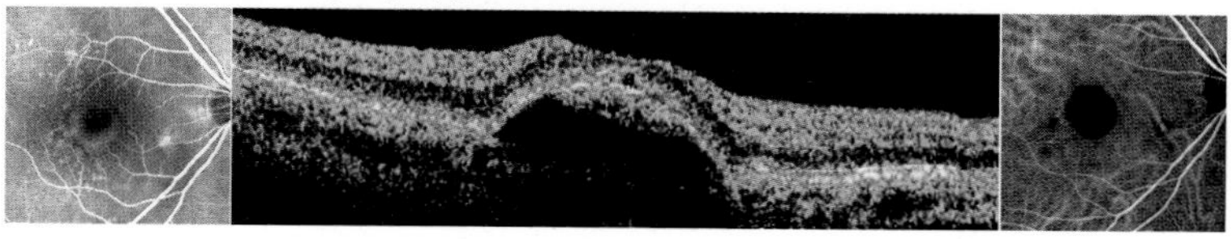

CLINICAL CASE No. 12: LARGE, ADVANCED, OCCULT CNV
Longstanding vascularized PED, *present for more than one year* .... Page 260

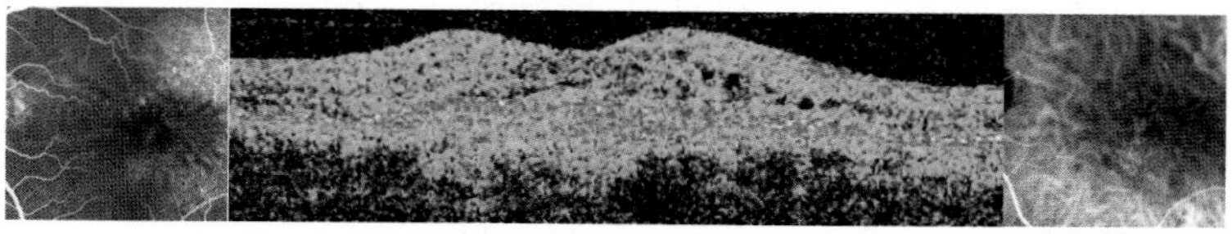

CLINICAL CASE No. 13: HEMORRHAGIC COMPLICATIONS OF OCCULT CNV
Vast macular hemorrhage *and intraretinal hemorrhage* .... Page 264

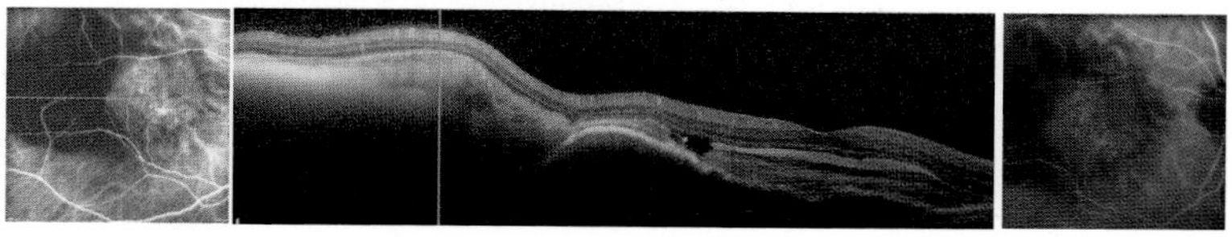

CLINICAL CASE No. 14: ADVANCED CNV WITH HEMORRHAGIC COMPLICATIONS
Vast macular hemorrhage *around and away from CNV* .... Page 266

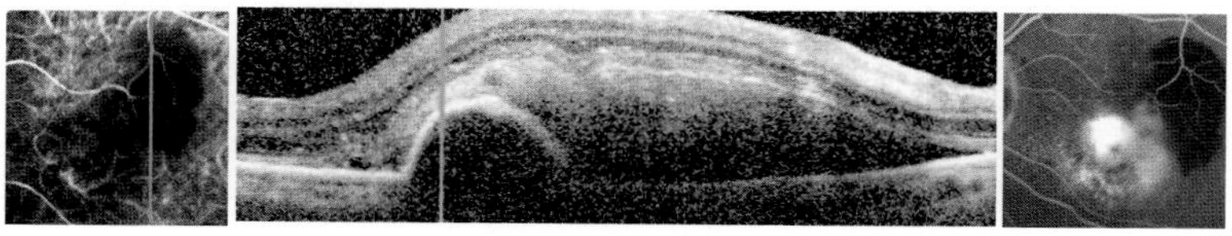

CLINICAL CASE No. 15: ADVANCED OCCULT CNV
Longstanding extensive lesion, *continuing to progress with persistent symptoms* .... Page 268

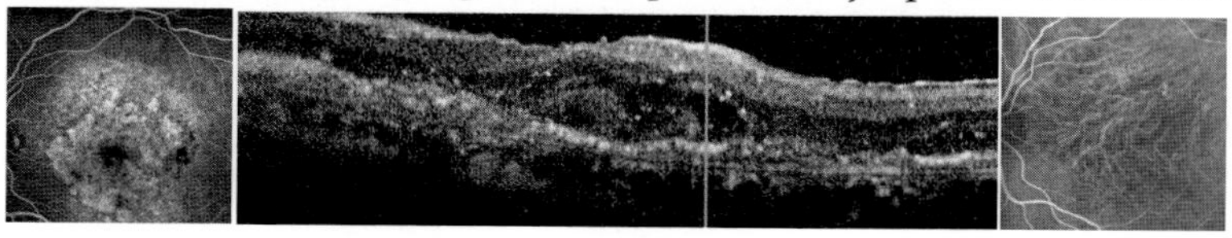

CLINICAL CASE No. 01: Occult CNV – Initial Stage, Asymptomatic

Initial, dormant lesion *discovered on complete clinical examination of the fellow eye in a woman with wet AMD. Natural history of the lesion during 3 year's follow-up without treatment.*

Clinical and Biomicroscopic Signs

A 72-year-old woman treated for wet AMD in her left eye reported no symptoms in her right eye.

Both eyes were regularly examined.

VA RE: 20/20 – VA LE: 20/40.

Clinical examination revealed a few, medium-sized soft drusen, predominantly perifoveal with no SRF or hemorrhage.

Autofluorescence Image

No alteration in the foveal area (of xanthophyll pigment). Presence of a minimal hyper-fluorescence in the temporal macular area with no signs of SRF (**Figure 2**).

Angiography (Figure 2)

Fluorescein angiography: progressive, irregular, poorly-delineated, temporal macular hyper-fluorescence over 1 disc diameter with several sites of fluorescein leakage and pinpoints. There is also central masking by xanthophyll pigment, which represents a false image of foveal sparing.

ICG angiography: multiple irregular hyper-fluorescence zones within the dark background of the PED occupying the subfoveal macula. This lesion was suggestive of a barely visible neovascular network. Presence of a poorly-delineated plaque in the late phase.

Suggested Angiographic Diagnosis:
Area of occult CNV in a very small PED without hemorrhage (dormant), with no signs of decompensation and no symptoms.

Contribution of OCT

OCT showed a minimal, regular, thin PED.

However, separation of the RPE from Bruch's membrane (BM) that became clearly visible, confirmed the presence of a PED with a homogeneous, moderately reflective cavity and minimal shadowing.

The exudative reaction was very minor, causing only a slight increase in retinal thickness, but no SRF or cysts (**Figure 3**).

The outer nuclear layer was also thinned over the juxtafoveal PED, which extended as far as the center of the fovea.

The other retinal layers were not altered.

The foveal depression remained unchanged and preserved its normal profile (**Figure 3**).

Diagnosis

In this clinical case, whereby ophthalmological examination was performed in the context of follow-up of the fellow eye, imaging demonstrated an early stage of asymptomatic and uncomplicated CNV.

Fluorescein angiography demonstrated a limited area of irregular hyper-fluorescence with pinpoints, suggesting occult CNV with false image of foveal sparing due to xanthophyll pigment.

SLO-ICG angiography confirmed the presence of subfoveal CNV measuring 1.5 DD. It was characterized by clearly visible hyper-fluorescence which contrasted with the dark and hypo-fluorescent PED.

The diagnosis was therefore confirmed: recent, isolated ***occult choroidal neovascularization or vascularized PED*** without signs of decompensation and asymptomatic.

There was no indication for treatment at this stage (particularly at the time of the initial diagnosis, when PDT was the only available treatment modality).

The patient was reassessed every six months.

CLINICAL CASE No. 01: OCCULT CNV – INITIAL STAGE, ASYMPTOMATIC

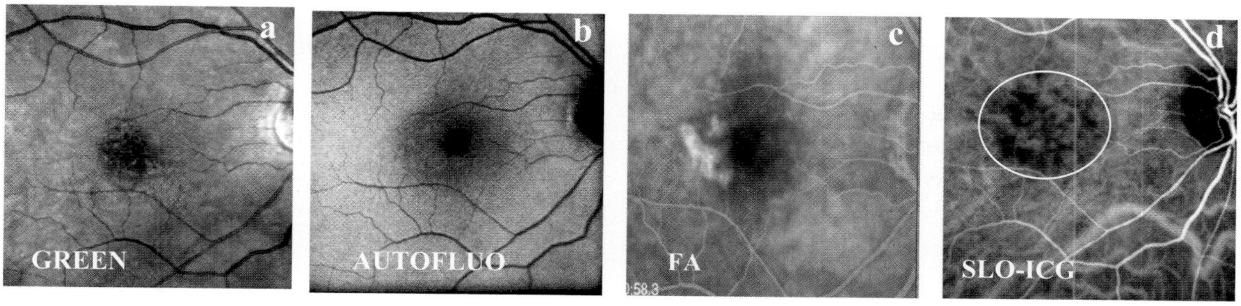

Figure 2: Occult CNV: initial, dormant stage. a): Red-free photograph: a few soft drusen. **b): Autofluorescence**: small temporal hyper-fluorescence. **c): Fluorescein angiography**: delayed, localized, temporal hyper-fluorescence. **d): SLO-ICG angiography:** poorly-defined, subfoveal neovascular membrane against the dark PED.

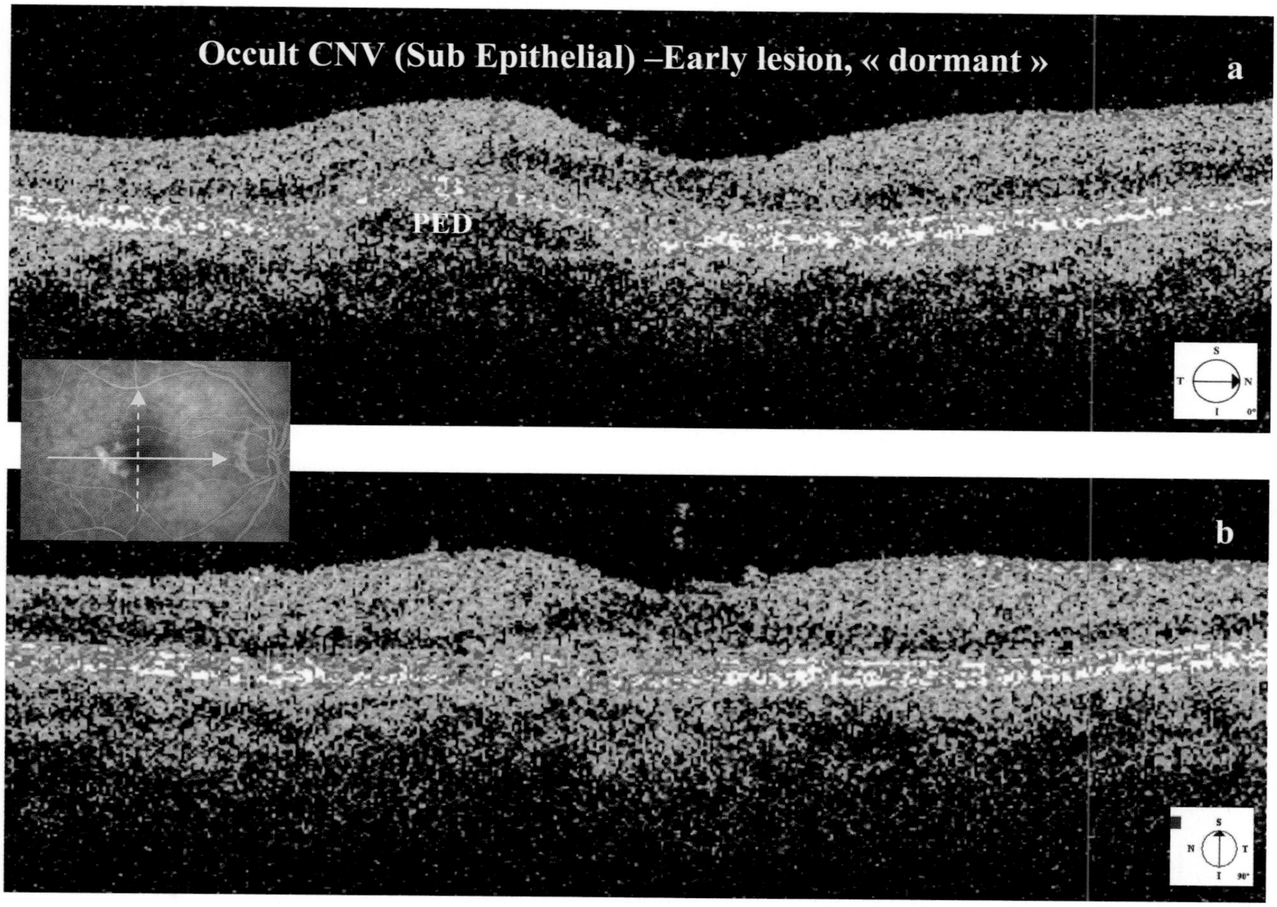

Figure 3: Occult CNV in the initial, dormant stage.

a): Stratus* horizontal section: minimal, localized, juxtafoveal and subfoveal elevation of the RPE with no irregularities of the RPE. The cavity is slightly reflective, homogeneous and allows Bruch's membrane to be visible with only minimal shadowing. No fluid accumulation anterior to the RPE. Retinal thickness remains unchanged and the foveal depression is preserved.

b) Stratus* vertical section: Slightly increased retinal thickness and irregularities of the outer nuclear layer.

CLINICAL CASE No. 01: Occult CNV – Initial Stage, Asymptomatic

3 Year Follow-Up

Follow-up of the natural history of this lesion was obtained in the context of observation of the fellow eye over a period of 30-months by evaluation of visual acuity and imaging by OCT, fluorescein angiography, and ICG angiography.

The natural history was initially reassuring with relatively minor and slowly progressive changes and maintenance of almost normal visual acuity, perceived as comfortable by the patient.

The decision to treat this fellow eye was taken after a decline in visual acuity (5/10) experienced at the 30th month, especially as imaging confirmed the deterioration.

On OCT, the initially minimal PED gradually spread over a larger area and became thicker with a more irregular and wavy appearance.

The RPE did not appear to be thickened or fragmented, and the cavity remained moderately reflective.

On the other hand, the moderate intraretinal fluid persisted and then increased with alteration of the outer nuclear layer (**Figure 4a**).

OCT showed diffuse intraretinal fluid that appeared to slightly dissociate the various retinal layers, even affecting the inner plexiform layer with a layer of subretinal fluid (**Figure 4b**).

At the fifth examination, this serous SRF had become larger, involving almost all of the foveal region. This major change associated with the loss of visual acuity led to the decision to initiate treatment.

On the first **fluorescein angiography** examination, the hyper-fluorescent zone appeared to remain unchanged and was only visible in the temporal macular zone.

However, at the fourth and especially the fifth examination, it occupied 2/3 of the foveal area but always with slow and late fluorescein leakage from occult choroidal neovascularization (**Figure 4c**).

On **ICG angiography**, the image of occult CNV contrasting with the dark PED changed very little, but each examination confirmed that the lesion was subfoveal and occupied all of the fovea.

At the last examination, the lesions had clearly worsened on all three imaging modalities in parallel with loss of visual acuity (**Figure 4d**).

Conclusion

This lesion consisted of occult CNV detected during systematic examination of the fellow eye. There was an absence of any symptoms, which had remained dormant and stable for more than two years.

The diagnosis was confirmed by the various imaging modalities, despite the absence of symptoms.

A wait-and-see approach, requested by the patient, appeared justified in view of the excellent quality of vision and the limited treatment available at that time.

However, clinical observation subsequently demonstrated deterioration allowing rapid introduction of intravitreous anti-VEGF therapy.

The immediate result, with improvement of visual acuity and resolution of symptoms, reassured the patient to such a degree that she wanted to stop injections after the first session.

The persistence of several abnormalities on the various imaging modalities justified maintenance of regular observation, at least every three months (or more frequently, if new symptoms developed).

CLINICAL CASE No. 01: OCCULT CNV – INITIAL STAGE, ASYMPTOMATIC
3 Year Follow-up

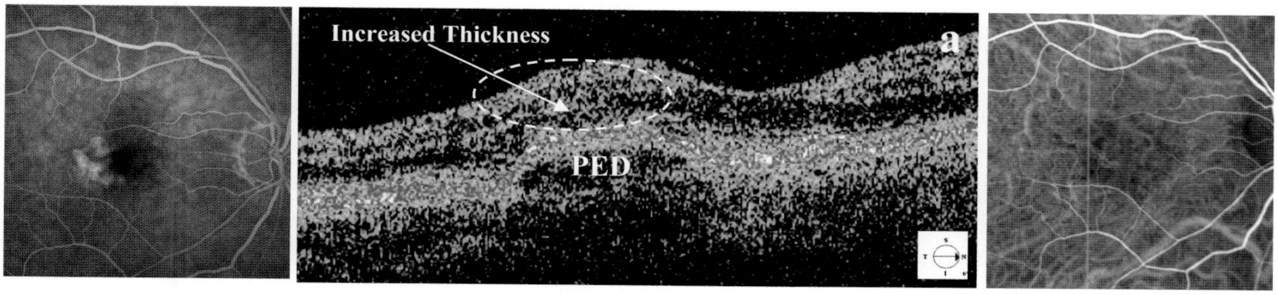

Figure 4: Occult CNV at the initial, dormant stage.
a:) 6th month: notice the identical appearance. Alteration of the outer nuclear layer just over the PED with increased retinal thickness. Normal visual acuity: 20/20.

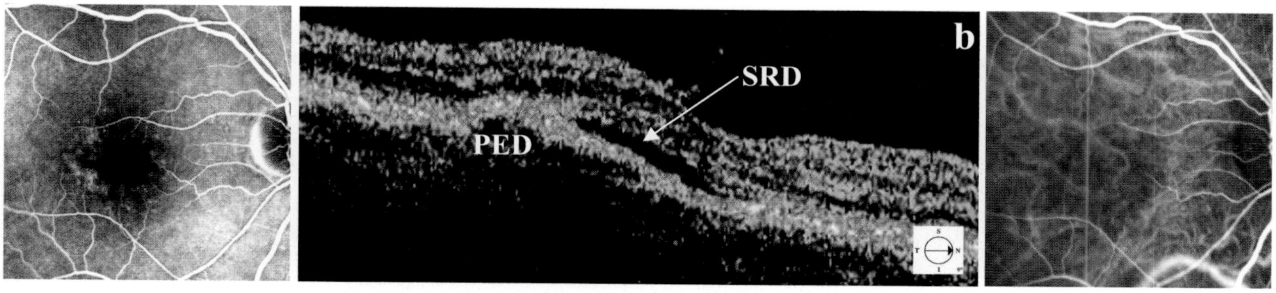

Figure 4: Occult CNV at the initial, dormant stage.
b): At 12th month: marked accentuation of exudation with intraretinal fluid and especially SRF VA: 20/30.

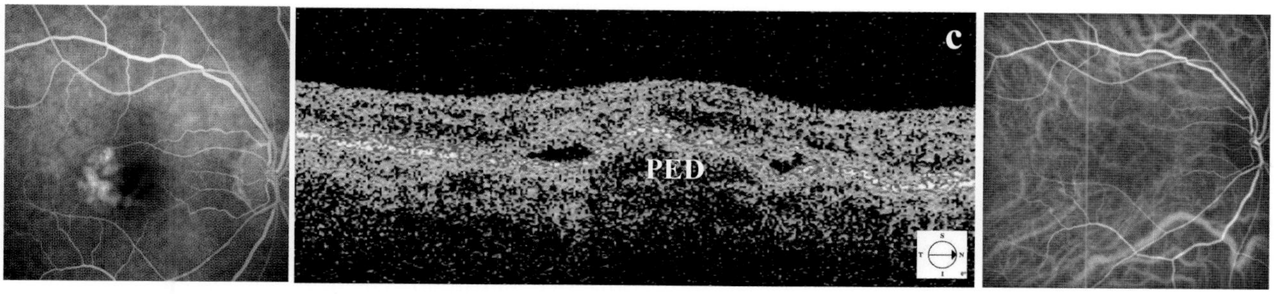

Figure 4: Occult CNV at the initial, dormant stage.
c): At 18th month: almost stable appearance of the PED and SRF. Treatment not yet initiated (at the patient's request). VA: 20/25.

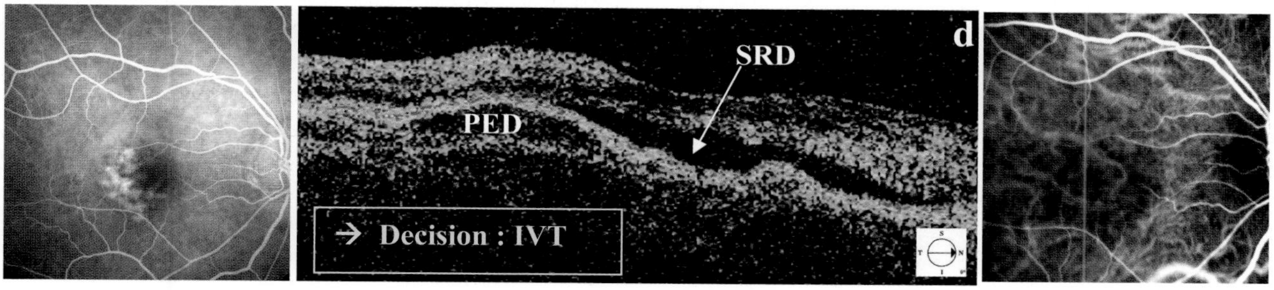

Figure 4: Occult CNV at the initial, dormant stage.
d): At 30th month: slight extension of the lesion and marked deterioration of the SRF and the PED. VA: 20/40 → **Decision to initiate intravitreal anti-VEGF therapy**.

CLINICAL CASE No. 02: Occult CNV – Initial Stage, Symptomatic

Lesion at initial stage, after onset of the first symptoms, leading to the discovery of occult CNV. Course in response to PDT, 2 year follow-up.

Clinical Signs

A 72-year-old woman experienced loss of visual acuity in the left eye to 20/50 about three weeks prior to presentation, associated with worrisome metamorphopsias.

Vision in the other eye was normal at this stage.
VA RE: 20/20 - VA LE: 20/50.

Biomicroscopic examination showed a few soft drusen and a small SRF about 1 DD, without hemorrhage or exudate.

Fluorescein angiography: Progressive, heterogeneous and poorly-delineated temporal macular hyper-fluorescence measuring about 1 DD with diffuse and pinpoint leakage. Central masking by xanthophyll pigment.
SLO-ICG angiography: Irregular subfoveal area of hyperfluorescence within the dark PED, suggesting occult CNV (**Figure 5**).

Suggested Angiographic Diagnosis:
Occult CNV within a small PED.

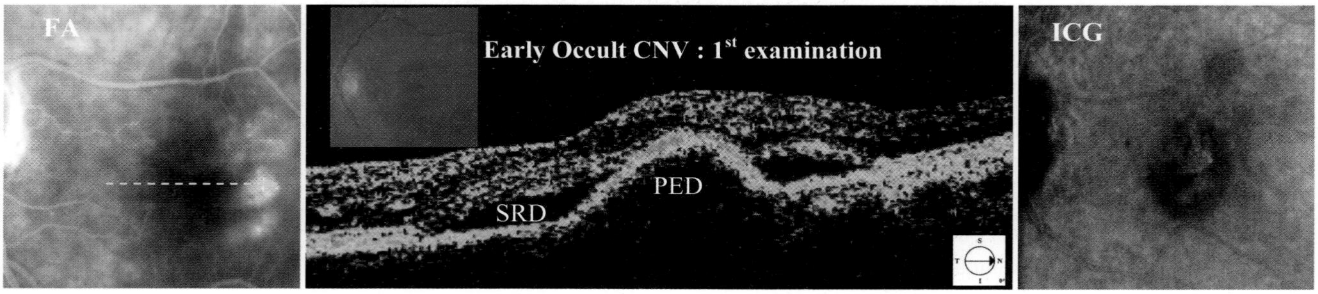

Figure 5: Occult CNV, initial stage after onset of the first symptoms.
Horizontal section (Stratus) correlated with fluorescein and SLO-ICG angiography.* Presence of a fairly prominent, rounded, regular, juxtafoveal PED associated with SRF (surrounding the PED) and slightly increased retinal thickness.

Diagnosis and Follow-Up

OCT confirmed the diagnosis suggested by angiography by showing diffuse intraretinal fluid with increased retinal thickness.
A serous retinal detachment was also clearly visible on OCT but with no disorganization of retinal layers.
The RPE was slightly irregular and thinned with a rounded, regular but fairly prominent PED displacing the retina and SRF surrounding the PED (**Figure 5**).
The diagnosis of occult choroidal neovascularization with PED and SRF was confirmed, consistent with the patient's loss of visual acuity (4/10) experienced for several weeks. Photodynamic therapy, the only available treatment at that time, was initiated immediately. The response to treatment was immediately favorable with resolution of the SRF and improvement of VA, despite persistence of the unchanged PED. Subsequent follow-up at the 6th month, one year, and two years showed remarkable stabilization of the lesion and VA at 20/32-20/40.
There was little change in the angiographic signs, but the lesion also did not deteriorate (**Figure 6a, b, and c**).
On OCT, the PED was flat but hypo-reflective with no signs of fibrosis. The neurosensory retina had a normal architecture with good visibility of the IS/OS interface and no SRF (**Figure 6d**).

Conclusion: Initial stage of occult CNV at the time of the first symptoms, leading to the detection of the occult CNV. The response to PDT was favorable. At the 2-year examination, the lesions had remained stable with satisfactory visual acuity.

CLINICAL CASE No. 02: OCCULT CNV – INITIAL STAGE, SYMPTOMATIC
Post PDT follow-up

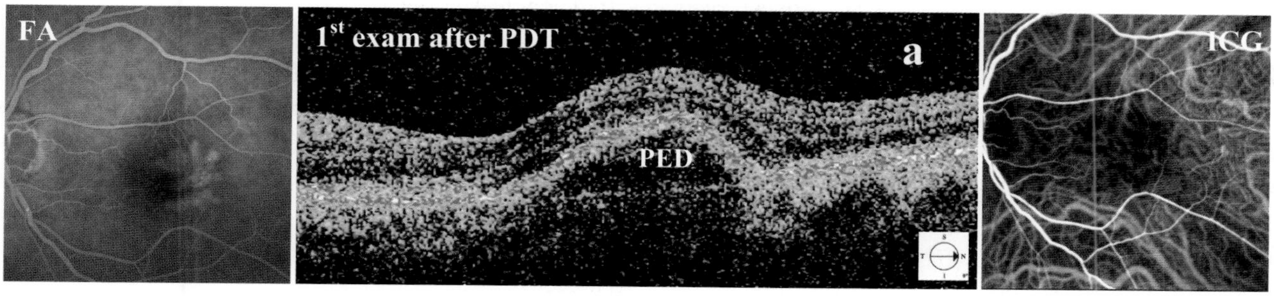

Figure 6: Initial stage of occult CNV after photodynamic therapy.
a): Three months after the first PDT session: marked improvement of intraretinal fluid and SRF almost identical appearance of the PED. VA: 20/40.

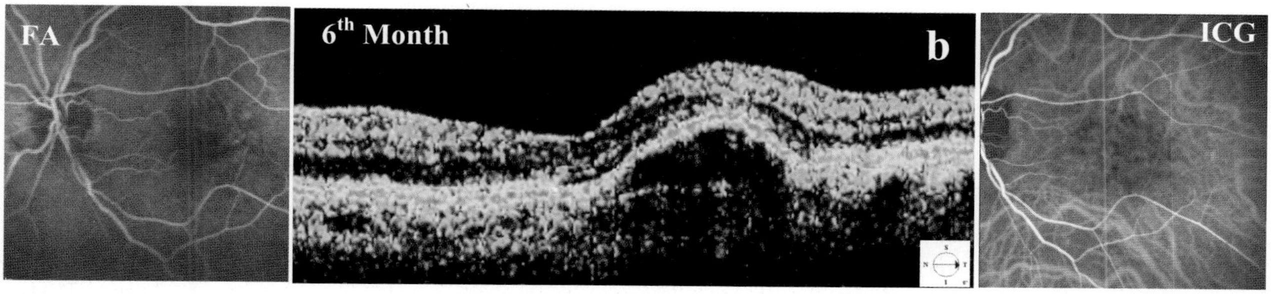

Figure 6: Initial stage of occult CNV after photodynamic therapy.
b): Six months later: almost identical appearance. Persistence of the PED. VA: 20/40 stable. → **No further treatment.**

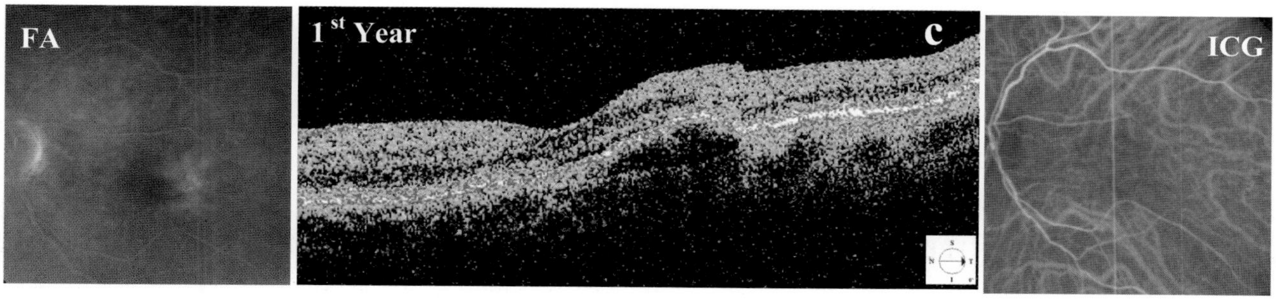

Figure 6: Initial stage of occult CNV after photodynamic therapy.
c): One year later: Stabilization of angiographic and OCT signs. VA: 20/40 → **No further treatment.**

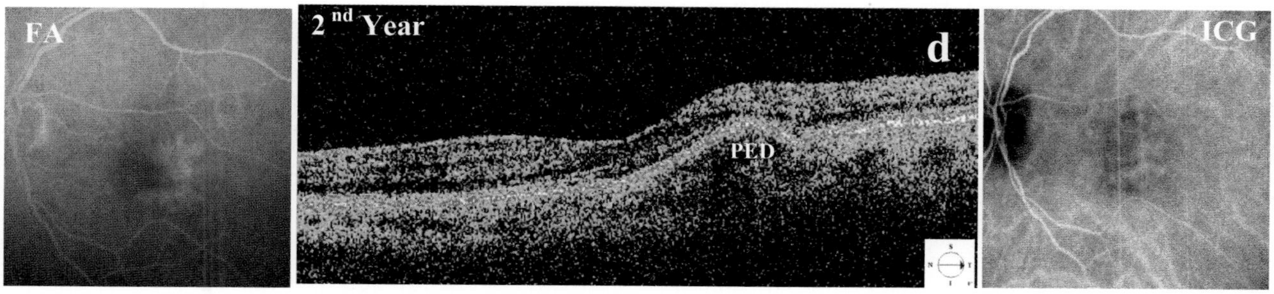

Figure 6: Initial stage of occult CNV after photodynamic therapy.
d): Two years later: few changes of the lesion. Persistence of the PED with minimal fibrosis (demonstrated on SLO-ICG). No symptoms. VA: 20/32 → **Observation.**

CLINICAL CASE No. 03: Early, Small Occult CNV

Typical early form, present for several months. Natural history without treatment (at the patient's request) during treatment of the first eye.

Clinical and Biomicroscopic Signs

A 73-year-old woman presented with minor symptoms in the right eye and a slight relative reduction of visual acuity. VA RE: 20/40 - VA LE: 20/80.

Biomicroscopic examination revealed several medium-sized soft drusen, predominantly perifoveal, but no SRF, hemorrhage, or hard exudates.

Autofluorescence Reference Image

No alteration of xanthophyll pigment. Presence of a minimal, oval-shaped, hyper-fluorescence at the temporal macular area suggesting a macular lesion.

Fluorescein Angiography

Progressive, heterogeneous, and poorly-delineated macular hyper-fluorescence over 2 DD, masked in its center by xanthophyll pigment with late fluorescein leakage and pinpoints.

SLO-ICG Angiography

Vast, rounded, poorly-delineated hyper-fluorescent area occupying the entire subfoveal zone and suggesting a neovascular network within the dark PED (**Figure 7**).

Suggested Angiographic Diagnosis:
Small area of occult CNV within a vascularized PED.

Contribution of OCT: *Stratus** Horizontal and Vertical Sections (Figure 8)

At the RPE Level

Presence of a regular, moderately large elevation, composed of multiple flat domes with a wavy appearance, suggestive of fairly extensive flat PED in the fovea.

This PED was relatively flat, allowing good visibility of Bruch's membrane. The RPE band was occasionally slightly thinned.

The PED cavity was hypo-reflective and almost optically empty and slightly more organized in the nasal sector. The PED had induced partial and moderate posterior shadowing.

Anterior to the RPE

The neurosensory retina was only slightly altered with good preservation of retinal structure.

The foveal depression was almost normal, confirming the recent nature of the lesion, with preservation of good visual acuity.

There was intraretinal fluid with slightly increased retinal thickness, subretinal fluid, and a subfoveal SRF.

As expected, the CNV itself was barely visible on OCT.

Diagnosis

OCT examination demonstrated a relatively small, wavy pigment epithelium detachment with a slightly reflective cavity, especially just underneath the RPE, indicating the presence of low-density fibrovascular tissue. Adjacent to the PED, an exudative reaction with diffuse infiltration (moderate retinal thickening) and an SRF. The retinal layers were not disorganized.

Fluorescein angiography immediately demonstrated irregular hyper-fluorescence with pinpoints, suggestive of occult neovascularization with a false image of foveal sparing due to xanthophyll pigment.

SLO-ICG angiography confirmed the presence of choroidal neovascularization and localized it to the subfoveal area, approximately 1.5 DD in size.

The diagnosis was therefore confirmed: recent **occult choroidal neovascularization** or **vascularized PED** with no signs of decompensation and only moderate symptoms at this stage (**Figures 7 and 8**).

Treatment was offered, but the patient preferred to wait until completion of treatment of the other much more severely affected eye.

CLINICAL CASE No. 03: EARLY, SMALL OCCULT CNV

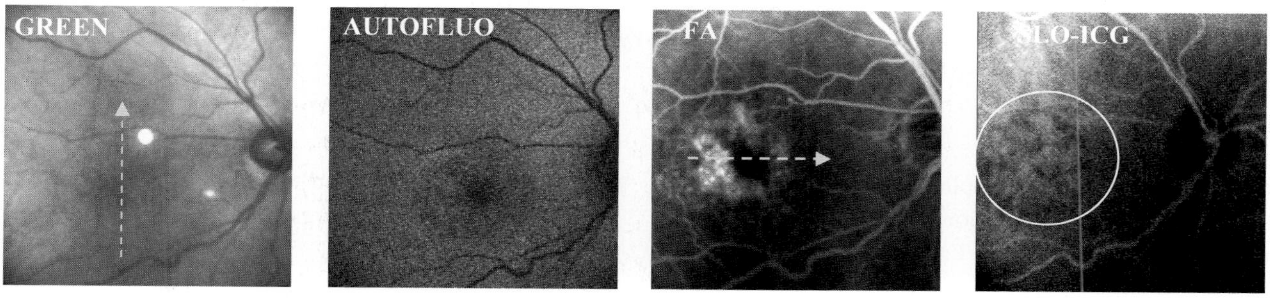

Figure 7: Typical early occult CNV–First examination. VA: 20/40.

Autofluorescence: minimal oval-shaped temporal macular zone of hyper-fluorescence. **Fluorescein angiography**: progressive, poorly-delineated hyper-fluorescence over an area of 2 DD with pinpoint leakage. **ICG angiography:** neovascular membrane visible against the dark PED.

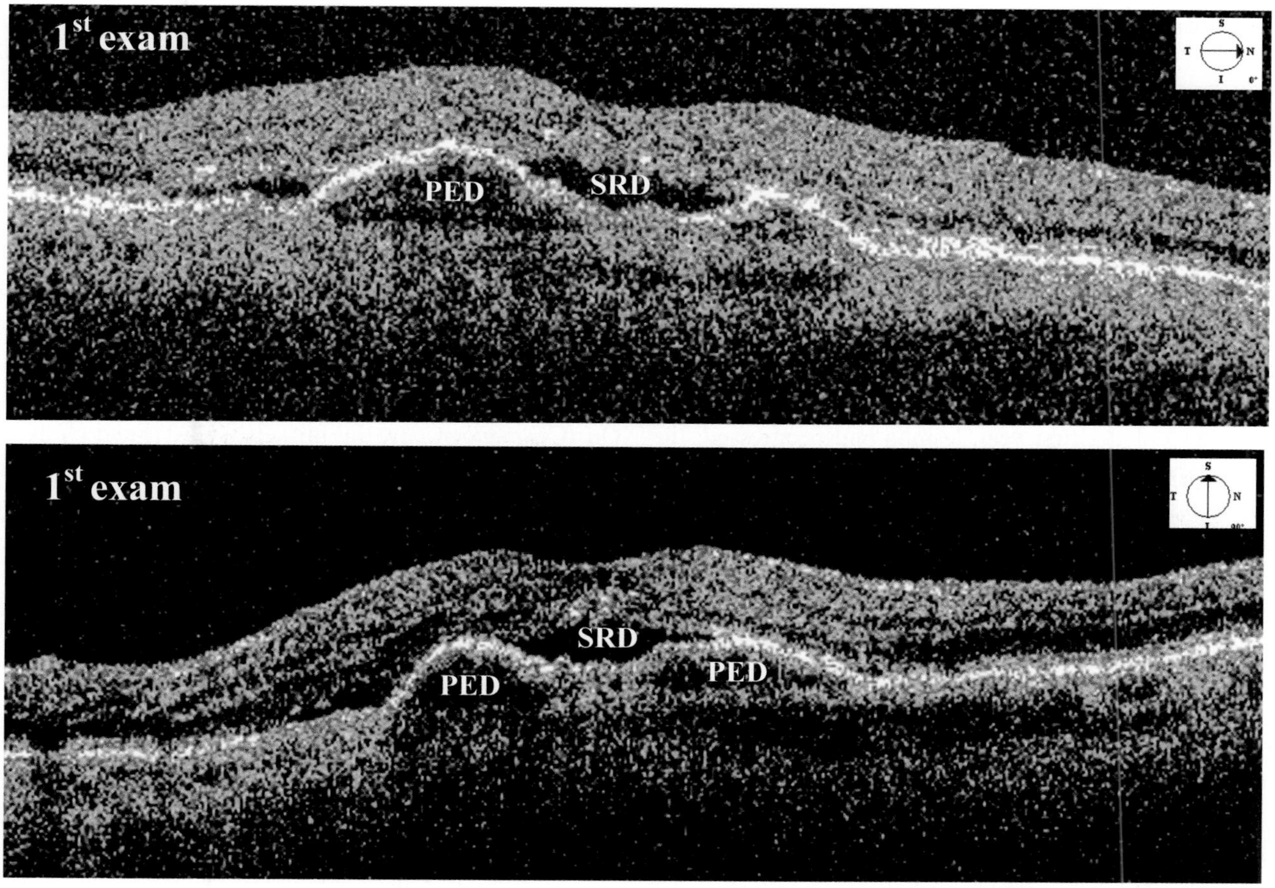

Figure 8: Typical early occult CNV.

Stratus* horizontal and vertical sections: moderate, regular flat with multiple domes of elevation, giving a wavy appearance and suggesting PED. The PED cavity is hypo-reflective and almost optically empty.
Intraretinal fluid infiltration, causing slightly increased retinal thickness and subretinal fluid with a subfoveal SRF.

CLINICAL CASE No. 03: Early, Small Occult CNV

Natural History over 3 Years

The **natural history** was followed routinely, assessing the usual functional and morphological parameters for almost 3 years.

Visual acuity, initially considered to be satisfactory, slowly deteriorated, causing increasing disability.

However, this vision loss was well-tolerated and accepted by the patient over time, as this eye was always better than the fellow eye.

OCT examinations demonstrated relatively minor and moderate changes with no sudden complications.

Serial OCT examinations remained essentially stable, not revealing any convincing signs of marked deterioration (**Figure 9a-d**).

At the third month, the PED had spread with the formation of a few cystic spaces but remained relatively flat, moderately reflective, with a small SRF and a small amount of intraretinal fluid with no loss of the foveal depression (**Figure 9a**).

At the end of the first year, lesions had progressed: the PED was more prominent, the SRF was more extensive with diffuse intraretinal fluid causing loss of the foveal depression (**Figure 9b**).

However, this deterioration was only limited, as the retinal layers remained well-organized and not dissociated.

The OCT findings were practically unchanged at the end of the second year (**Figure 9c**).

However, at the third year, the OCT features, although similar to those of previous examinations, showed worsening of the lesions: the PED was much more extensive and had become wavy with several cysts and moderate hyper-reflectivity.

These findings were suggestive of *fibrosis underneath the pigment epithelium* but with no exudative reaction or disorganization of retinal layers (**Figure 9d**).

On angiography, the lesions remained relatively stable over time.

On fluorescein angiography, the shape of the lesion and its overall surface area, as well as pinpoint leakage remained almost unchanged with no complications, no classic CNV, and no hemorrhage.

On ICG angiography, the initially well-defined choroidal neovascularization, gradually spread to invade all of the surface area of the PED but without causing any other complications.

Conclusion

This is a typical case of slowly progressing occult choroidal neovascularization with all the typical clinical signs of the disease but with no complications apart from moderate fibrosis underneath the RPE.

Visual acuity declined slowly, but finally caused functional disability, interfering with reading, and with the potential to be permanent. This relatively severe, although slow natural progression, constitutes an indication for current treatments.

Treatment must be considered at the first signs of decompensation, either loss of visual acuity, hemorrhagic complications, or extension of the lesions, even if these changes do not always occur simultaneously or suddenly.

CLINICAL CASE No. 03: EARLY, SMALL OCCULT CNV
Natural history

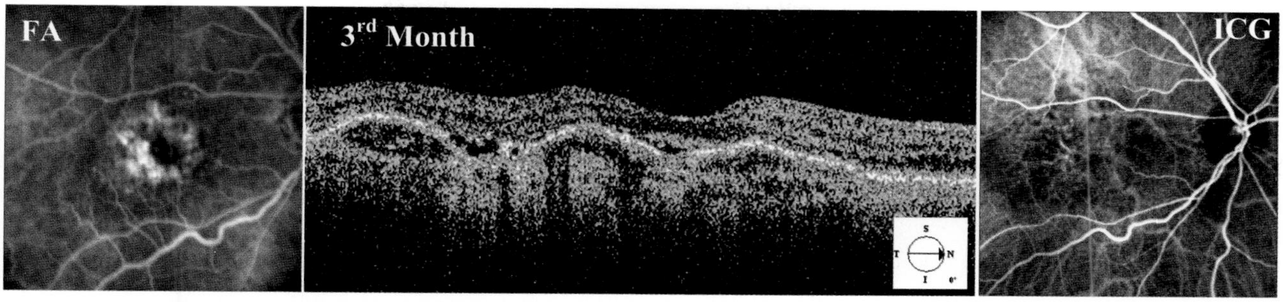

Figure 9: Typical early occult CNV–Natural history.
Stratus* horizontal section correlated with fluorescein angiography and SLO-ICG angiography:
a): Third month: limited zone of hyper-fluorescence. CNV visible on ICG angiography. Wavy PED with a slight exudative reaction. **VA: 20/50.**

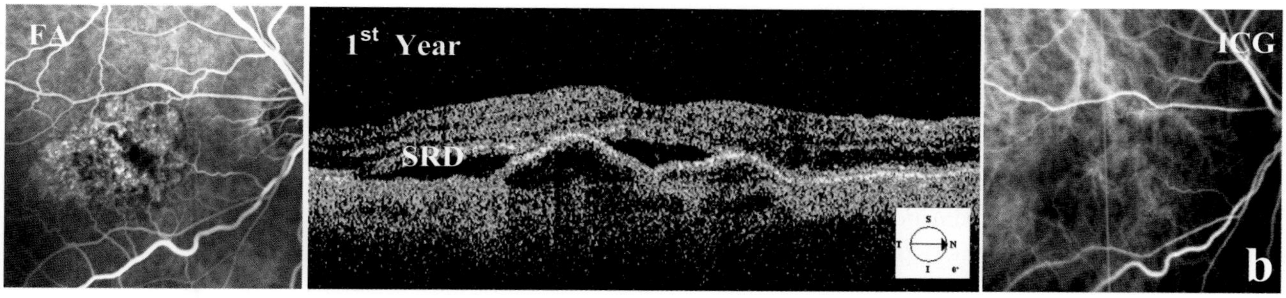

Figure 9: Typical early occult CNV–Natural history.
b): One year: extension of the lesion on fluorescein angiography but stable on ICG angiography. Marked accentuation of the leakage. **VA: 20/80.**

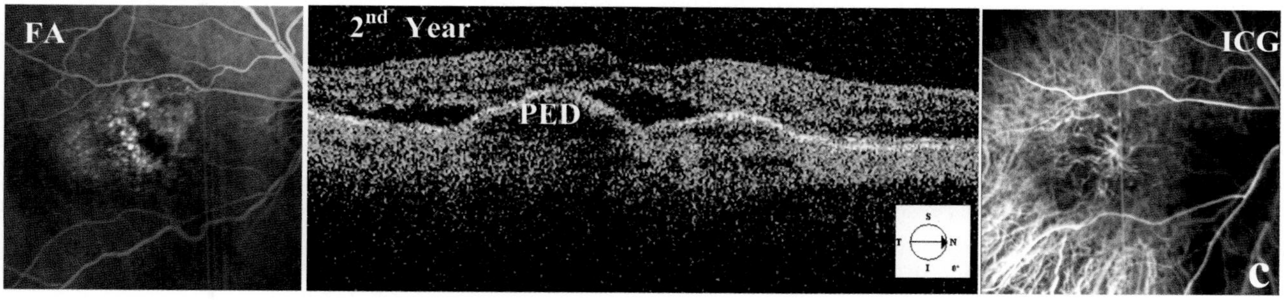

Figure 9: Typical early occult CNV–Natural history.
c): Twp years: virtually stable appearance on angiography and OCT. Decline of visual acuity. **VA: 20/100.**

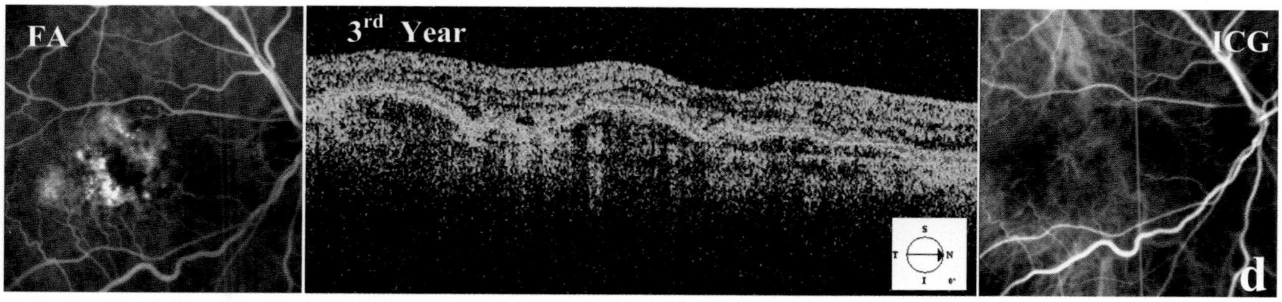

Figure 9: Typical early occult CNV–Natural history.
d): Three years: extension of the lesion on fluorescein angiography. CNV visible on ICG angiography, invading all of the PED. **OCT** shows progressive fibrosis of the PED with no leakage. **VA: 20/100.**

CLINICAL CASE No. 04: Moderately Large Occult CNV

Moderately large occult CNV, with symptoms present for more than 6 months. Course during anti-VEGF therapy with stabilization and prolonged treatment.

Clinical Signs

A 79-year-old patient presented with progressive and moderate decline of visual acuity in the left eye that was immediately worrying due to a longstanding fibrovascular lesion in the right eye.
VA RE: 20/640 - VA LE: 20/63.

Biomicroscopic Examination

Biomicroscopic examination showed few changes in the macular region, limited to a few soft drusen in the temporal macular zone.

Autofluorescence

Autofluorescence visualized reticular drusen in the region of the superior temporal arcade and a small inferior juxtafoveal hyper-fluorescent zone (**Figure 10**).

Fluorescein and ICG Angiography

Fluorescein angiography: progressive hyper-fluorescence with pinpoint fluorescein leakage in the inferior and temporal region, masked by xanthophyll pigment in its center.

SLO-ICG angiography: vast hypo-fluorescent area, suggesting the presence of a heterogeneous, irregular, subfoveal PED, but well-delineated on late phases and surrounded by several soft drusen (**Figure 10**).

Suggested Angiographic Diagnosis:
Recent decompensation of a vascularized PED with the characteristic appearance of small occult CNV without hemorrhage on fluorescein angiography.

Contribution of OCT

_Stratus_* horizontal section

At the RPE level, a small temporal PED is present, extending as far as the fovea. This PED had an irregular appearance with several cysts. The PED cavity was moderately reflective but homogeneous.

Anterior to the RPE, the neurosensory retina was only slightly modified with relative preservation of the retinal structure. However, it was diffusely thickened by intraretinal fluid predominantly in the outer layers and also subretinal fluid

Vertical section

The PED was visible but appeared to be fairly flat on the vertical section.

In contrast, the SRF was more extensive with marked settling of intraretinal fluid (**Figure 11**).

The foveal depression was relatively unchanged, confirming the recent nature of the lesion with preservation of good visual acuity.

Diagnosis

The OCT examination demonstrated a small, irregular, heterogeneous, and fairly flat pigment epithelium detachment with a moderately reflective cavity.

An exudative reaction with moderately increased retinal thickness and a small subfoveal SRF was demonstrated adjacent to the PED, and the retinal layers were not disorganized.

These features are typical of **recent small occult CNV**.

Fluorescein angiography was highly suggestive of this lesion, indicating early decompensation in this eye.

SLO-ICG angiography confirmed these findings and reaffirmed the diagnosis.

This recent lesion with moderate symptoms justified immediately anti-VEGF therapy in an attempt to prevent progression.

CLINICAL CASE No. 04: MODERATELY LARGE OCCULT CNV: Prolonged anti-VEGF therapy

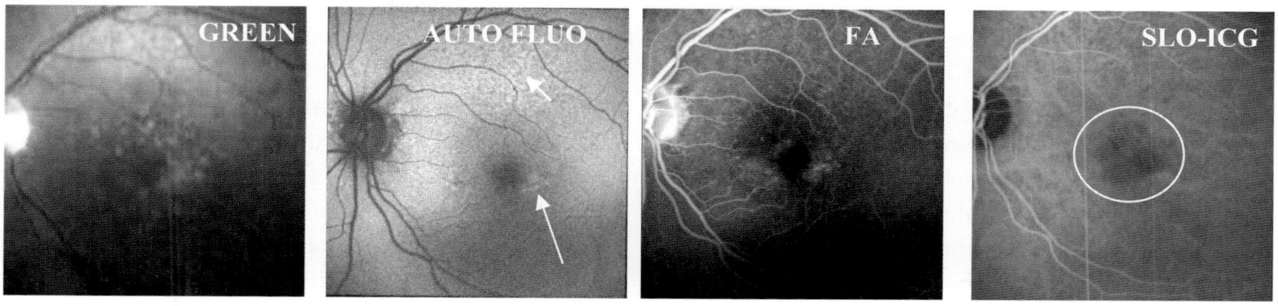

Figure 10: Moderately large occult CNV–First examination. VA: 20/63.
Red-free fundus photograph: soft drusen, mainly in the temporal macular zone.
Autofluorescence: reticular drusen (*small arrow*). Inferior juxtafoveal hyper-fluorescence (*arrow*).
Fluorescein angiography: irregular hyper-fluorescence and pinpoint leakage; central masking by xanthophyll pigment.
ICG angiography: hypo-fluorescent area suggesting the presence of a heterogeneous and irregular subfoveal PED (*circle*).

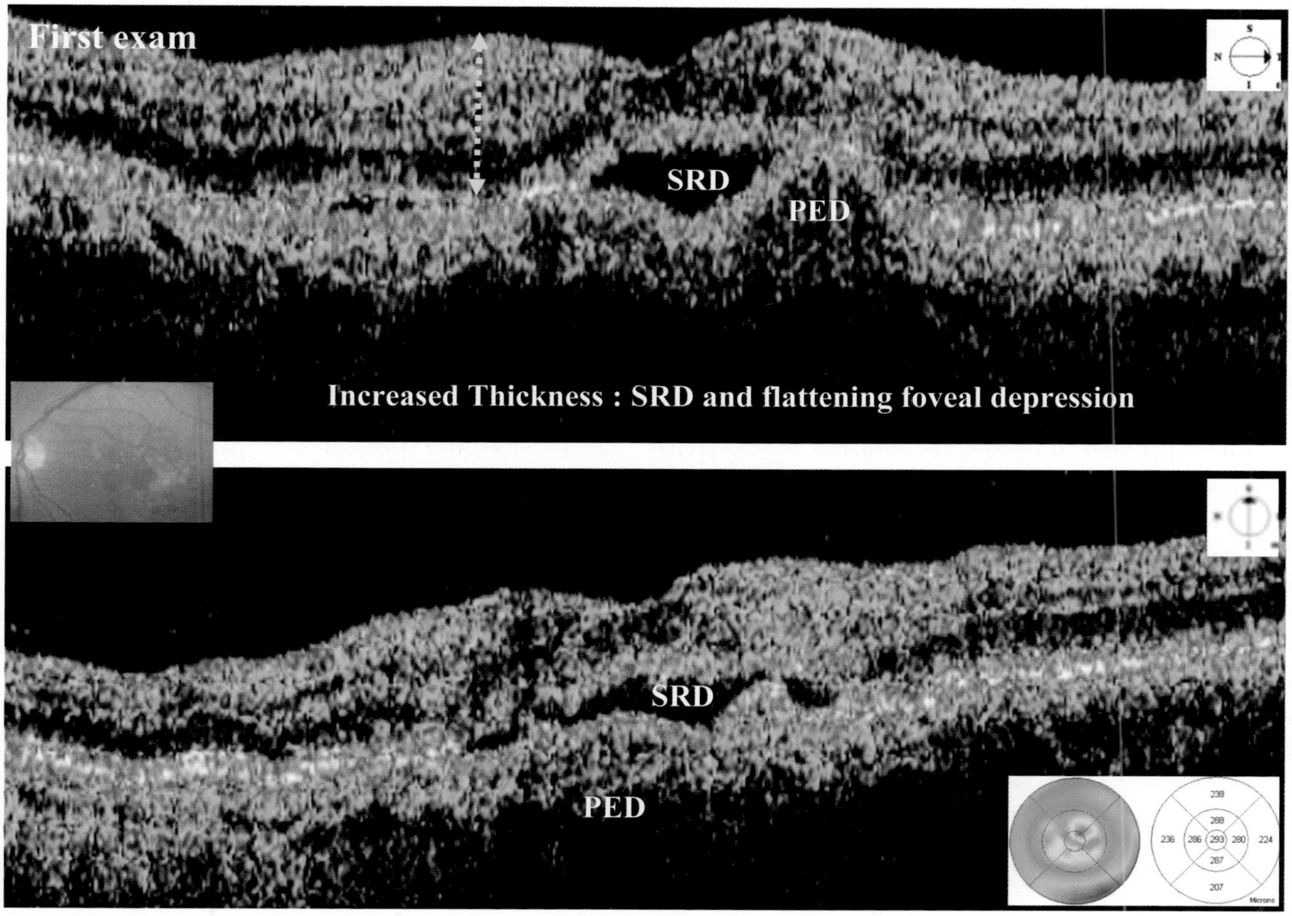

Figure 11: Moderately large occult CNV – First examination. VA: 20/63.
Stratus* horizontal and vertical sections: irregular, moderately reflective PED with several cysts.
Intraretinal fluid more marked in the dependent part and mainly subfoveal SRF

CLINICAL CASE No. 04: Moderately Large Occult CNV: Prolonged Anti-VEGF Therapy

Anti-VEGF therapy was administered by repeated intravitreal injections over a period of 18 months due to persistent PED and downward shifting SRF. There was a certain degree of extension of the angiographic lesions contrasting with slow improvement and stabilization of the symptoms Visual acuity varied in parallel with treatment: several moderate variations with initial improvement followed by slight deterioration, each time that treatment was stopped. Treatment was therefore administered every 2 months to restore visual acuity to 20/40.

Clinical Features

Lesions slowly deteriorated: **autofluorescence photographs** showed extension of the lesion and the hyper-fluorescent halo (**Figure 12a**).

TD-OCT examinations (using the *Stratus** during the first year) demonstrated the course of intraretinal and subretinal fluid and the PED.

- The overall aspect of OCT sections appeared to accurately reflect partial resolution of exudation during the first 3 months but with persistence of shifting fluid (**Figure 12b**).
- After a brief phase of paradoxical deterioration, the third injection provided marked improvement.
- Injections were subsequently performed every 2 to 3 months due to recurrence of symptoms or morphological changes on the various imaging modalities.
- At the end of the first year and after 6 intravitreal injections, the retina had normal thickness and organization (contrasting slightly with the angiographic appearance). The PED had collapsed with slight fibrosis and moderate reflectivity (**Figure 12c**).
- However, during the second year, although the lesions appeared to be stabilized, the patient experienced a relapse marked by recurrence of intraretinal fluid.

Spectralis** SD-OCT demonstrated changes such as: *alterations of the IS/OS interface and external limiting membrane*, disrupted or thickened in various places over the vascularized PED.

The outer nuclear layer was invaded by a denser material and bright hyper-reflective spots suggesting recurrent CNV (**Figure 12d**).

Anti-VEGF therapy was therefore continued with one injection every 2 months allowing functional (VA: 20/40) and morphological stabilization.

On **fluorescein angiography**, the irregular hyper-fluorescence and pinpoints became increasingly visible, occupying all of the foveal region but with no increase of its overall surface area. All the occult CNV persisted and appeared to become stabilized during treatment with neither complications nor new hemorrhages.

On **ICG angiography**, the overall surface area of the vascularized PED remained stable. The CNV was increasingly visible and gradually occupied all of the PED.

This persistence of the PED did not appear to be due to a new complication, but rather to slow scarring.

> Overall, this case presented a favorable course, despite recurrences and persistence of the PED, with shifting SRF and slight extension of the angiographic lesions. These features indicated the need for prolonged treatment with repeated anti-VEGF IVT injections for 18 months.

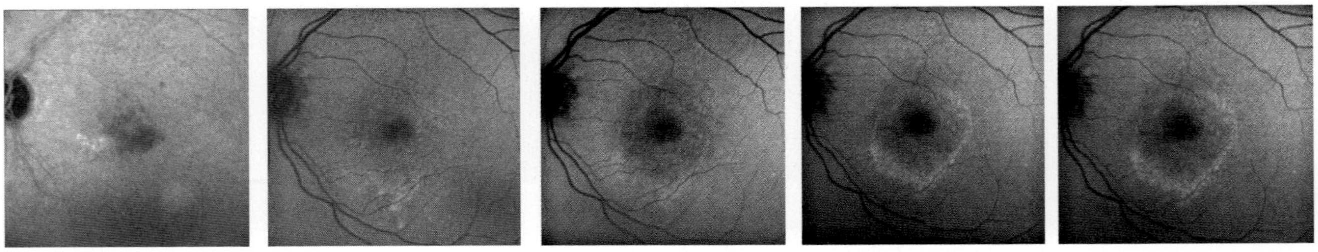

Figure 12a): Moderately large occult CNV: autofluorescence appearance during follow-up after treatment (repeated IVT injections every 2 months for 18 months). Extension of the hyper-fluorescent halo with no alteration of the central zone.

CLINICAL CASE No. 04: MODERATELY LARGE OCCULT CNV: Prolonged anti-VEGF therapy

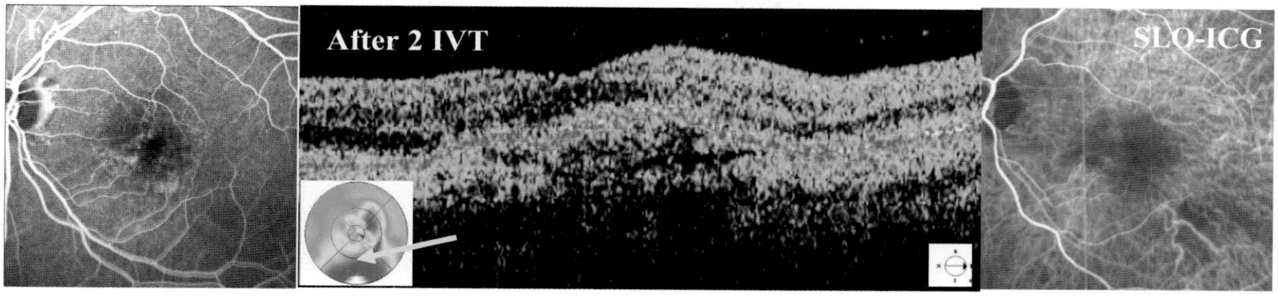

Figure 12b): Moderately large occult CNV–Examination after the second injection. VA: 20/80.

Brief paradoxical phase of deterioration with loss of visual acuity and persistence of shifting fluid (*arrow*) despite partial resolution of leakage.

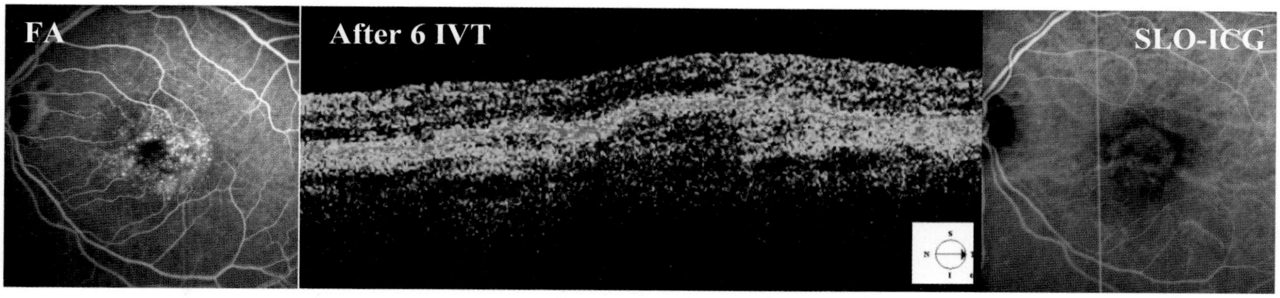

Figure 12c): Moderately large occult CNV–Examination after the sixth injection. VA: 20/40.

Marked improvement of visual acuity, resolution of intraretinal fluid, and collapse of the PED. Note the good visibility of angiographic signs and the CNV on ICG angiography, which persisted but with no signs of worsening.

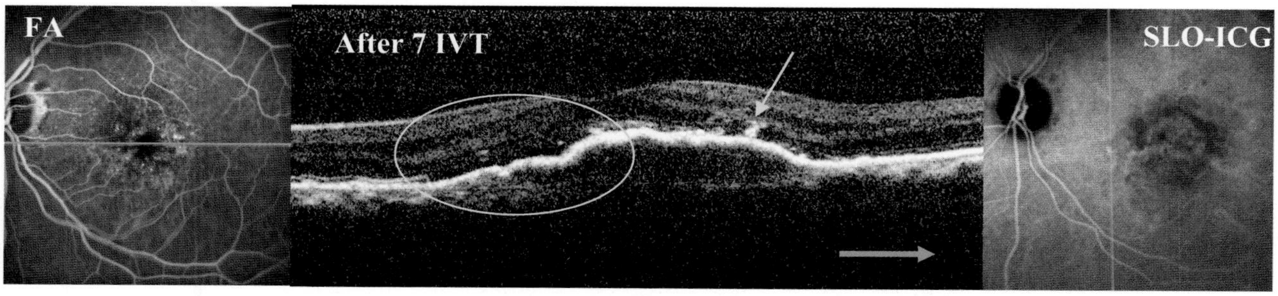

Figure 12d): Moderately large occult CNV–Examination after the 7th injection. VA: 20/40.

Relapse marked by recurrence of intraretinal fluid, clearly visualized on *Spectralis** OCT: the IS/OS interface and external limiting membrane are disrupted or thickened in some places (*yellow circle*) over the vascularized PED. The outer nuclear layer is invaded by a denser material and bright hyper-reflective spots (*yellow arrow*).

CLINICAL CASE No. 04: Moderately Large Occult CNV: Prolonged Anti-VEGF Therapy

Spectral-Domain OCT

Spectral-Domain OCT analysis of the outer retinal layers allowed monitoring of the course of this clinical case and the effects of choroidal neovascularization and the vascularized PED on the photoreceptors themselves.

Signs of recurrence were observed at the time of the 7th injection:

- The IS/OS interface was no longer visible over the dome of the PED.
- In the subfoveal region, the IS/OS interface was replaced by a zone of hyper-reflectivity and several temporal bright hyper-reflective spots (**Figure 13a**).

After each of the following injections:

- These abnormalities gradually resolved with return of a continuous IS/OS *interface* (**Figure 13b**).
- **Bright hyper-reflective spots** became smaller and less numerous and then became considerably rarer (**Figure 13b, c, and d**).
- The *outer nuclear layer* gradually regained almost normal thickness and reflectivity (**Figure 13d**). [Note that the fourth section is slightly eccentric downwards, which gives a false impression of regression of the PED itself].
- The **PED** persisted, but was flatter, wavy, and hypo-reflective.
- A small SRF persisted and remained detectable throughout the course, but all retinal layers regained an almost normal organization (**Figure 13d**).
- The vitreous appeared to be detached at this stage of the disease (**Figure 13d**).

Conclusion

This typical, moderately large, **occult CNV lesion** with recent decompensation marked by loss of visual acuity and subretinal and intraretinal fluid, justified treatment with repeated IVT injections of anti-VEGF.

Throughout the course, with a current follow-up of 18 months, the response to treatment was generally satisfactory but always partial and incomplete, marked by several recurrences.

Treatment corresponded to the usual regimen: first a series of 3 injections followed by injections as required, according to the imaging findings and visual acuity.

Injections were therefore repeated every 2 to 3 months, depending on the results of these examinations. The current result is overall satisfactory with visual acuity maintained at 20/40.

However, the PED, although flattened, still persisted with a characteristic wavy profile and no marked fibrosis.

A layer of subretinal fluid remains visible and has never completely resolved.

Analysis of the outer retinal layers demonstrated marked changes during active phases (disruption of the IS/OS interface, bright hyper-reflective spots and progressive return to normal with successive treatment sessions in parallel with improvement of visual acuity, indicating a favorable prognosis at this stage.

However, persistence of intraretinal fluid and the PED justifies prolonged observation for a currently undefined duration.

CLINICAL CASE No. 04: MODERATELY LARGE OCCULT CNV: Prolonged anti-VEGF therapy

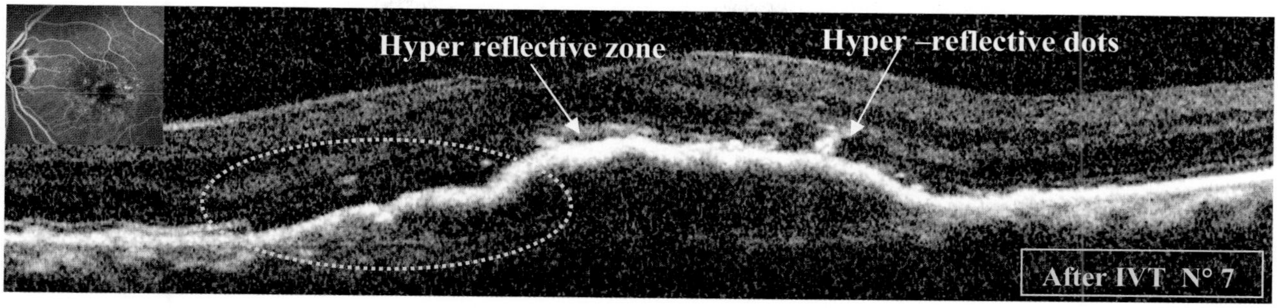

Figure 13a): Moderately large occult CNV. Recurrence. Examination after the 7th injection. VA: 20/40.
Loss of the IS/OS interface over the PED; a zone of hyper-reflectivity and several subfoveal bright hyper-reflective spots.

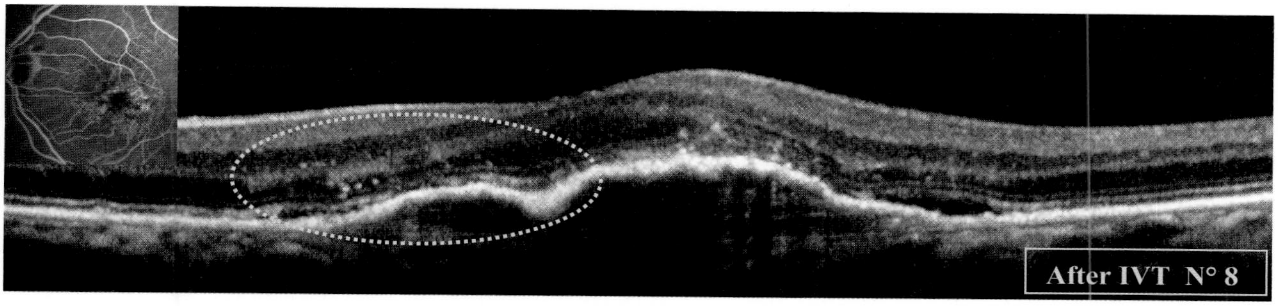

Figure 13b): Moderately large occult CNV–Examination after the 8th injection. VA: 20/63.
Persistence of leakage, but the IS/OS interface is now visible and continuous.

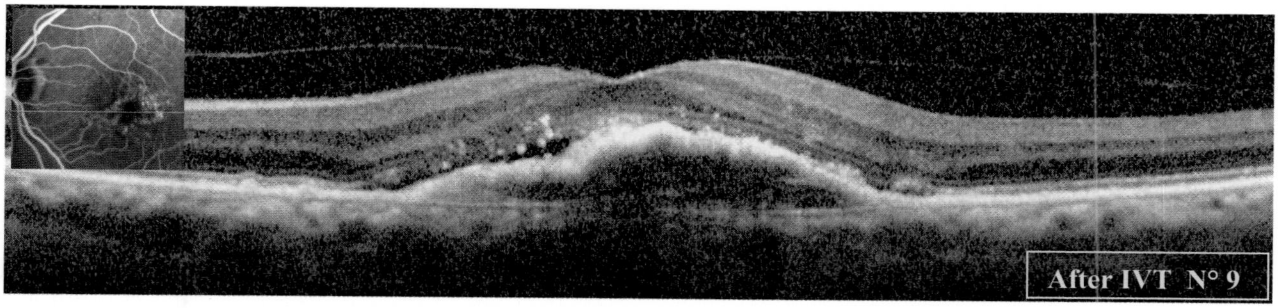

Figure 13c): Moderately large occult CNV–Examination after the 9th injection. VA: 20/40.
Progressive improvement with reduction of the bright hyper-reflective spots which are smaller and less numerous.

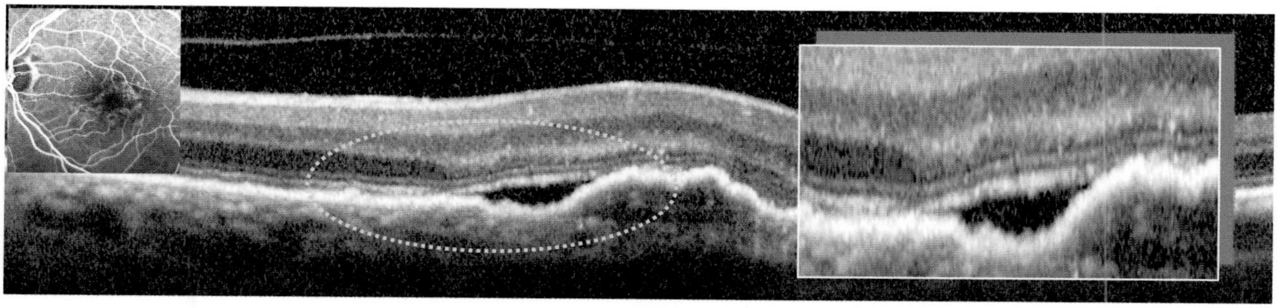

Figure 13d): Moderately large occult CNV–Examination 2 months after the 9th injection. VA: 20/40.
Almost normal organization of the retinal layers. A small SRF remains visible with a few irregularities of the outer segments. The residual PED is wavy and weakly reflective. The vitreous appears to be detached at this stage.

CLINICAL CASE No. 05: Minimally Classic CNV

Occult CNV associated with a small zone of minimally classic CNV.
Response to treatment by PDT followed by intravitreal anti-VEGF injections.

Clinical and Biomicroscopic Signs

A 72-year-old woman presented with slowly declining visual acuity and metamorphopsias mainly in the left eye, experienced for several months prior to examination.

VA LE: 20/80 – VA RE 20/40.

Biomicroscopic examination revealed several, medium-sized perifoveal drusen associated with a central SRF measuring 2 DD.

Autofluorescence images showed the presence of a regular, circular halo with no alteration of xanthophyll pigment.

Fluorescein and SLO-ICG Angiography

Fluorescein angiography: irregular, progressive 2 DD hyper-fluorescence with leakage and pinpoints. This zone comprised a clearly-delineated area of marked hyper-fluorescence with fluorescein leakage.
ICG angiography: the small area of classic CNV was rapidly stained and surrounded by a dark border (**Figure 14**). Occult CNV was observed later, forming a poorly-defined subfoveal neovascular network within the dark PED.

Suggested Angiographic Diagnosis:
Occult CNV associated with a small area of classic CNV (minimally classic).

Contribution of OCT: *Stratus** Horizontal and Vertical Sections (Figure 15)

At the RPE Level

Several undulations and elevations were observed within the RPE, delineating multiple pockets of relatively flat, irregular, and wavy PED.

The RPE was irregular with thinner and thicker zones delineating the vascularized PED.

The PED cavity was hypo-reflective allowing visualization of Bruch's membrane.

A moderately reflective (green) band was visible posterior to the RPE, with an optically empty zone situated even more posteriorly.

Anterior to the RPE

The neurosensory retina was thickened with diffuse intraretinal fluid and loss of the foveal depression.

A small SRF was visible between the pockets of the PED and especially around the PED (clearly visible on the vertical section).

In particular, a zone of subfoveal hyper-reflectivity was contiguous with the RPE, caused disorganization of the outer layers, and represented classic CNV.

Diagnosis

The **clinical features** corresponded to moderately large occult CNV evolving slowly, over several months.

The course was recently complicated by a small juxtafoveal and subfoveal zone of classic CNV with fluorescein leakage, accounting for the patient's symptoms and recent loss of visual acuity.

These features are often called ***minimally classic CNV***. Development of this complication, even in the absence of hemorrhage, justifies treatment.

The only treatment available at that time was photodynamic therapy, which was delivered to all of the surface of the lesion detected by angiography.

CLINICAL CASE No. 05: MINIMALLY CLASSIC CNV

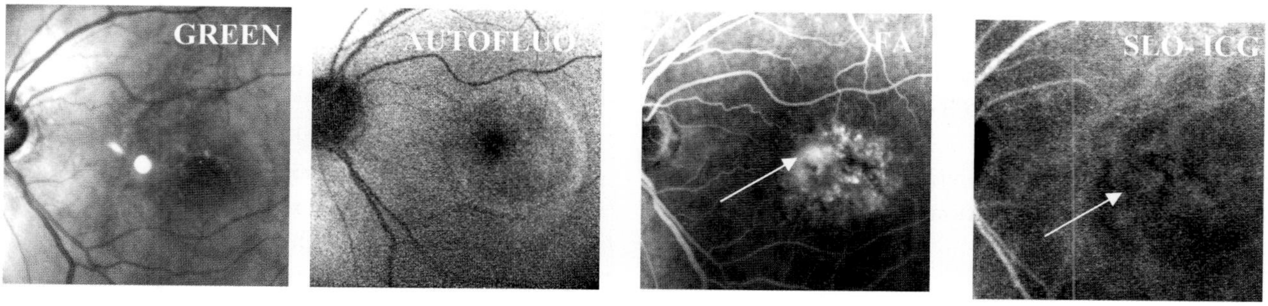

◘ Figure 14: *Minimally classic* **CNV – First examination. VA: 20/80.**
Autofluorescence: SRF and regular, circular halo. **Fluorescein angiography:** *irregular hyper-fluorescence and pinpoints with a well-delineated area of more intense hyper-fluorescence (arrow).* **ICG angiography**: *clearly visible subfoveal CNV (arrow).*

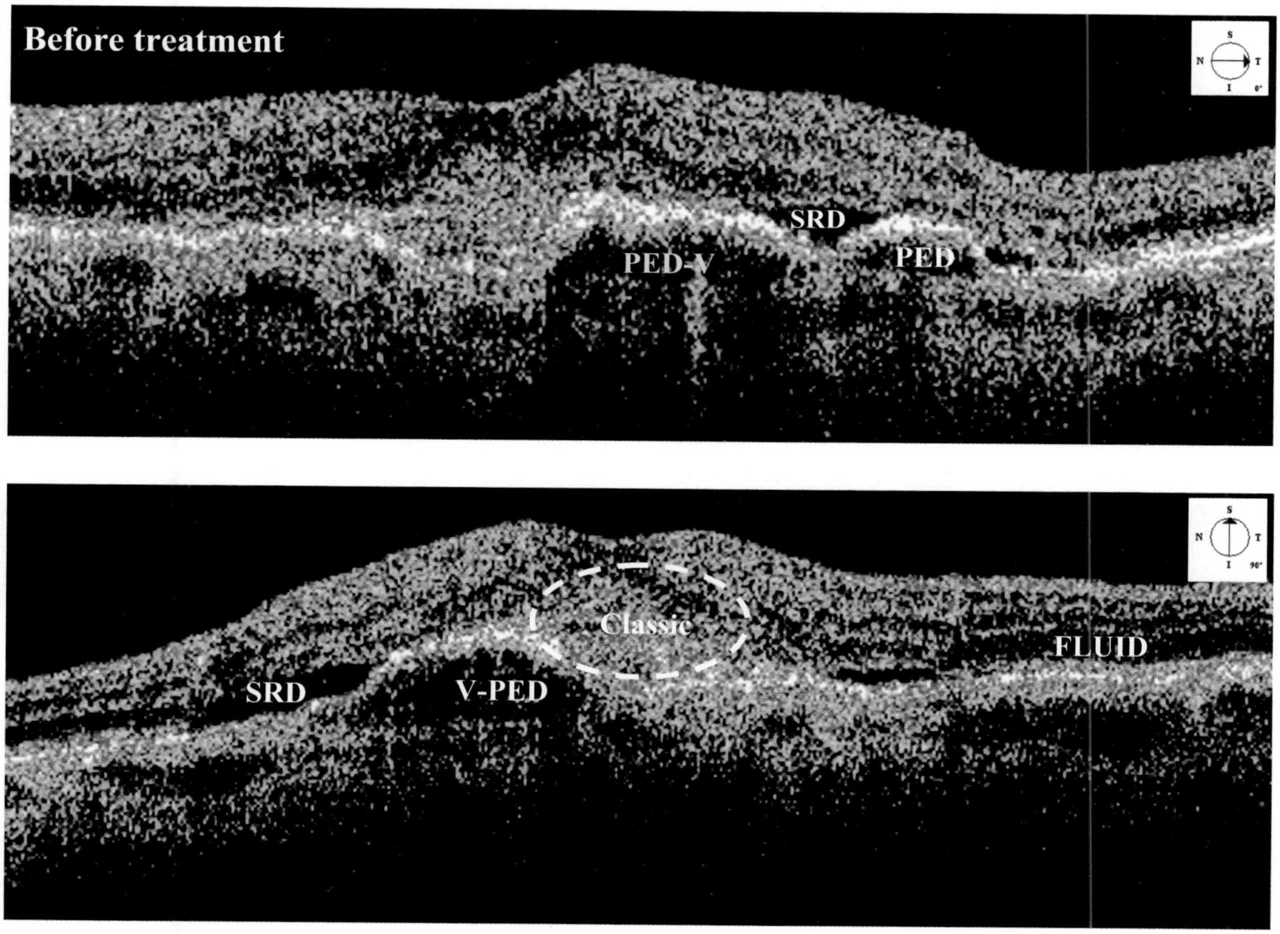

◘ Figure 15: ***Minimally Classic*** **CNV. VA: 20/80.**
Stratus* **horizontal and vertical sections:** irregular, moderately reflective PED composed of 3 pockets with intraretinal fluid and SRF more marked at the perifoveal region. A juxtafoveal or subfoveal hyper-reflective area (classic CNV) can be seen in this area.

CLINICAL CASE No. 05: Minimally Classic CNV Follow-Up Post Treatment (PDT plus Anti-VEGF)

Treatment consisted of verteporfin photodynamic therapy (PDT), the standard treatment at that time, followed by IVT injections of anti-VEGF for a recurrence.

These treatments initially provided a functional improvement, followed by stabilization of visual acuity, except during the recurrence.

Clinical Features

Autofluorescence photographs showed extension of the lesion with early changes in the central zone (**Figure 16**).

TD-OCT examinations demonstrated changes of the zone of hyper-reflectivity corresponding to classic CNV during this follow-up (**Figure 17a-d**).

The overall appearance on OCT sections appeared to fairly accurately reflect the progression, resolution, and then recurrence of classic CNV and intraretinal fluid, although the subretinal component was only slightly detectable.

- A marked improvement was observed by the second PDT session, but the hyper-reflective zone of classic CNV was still visible.
- One year later, after 3 PDT sessions, the hyper-reflective classic CNV had resolved but a minimal SRF still remained.
- Two years later, although the lesions appeared to be stable, the patient developed a recurrence marked by return and marked extension of a preretinal zone of hyper-reflectivity with leakage, extensive SRF and increased retinal thickness.

Complementary PDT and IVT injections of anti-VEGF (a single session) were therefore performed.

- After 3 years of follow-up, marked improvement with stabilization, reapplication, and preservation of normal retinal thickness.

On **fluorescein angiography**, the improvement mainly involved the classic CNV component, which initially resolved and then recurred. Treatment appeared to have little effect on the zone of occult CNV, which remained stable with no signs of deterioration (**Figure 17c**).

On **ICG angiography**, the CNV appeared to become atrophied and limited to large draining vessels. The outline of PDT was clearly visible.

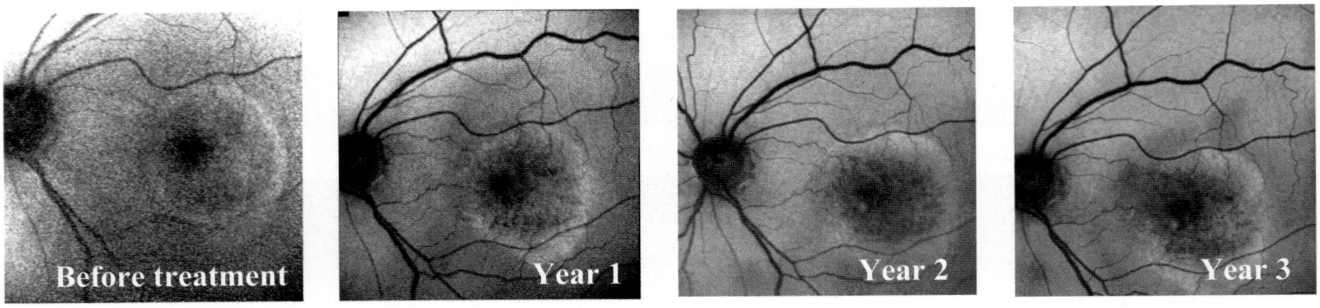

Figure 16: Minimally classic CNV: autofluorescence appearance.
During post treatment follow-up (PDT plus intravitreal injection): progressive extension of the hyper-fluorescent halo and alteration of the central area.

Conclusion

This occult CNV with subsequent development of minimally classic CNV remained stable for almost two years after PDT with maintenance of VA at 20/50.

However, a fairly severe late recurrence occurred after 2 years of clinical follow-up with deterioration of all signs, especially on OCT, requiring combined treatment by PDT and IVT injection of anti-VEGF with rapid improvement after a single session.

The current persistence of several abnormalities on the various imaging modalities justifies maintenance of regular observation, every 3 months and then at longer intervals (or earlier in the event of recurrent symptoms).

CLINICAL CASE No. 5: MINIMALLY CLASSIC CNV
Post treatment follow-up (PDT plus Anti-VEGF)

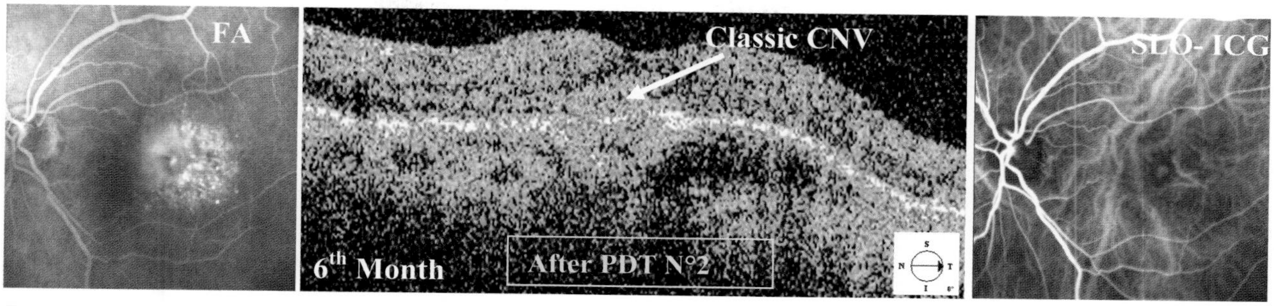

Figure 17: Minimally classic CNV. VA LE: 20/50.
a): Six months later: after 2 PDT sessions, regression of the SRF partial regression of the hyper-reflectivity of classic CNV.

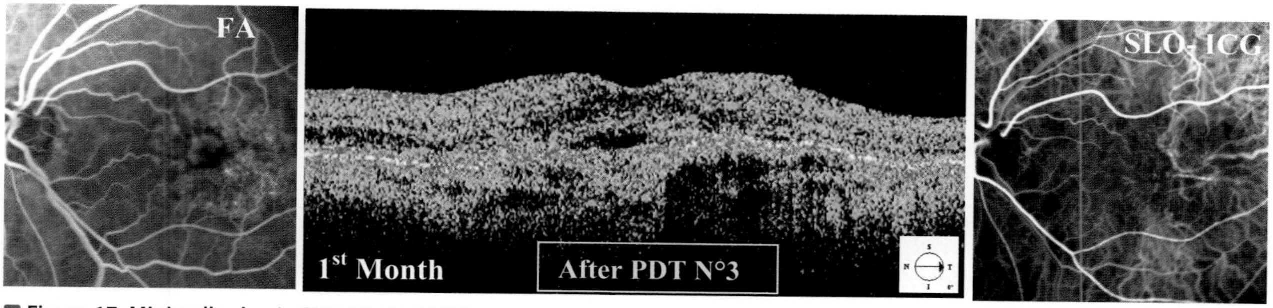

Figure 17: Minimally classic CNV. VA LE: 20/50.
b): One year later after 3 PDT sessions: progressive improvement. Regression of classic CNV but persistence of a minimal SRF Occult CNV are still perfused on angiography, and OCT shows a flat, wavy, vascularized PED.

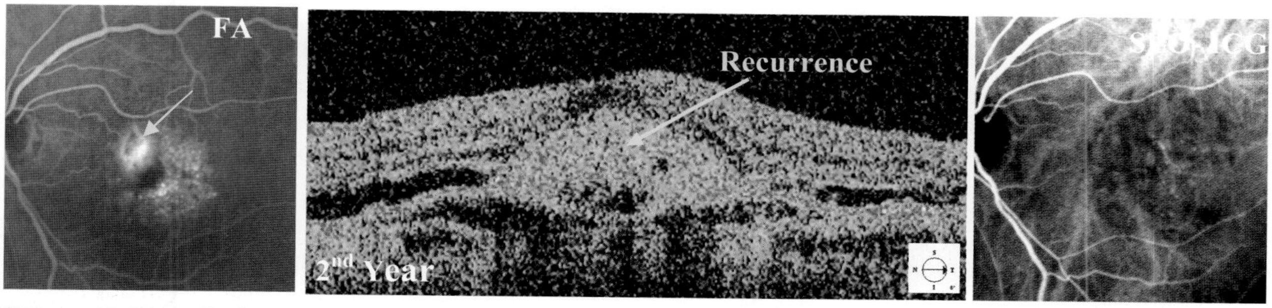

Figure 17: Minimally classic CNV- VA LE: 20/80.
c): After 2 years: recurrence: subretinal and intraretinal fluid; revascularization of classic CNV → extension of occult CNV and extension of intraretinal hyper-reflectivity → **New course of treatment with PDT plus intravitreal injections of anti-VEGF.**

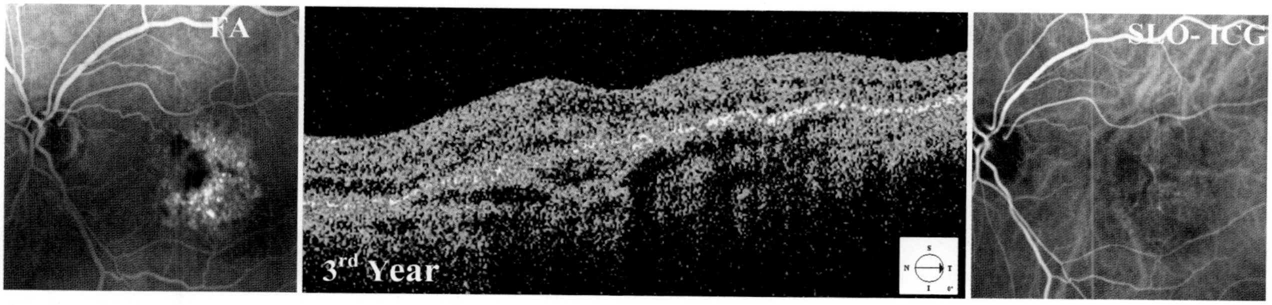

Figure 17: Minimally classic CNV. VA LE: 20/50.
d): After 3 years: at the end of follow-up, marked improvement: stabilization, reapplication, and preservation of almost normal retinal thickness. Persistence of a relatively flat and organized fibrovascular PED.

CLINICAL CASE No. 06: Occult CNV (Minimally Classic)

Recently decompensated occult CNV with symptoms related to classic CNV. Response to treatment by anti-VEGF and SD-OCT follow-up.

Clinical Signs

A 60-year-old man presented with visual discomfort in the right eye with a few micropsias and deformed images, with normal visual acuity and no symptoms in the left eye.
VA RE: 20/32 - VA LE: 20/20.

Biomicroscopic Examination and Autofluorescence

Biomicroscopic examination demonstrated numerous soft drusen of various sizes, sometimes clustered or confluent forming a superior and temporal crown.

All of the inferior macular region was raised and blurred with a **grayish** inferior nasal zone but without hemorrhage and/or lipid exudates (**Figure 18**).

Autofluorescence photographs did not show any abnormal hyper-fluorescence but the presence of an oval-shaped zone of hypo-fluorescence corresponding to the raised zone.

Fluorescein and ICG Angiography

Progressive hyper-fluorescence and pinpoints in the inferior and temporal region with slow fluorescein leakage. A localized inferior nasal lesion with much more intense fluorescein leakage was visualized in this zone (**Figure 18**, *arrow*).

SLO-ICG angiography showed a vast hypo-fluorescent oval-shaped subfoveal PED, well-delineated on the late phases. A small hyper-fluorescent zone was clearly visualized within the PED, suggesting occult CNV that had become visible (**Figure 18**, *arrow*).

Suggested Angiographic Diagnosis:
Recent decompensation of a vascularized PED with juxtafoveal choroidal neovascularization, corresponding to *minimally classic* CNV.

Contribution of OCT (*Stratus**)

Horizontal section

At the RPE level, presence of a relatively small PED, mainly temporal but extending as far as the fovea. This PED was relatively flat with good visibility of Bruch's membrane. The PED cavity was hypo-reflective and almost optically empty.

Anterior to the RPE, the neurosensory retina was only slightly modified with good preservation of retinal structure and minimal intraretinal fluid. CNV were barely visible on this section.

Oblique section

The PED was not visible on this section, which demonstrated hyper-reflectivity related to the presence of juxtafoveal classic CNV anterior to the RPE with adjacent retinal thickening (**Figure 19**).

The foveal depression was only slightly modified, confirming the recent onset of the lesion explaining the good visual acuity.

Diagnosis

*Stratus** **TD-OCT** demonstrated a relatively flat pigment epithelium detachment. The PED cavity was almost optically empty. An adjacent hyper-reflective lesion, anterior to the RPE, associated with a limited exudative reaction and moderate retinal thickening was also demonstrated with no disorganization of retinal layers.

This combination of signs was suggestive of occult choroidal neovascularization with recent appearance of a small area of juxtafoveal classic choroidal neovascularization, often called ***minimally classic***.

Fluorescein angiography was suggestive of this lesion, occurring at a relatively young age and accompanied by numerous drusen.

SLO-ICG angiography confirmed these findings and clearly confirmed the diagnosis.

This lesion was recent with moderate symptoms. A diagnosis of drusenoid PED could be considered, but the presence of an exudative reaction confirmed the diagnosis and justified immediate anti-VEGF therapy to prevent progression.

CLINICAL CASE No. 06: MINIMALLY CLASSIC CNV
Spectral-Domain OCT follow-up post anti-VEGF therapy.

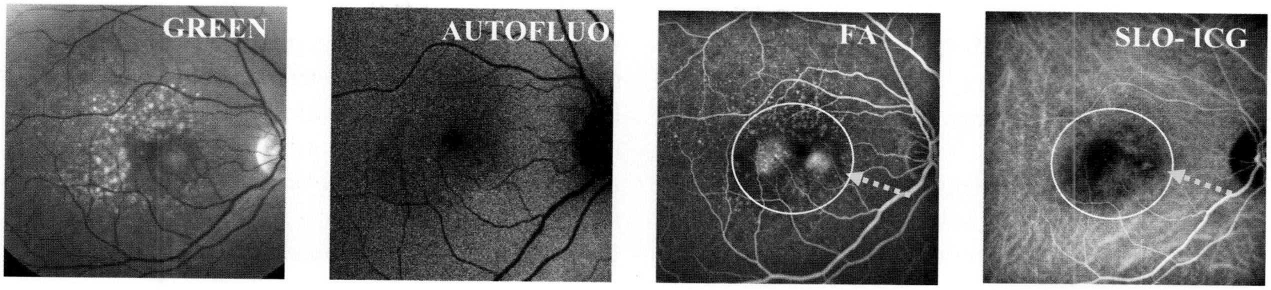

Figure 18: Occult CNV with small area of minimally classic CNV. VA: 20/32.
Red-free: numerous soft drusen, sometimes confluent. **Autofluorescence**: extensive hypo-fluorescence related to the poorly visible SRF. **Fluorescein angiography:** *inferior temporal hyper-fluorescence and pinpoints, and the presence of a small localized inferior nasal lesion with intense fluorescein leakage (yellow arrow).* **SLO-ICG angiography**: *well-delineated, hypo-fluorescent subfoveal PED. Small hyper-fluorescent zone, suggestive of occult CNV that has become visible (yellow arrow).*

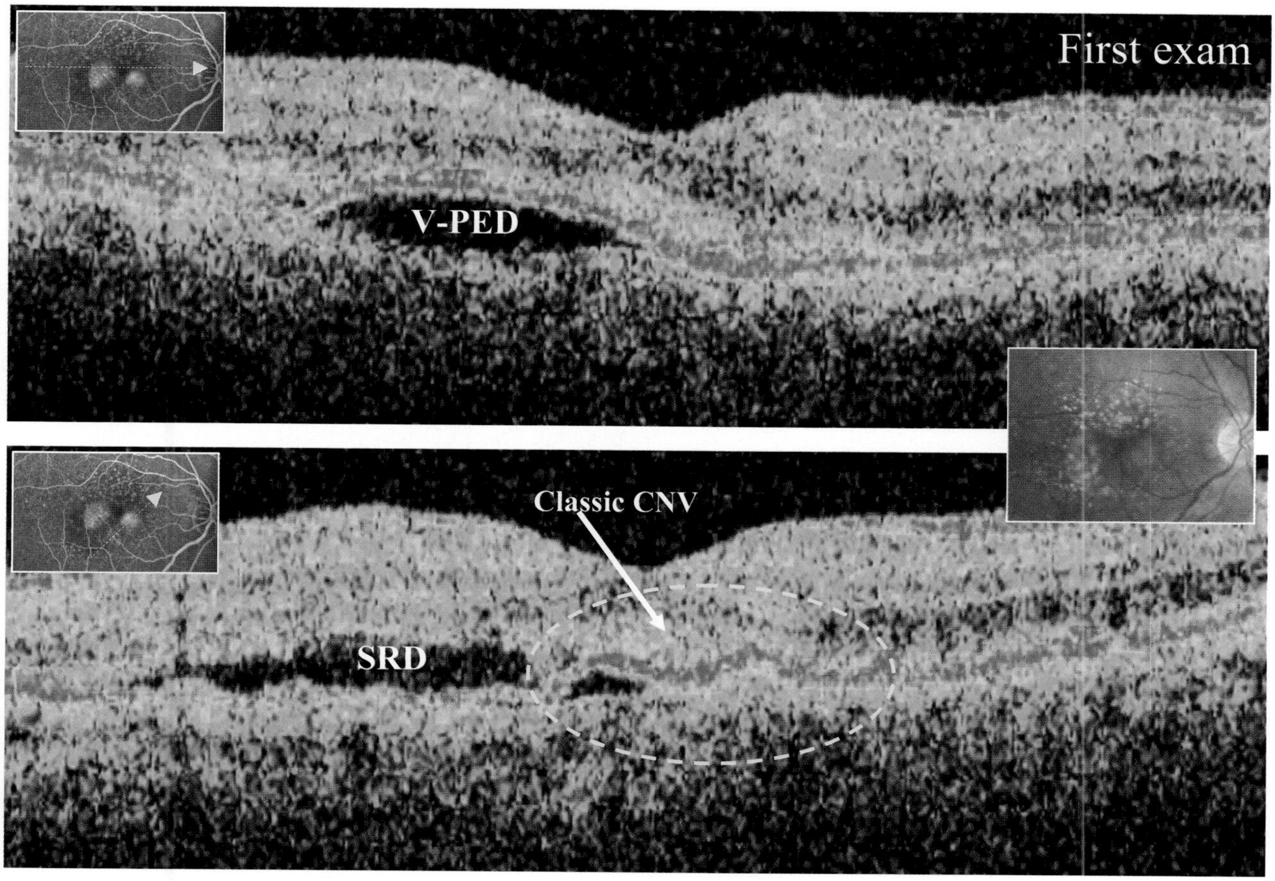

Figure 19: Occult CNV with small area of minimally classic CNV. VA: 20/32.
Stratus* Horizontal section: relatively flat temporal PED extending as far as the fovea; the PED cavity is almost optically empty allowing good visibility of Bruch's membrane. Good preservation of retinal structure anterior to the RPE.
Stratus* oblique section: the PED is not visible on this section, which demonstrates clearly visible *hyper-reflectivity* related to the presence of juxtafoveal classic CNV anterior to the RPE with adjacent retinal thickening. The foveal depression is only slightly modified, confirming the recent onset of the lesion and accounting for maintenance of good visual acuity.

CLINICAL CASE No. 06: Minimally Classic CNV

Follow-up during anti-VEGF therapy

The response to treatment by monthly intravitreal anti-VEGF injections (*Lucentis**) was monitored by visual acuity, OCT, FA, and ICG angiography.

Satisfactory results were rapidly obtained with subjective improvement of symptoms and restoration of normal VA by the second month, leading the patient to request suspension of treatment for 1 month.

However, a third injection to consolidate the results was performed after the fourth follow-up visit.

Since this time, the patient has been followed by VA, which has remained satisfactory despite two recurrences, rapidly resolving after intravitreal injections.

On **TD-OCT**, the moderate intraretinal fluid resolved rapidly, but returned at each recurrence.

- *On the first follow-up examination*, the PED remained unchanged, but retinal thickening had clearly decreased (but persisted over the classic CNV) with localized alteration of the outer nuclear layer (**Figure 19a**).
- *On the second follow-up examination* (1 month after the first IVT injection), the serous retinal detachment had collapsed and was no longer visible (**Figure 19b**).

The zone corresponding to rapid and intense fluorescein leakage was less hyper-reflective and almost undetectable on conventional Time-Domain OCT and remained unchanged on the second and third examinations.

Spectral-Domain OCT (*Spectralis**) demonstrated a relatively flat residual hypo-reflective lesion anterior to the RPE with no exudative reaction. The neurosensory retina had regained an almost normal organization with a homogeneous, symmetrical foveal depression.

Detailed image analysis showed a very flat PED outlined by Bruch's membrane. The external limiting membrane was continuous with a normal appearance. Several alterations of the IS/OS interface and outer nuclear layer are visible with a few bright hyper-reflective spots (**Figure 19c**).

Several recurrences with SRF and loss of VA were treated with further injections (**Figure 19d**). The patient has now been followed for one year with injections at each episode (5 injections).

At the last examination, the lesions appeared to have considerably regressed with good stabilization. Outer retinal layers, well visualized by *Spectralis**, showed few alterations with persistence of slight fibrosis underneath the RPE (**Figure 19e**).

On **fluorescein angiography**, by the first follow-up examination, the fluorescein leakage suggestive of classic CNV remained visible but had decreased in size and intensity, with late staining and without completely disappearing. The PED was virtually no longer visible.

On **ICG angiography**, the zone corresponding to CNV had become hypo-fluorescent, even at late phases, and smaller. The hypo-fluorescent image of the PED faded and regressed by the 2nd examination.

Conclusion

This case of occult CNV associated with active juxtafoveal and subfoveal classic CNV was examined at a very early stage. The clinical course in response to treatment was favorable with recovery and maintenance of normal visual acuity.

This emphasizes the value of early diagnosis to allow treatment as early as possible.

Visual acuity was restored even more rapidly than all of the imaging signs, which nevertheless resolved in parallel.

Despite persistence of minor alterations on both types of angiography and minimal PED on OCT, the normal appearance of the external limiting membrane and IS/OS interface indicated a good visual prognosis (**Figure 19e**).

Regular follow-up during the second year, at least every 3 months (or more frequently in the case of symptoms) remained essential.

The place of maintenance therapy has not yet been clearly defined and must be considered case-by-case during follow-up.

CLINICAL CASE No. 06: MINIMALLY CLASSIC CNV: Post treatment follow-up

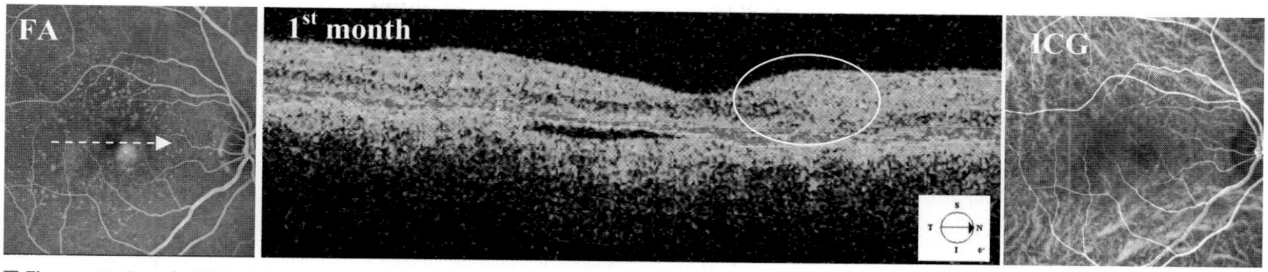

Figure 19: Occult CNV with serous PED and minimally classic CNV. VA RE: 20/25.
a): One month after the first intravitrael injection: rapid resolution of the SRF. Collapse of the PED. Persistence of retinal thickening (*circle*).

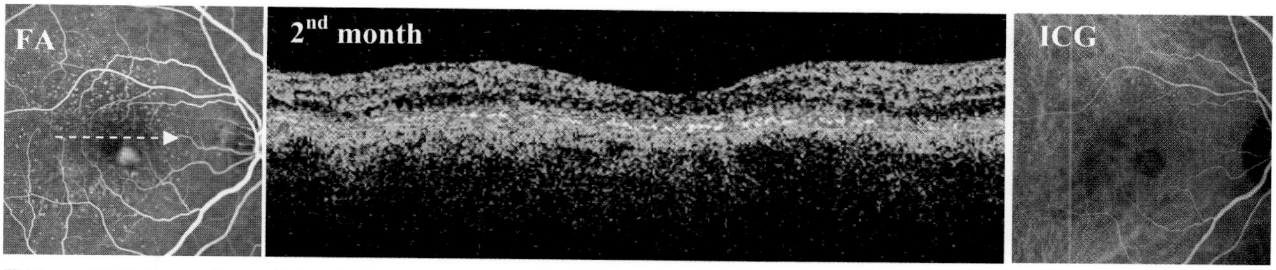

Figure 19b): Second month just before the second intravitrael injection. VA: 20/25. Marked improvement. No fluorescein leakage and no signs of SRF.

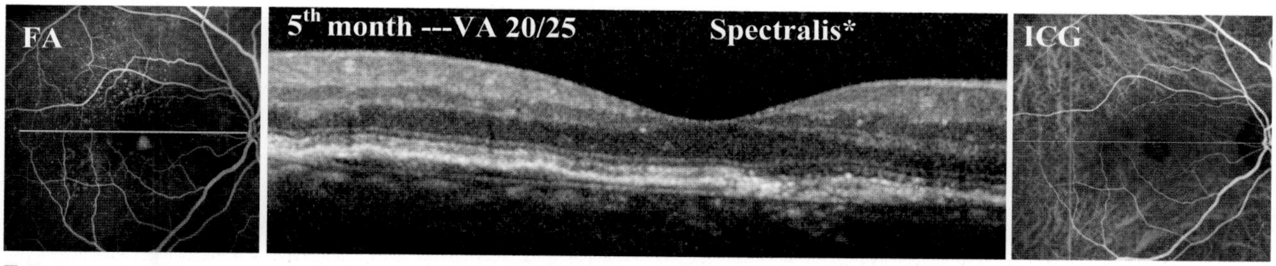

Figure 19c): Fifth month. VA: 20/25. No recurrence. Persistent but minimal alterations of the RPE and PED and no signs of SRF.

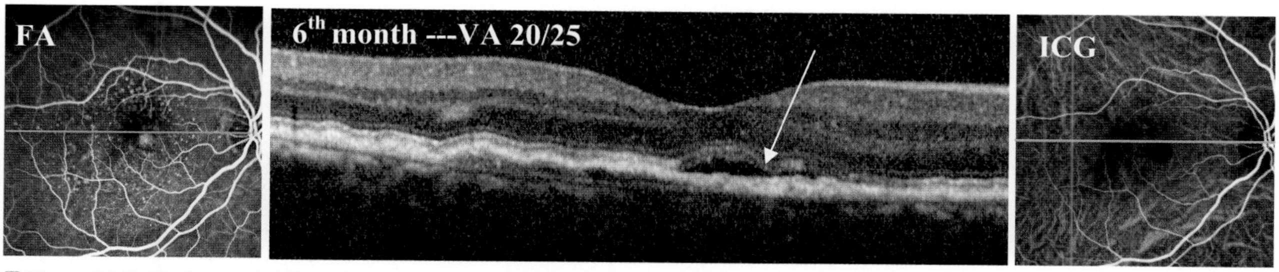

Figure 19d): Sixth month. VA: 20/25. Recurrence of symptoms and subfoveal SRF.

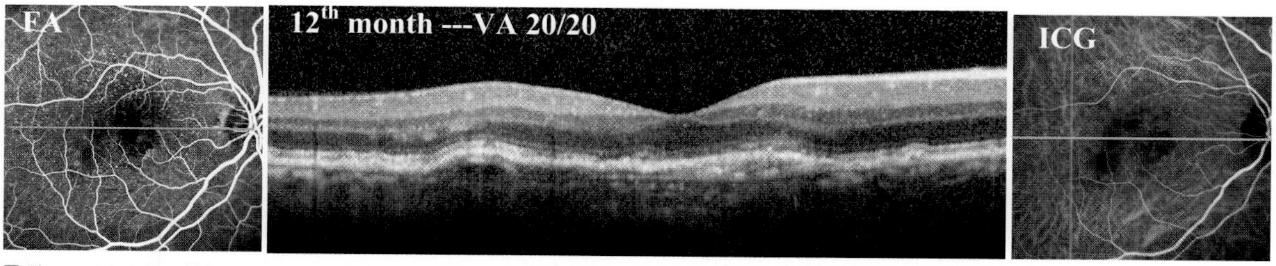

Figure 19e): Twelfth month. VA: 20/20. Regression of all lesions with stabilization over a period of 6 months. Minor changes of outer retinal layers and persistence of slight fibrosis underneath the RPE.

CLINICAL CASE No. 06: Minimally Classic CNV

SD-OCT follow-up during anti-VEGF therapy

*Spectralis** **SD-OCT** illustrates the ability to detect minimal but clinically significant changes.

At the initial stage, with minimal symptoms and almost normal visual acuity, SD-OCT demonstrates the initial PED from Bruch's membrane as well as any early changes of photoreceptors (**Figure 20a**).

The **course of the lesions and the results of treatment** can be followed, not only in terms of the usual criteria of intraretinal fluid and retinal thickness, but also in terms of the first alterations of the retinal layers and probably inflammatory reactive signs (bright hyper-reflective spots and intraretinal denser zones).

These various structures are visible on standard sections of the posterior pole, but are particularly well-visualized on enlarged images despite slightly accentuated noise.

These lines are generally more clearly visible on a black (or white) background than on color images (**Figure 20a-d**).

On the first examination and during follow-up, the first step therefore consists of looking for Bruch's membrane separated from the RPE, suggesting a PED and the presence of occult CNV.

The course of the PED is studied by analyzing the RPE and the more or less prominent dome-shaped or wavy pigment epithelium detachment, and the extent of the exudative reaction or fibrosis.

Analysis of the inner and outer segments and the IS/OS interface and external limiting membrane that delineate them, is just as important as evaluation of subretinal and intraretinal fluid.

In this Patient,
The *first recurrence* was marked by a small subfoveal SRF associated with thickening and irregularity of the RPE, especially marked in the central zone.

Photoreceptor outer segments presented a jagged and irregular appearance, suggesting possible photoreceptor damage in the zone where they are separated from the RPE.

The **IS/OS interface** was much thicker and hyper-reflective but remained intact, like the external limiting membrane.

The **outer nuclear layer** was also slightly modified, thinned, and more reflective than in normal zones. Several bright hyper-reflective spots were also observed adjacent to the lesion and on the edges of the SRF.

All these changes were moderate, as the recurrence was only very recent (**Figure 21**).

- During the *second recurrence*, all these signs were accentuated: vascularized PED, accumulation of bright hyper-reflective spots and dense zones. However, the absence of disorganization of retinal layers indicated a good prognosis (**Figure 22**).

- *At the last examination*, after a stable period lasting 6 months, the prognosis was fairly easily established on the basis of:

- Classical criteria (absence of intraretinal fluid and normal thickness),

- As well as additional SD-OCT criteria:

- persistence of a few rare bright hyper-reflective spots,

- IS/OS interface, external limiting membrane, and outer nuclear layer continuous and clearly visible.

Note the moderate localized altèration at the site of classic CNV (**Figure 23**).

During obligatory long-term observation, these criteria can be easily compared by using an eye-tracking system.

CLINICAL CASE No. 06: MINIMALLY CLASSIC CNV
SD-OCT post treatment follow-up

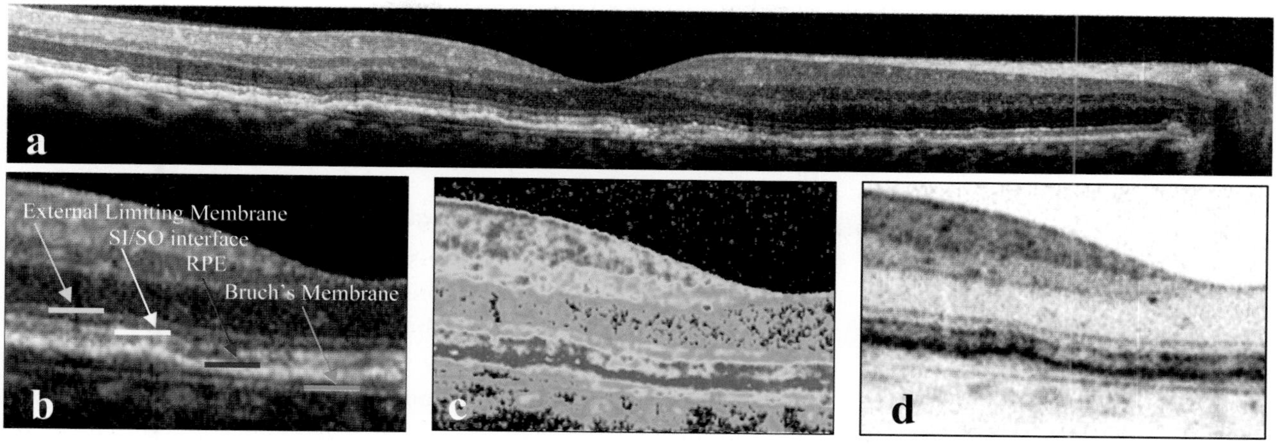

Figure 20: Occult CNV with serous PED and minimally classic CNV: black and white background and color enlargements.

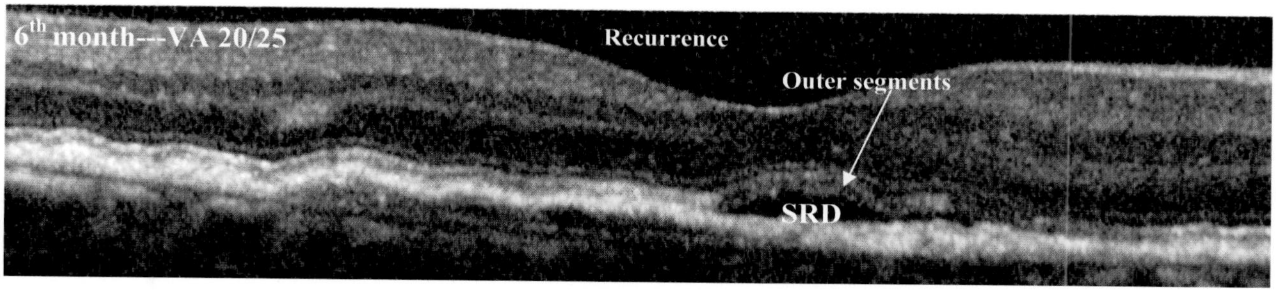

Figure 21: First recurrence with SRF: alterations of outer segments and the outer nuclear layer.

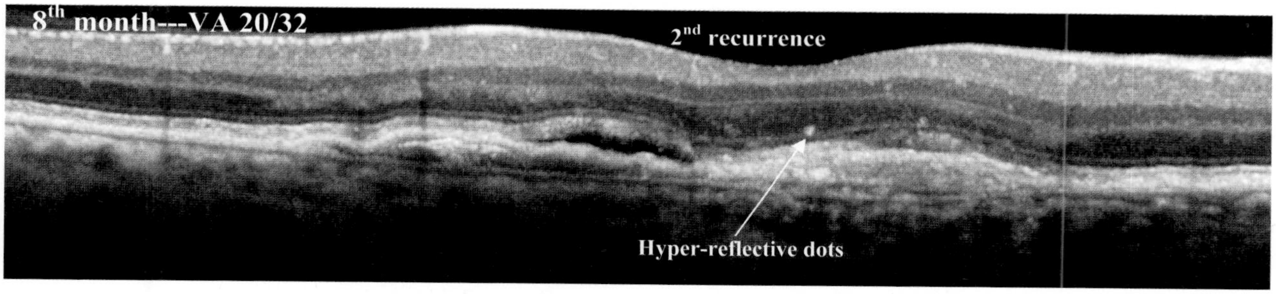

Figure 22: Second recurrence with SRF and PED: multiplication of bright hyper-reflective spots, thickening of the IS/OS interface, and extensive alterations of the outer nuclear layer.

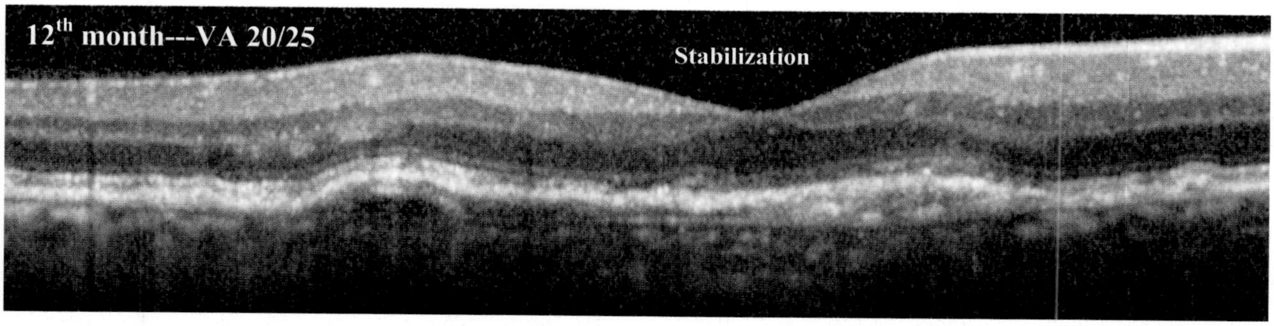

Figure 23: Twelfth month: stabilization. Resolution of bright hyper-reflective spots and normal appearance of outer layers.

CLINICAL CASE No. 07: Large Occult CNV

Occult choroidal neovascularization, progressing over many months, with moderate symptoms. Follow-up by Time-Domain OCT and Spectral-Domain OCT after anti-VEGF therapy.

Clinical signs

A 75-year-old man presented for the first time with a slowly progressive decline of vision in his right eye without complaints of metamorphopsias. He did not notice the symptoms initially because of good vision in his fellow eye.
VA RE: 20/32 - VA LE: 20/25.
Biomicroscopic examination: demonstrated an oval-shaped, relatively flat macular elevation with several poorly visible juxtafoveal hemorrhages (**Figure 25**) and numerous, non-confluent soft drusen. They were especially noticeable in the temporal macular zone and there were no associated lipid exudates.
Autofluorescence showed a very extensive, clearly demarcated, intensely hyper-fluorescent oval-shaped lesion with little alteration of xanthophyll pigment. This autofluorescent zone extended inferiorly, suggesting an alteration of the RPE and the presence of SRF.

Fluorescein Angiography

Relatively early, heterogeneous hyper-fluorescence with several areas of pinpoint leakage in the macular region. This zone, slightly over 3 DD, gradually stained with late and moderate leakage (**Figure 24**).

SLO-ICG Angiography

(a) Early phase: vast, rounded, well-delineated, subfoveal hypo-fluorescent lesion, indicating a pigment epithelium detachment. A choroidal neovascular membrane was clearly visible against this dark background, which occupied almost the entire surface of the lesion (**Figure 24**).
(b) Late phase: this neovascular membrane became clearly visible on ICG angiography and was drained by several inferior vessels encroaching in the center.

Suggested Diagnosis:
Large, isolated subfoveal occult choroidal neovascularization.

Contribution of OCT (*Stratus**)

Horizontal section
In the RPE, presence of moderate but fairly wide elevation with thickening. This PED was irregular, bi-lobed, with a central hyper-reflective area.
The PED cavity was hypo-reflective but not optically empty with several more reflective irregularities posterior to the RPE and in the center, at the site of neovascularization. Bruch's membrane was poorly visualized. There was moderate posterior shadowing (**Figure 25a**).
Anterior to the RPE, the neurosensory retina was slightly thickened with partial disorganization of retinal layers that were poorly distinguished. Slight intraretinal fluid caused partial loss of the foveal depression. A **hypo-reflective SRF** was visible at the edge of the lesion with no cysts and no intraretinal hyper-reflective structures.

Vertical and oblique sections
The appearance was almost identical, suggesting that the PED and neovascularization occupied a regular, rounded zone (**Figure 25b and c**).
The hyper-reflectivity, more intense in the center, was probably related to neovascularization and associated fibrosis.

Diagnosis
OCT examination demonstrated a relatively flat but fairly extensive, irregular, and bi-lobed **fibrovascular pigment epithelium detachment** with a moderately reflective cavity.
The **exudative reaction** was limited, with subretinal and intraretinal fluid predominantly in the inferior nasal sector (thickness: 240 microns). These signs suggested the presence of **occult choroidal neovascularization.**
Angiography confirmed the presence of **subfoveal occult CNV** with a well-defined membrane on SLO-ICG, inducing leakage and progressive fibrosis.
This slowly progressive lesion had only recently caused symptoms, although the lesion was already 3 DD with the early signs of fibrosis.
These first signs of decompensation justified initiation of anti-VEGF therapy.

CLINICAL CASE No. 07: LARGE OCCULT CNV

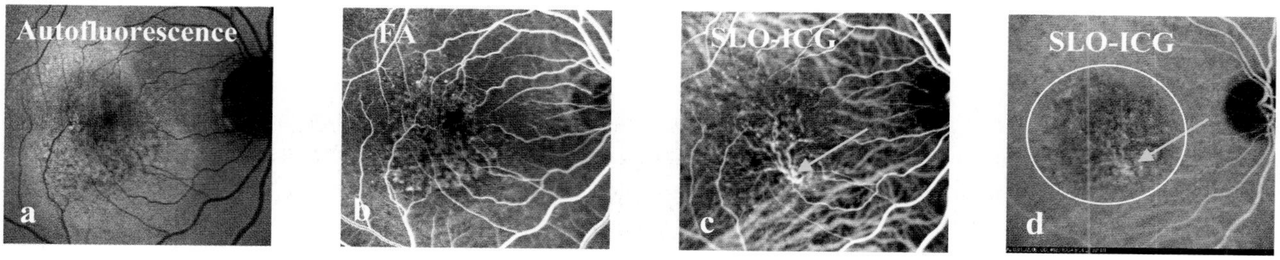

Figure 24: Large occult CNV. VA: 20/32.

a): Autofluorescence: oval-shaped, relatively flat macular elevation. Very extensive, clearly demarcated autofluorescent zone extending inferiorly, suggesting alteration of the RPE and the presence of SRF. Xanthophyll pigment is slightly altered.
b): Fluorescein angiography: relatively early, heterogeneous, discrete hyper-fluorescence with several areas of pinpoint leakeage occupying the macular region. The lesion is slightly over 3 DD with late and moderate fluorescein leakage.
c): SLO-ICG angiography, early phase: vast, rounded, well-delineated, subfoveal hypo-fluorescent lesion, indicating pigment epithelium detachment. A choroidal neovascular membrane is clearly visible against this dark background, occupying almost the entire surface of the lesion (*yellow arrow*).
d): Late phase: the neovascular membrane remains clearly visible on ICG angiography and is drained by several inferior vessels encroaching the center in the late image (*circle*).

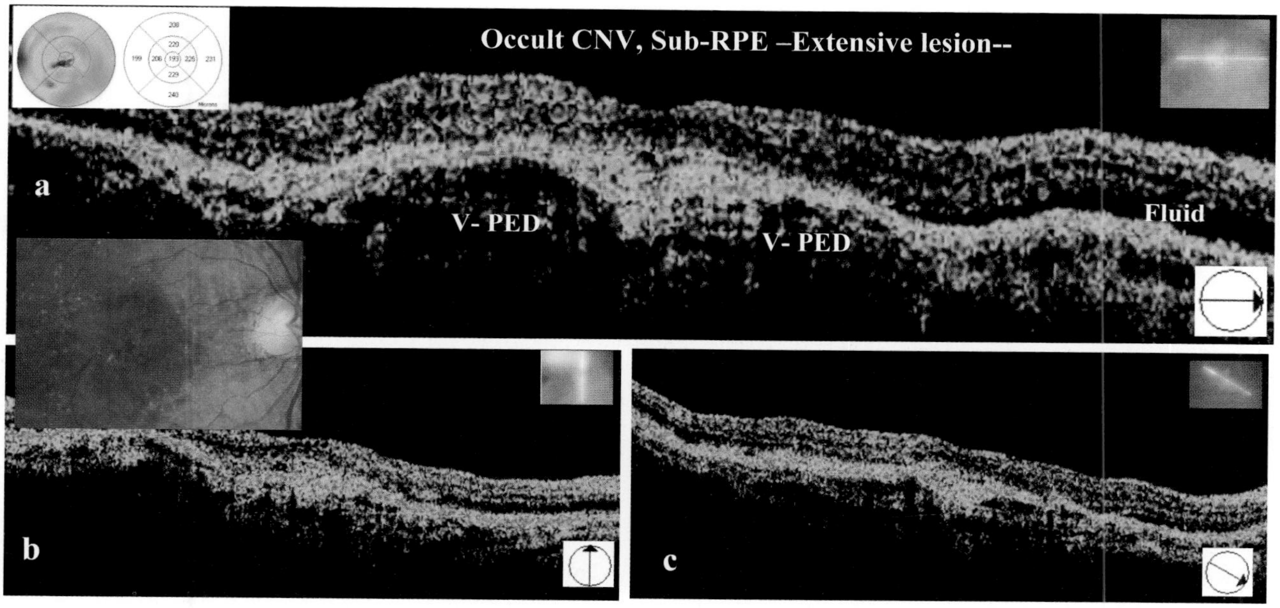

Figure 25: Large occult CNV. VA: 20/32.

a): *Stratus horizontal sections:** irregular, bi-lobed PED with central hyper-reflectivity at the site of neovascularization.
The RPE is thickened and irregular with moderate but fairly wide elevation. The PED cavity is hypo-reflective but not optically empty, with moderate posterior shadowing. Bruch's membrane is poorly visualized.
Anterior to the RPE, slight retinal thickening and loss of the foveal depression; partial disorganization of retinal layers, which are poorly distinguished. A **hypo-reflective SRF accumulation** is visible at the edge of the lesion, with no cysts and no intraretinal hyper-reflective structures.
b and c): Vertical and oblique sections: the appearance is almost identical, suggesting that the PED and CNV occupy a regular, rounded zone.

CLINICAL CASE No. 07: Large Occult CNV Follow-Up after Treatment

The response to treatment of monthly intravitreal injections of anti-VEGF (*Lucentis**) was monitored with visual acuity, OCT, fluorescein angiography, and ICG angiography.

During the first year, the patient was followed by conventional imaging and *Stratus** TD-OCT (**Figure 26**).

During the second year, follow-up imaging was performed with simultaneous angiography and SD-OCT (*Spectralis**) (**Figure 27**).

Follow-Up during the First Year

Visual acuity initially declined and then improved after the second injection, before stabilizing at 20/25 throughout this initial period.

TD-OCT

On the first follow-up examination
Retinal thickness gradually decreased and intraretinal fluid resolved. The foveal depression became more clearly visible and retinal layers became more distinct (**Figure 26a**).

After the second injection
A layer of subretinal fluid was observed that persisted and increased despite improvement of visual acuity (**Figure 26b-e**).

The pigment epithelium detachment became flatter, more irregular, and wavy, with a moderately reflective cavity (false green color) suggesting progressive organization with no intraretinal fluid.

After the fourth injection
The imaging signs remained stable and visual acuity remained normal (**Figure 26c and d**).

IVT injections were therefore stopped, while maintaining follow-up imaging every two months for the first year.

Fluorescein Angiography

The irregularly hyper-fluorescent lesion remained almost stable with the appearance of a few hypo-fluorescent defects.

However, the lesion did not increase in size and did not present any signs of new hemorrhage (**Figure 26c, d, and e**).

ICG Angiography

The neovascular membrane remained visible, and large vessels were well perfused at each examination.

However, the membrane appeared to be thinner and limited to the two inferior draining vessels (**Figure 26c, d, and e**).

At this Stage
The lesion appeared to be stabilized with good VA. This improvement justified suspension of IVT injections (**Figure 26e**).

Subjective and objective improvement was obtained rapidly after the second injection, with restoration of visual acuity to 20/25 that remained stable on several successive examinations. Suspension of treatment is temporary and can only be considered to be definitive after long-term follow-up.

This functional improvement contrasted with the persistent SRF visualized by OCT, which may correspond to transient intraretinal fluid before complete resorption.

This contrast between clinical and OCT signs required a very cautious attitude during the second year. Follow-up was maintained and subsequently used SD-OCT.

CLINICAL CASE No. 07: LARGE OCCULT CNV
Follow-up after treatment

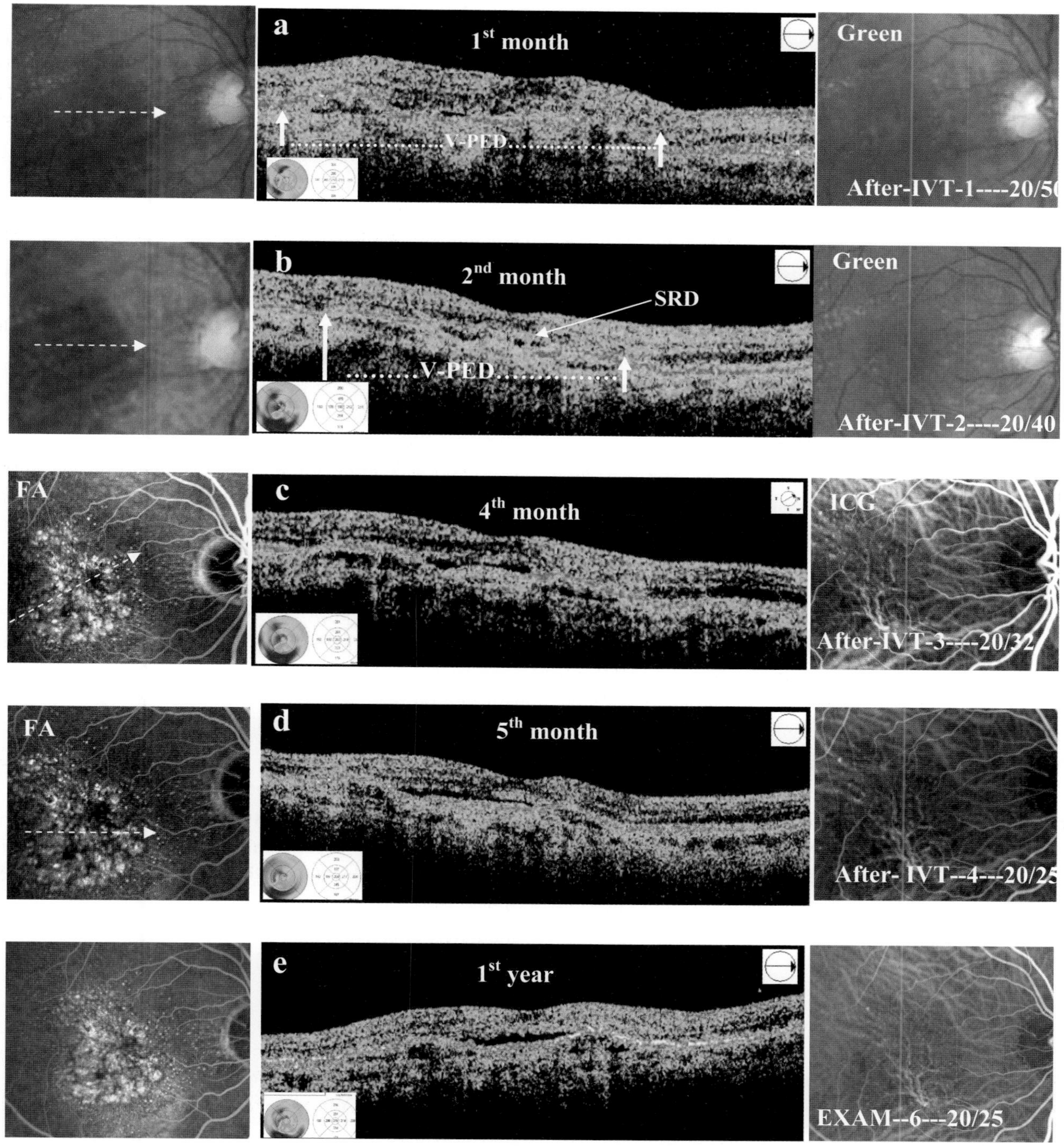

Figure 26: Large occult CNV. VA: 20/50.

a): After the first IVT injection: slight improvement on OCT despite a relative decline in visual acuity.
b): Functional improvement, decreased retinal thickness, minimal subretinal fluid.
c): After the third IVT injection: improvement of visual acuity; persistence of SRF. VA: 20/32.
d): After the fourth IVT injection: stable appearance with persistence of SRF but normal VA. Treatment was suspended.
e): Seven months later: stable lesion with normal VA despite persistence of a small amount of SRF, with no IVT injections for 7 months.

CLINICAL CASE No. 07: Large Occult CNV

SD-OCT Follow-Up during the Second Year of Anti-VEGF Therapy

Due to the **discordant** course of morphological changes and symptoms, treatment was guided by detailed analysis and comparison of the various signs.

The clinical course and response to treatment can be followed in terms of the usual criteria of intraretinal fluid but also **alterations of the neurosensory retina** and other **reactive signs** (bright hyper-reflective spots and intraretinal dense zones). These various features are more clearly visible on enlarged views.

Spectralis * **SD-OCT** allowed long-term follow-up of the effects of neovascularization on the outer retinal layers (**Figure 27a-d**).

Due to the persistence of limited changes on OCT (small amount of SRF, predominantly shifting) with almost normal visual acuity and no metamorphopsias, close monitoring was performed without injections.

After one year of follow-up

- *Symptoms* remained minimal with normal visual acuity.
- However, *detachment of the RPE* from Bruch's membrane remained clearly visible with a wavy appearance composed of several fluid pockets, but it remained relatively flat with only a small amount of intraretinal fluid. Several signs of *fibrosis* and early organization, as well as multiple irregularities of the RPE, were observed (**Figure 27**).
- The *outer nuclear layer* was constantly visible, but thinned, as if displaced by the dome of the PED, with localized areas of increased density (**Figure 27a), (*circle***).
- The *external limiting membrane* was clearly visible in the central zone.
- The *IS/OS interface* between outer segments and inner segments was markedly altered in the zone of the SRF, with the presence of several bright hyper-reflective spots and irregularities of the outer segments (**Figure 27a**) (***arrow***).

Four months later

The situation appeared to be stable with no new symptoms and very little alteration of the angiographic or SD-OCT signs (**Figure 27b**). However, another intravitreous injection of anti-VEGF was administered due to persistence of a marked shifting SRF and the presence of active lesions in the fellow eye.

Subsequent examinations showed a satisfactory appearance that remained stable for the following three months (no symptoms, stability of fundus, and OCT images) (**Figure 27c**).

At the end of the second year

The patient experienced a symptomatic recurrence over several days with loss of visual acuity and changes of the outer retinal layers and RPE (**Figure 27d**). This recurrence was treated by another IVT injection that was immediately effective, providing functional recovery.

In this Patient

The course initially appeared to be stabilized for more than a year, and any further treatment was not justified, apart from a "maintenance" injection. However, persistence of SRF and alterations of the outer retinal layers required long-term follow-up. The patient experienced a recurrence at the end of the second year, with loss of VA and metamorphopsias without obvious angiographic changes.

However, at the time of the recurrence, detailed analysis of OCT showed almost complete loss of the outer nuclear layer in the central zone with the appearance of hyper-reflective material anterior to the RPE and an increased number of bright hyper-reflective spots. The PED cavity was invaded by hyper-reflective material, suggestive of progressive fibrosis (**Figure 27d**).

Immediate treatment led to rapid resolution of all of these signs, and this recurrence justified observation for at least another year.

CLINICAL CASE No. 07: LARGE OCCULT CNV
SD-OCT follow-up during the second year of anti-VEGF therapy

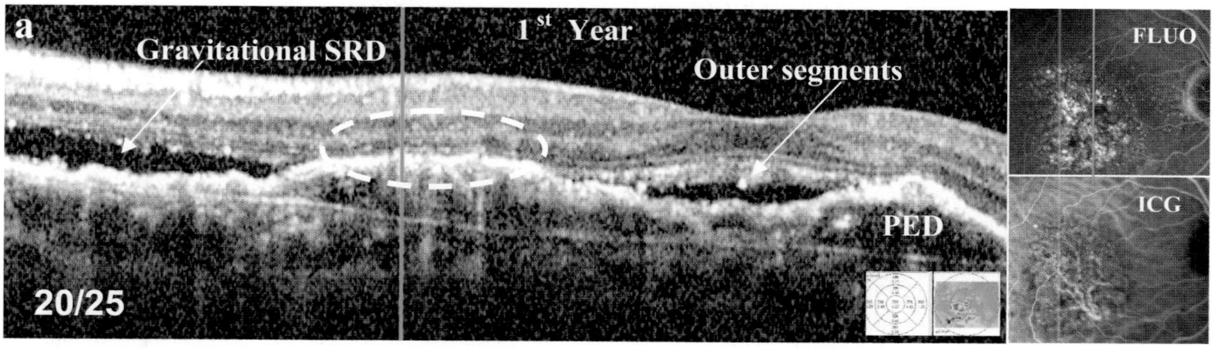

Figure 27a): SD-OCT follow-up: detachment of the RPE from Bruch's membrane, with a wavy appearance, a small amount of intraretinal fluid and early fibrosis. The *outer nuclear layer* is displaced by the dome of the PED.

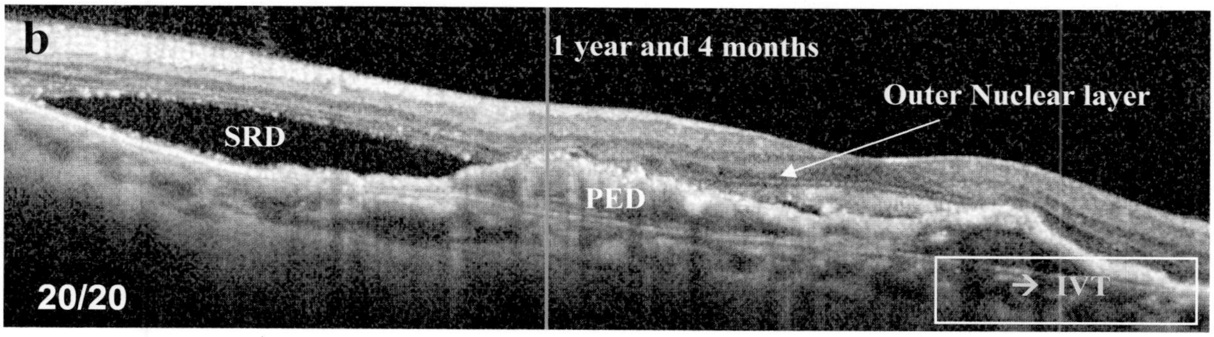

Figure 27b): SD-OCT follow-up: four months later, persistence of a marked shifting SRF → IVT injection.

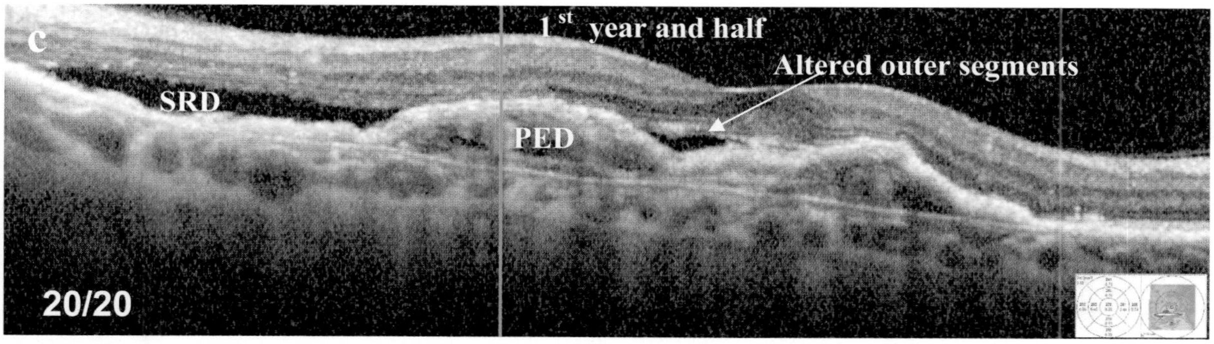

Figure 27c): SD-OCT follow-up: Eighteenth months: persistent alterations of the outer retinal layers.

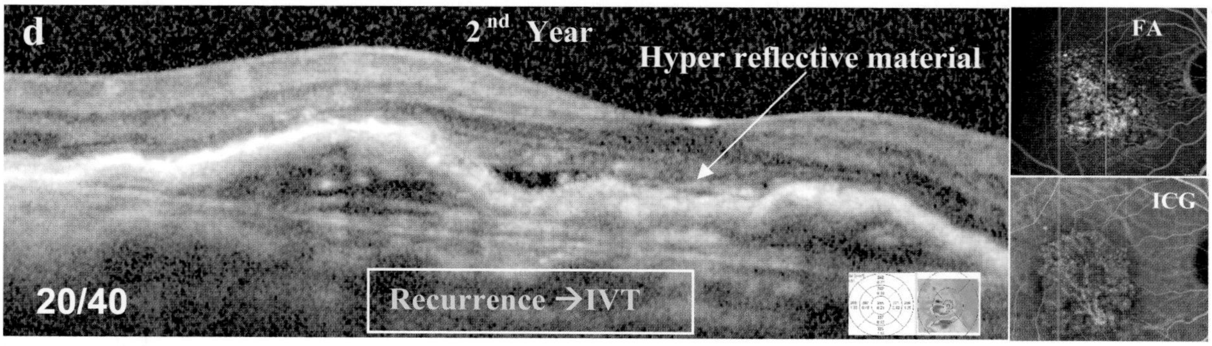

Figure 27d): SD-OCT follow-up: Recurrence at two years: loss of the *outer nuclear layer* in the central zone. Presence of hyper-reflective material anterior to the RPE. Increased number of bright hyper-reflective spots. Progressive fibrosis of the PED.

CLINICAL CASE No. 07: LARGE OCCULT CNV

SD-OCT analysis of the changes induced by the presence of occult choroidal neovascularization demonstrated by SLO-ICG

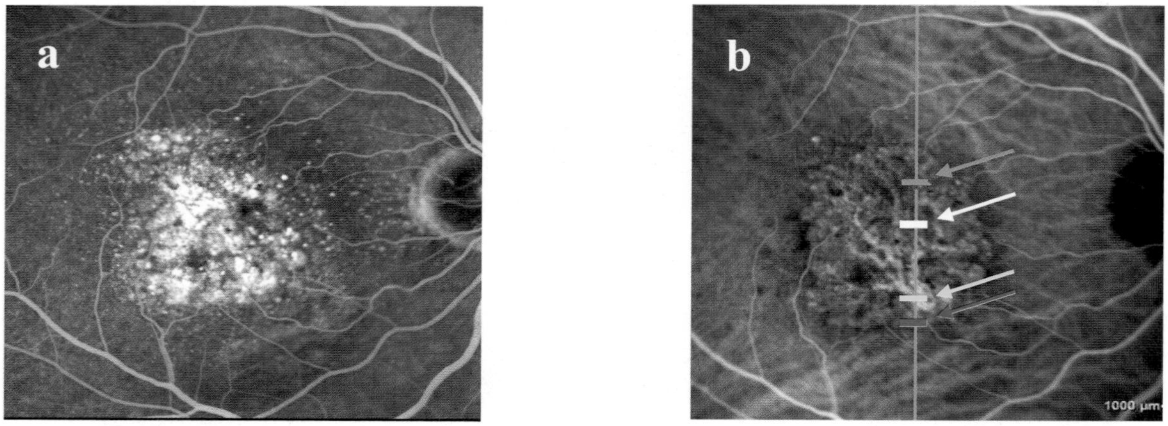

Figure 28: Correlation between angiography and OCT at various points of the lesion.

a): Typical fluorescein angiography image of occult choroidal neovascularization, on which the vessels remain invisible.
b): ICG angiography demonstrating all of the CNV vessels.

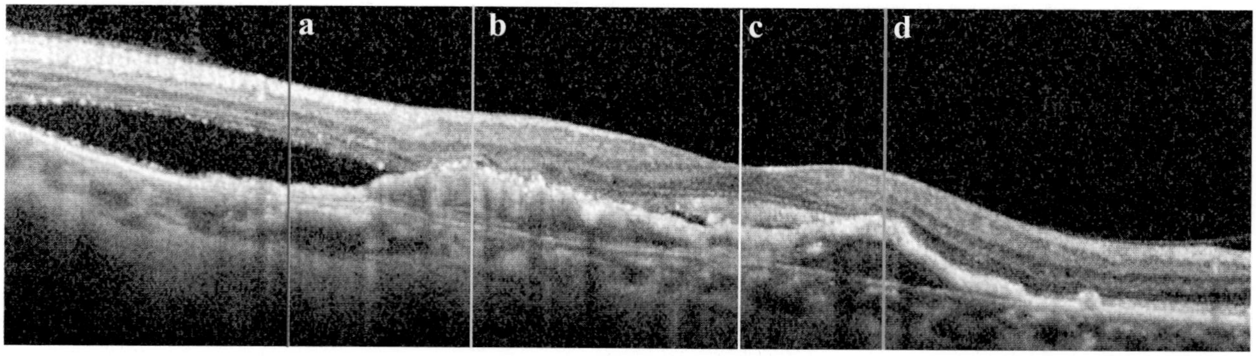

Figure 29: Correlation between angiography and OCT at various points of the lesion.

The OCT features corresponding to these angiographic signs can be studied by placing the calliper at various points of the lesion and neovascular membrane (the corresponding angiographic signs can also be displayed from the OCT section).
a): Inferior part of the lesion, just beyond the PED and CNV with a shifting SRD on OCT.
b): Confluence of very large draining vessels, localized by OCT in the most prominent zone of the PED with more intense hyper-reflectivity.
c): Zone of medium-sized draining vessels, corresponding to a flattened zone of the PED.
d): Zone of small branches of the neovascular membrane corresponding to a zone of the PED with an exudative appearance.
The choroidal neovascularization itself is not visualized.

CLINICAL CASE No. 07: LARGE OCCULT CNV

Automatic SD-OCT evaluation of thickness variations

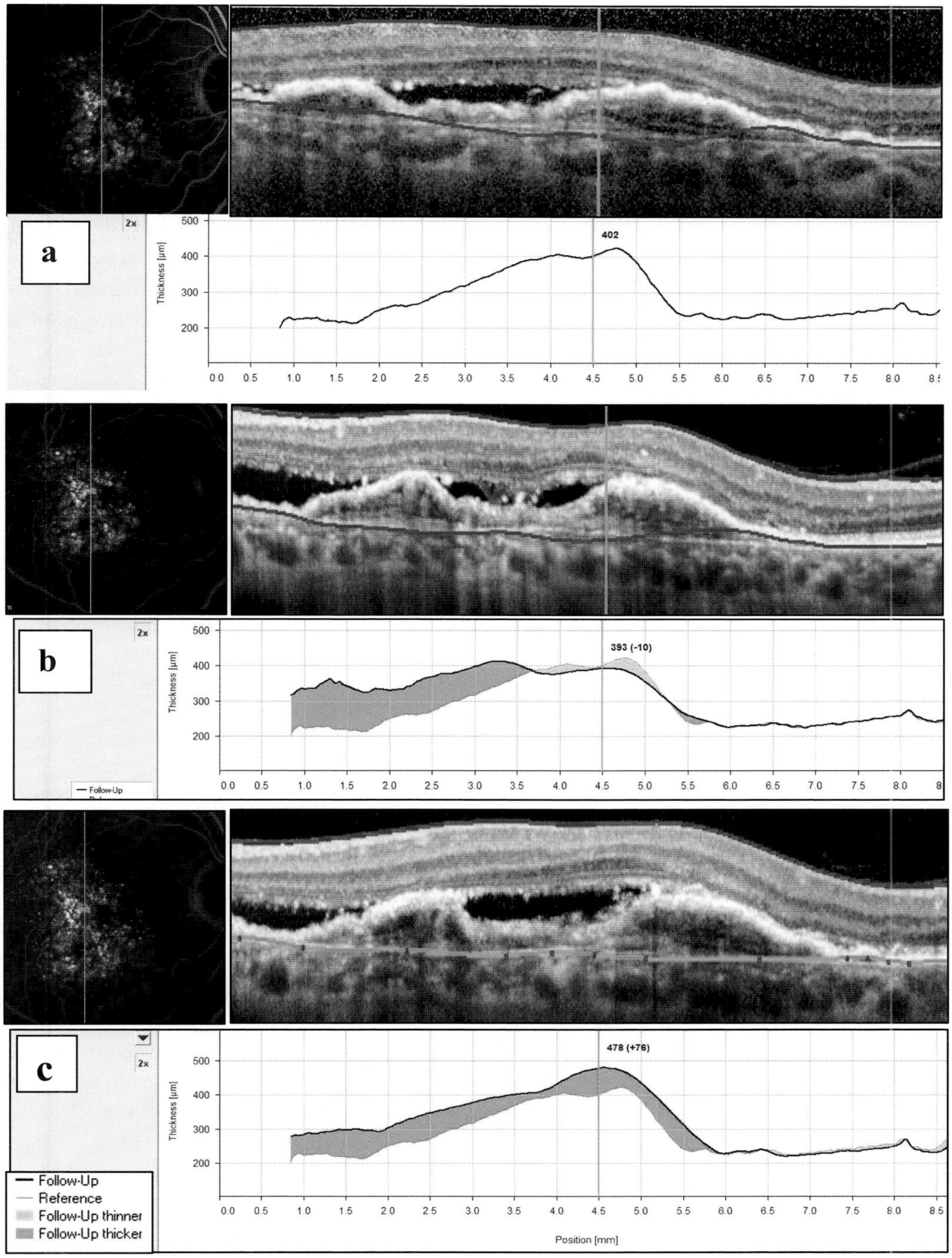

◘ Figure 30: Automatic comparative graphs of thickness variations induced by occult CNV compared to the same place on the initial examination.
a): Initial image: simultaneous fluorescein angiography and *Spectralis** OCT with reference plot.
b): Four months later: with map representation of increased (pink) or decreased (green) retinal thickness.
c): Six months later: Recurrence: automatic retinal thickness comparison graph.
Note that any variations must be confirmed and corrected manually on the images.

CLINICAL CASE No. 08: Mixed (Classic and Occult) CNV of Equal Dimensions

Mixed choroidal neovascularization progressing over several months with moderate symptoms.
Follow-up by TD-OCT and SD-OCT after anti-VEGF therapy.

Clinical Signs

A 79-year-old man presented for the first time with moderate, progressive, unilateral vision loss in his right eye, which was associated with metamorphopsias.
VA RE: 20/50 - VA LE: 20/25.
Biomicroscopic examination showed an oval-shaped, relatively flat, macular and temporal elevation with a grayish rim and two small poorly visible juxtafoveal hemorrhages. Several soft drusen were seen at the edge of the lesion with no lipid exudates.
Autofluorescence showed poorly-demarcated slight hyper-fluorescence in the temporal part of the macula, sparing the central zone and xanthophyll pigment.

8

Fluorescein Angiography

- ***In the superior half of the lesion***, a juxtafoveal and subfoveal zone of early, intense, and well-delineated hyper-fluorescence suggested classic CNV with intense and rapid fluorescein leakage and very large cysts at the late phase.
- ***In the inferior half of the lesion***, an area of slightly heterogeneous, gradually staining hyper-fluorescence with several pinpoint leaks and late and moderate fluorescein leakage (**Figure 31**).

SLO-ICG Angiography

a) Early phase: narrow juxtafoveal and superior temporal vessels with rapid circulation. This neovascular membrane was drained by a larger vessel which coursed towards the inferior macular sector.
b) Late phase: extensive, oval-shaped, well-demarcated, hyper-fluorescent lesion. The inferior and superior parts presented different structures (**Figure 31**).

Suggested Diagnosis:
Mixed juxtafoveal and subfoveal classic and occult CNV.

Contribution of OCT (*Stratus** and *Spectralis**)

On the *horizontal section* in the center the fovea
***Stratus** TD-OCT** showed irregular thinning without elevation of the RPE in the juxtafoveal and temporal zones.

Anterior to the RPE
- Zone of hyper-reflectivity extending as far as the fovea (arrows) with slight shadowing.
- Beyond, intraretinal cysts with markedly increased retinal thickness (**Figure 31**).

***Spectralis** SD-OCT**
- The same signs were clearly visible, with intraretinal fluid, cysts, and numerous bright hyper-reflective spots. The limits of the juxtafoveal and subfoveal lesion were more clearly defined.
- The *external limiting membrane* and IS/OS interface were altered over the zone of hyper-reflective CNV.
- The *outer nuclear layer* was thinned and invaded by a hyper-reflective zone (**Figure 31**).

On the vertical section through the inferior lesion
***Stratus** TD-OCT**
- The moderately reflective vascularized PED was well demonstrated from below to upwards, and
- Hyper-reflectivity anterior to the RPE and cysts corresponding to classic CNV (**Figure 32**).

***Spectralis** SD-OCT**
- The appearance on SD-OCT was identical, but SD-OCT provided good visibility of the vascularized PED and subfoveal classic CNV.
- A small SRF accumulation was demonstrated all around the lesion with numerous bright hyper-reflective spots, as well as alteration of the outer segments and outer nuclear layer (**Figure 32**).

Note the persistence of foveal vitreoretinal adhesions.

Diagnosis
OCT confirmed the presence of a mixed lesion with:
- An extensive subfoveal vascularized PED with a moderately reflective cavity, and
- An area of active classic CNV with alteration of outer layers, intraretinal fluid, and temporal, subfoveal, and juxtafoveal cysts.

These findings confirmed and refined the diagnosis suggested by fluorescein angiography (classic CNV) and ICG angiography (vascularized PED and draining vessels), justifying immediate anti-VEGF therapy.

CLINICAL CASE No. 08: MIXED (CLASSIC AND OCCULT) CNV OF EQUAL DIMENSIONS

Horizontal section through classic CNV

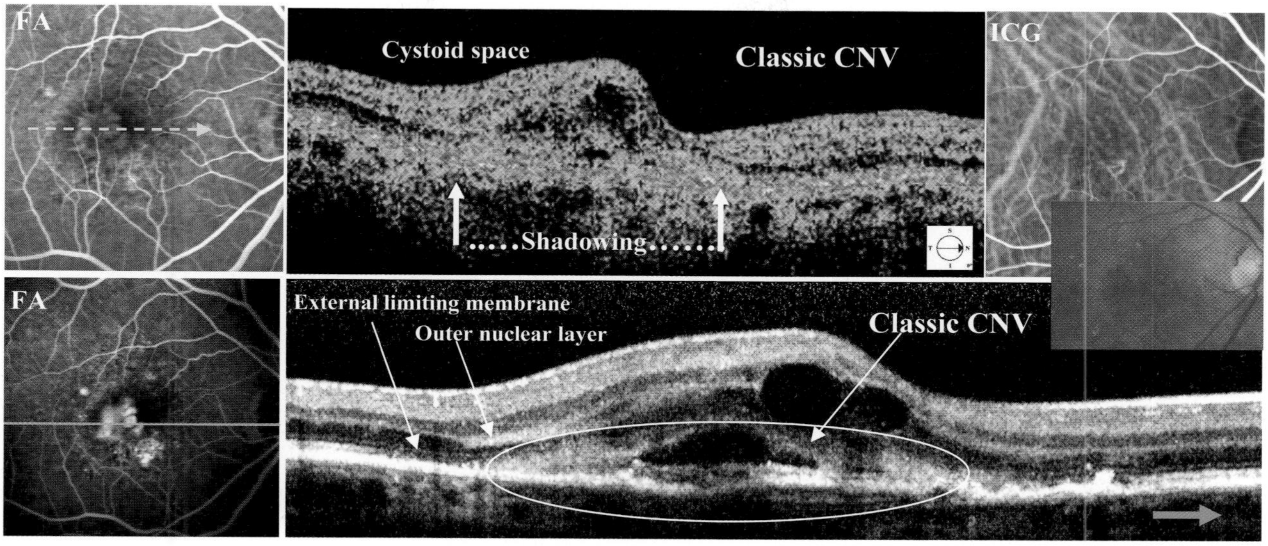

Figure 31: Mixed (Classic and occult) choroidal neovascularization of equal dimensions. VA: 20/50.
***Stratus** and *Spectralis** horizontal sections correlated with fluorescein angiography and SLO-ICG angiography.**
The ***Stratus**** horizontal section does not show the PED. *Anterior to the RPE*, localized hyper-reflectivity and slight shadowing (*arrows*).
Note the increased retinal thickness and intraretinal cysts.
On *Spectralis,** thinning of the RPE, clearly visible shadowing, hyper-reflectivity anteriorly, intraretinal fluid, and cysts with numerous bright hyper-reflective spots.
The external limiting membrane and IS/OS interface are altered over the zone of hyper-reflective CNV. The outer nuclear layer is thinned.

Vertical section through occult CNV

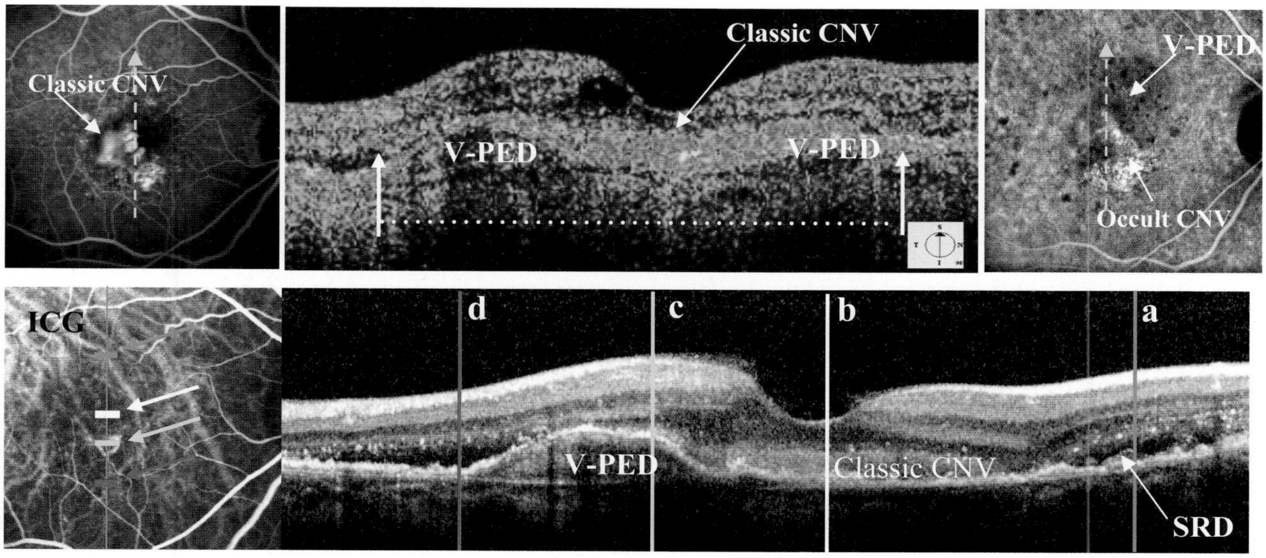

Figure 32: Mixed, classic, and occult choroidal neovascularization of equal dimensions. VA: 20/50.
***Stratus** and *Spectralis** vertical sections correlated with fluorescein angiography and SLO-ICG angiography.**
The ***Stratus**** vertical section clearly shows the moderately reflective subfoveal vascularized pigment epithelium detachment. Hyper-reflectivity anterior to the RPE (classic CNV) and intraretinal fluid and cysts.
On ***Spectralis****, vascularized PED and subfoveal classic CNV. Numerous bright hyper-reflective spots, alterations of outer segments and outer nuclear layer. Note the persistence of vitreoretinal adhesions.

CLINICAL CASE No. 08: Mixed (Classic and Occult) CNV of Equal Dimensions

Follow-Up after Treatment

The response to treatment of monthly intravitreal injections of anti-VEGF (*Lucentis**) was monitored with visual acuity, OCT, fluorescein angiography, and ICG angiography.

Each injection was administered as indicated, which was followed by an immediate and dramatic improvement in retinal architecture (**Figure 33**).

After the first injection, visual acuity was moderately improved but with a marked improvement of visual symptoms.

OCT

By the first examination, dramatic improvement was demonstrated, with reduction of retinal thickness and a complete and rapid resolution of the large foveal and juxtafoveal intraretinal cysts.

On the **horizontal section**, resolution of intraretinal fluid and restoration of a normal and symmetrical foveal depression.

The inner and outer retinal layers became clearly visible. The outer nuclear layer was constantly visible and was only thinned over the classic CNV. The external limiting membrane was distinguishable with a normal appearance.

The only residual sign after resolution of classic CNV was the localized zone of hyper-reflectivity between the external limiting membrane and the IS/OS interface with thickening of the IS/OS interface (**Figure 33**).

In the inferior part of the **vertical section**, persistence of the vascularized PED still extended as far as the foveal region, but with a normal appearance of retinal layers.

Fluorescein Angiography and ICG Angiography

On fluorescein angiography, classic CNV regressed immediately with only minimal fluorescein leakage.

ICG angiography showed low perfusion of the classic CNV, but the occult CNV remained clearly visible and appeared to have become larger, justifying a second IVT injection.

Six Months Later

The situation remained stable and did not warrant any further IVT injections. VA had improved to 20/32.

***Spectralis** OCT** examinations confirmed resolution of intraretinal fluid and normalization of outer retinal layers.

Only the persistence of a hyper-reflective band anterior to the RPE suggested residual fibrosis of classic CNV.

The external limiting membrane was clearly visible with no hyper-reflective bright spots (**Figure 34**).

However, **the vertical section** showed a wavy, irregular, and relatively flat residual PED with a moderately reflective cavity, suggesting partial organization.

The external limiting membrane was normal but several irregularities were visible in the outer nuclear layer, which was thinned over the dome of the PED.

Autofluorescence photographs showed persistence of a superior temporal lesion but sparing the central macula.

Angiography confirmed the stabilized and scarred appearance of the lesion (**Figure 34**).

At this Stage

This mixed lesion comprising an extensive subfoveal vascularized pigment epithelium detachment and a zone of classic choroidal neovascularization appeared to be stabilized with good VA. This improvement justified suspension of IVT injections (**Figure 34**).

This subjective and objective improvement was obtained rapidly, by the first injection, with restoration of visual acuity to 20/50 then to 20/32, which remained stable on several successive examinations and for more than 6 months after the last injection. Suspension of treatment is only temporary and prolonged monitoring is essential.

The course can be easily assessed by the automatic retinal thickness (and volume) graph technique comparing the same site to the initial examination using the eye-tracking system.

CLINICAL CASE No. 08: MIXED (CLASSIC AND OCCULT) CNV OF EQUAL DIMENSIONS

Follow-up after treatment

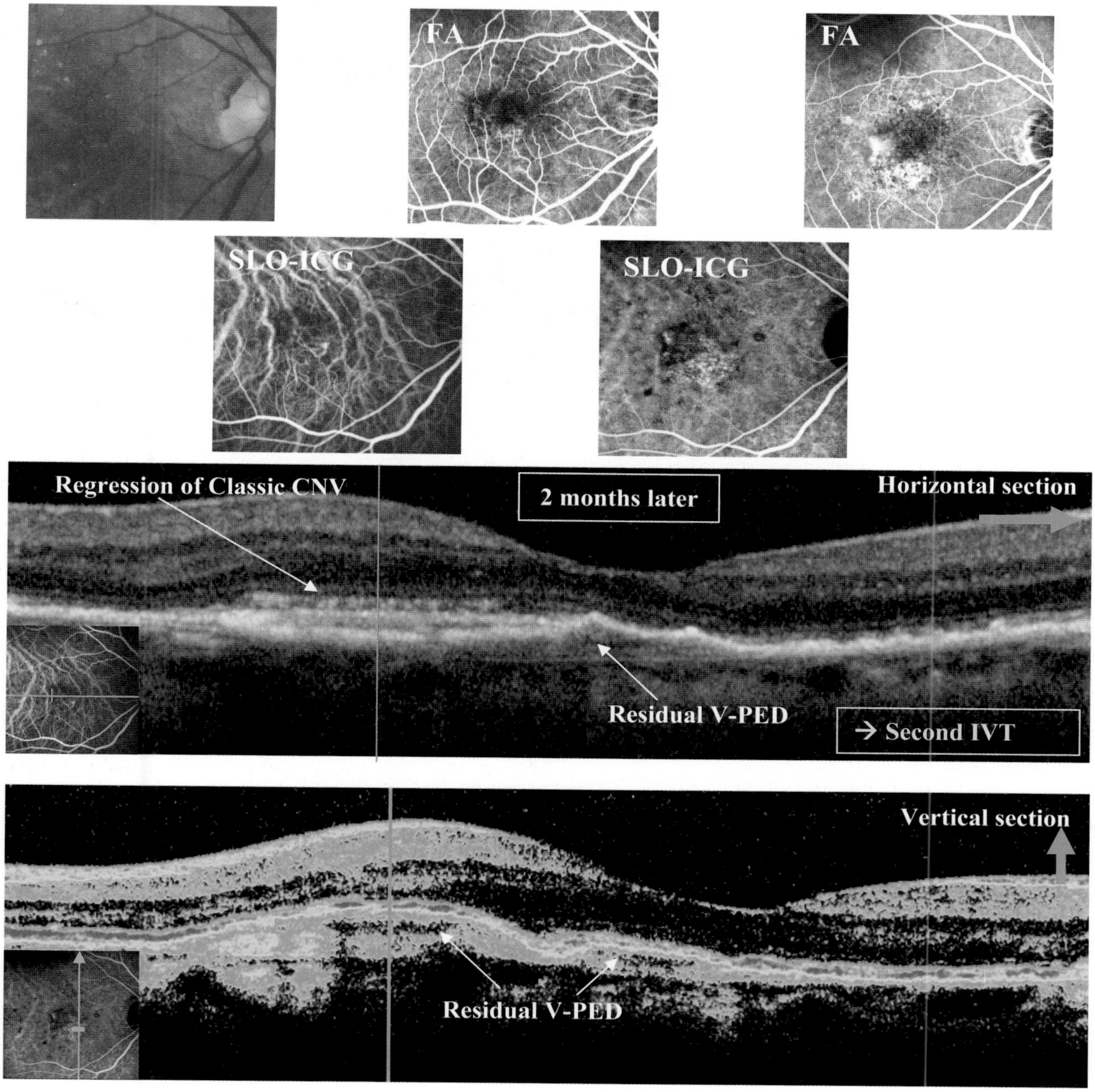

Figure 33: Mixed (classic and occult) CNV of equal dimensions of equal dimensions. Two months after the first IVT injection. VA: 20/50.

***Spectralis** horizontal and vertical sections correlated with color fundus photographs and angiography**: rapid regression of classic CNV and fluorescein leakage with persistence of the occult CNV.

***Spectralis** horizontal section**: dramatic improvement, with regression of intraretinal fluid and cysts, normal appearance of the outer nuclear layer and external limiting membrane; persistent thickening of the IS/OS interface over the site of the classic CNV.

***Spectralis** vertical section**: persistence of the flatter vascularized PED, which extends subfoveally. Normal appearance of the outer layers and foveal region.

CLINICAL CASE No. 08: : MIXED (CLASSIC AND OCCULT) CNV OF EQUAL DIMENSIONS

6 month follow-up after treatment

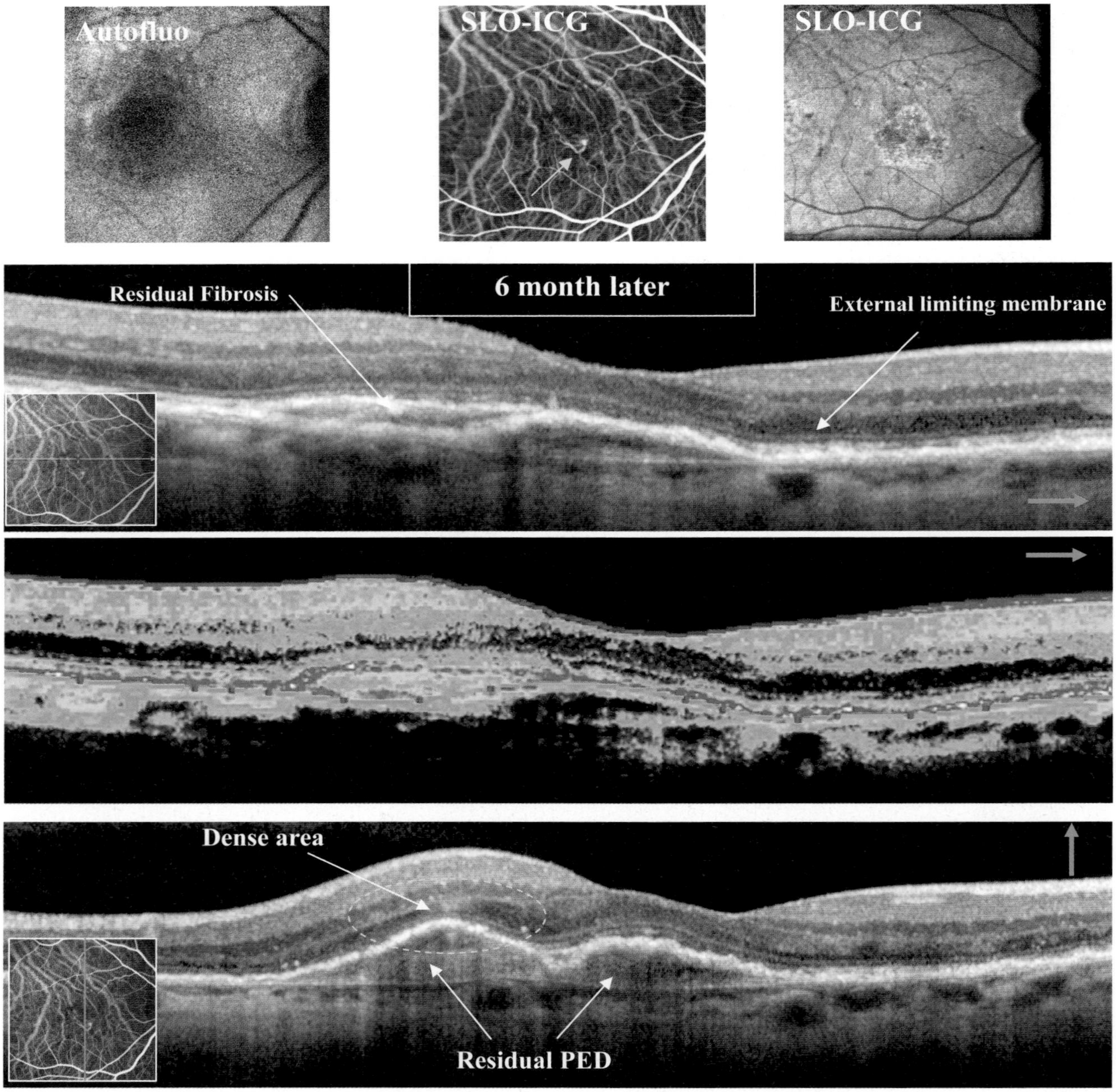

Figure 34: Mixed (classic and occult) CNV of equal dimensions. 6 months later. VA: 20/32.

***Spectralis** horizontal and vertical sections correlated with autofluorescence images and SLO-ICG angiography**: *resolution of all CNV with persistence of an inferior draining vessel (arrow).*

***Spectralis** horizontal section (black and white and color)**: confirmation of resolution of intraretinal fluid and normal appearance of the outer layers despite persistence of a hyper-reflective band, suggesting residual fibrosis of classic CNV. The external limiting membrane is clearly visible. Note also regression of bright hyper-reflective spots.

***Spectralis** vertical section:** persistence of a residual, wavy, irregular, and partially organized PED with almost complete resolution of its superior extension. Several irregularities of the outer nuclear layer over the dome of the PED.

CLINICAL CASE No. 08: : MIXED (CLASSIC AND OCCULT) CNV OF EQUAL DIMENSIONS

2-month follow-up after treatment

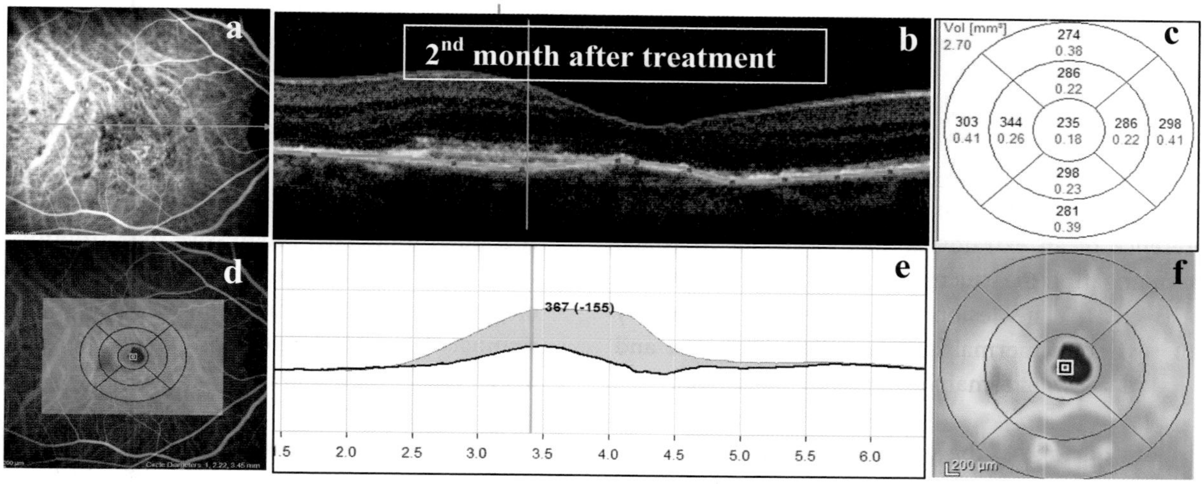

Figure 35: Mixed (classic and occult) CNV of equal dimensions. Two months after the first IVT injection. VA: 20/50.

Demonstration of retinal thickness variations related to regression of classic CNV and the associated fluorescein leakage: **a):** ICG angiography. **b):** *Spectralis** horizontal section with contouring of the inner profile (red) and outer profile (including the RPE) (green). **c):** ETDRS target with thickness figures in 9 sectors. **d):** Overlay of the target onto the fluorescein angiography image. **e):** Automatic graphic comparison of retinal thickness compared to the same site as the initial examination by means of the eye-tracking system. **f):** False color ETDRS target showing the normal appearance of the macula and persistence of the inferior temporal lesion.

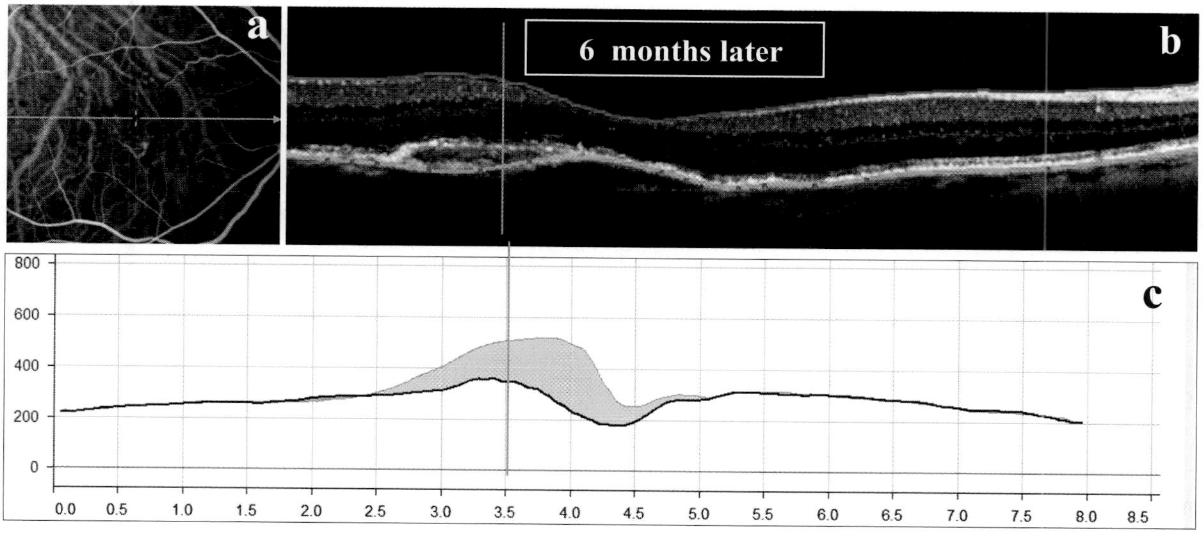

Figure 36: Mixed (classic and occult) CNV of equal dimensions. Six months later. VA: 20/32.

a): ICG angiography. **b):** *Spectralis** horizontal section. c): Automatic graphic comparison of retinal thickness compared to the same site as the initial examination.

CLINICAL CASE No. 09: Progressive Proliferation of Occult CNV

Occult CNV gradually deteriorating and recurring on an old laser scar.
Follow-up by TD-OCT and SD-OCT after anti-VEGF therapy.

The response to treatment by monthly intravitreous injections of anti-VEGF (*Lucentis**) was monitored with visual acuity, OCT, fluorescein angiography, and ICG angiography.

The decision to inject was made according to the clinical presentation and resulted in an immediate improvement of VA to 20/25 that was maintained throughout the 15 months of follow-up (**Figure 39**).

OCT

By the first follow-up examination, there was reduction of retinal thickness with almost complete resolution of the large intraretinal cysts, but persistence and even enlargement of the inferior foveal and juxtafoveal SRF on the vertical section (*Stratus OCT*).

The *third and fourth intravitreous injections* were therefore performed due to persistence of this intraretinal fluid (**Figures 39a and b**).

The *Spectralis* vertical section* showed marked improvement with normal retinal thickness, but persistence of numerous bright hyper-reflective spots in the outer layers and at the edge of the inferior SRF (**Figures 39b and c**).

At the ninth month, the examination appeared to be almost normal with a very flat PED and good visibility of the external limiting membrane and IS/OS interface. Almost all of the outer nuclear layer had become regular despite scattered bright hyper-reflective spots (**Figure 39c**).

However, one month later, the patient experienced a recurrence with no loss of visual acuity but with multiple changes on OCT.

OCT demonstrated accentuation of the PED, a dense hyper-reflective zone anterior to the RPE, disruption of the external limiting membrane, and numerous subfoveal bright hyper-reflective spots at the edge of the recurrent SRF (**Figures 39d and 40**).

A fifth injection (*Macugen**) was therefore performed and was rapidly effective, restoring normal morphology (**Figures 39e and 41**).

At the last Examination

Fifteen months after the first visit, retinal morphology was almost normal, despite a small amount of subretinal fluid, slight thickening of the IS/OS interface, and several subfoveal alterations of the outer segments with a concomitant decrease of VA to 20/32.

Angiography

Only minor lesions were observed: the area of occult CNV was still visible in the form of several pinpoint leaks with slight diffuse leakage.

On **SLO-ICG**, the zone of the PED remained dark but had low contrast and was poorly-delineated. The neovascular membrane was barely visible (**Figure 39**).

At this Stage

This post-laser recurrence in the form of occult CNV, after a remission interval of six months, evolved very slowly and progressively with preservation of fairly good VA due to its initially extrafoveal site.

The intraretinal fluid and cysts resolved slowly in response to treatment with return of almost normal morphology after 3 or 4 months (**Figure 39**).

This improvement persisted for several months, but another recurrence was observed on OCT and angiography after 9 months at the monthly follow-up with return of all signs but with no loss of VA. This emphasized the importance of follow-up imaging.

Another IVT injection was again effective, throughout 15 months of follow-up.

This suspension of treatment is probably only temporary. Persistence of the several alterations of the outer retinal layers, bright hyper-reflective spots, and a small SRF indicate the need for long-term follow-up.

CLINICAL CASE No. 09: PROGRESSIVE PROLIFERATION OF OCCULT CNV

Occult CNV gradually deteriorating and recurring on an old laser scar.
Follow-up by TD-OCT and SD-OCT after anti-VEGF therapy.

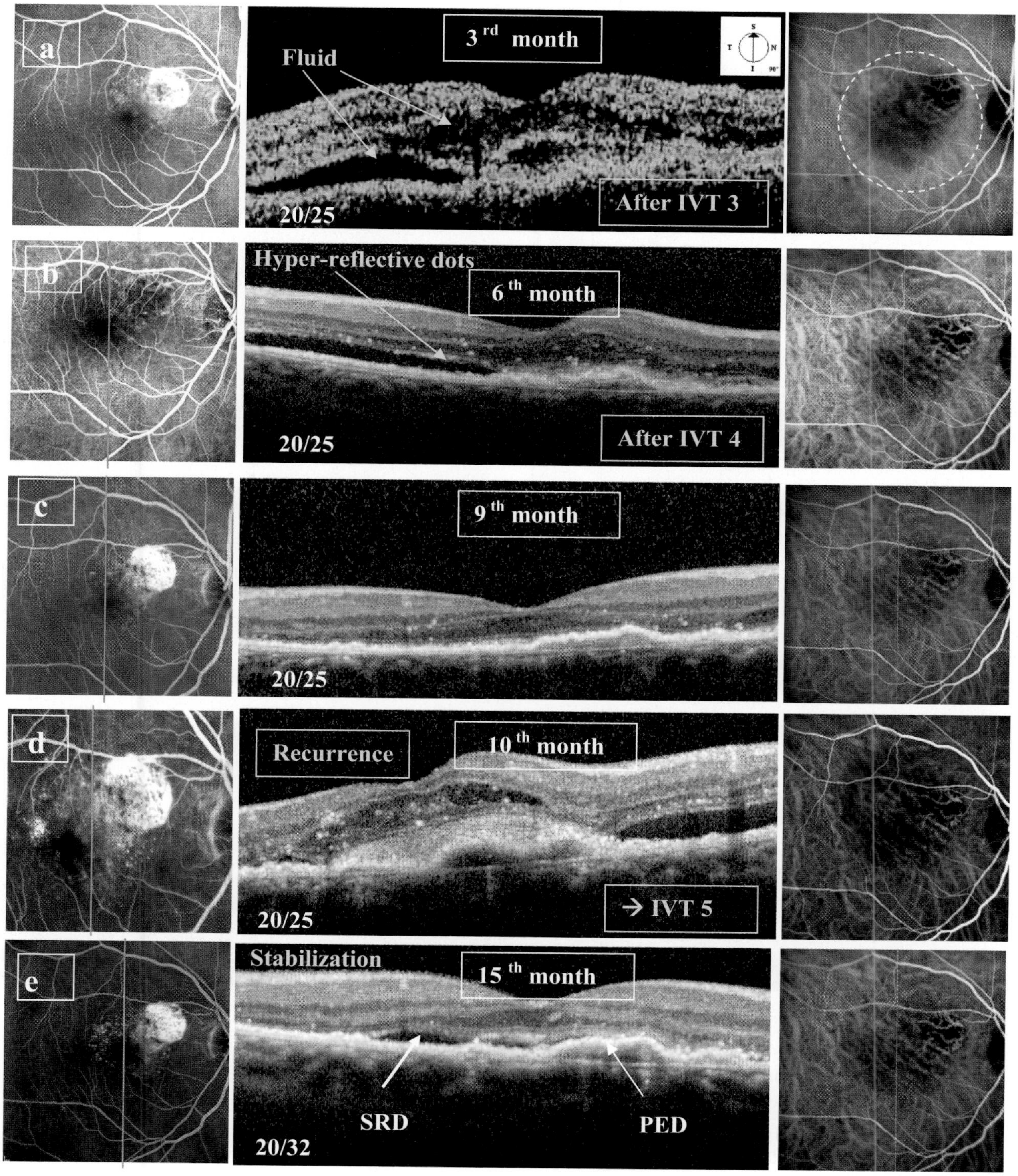

Figure 39: Occult choroidal neovascularization: recurrence on an extrafoveal laser scar. VA: 20/32.
Follow-up during treatment with:
a): improvement, **b)**: stabilization, **c)**: almost complete return to normal,
d): then recurrence requiring another injection, followed by **e)**: stabilization until 15th months later.

CLINICAL CASE No. 09: PROGRESSIVE PROLIFERATION OF OCCULT CNV

Occult CNV gradually deteriorating and recurring on an old laser scar.
Follow-up by TD-OCT and SD-OCT after anti-VEGF therapy.

ENLARGED IMAGES

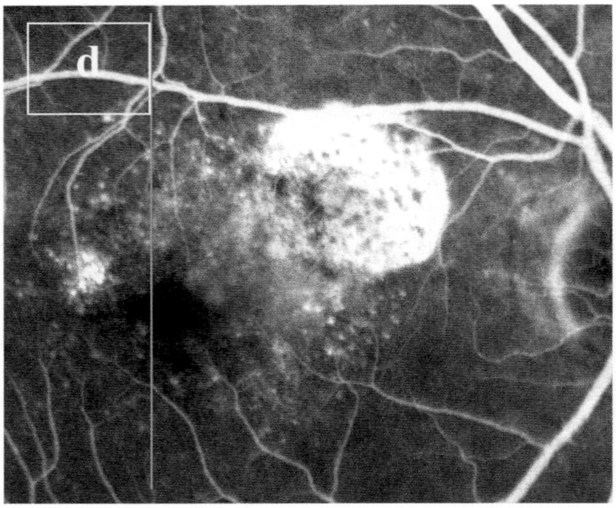

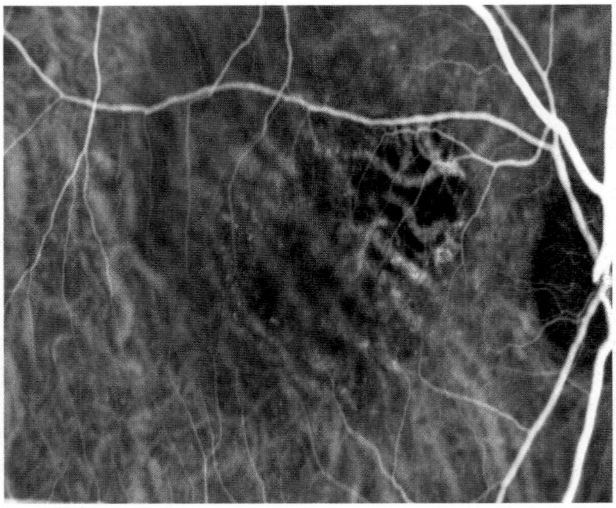

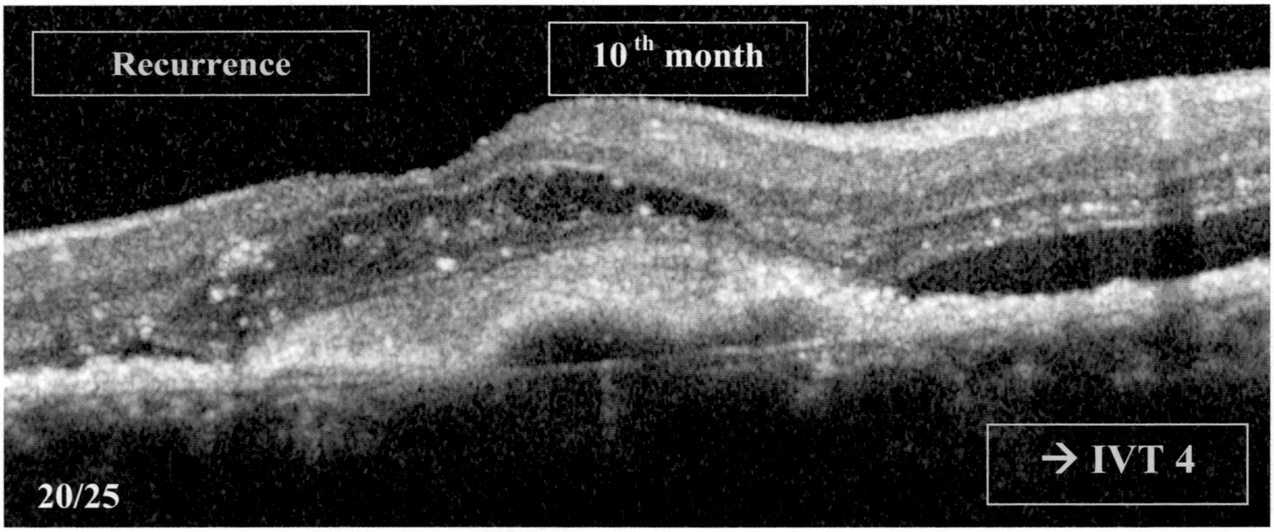

Figure 40: Occult choroidal neovascularization: recurrence at an extrafoveal laser scar. VA: 20/32.
d): Recurrence during follow-up of treatment:

- Within and posterior to the RPE:
  Accentuation of the PED;
  Irregularity of the RPE.
- Anterior to the RPE:
  Dense hyper-reflective zone;
  Disruption of the external limiting membrane; poorly-defined and thickened IS/OS interface;
  Numerous subfoveal bright hyper-reflective spots on the edge of the recurrent SRF;
  Poorly-defined and severely altered outer nuclear layer.

CLINICAL CASE No. 09: PROGRESSIVE PROLIFERATION OF OCCULT CNV

Occult CNV gradually deteriorating and recurring on an old laser scar.
Follow-up by TD-OCT and SD-OCT after anti-VEGF therapy.

ENLARGED IMAGES

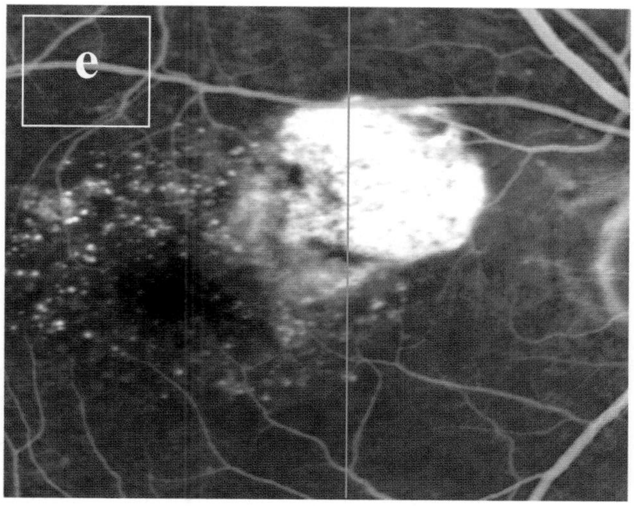

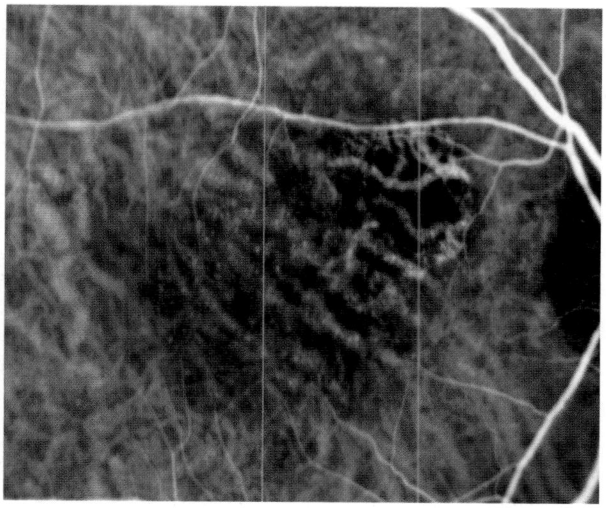

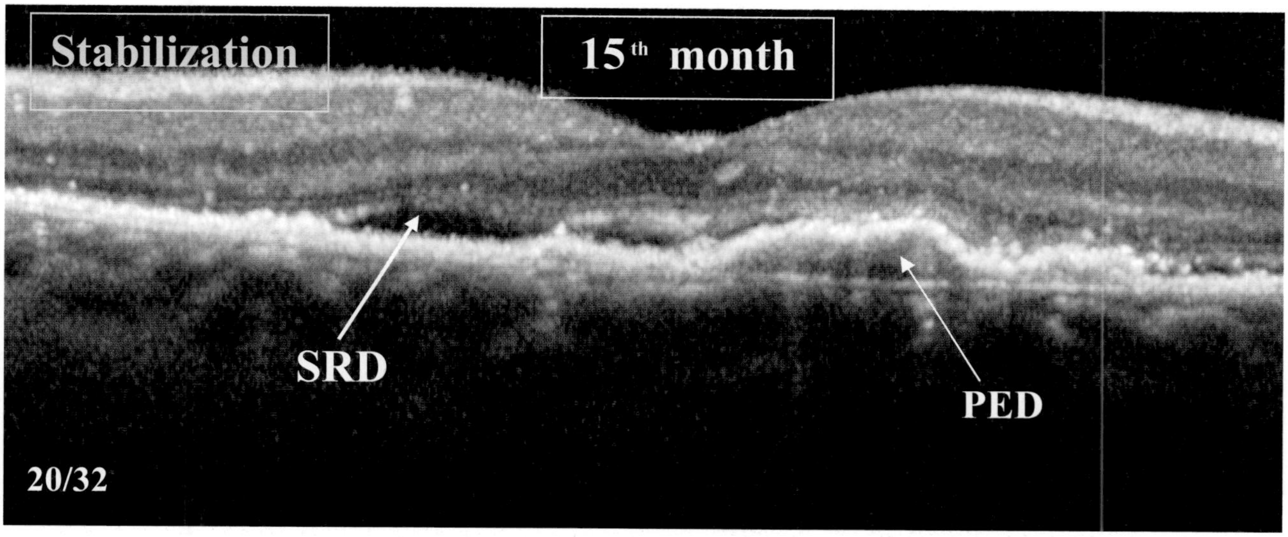

Figure 41: Occult choroidal neovascularization: recurrence at an extrafoveal laser scar. VA: 20/32.
e): Stabilization at the 15th month: almost normal morphology.

- Within and posterior to the RPE:
  Persistence of a wavy, relatively flat PED;
  Regular band of RPE.
- Anterior to the RPE:
  Subretinal fluid;
  Slight thickening of the IS/OS interface, but the external limiting membrane is clearly visible;
  Subfoveal alterations of the outer segments and several bright hyper-reflective spots;
  Clearly visible and regular outer nuclear layer with good organization of retinal layers.

CLINICAL CASE No. 10: Occult CNV with Serous PED

Typical occult CNV, moderately large with leakage and a dome-shaped PED. Follow-up by TD-OCT and SD-OCT after anti-VEGF therapy.

Clinical Signs

A 67-year-old woman was followed for recently decompensated wet AMD of the left eye.

The visual acuity in the left eye was slightly decreased with poorly-defined symptoms. The fellow eye (right eye) was asymptomatic with satisfactory visual acuity.

VA RE: 20/32 - VA LE: 20/50.

Biomicroscopic Examination

Presence of a central translucent serous elevation extending temporally over about 2 DD with no hemorrhage or lipid exudates. A small number of perifoveal soft drusen were observed in the right eye.

Autofluorescence:
A perimacular hyper-fluorescent halo was visible, predominantly in the temporal and inferior sectors with alteration of xanthophyll pigment in the same region (**Figures 42a-c**).

Fluorescein angiography (Figures 42d and e)

- *In the early phases*, dotted hyper-fluorescence visible against the dark background of the inferior 2/3 of the lesion.
- Gradual appearance of a circular macular zone of hyper-fluorescence with slight fluorescein leakage and numerous pinpoint leaks, partially masked by xanthophyll pigment in the superior part of the macula.

SLO-ICG angiography (Figures 42e and f)
a): *Early phase*: vast zone of central macular hypo-fluorescence, masking the choroidal vessels with no detectable neovascular membrane.
b): *Late phase*: the well-delineated zone of hyper-fluorescence was confirmed, suggesting a vascularized PED comprising an area of moderate, cloudy hyper-fluorescence with no well-defined neovascular membrane.

Suggested Diagnosis:
*Round, clearly demarcated, **vascularized pigment epithelium detachment** with hyper-fluorescence suggestive of occult CNV. Recently developed lesion without fibrosis.*

Contribution of OCT (*Stratus**)

***Stratus** horizontal section**
The exudative reaction was essentially visualized posterior to the RPE.
The RPE was raised to form a prominent **bullous cavity** with almost completely optically empty contents and slight shadowing, leaving Bruch's membrane visible.
On either side of this bullous cavity, the RPE was separated from Bruch's membrane with a flat, partially organized and moderately reflective (false green color) detachment, suggesting the presence of *fibrovascular tissue*.

Anterior to the RPE

There were no signs of SRF and only minimal intraretinal fluid on either side of the bullous PED (**Figure 43a**).

***Stratus** vertical section**
The appearance was essentially the same, suggesting a regular, dome-shaped vascularized PED with a rounded shape in all directions (**Figure 43b**).

Diagnosis
The OCT examination demonstrated that most of the lesion was situated underneath the retinal pigment epithelium with a fine layer of deep neovascularization and a marked serous exudative reaction due to the presence of typical occult choroidal neovascularization with a subfoveal **vascularized pigment epithelium detachment**.
No hemorrhage or classic choroidal neovascularization was observed and only minimal intraretinal fluid.
This **recent decompensation** had a limited clinical impact with relative foveal sparing, explaining maintenance of useful visual acuity.
OCT confirmed and refined the diagnosis suggested by angiography.
All these features justified immediate anti-VEGF therapy.

CLINICAL CASE No. 10: OCCULT CNV WITH SEROUS PED

Typical occult CNV, moderately large with leakage and a dome-shaped PED.
Follow-up by TD-OCT and SD-OCT after anti-VEGF therapy.

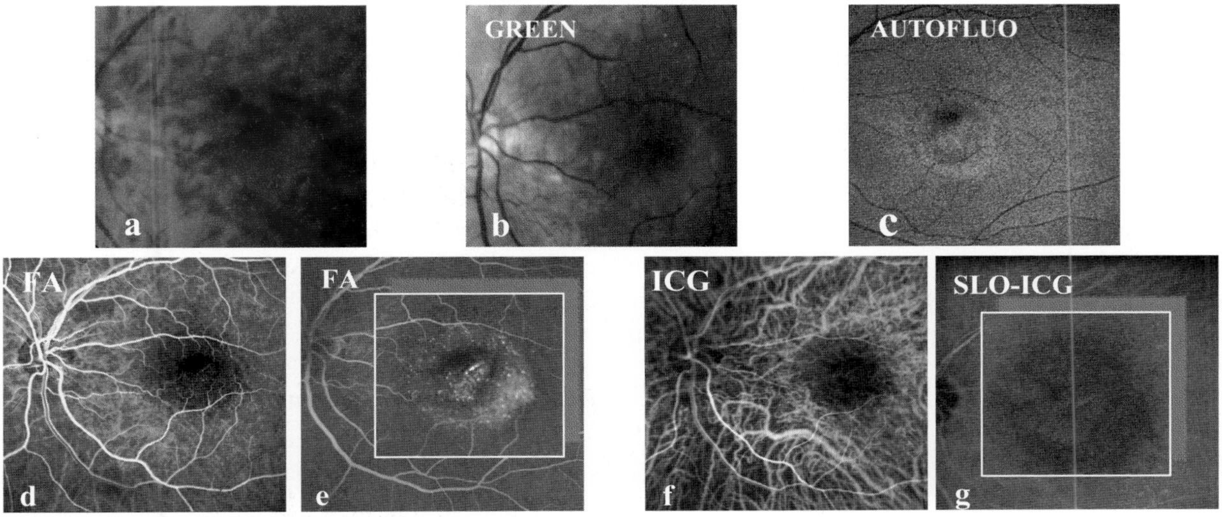

Figure 42: Occult choroidal neovascularization with exudative reaction and large PED. VA: 20/50.
a to c): Color, red-free, and autofluorescence: Central, translucent serous PED with a hyper-fluorescent halo.
d and e): Fluorescein angiography: *Early and progressive dotted hyper-fluorescence with slight fluorescein leakage and numerous pinpoint leaks, partially masked by xanthophyll pigment in the superior part of the lesion.*
f and g): SLO-ICG angiography: *Central macular hypo-fluorescence with no detectable neovascular membrane, suggesting a well-demarcated vascularized PED in the late phase with a central hyper-fluorescent area but no well-defined neovascular membrane.*

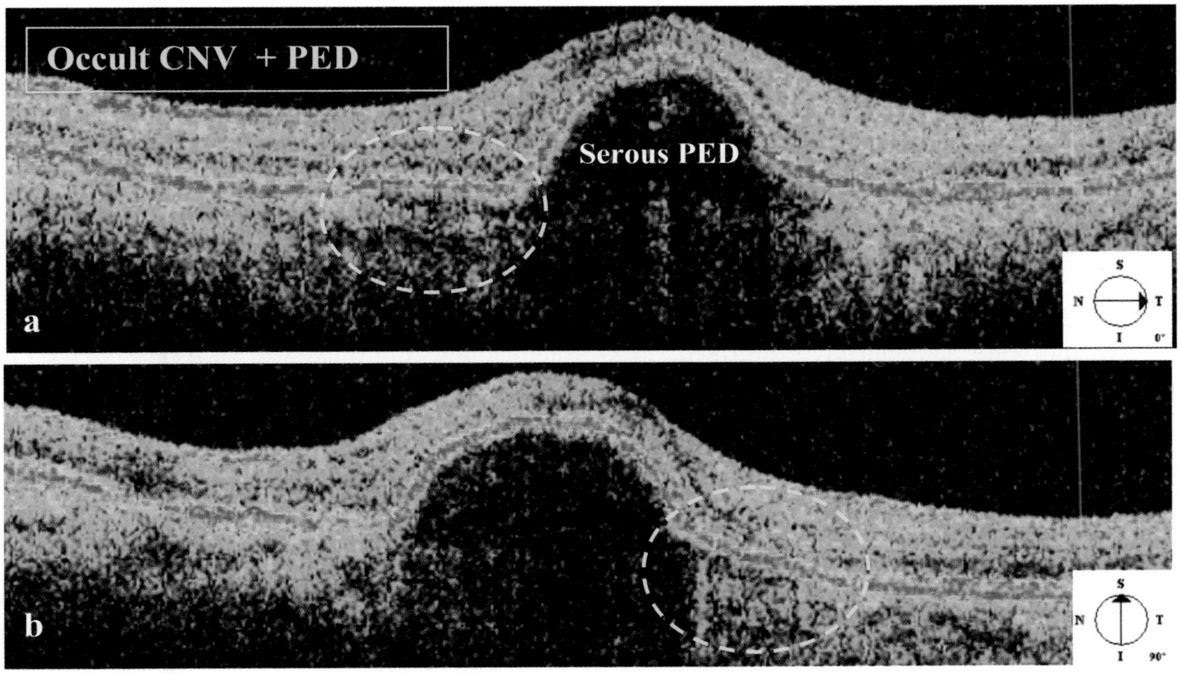

Figure 43: Occult choroidal neovascularization with exudative reaction and PED. VA: 20/50.
a): *Stratus horizontal section**: Exudative reaction posterior to the RPE. Bullous cavity causing dome-shaped elevation of the RPE with slight shadowing, allowing visualization of Bruch's membrane.
On either side of this bullous cavity, the RPE is separated from Bruch's membrane with a flat, partially organized, and moderately reflective (false green color) detachment.
b): *Stratus vertical section**: relatively flat, regular, dome-shaped, rounded vascularized PED, partially organized at its edges.

CLINICAL CASE No. 10: Occult CNV with Serous PED

Typical occult CNV, moderately large with leakage and a dome-shaped PED.
Follow-up by TD-OCT and SD-OCT after anti-VEGF therapy.

The response to treatment by monthly intravitreous injections of anti-VEGF (*Lucentis**) was monitored with visual acuity, OCT, fluorescein angiography, and ICG angiography.

Visual acuity improved to 20/40 after the first injection and this immediate response was accentuated and then maintained throughout the 2 years of follow-up. Each injection was decided according to the clinical presentation (**Figure 44**).

OCT

At the First Follow-up Examination

The pigment epithelium detachment was considerably flattened. The RPE was still separated from Bruch's membrane, but this elevation was much less marked.

The *PED cavity* was globally hypo-reflective, except in the periphery which remained moderately reflective.

The PED had a *wavy surface*, but the RPE itself had a regular appearance with no thickness variations.

Anterior to the RPE, retinal thickness was almost normal, but the retina remained raised with loss of the foveal depression (**Figures 44a and b**).

The first signs of improvement were observed after the first injection and were subsequently confirmed. Repeated IVT injections were performed due to persistence of the PED but were suspended *after the fourth injection* due to nonresponse.

Subsequent examinations performed every 3 months, demonstrated remarkably stable features with good visual comfort and few changes on OCT: the flat, wavy PED persisted. Outer retinal layers gradually became more distinct (**Figure 44c**).

At the last Examination

The IS/OS interface was constantly visible with slight subfoveal thickening. The external limiting membrane was visible, linear, and continuous. The outer nuclear layer became regular with a homogeneous thickness. The foveal depression became visible with an almost normal profile (**Figure 44d**).

Angiography

The global appearance was favorable with marked regression of the lesions but without complete resolution of the angiographic abnormalities.

On **fluorescein angiography**, the zone of hyper-fluorescence decreased gradually at each examination, but persisted in the inferior temporal zone.

SLO-ICG angiography did not reveal any abnormal neovascular membranes, but the dark PED persisted on all examinations, confirmed with persistence of the PED on SD-OCT (**Figure 44**).

At this Stage

This case of **occult choroidal neovascularization** was associated with a prominent, dome-shaped, mostly serous (no detectable neovascular membrane) **bullous PED**. It was identified and treated at a relatively early stage with marked intraretinal fluid but no hemorrhage.

The response to treatment was immediately favorable, but persistence of the PED justified repeated intravitreous injections until stabilization, obtained after the third or fourth injection.

Treatment was then suspended with follow-up every 3 months for 2 years.

At the last examination, retinal morphology was almost normal despite persistence of a relatively flat PED with no intraretinal fluid and no marked alterations of the outer retinal layers.

The prognosis was good in this case, but follow-up every 3 months and then every 6 months remained essential.

CLINICAL CASE No. 10: OCCULT CNV WITH SEROUS PED

Typical occult CNV, moderately large with leakage and a dome-shaped PED.
Follow-up by TD-OCT and SD-OCT after anti-VEGF therapy.

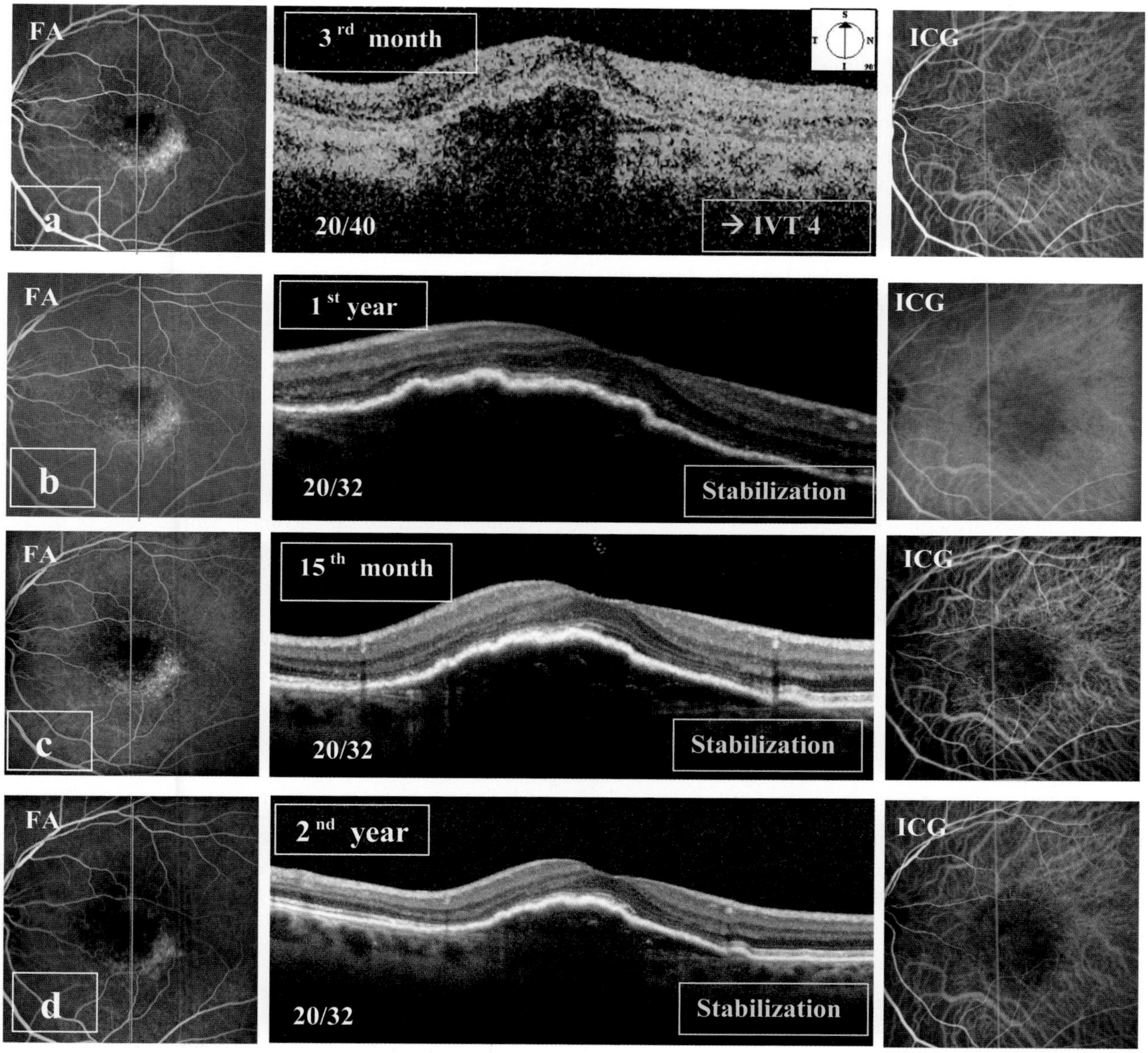

Figure 44: Occult choroidal neovascularization with exudative reaction and predominantly serous PED.

a and b): Flattening of the PED. The cavity is globally hypo-reflective, except in the periphery. The PED has a wavy surface. The RPE appears regular with no thickness variations.
Anterior to the RPE, the retina has a normal thickness, but is raised by the RPE with loss of the foveal depression.

c and d): The flat PED with a wavy surface is still visible. The outer retinal layers have gradually become more clearly distinguished. The subfoveal IS/OS interface is slightly thickened. The external limiting membrane is linear and continuous. The outer nuclear layer has a homogeneous thickness. The foveal depression is now visible.

CLINICAL CASE No. 11: Occult CNV at the Edge of a Serous PED

Follow-up by TD-OCT and SD-OCT after anti-VEGF therapy.

Clinical Signs

A 70-year-old woman presented with a few soft drusen in her *right* eye that were confluent in some areas, with almost normal visual acuity (20/32) **(Figure 45).**

Initially followed during the last several years for wet AMD in the *left* eye, she had developed a vascularized PED and had stabilized with visual acuity of 20/100.

Six months later, visual acuity in her *right* eye declined to 20/50 and remained at 20/100 in her left eye. Major clinical changes were noted in her right eye.

Biomicroscopic examination
A central, round, translucent, serous elevation measuring 1 DD with no hemorrhage was seen.

Autofluorescence: A small temporal macular hyper-fluorescent zone was present.

Fluorescein angiography (Figure 46a and b)
a) *Early phase*: temporal and extrafoveal zone of heterogeneous hyper-fluorescence.

b) *Late phase:* progressive pooling of fluorescein in the macular region and staining of the central PED cavity with no fluorescein leakage.

SLO-ICG angiography (Figures 46c and d)
c) *Early phase*: dark central macular hypo-fluorescence without evidence of a neovascular membrane.

d) *Late phase*: the hypo-fluorescence of the well-demarcated PED persisted. An irregular area of moderate hyper-fluorescence appeared in the periphery, at 7 o'clock, suggesting a limited zone of occult CNV.

Suggested Diagnosis:
Recent onset of a well-demarcated, round, vascularized pigment epithelium detachment with a zone of occult CNV at its inferior temporal edge.

Contribution of OCT (*Stratus**)

***Stratus** horizontal section**
The RPE was elevated, forming a rounded and regular dome and delineating a bullous cavity with Bruch's membrane underneath. There was also slight shadowing posteriorly.

A moderately reflective band (false green color) was visualized posterior to the PED. Further posteriorly, the cavity was optically empty, suggesting a space filled with serous fluid.

The PED displaced the neurosensory retina, causing loss of the foveal depression. The retina was slightly thickened and with a small cystoid space, but there was no disorganization of the retinal layers (**Figure 46e**).

***Stratus** vertical section**
The appearance was almost identical on the vertical section, suggesting that the lesion had a symmetrical rounded shape in all axes (**Figure 46f**).

Diagnosis
OCT confirmed the diagnosis suggested by biomicroscopy and angiography: a *serous PED arising adjacent to a small zone of occult CNV.*

This recently symptomatic lesion was a **complication of high-risk drusen** with:

- Proliferation of occult CNV, associated with an intense exudative reaction, and a
- Bullous PED but with no hemorrhage or classic CNV.

The functional repercussions were still moderate but of concern, due to the severe lesion in the other eye. These features justified *initiation anti-VEGF therapy*.

CLINICAL CASE No. 11: OCCULT CNV AT THE EDGE OF A SEROUS PED
First examination: soft drusen

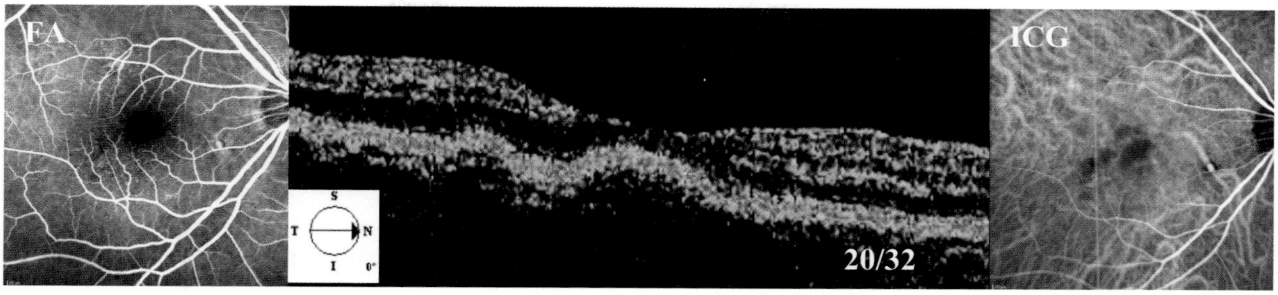

Figure 45: Confluent high-risk soft drusen. VA: 20/32.
Limited number of soft drusen but sometimes confluent and fairly large. No intraretinal fluid or SRF.

Six months later: serous PED

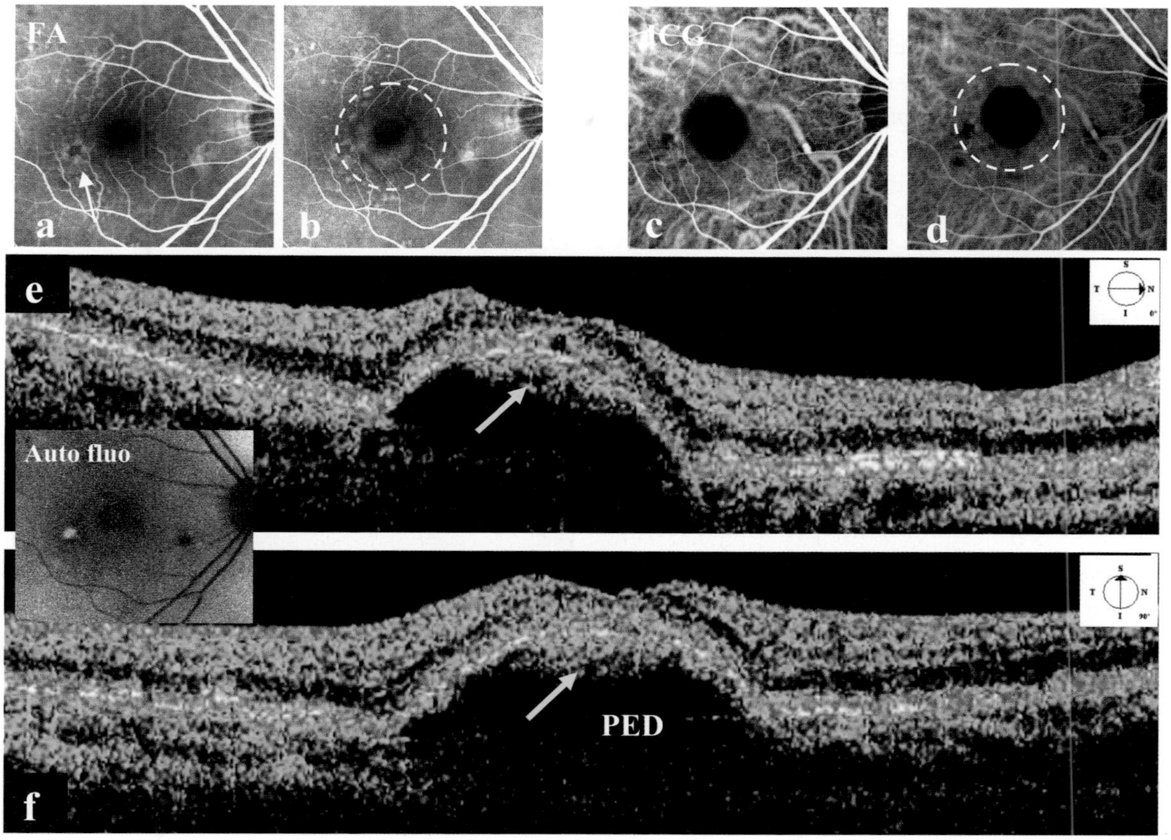

Figure 46: Occult CNV at the edge of a serous PED. VA: 20/50 (same patient as Figure 45).
a and b): Fluorescein angiography: temporal and extrafoveal zone of heterogeneous hyper-fluorescence (*arrow*) with progressive pooling of fluorescein in the macular region. Note also, staining of the central cavity with no fluorescein leakage *(circle)*.
c and d): SLO-ICG angiography: precisely demarcated PED. Zone of hyper-fluorescent and irregular occult CNV, at 7 o'clock.
e and f): *Stratus TD-OCT:** regular, dome-shaped elevation of the RPE. The bullous cavity between the RPE and Bruch's membrane is clearly visible with slight posterior shadowing.
Note, posterior to the RPE, the moderately reflective band (*yellow arrow*) and otherwise optically empty cavity. Loss of the foveal depression, small amount of intraretinal fluid with a small cyst, but no disorganization of the retinal layers.

CLINICAL CASE No. 11: Occult CNV at the Edge of a Serous PED

The response to treatment by monthly intravitreous injections of anti-VEGF (*Lucentis**) was monitored by visual acuity, OCT, fluorescein angiography, and ICG angiography.

Visual acuity improved immediately to 20/32 and then remained stable for the 15 months of follow-up. However, due to the subjective variations reported by the patient, maintenance injections were administered every 3 to 6 months according to imaging and clinical examination (**Figure 47**).

OCT

At the First Follow-up Examination

The RPE remained regular with normal thickness and the PED cavity was still optically empty. The pigment epithelium detachment slightly decreased in size but with persistent loss of the foveal depression.

In contrast, the SRF over the dome of the PED deteriorated with marked alteration of the outer retinal layers.

The *outer nuclear layer* was displaced and relatively thinned (**Figure 47a**).

Intravitreal injections were repeated due to persistence of the SRF. They were suspended after the third injection due to partial improvement and good visual acuity.

Subsequent follow-up examinations, performed every 3 months, demonstrated remarkably stable features with good visual function and relatively constant OCT findings.

The less prominent and regular PED persisted. The outer layers were much more clearly visualized and regular despite persistent thickening of the IS/OS interface and thinning of the outer nuclear layer (**Figure 47b**).

After the 12th month, a slight decline in visual acuity (20/40) was observed, in parallel with slight extension of the lesions and appearance of a moderately reflective band, just posterior to the RPE.

The outer retinal layers were not altered and the SRF had decreased, but changes of the outer segments were clearly visible (**Figure 47c**).

At the last Examination (15th Month)

The external limiting membrane was constantly visible. The IS/OS interface was visible, still thickened subfoveally, with numerous bright hyper-reflective spots and irregularities of outer segments. The foveal depression was again visible and with an almost normal profile (**Figures 47d and e**).

Angiography

The area of occult CNV markedly regressed with no visible neovascular membrane and an overall improved appearance.

However, on both **fluorescein angiography** and **SLO-ICG angiography**, the PED became slightly larger and then stabilized. (**Figure 47**).

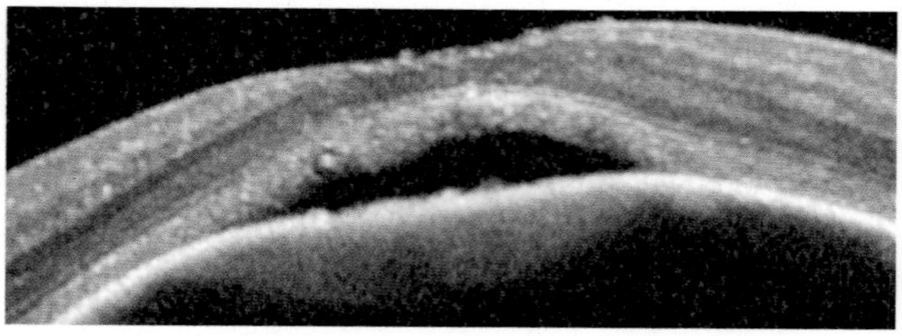

Figure 47e: Occult CNV after treatment. Enlarged image.

At this Stage

This case of **bullous PED** arising at the edge of a small area of occult choroidal neovascularization was identified and treated at a very early stage, before marked extension of the CNV and in the absence of hemorrhage.

The **response to treatment** was favorable by the 3rd intravitreal injection, but treatment was continued due to persistence of the PED and a slight recurrence, until stabilization of the lesions after the 5th injection.

At the last examination, the neurosensory retina retained almost normal morphology, despite alterations of outer segments, as usually observed in the case of persistent SRF. **The PED remained almost unchanged**, but without fibrosis, which explained the good visual acuity. Outer and inner retinal layers were clearly visible and well-organized.

The prognosis was favorable in this case, but quarterly, then half-yearly **observation** remained essential.

CLINICAL CASE No. 11: OCCULT CNV AT THE EDGE OF A SEROUS PED

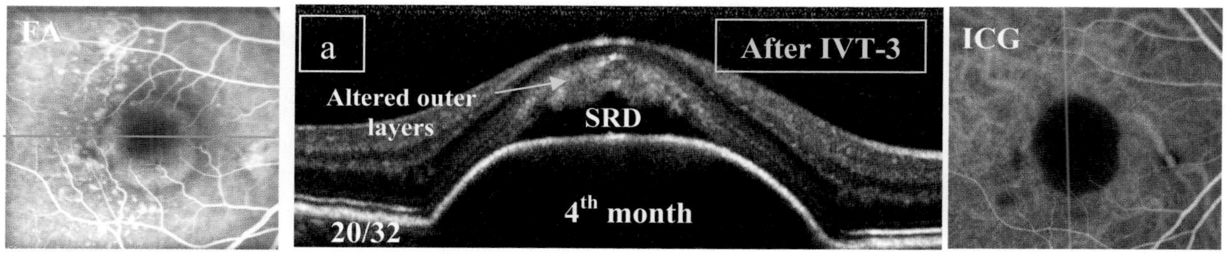

Figure 47: Occult CNV at the edge of a serous PED.
a): At the 4th month. VA: 20/32: the PED is less prominent but with persistent loss of the foveal depression. The RPE remained regular with normal thickness and an optically empty cavity. However, the SRF has increased over the dome of the PED with marked alteration of outer retinal layers. The external limiting membrane is almost no longer visible, nor is the IS/OS interface, which appears to be replaced by a dense hyper-reflective zone containing numerous bright hyper-reflective spots. There is displacement and relative thinning of the outer nuclear layer.

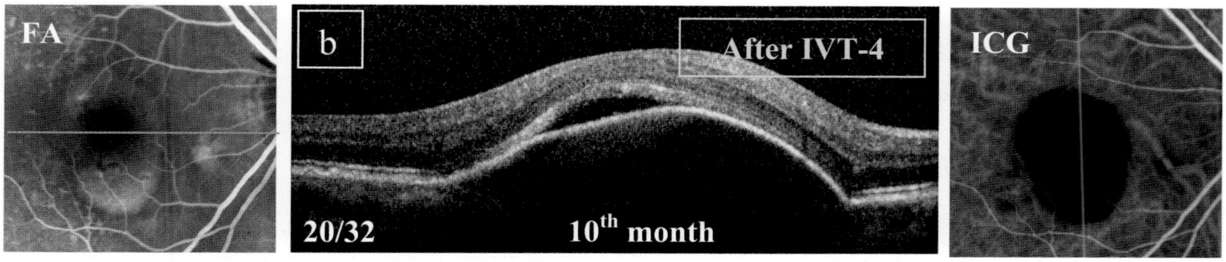

Figure 47: Occult CNV at the edge of a serous PED.
b): At the 10th month. VA: 20/32: persistent, but less prominent and more regular PED. The outer retinal layers are normal and much more clearly individualized. Persistent thickening of the IS/OS interface and thinning of the outer nuclear layer.

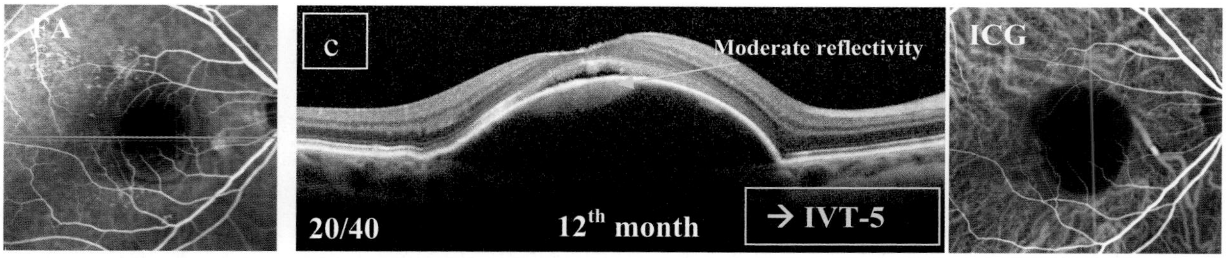

Figure 47: Occult CNV at the edge of a serous PED.
c): At the 12th month. VA: 20/40: slight decline of visual acuity with slight extension of the lesions. Appearance of a moderately reflective band, just posterior to the RPE. The outer retinal layers are well-organized, and the SRF has decreased, but alterations of the outer segments are clearly visible.

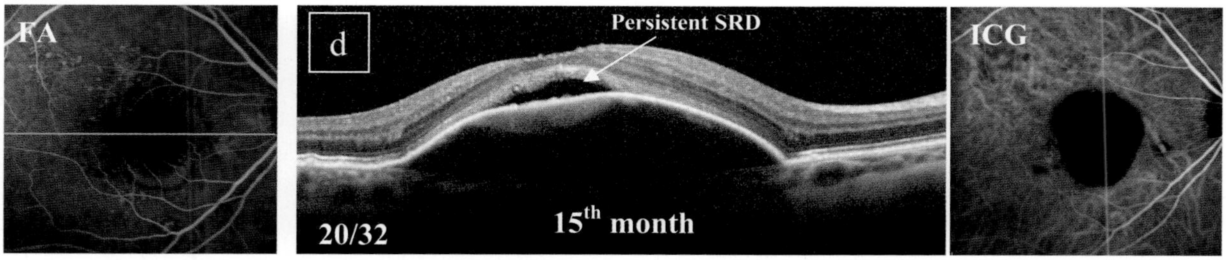

Figure 47: Occult CNV at the edge of a serous PED.
d): At the 15th month: VA: 20/32: the external limiting membrane is still visible. The IS/OS interface is also visible but remains thickened subfoveally with numerous bright hyper-reflective spots and irregularities of the outer segments. The foveal depression has become defined again with an almost normal profile. Note persistence of the PED on angiography and SD-OCT.

CLINICAL CASE No. 12: Large, Advanced, Occult CNV

Longstanding vascularized PED.
Follow-up by TD-OCT and SD-OCT, treated by PDT then anti-VEGF therapy.

Clinical Signs

A 77-year-old woman was already followed for AMD and had been treated by PDT first in the right eye and then in the left eye, with temporary improvement.

She presented with recent loss of visual acuity in the left eye, which had been the better of the two eyes up until that point.

VA RE: 20/160 - VA LE: 20/100.

Biomicroscopic Examination

The **first examination** of the **left eye** showed a small paracentral hemorrhage, a more marked retinal detachment, and several radial folds in the temporal region.

Autofluorescence

A vast hyper-fluorescent halo was visible, occupying almost all of the posterior pole, but sparing the zone of xanthophyll pigment.

Fluorescein angiography (Figures 48a and b)

In early phases, a very large area of progressive hyper-fluorescence with pinpoint leakage seen superiorly, inferiorly, and temporally, suggesting progressive filling of a vast PED with irregular margins. This hyper-fluorescence was heterogeneous with several temporal radial folds in the macula.

SLO-ICG angiography (Figures 48c and d):

Early phase: vast hypo-fluorescent area measuring 3 DD with irregular margins, occasionally retracted.

Late phase: the well-delineated hypo-fluorescence of the PED was confirmed with a poorly visible, small neovascular membrane in the central region.

Suggested Diagnosis:
Irregular, partially retracted vascularized PED with radial folds, invaded by a vast neovascular membrane.

Contribution of OCT (*Stratus**)

***Stratus** horizontal section**

The *RPE* was markedly elevated, especially in the temporal macular region, with a moderately reflective cavity, allowing partial visualization of Bruch's membrane. A hyper-reflective band (green) was present in the foveal region.

Anterior to the RPE, a large hyper-reflective band was suggestive of fibrosis. All of the neurosensory retina was thickened with poor visibility of retinal layers (**Figure 48e**).

***Stratus** vertical section**

The section passing directly through the foveal region clearly visualized the central depression, despite the presence of cysts in the plexiform layers.

The RPE appeared to be more or less merged with a hyper-reflective zone that appeared to occupy almost all of the cavity of the flat vascularized PED (**Figure 48f**).

Diagnosis

The diagnosis suggested by biomicroscopy and angiography, and confirmed by OCT examination, was that of partially retracted **vascularized pigment epithelium detachment** with radial folds, largely invaded by an area of choroidal neovascularization with fibrosis.

This longstanding and advanced lesion was initially treated by PDT, with only partial resolution.

The patient presented with a recent **recurrence** associated with an exudative reaction and moderate fibrosis. The functional impact was considerable and of concern, in view of the severe lesion of the fellow eye.

These features justified *intravitreous anti-VEGF therapy*, although the functional prognosis remained poor for such an extensive lesion with signs of fibrosis and retraction.

CLINICAL CASE No. 12: LARGE, ADVANCED, OCCULT CNV

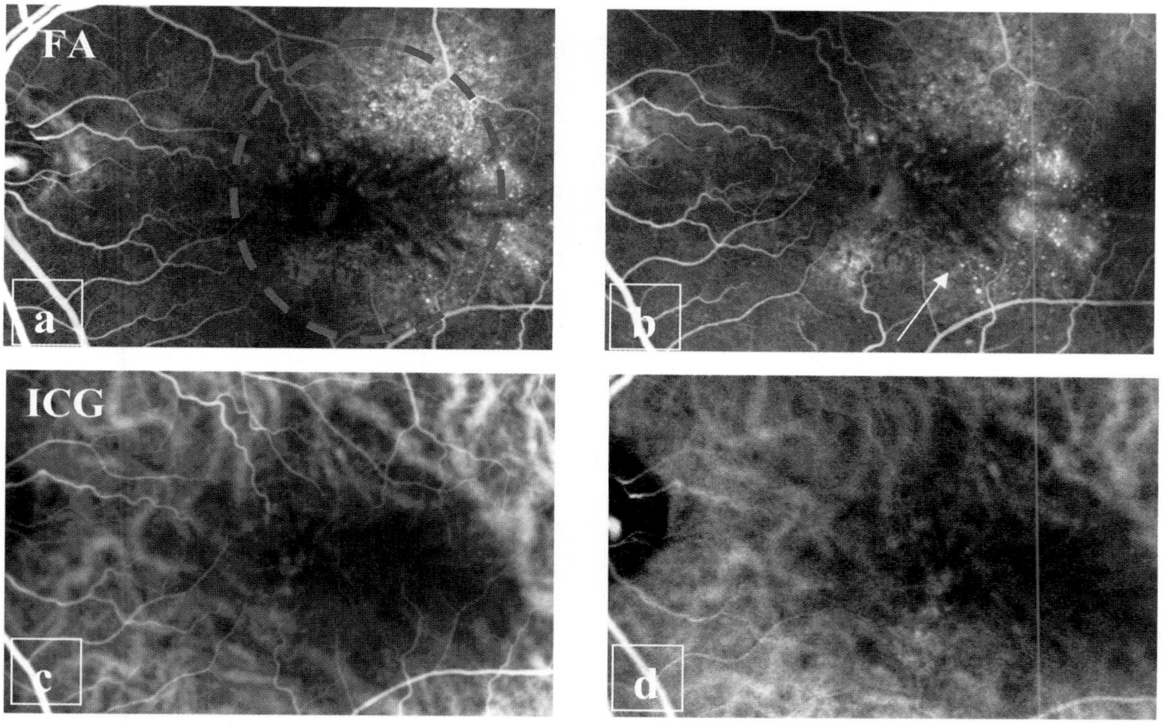

Figure 48: Large, advanced occult CNV. VA: 20/100.
a and b): Fluorescein angiography: vast area of progressive hyper-fluorescence with pinpoint leakage *(circle)*. Progressive filling of a vast PED with irregular margins and several temporal macular radial folds (*arrow*);
c and d): SLO-ICG angiography: hypo-fluorescent PED measuring 3 DD, with occasionally retracted contours, well-delineated in the late phase and with a poorly visible neovascular membrane.

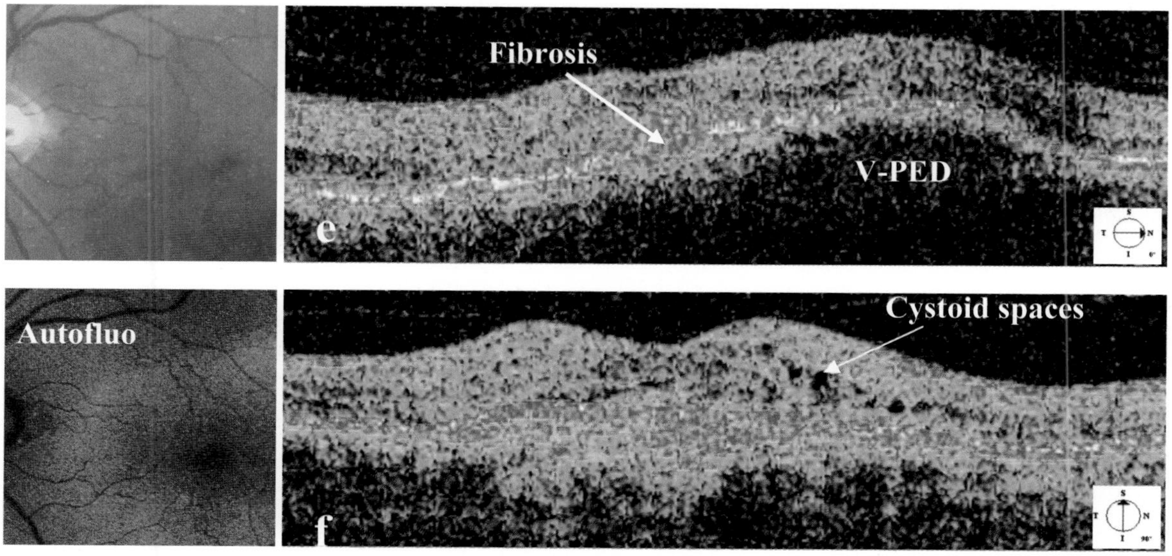

Figure 48: Large, advanced occult CNV. VA: 20/100.
e and f): *Stratus TD-OCT section**: temporal macular elevation of the RPE band with moderately reflective cavity allowing partial visualization of Bruch's membrane. Note the hyper-reflective band (*green*) in the foveal region.
Anterior to the RPE, a large hyper-reflective band is suggestive of fibrosis. The neurosensory retina is thickened with poorly distinguished retinal layers and several cysts in the plexiform layers.

CLINICAL CASE No. 12: Large, Advanced, Occult CNV

Intravitreal anti-VEGF therapy (*Lucentis**) was monitored for a period of almost two years.

Visual acuity improved progressively after each of the six intravitreal injections to reach 20/25 (score: 81), which remained stable over the next six months. The patient was again able to read, one year after starting treatment (**Figure 49**).

OCT

At the First Follow-up Examination

Despite functional improvement, the OCT remained relatively unchanged: the PED decreased, but the hyper-reflectivity anterior to the RPE and the moderate intraretinal fluid persisted (**Figure 49a**).

During the first year
The course was favorable, with slow, regular improvement of visual acuity from 20/63 to 20/50, and then to 20/40 and 20/32. The vascularized PED remained visible, fairly flat, and partially organized, while thickening of the RPE resolved.

The IS/OS interface and external limiting membrane were visible but disrupted. The outer nuclear layer remained very irregular, with denser and slightly hyper-reflective zones. Retinal thickness gradually decreased but did not return to normal (**Figure 49b**).

Subsequent follow-up examinations were performed every 3 months, or more frequently, often at the time of treatment of the fellow eye. The improvement of visual acuity was maintained and remained stable at 20/25. The OCT appearance improved.

At the 15th Month

The PED persisted with irregularities of the RPE and hyper-reflectivity of the PED cavity in the subfoveal zone. A small SRF remained visible on SD-OCT, possibly related to alterations of the RPE.

Outer retinal layers were clearly distinguishable and regular with persistent thickening of the IS/OS interface and jagged irregularities of the outer nuclear layer with a few rare bright hyper-reflective spots (**Figure 49c**).

At the last Follow-Up Examination

The OCT features remained stable 6 months after stopping intravitreal injections to the left eye.

The retinal layers had an almost normal appearance, apart from several irregularities of the outer nuclear layer and significant thickening of the IS/OS interface over the residual SRF with irregularities of outer segments (**Figure 49d**). Note that the posterior vitreous was detached.

Angiography

Fluorescein angiography: the radial folds became smaller and gradually faded. The hyper-fluorescent occult CNV and pinpoint leakage persisted but became smaller and less intense.

ICG angiography: the dark PED was replaced by a weakly fluorescent late plaque. The neovascular membrane was poorly visible and limited to large vessels (**Figure 49**).

At this Stage
This case of a partially retracted **vascularized pigment epithelium detachment** with radial folds, largely invaded by a neovascular membrane with fibrosis, was identified and treated at a very advanced stage.

The **response to treatment** was very slow but favorable, with more rapid improvement after the 3rd IVT, justifying continuation of treatment until stabilization, obtained after the 6th injection.

At the last examination, the morphology of the neurosensory retina was almost normal, despite persistence of a small SRF and several alterations of outer segments, probably related to the prolonged course.

The **PED persisted almost unchanged** with moderate fibrosis. Inner and outer retinal layers were clearly visible and well-organized, accounting for the good visual acuity.

The prognosis was favorable at this stage, but quarterly and half-yearly **observation** remained essential.

CLINICAL CASE No. 12: LARGE, ADVANCED, OCCULT CNV

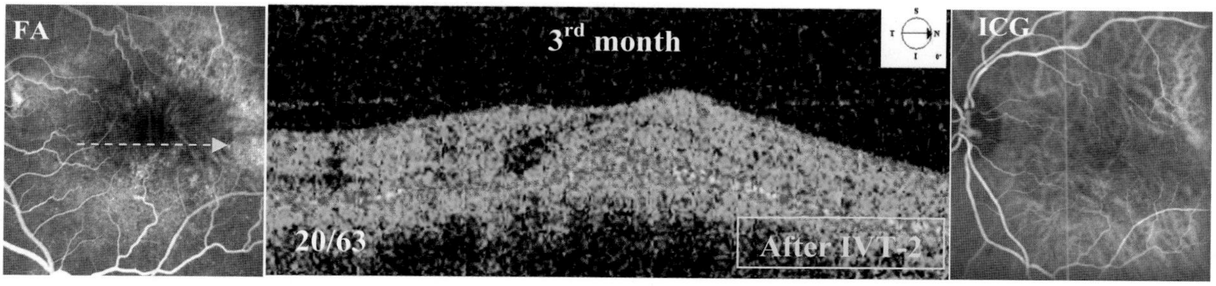

Figure 49: Large, advanced occult CNV.
a): At the 3rd month. VA: 20/63: decreased thickness of the RPE, but persistence of the hyper-reflectivity anterior to the RPE.

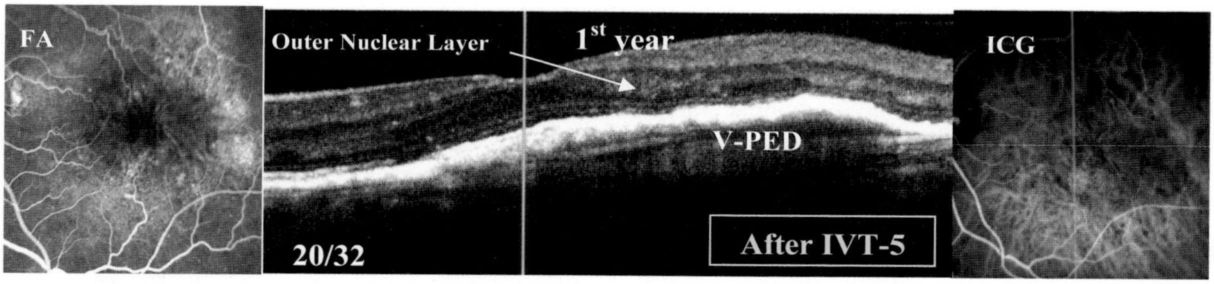

Figure 49: Large, advanced occult CNV.
b): At the 12th month. VA: 20/63: flat and partially-organized vascularized PED. The IS/OS interface and external limiting membrane are visible but disrupted. The outer nuclear layer remains irregular with more reflective zones.

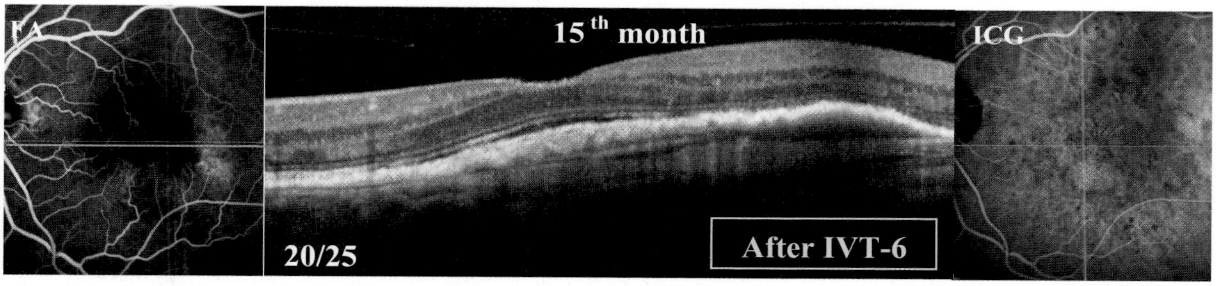

Figure 49: Large, advanced occult CNV.
c): At the 15th month. VA: 20/25: the PED persists with irregularities of the RPE and hyper-reflectivity of the cavity. A small SRF is still visible on SD-OCT, possibly related to alteration of the RPE. Outer layers are regular with thickening of the IS/OS interface and irregularities in the outer nuclear layer and a few rare bright hyper-reflective spots.

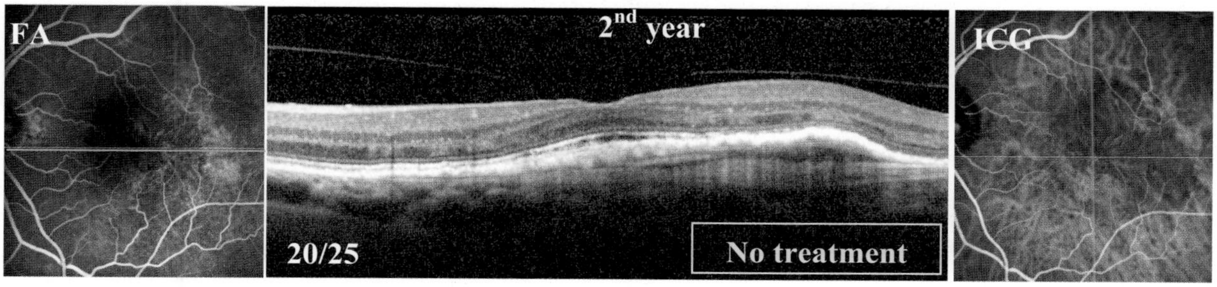

Figure 49: Large, advanced occult CNV.
d): At the 24th month. VA: 20/25: the vitreous is detached. The retinal profile is almost normal. Note several irregularities of the outer nuclear layer and thickening of the IS/OS interface over the residual SRF, with irregularities of the outer segments.

CLINICAL CASE No. 13: Hemorrhagic Complications of Occult CNV

Large sub-macular hemorrhage and intraretinal hemorrhage.
Follow-up by SD-OCT after anti-VEGF therapy.

Occult choroidal neovascularization can be associated with **major hemorrhagic complications** that can sometimes be the first signs of a lesion that has slowly advanced over a long period of time. These hemorrhagic complications can occur with no apparent cause. They often present as a sub-macular hemorrhage measuring several disc diameters and may sometimes be very extensive, extending as far as the temporal arcade or beyond, inducing sudden severe loss of visual acuity.

This **subretinal** hemorrhage can be treated surgically to slide the hematoma inferiorly (with air bubble and positioning), or it can be surgically evacuated, sometimes with useful results, but the indications have not been clearly defined. When the hemorrhage is behind the RPE, these treatments may be ineffective or even deleterious. In many cases, intraretinal and subretinal hemorrhage and hemorrhagic pigment epithelium detachment are related to an **RPE tear**, often in the temporal sector. In this situation, the hemorrhage usually has a suggestive **arcuate shape**, masking the tear and the associated choroidal neovascularization.

Fundus imaging is particularly useful in all of these cases, especially SLO-ICG angiography, which can cross a relatively thin layer of blood, and OCT, which can demonstrate the tear and the type of neovascularization (**Figures 50, 51, and 52**).

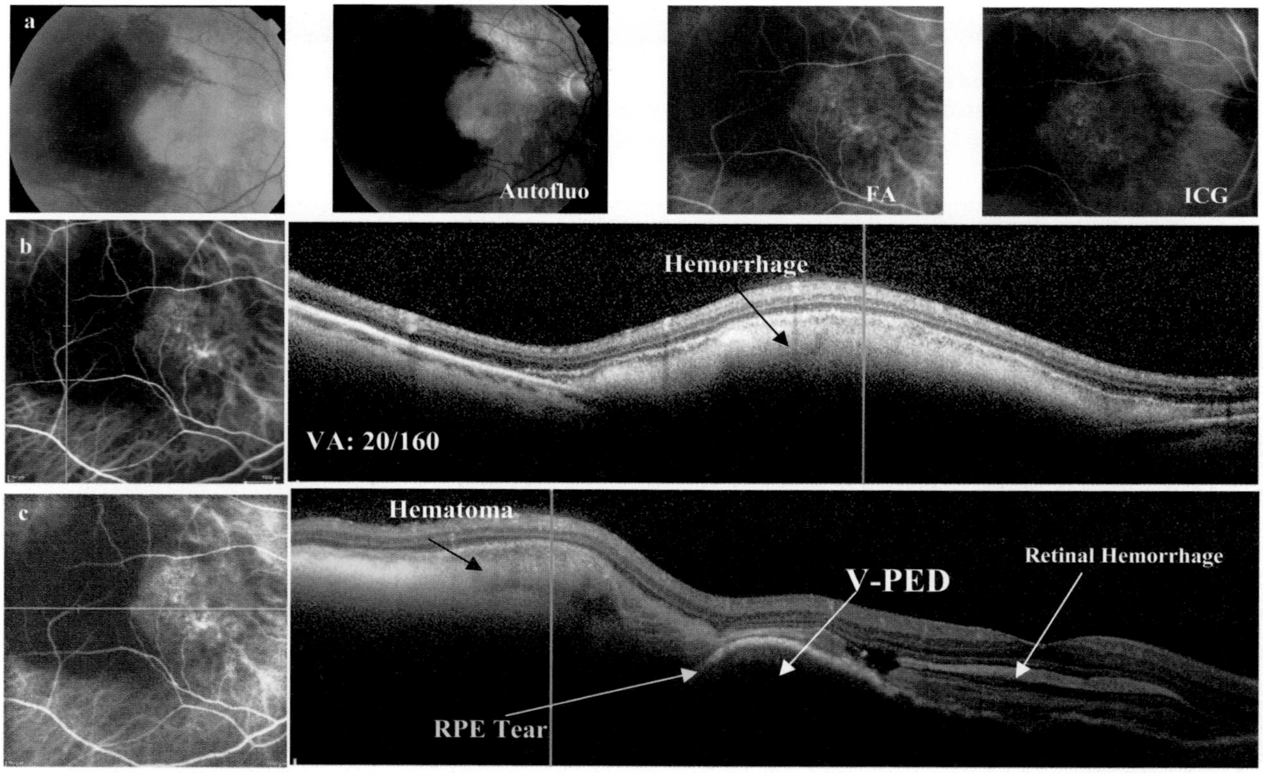

Figure 50: Submacular hemorrhage revealing slowly evolving occult CNV in a 77-year-old man. VA RE: 20/160, LE: 20/32.

a): Color fundus photograph, autofluorescence, and angiography: temporal arcuate hemorrhage with a dense deep zone and a lighter intraretinal zone adjacent to a vascularized PED, which is entirely invaded by occult CNV.

b): *Spectralis vertical section** through the subretinal hemorrhage, initially intensely hyper-reflective then completely blocking posterior passage of light with total masking. Note the thickening of the IS/OS interface but good preservation of the other retinal layers.

c): *Spectralis horizontal section**: the vascularized PED can be seen adjacent to the hematoma, with alteration of the RPE and presence of a fine layer of retinal hemorrhage, which extends almost as far as the optic disc. Note the apparent disruption of the RPE, suggesting a temporal tear.

CLINICAL CASE No. 13: HEMORRHAGIC COMPLICATIONS OF OCCULT CNV

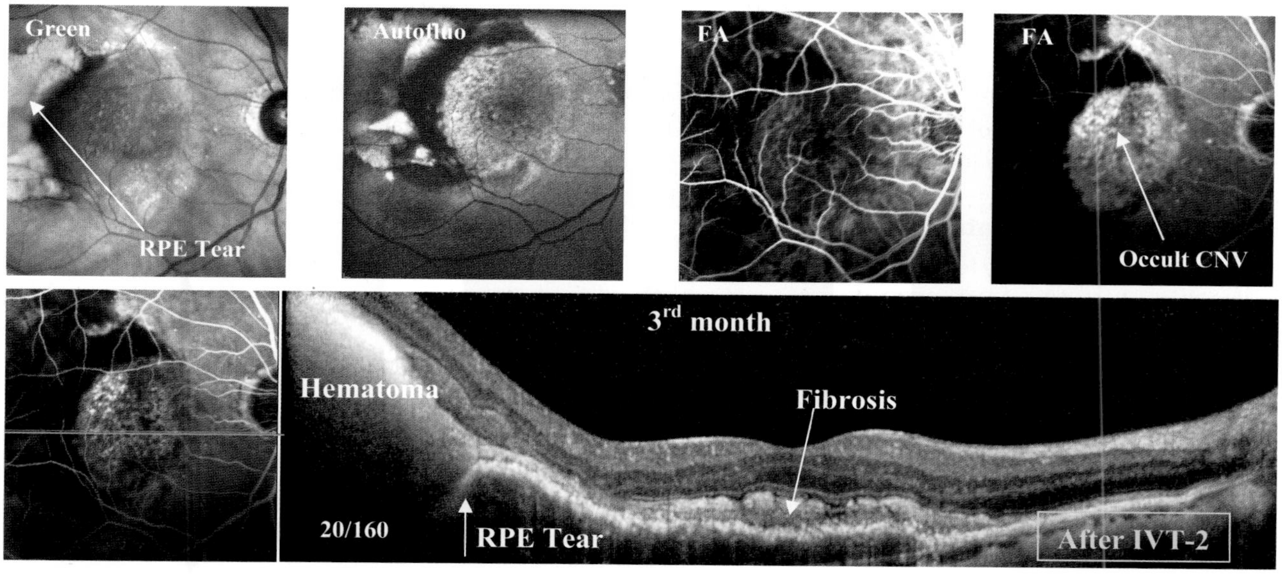

Figure 51: Submacular hemorrhage revealing slowly evolving occult CNV. Same patient as in Figures 50 and 51.

After 2 intravitreal injections of anti-VEGF at the 3rd month, the blood is still present and has become organized. The preretinal hemorrhage has resolved leaving a hyper-reflective structure suggestive of fibrosis anterior to the RPE. The vascularized PED remained unchanged.

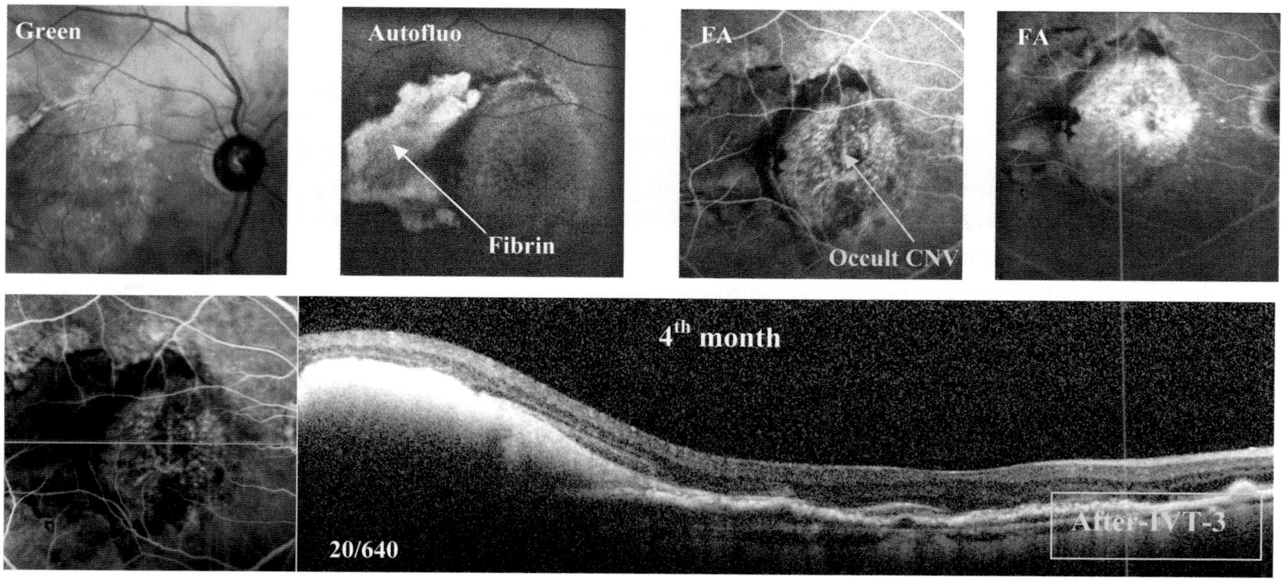

Figure 52: Submacular hemorrhage revealing a slowly evolving occult CNV. Same patient as in Figures 50 and 51.

At the 4th month, after 3 intravitreal injections of anti-VEGF, there was a dramatic loss of VA due to atrophy of all retinal layers of the fovea with loss of the outer nuclear layer. The PED is flat with subretinal fibrosis. The RPE is irregular and thinned, and the hemorrhage is still present and organized. The preretinal hemorrhage is no longer visible, leaving a fine hyper-reflective band anterior to the RPE.

CLINICAL CASE No. 15: Advanced Occult CNV

Longstanding extensive lesion continuing to progress with persistent symptoms.
Follow-up by SD-OCT after anti-VEGF therapy.

Clinical Signs

An 82-year-old woman had been followed previously for AMD for several years, with major changes in both eyes. Both eyes developed irreversible central scotomas despite various treatments.
The patient presented with progressive loss of visual acuity and with the hope of a new treatment.
VA RE: 20/800 - VA LE: 20/400.

Biomicroscopic Examination

Examination of the *left eye* revealed a poorly-demarcated, discolored, extensive 4 DD lesion with several peripheral retinal hemorrhages. The lesion was relatively flat except in the superior temporal sector (**Figure 54a**).
On **autofluorescence**, the lesion was dark, suggesting moderate but extensive *atrophy* with a large peripheral hyper-fluorescent halo and visible hemorrhages.

Fluorescein angiography (Figure 54b)

Fluorescein angiography showed an early and moderate hyper-fluorescent zone with progressive staining but limited fluorescein leakage except at the periphery. A central hypo-fluorescent zone was suggestive of accumulation of material.

Diffuse alterations of the RPE were also observed with abnormal transmission of fundus fluorescence all around the central area.

SLO-ICG angiography (Figure 54c)

The large choroidal vessels were abnormally visible. The lesion was extensive, hypo-fluorescent, and clearly demarcated, except in the peripheral active lesions, visible against the dark background of the PED.

Suggested Diagnosis:
Old, extensive lesion, essentially in the process of atrophy but with active lesions in the periphery and persistent symptoms.

Contribution of OCT (*Spectralis**)

*Spectralis** horizontal section

The RPE was irregular and thinned with zones of variable density. The RPE was separated from Bruch's membrane over the entire surface of the lesion with a flat, organized, moderately reflective vascularized PED.
Anterior to the RPE, the *external limiting membrane* and *IS/OS interface* were not visible. The *outer nuclear layer*, no longer visible in the foveal zone, appeared to be invaded by an irregular zone of increased density with scattered bright hyper-reflective spots.
Increased retinal thickness, intraretinal fluid, and cysts induced major disorganization of the retinal structure (**Figure 53d**).

*Spectralis** vertical section

This section visualized the flat and organized vascularized PED, the marked changes of the outer retinal layers with bright hyper-reflective spots, dense zones, cysts, and increased retinal thickness.

The inner retinal layers were only slightly altered (**Figure 53e**).

*Stratus** horizontal section

This section confirmed the increased retinal thickness, cysts, and SRF, but the flat vascularized PED was not visible (**Figure 53f**).

Diagnosis
The diagnosis of extensive, **longstanding occult CNV** in the process of atrophy but with active zones in the periphery, suggested by biomicroscopy and angiographies, was *confirmed* by SD-OCT.
This lesion continued to deteriorate despite various treatments, and the patient presented in the hope of a new treatment.
The visual prognosis was poor.
However, the presence of persistent intraretinal fluid, cysts, and increased retinal thickness appeared to justify another trial of treatment with a reserved functional prognosis due to disorganization of the retinal layers and loss of the outer nuclear layer.

CLINICAL CASE No. 15: ADVANCED OCCULT CNV

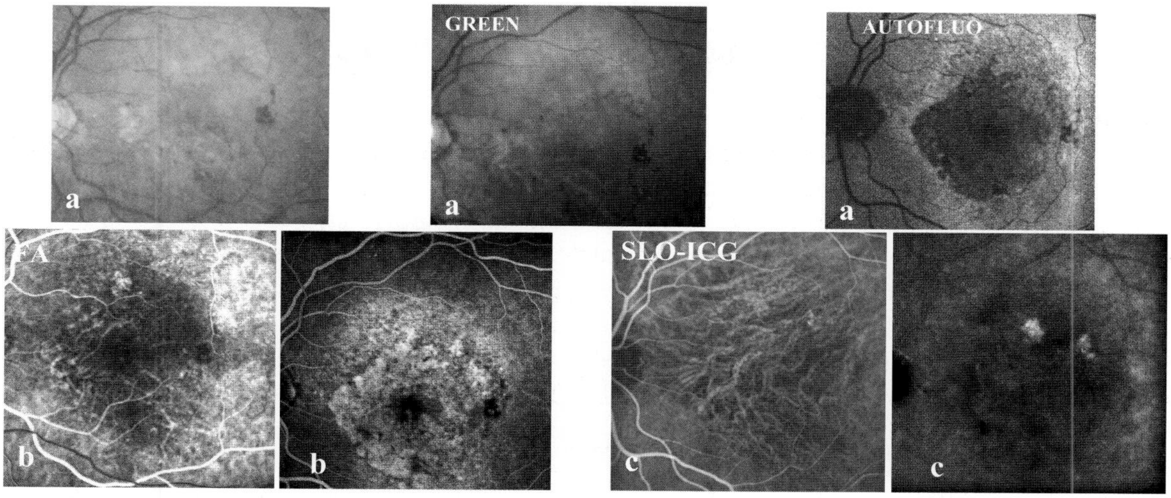

Figure 54: Old, extensive occult CNV in the process of healing and atrophy, still active in the periphery. VA RE: 20/800 - VA LE: 20/400.

a): Color, red-free, autofluorescence: extensive 4 DD lesion, partially atrophic with several hemorrhages.

b): Fluorescein angiography: moderate hyper-fluorescence with progressive staining but limited fluorescein leakage except in the periphery. Hypo-fluorescent deposits in the center. Diffuse changes of the RPE all around the lesion.

c): SLO-ICG angiography: large choroidal vessels are abnormally visible. Note the extensive, hypo-fluorescent lesion with two *active sites in the periphery, visible against the dark background of the PED.*

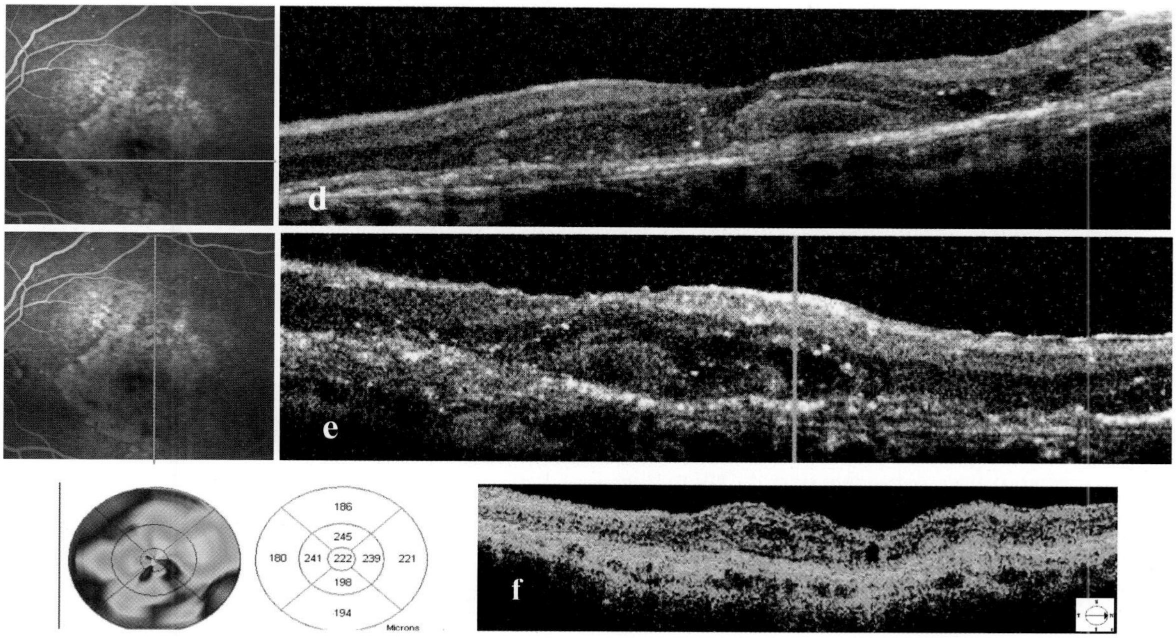

Figure 54: Old, extensive occult CNV in the process of healing and atrophy still active in the periphery. VA RE: 20/800 - VA LE: 20/400.

d): *Spectralis horizontal section**: flat, organized, and moderately reflective vascularized PED with an irregular RPE separated from Bruch's membrane over the entire surface of the lesion. The external limiting membrane and IS/OS interface are not visible. The outer nuclear layer is no longer visible in the foveal zone and appears to be invaded by an irregular zone of increased density with scattered bright hyper-reflective spots. Increased retinal thickness, intraretinal fluid, and cysts induce major disorganization of retinal structure.

e): *Spectralis vertical section**: flat, organized, vascularized PED with marked changes of the outer layers.

f): *Stratus TD-OCT section**: increased retinal thickness, cysts, and SRF are visible, but the flat vascularized PED is not seen.

CLINICAL CASE No. 15: Advanced Occult CNV

The response to treatment by intravitreous injections of anti-VEGF (*Lucentis**) was monitored in terms of functional results and imaging before each injection.

Unfortunately, visual acuity ended up stable at 20/320 despite a slight initial improvement.

The patient's metamorphopsias resolved, and she started low vision rehabilitation (**Figure 54**).

OCT

The first follow-up examination demonstrated a slight improvement and all of the outer nuclear layer was clearly visible, although displaced and raised by dense material with bright hyper-reflective spots and several cysts (**Figure 54a**).

At the 6th month, no functional improvement was observed despite a 4th injection. Bruch's membrane was clearly visible, and the flat, organized PED remained unchanged (**Figure 55b**).

Anterior to the RPE, the outer layers were disorganized and the IS/OS interface was only occasionally visible.

The outer nuclear layer was altered with numerous persistent bright hyper-reflective spots with a partially retracted epiretinal membrane.

At the 9th month (Figure 55c)
The OCT appearance was practically unchanged with decreased retinal thickness and bright hyper-reflective spots.

At the last examination (Figure 55d)
Six months after the last IVT injection, all of the retina was thinned, especially in the foveal region with thinning of the RPE and loss of the outer retinal layers.

The outer nuclear layer was in contact with the atrophic RPE, suggesting photoreceptor atrophy. These alterations were clearly visible on enlarged views (**Figures 56a and b**).

Angiography (Figure 55)
The lesion remained the same size, but fluorescein leakage and hemorrhages had resolved. Atrophy was clearly visible on ICG angiography.

At this Stage
This case of **longstanding, extensive occult CNV** in the process of atrophy, with active lesions at the periphery was treated due to the presence of several signs of activity, despite the long history of the lesions.

In view of the poor visual acuity in the fellow eye, *repeated intravitreous injections* were administered for 6 months.

No functional improvement was obtained. However, the intraretinal fluid and reactive inflammatory signs (bright hyper-reflective spots and dense zones) faded and then resolved.

The inner retinal layers regained a normal structure, but with thinning of all of the retina, corresponding to **atrophy of inner and outer segments**, clearly visible on SD-OCT and justifying discontinuation of treatment.

By stopping extension and exudation, treatment was nevertheless useful, but it did not provide any improvement of visual acuity due to the longstanding nature of the lesions.

Low vision rehabilitation would be considered useful for this patient.

CLINICAL CASE No. 15: ADVANCED OCCULT CNV

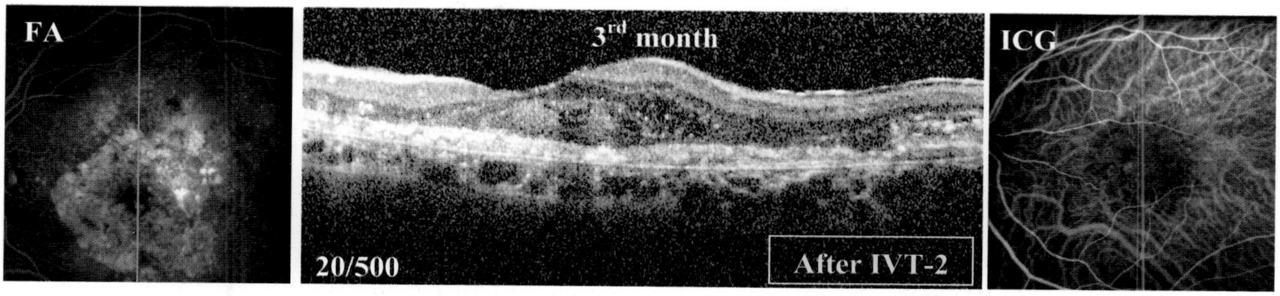

Figure 55: Old, extensive occult CNV in the process of healing and atrophy, still active in the periphery.
a): At the 3rd month. VA: 20/500: all of the outer nuclear layer is clearly visible, but displaced and raised by dense material. Note the bright hyper- reflective spots and several cysts.

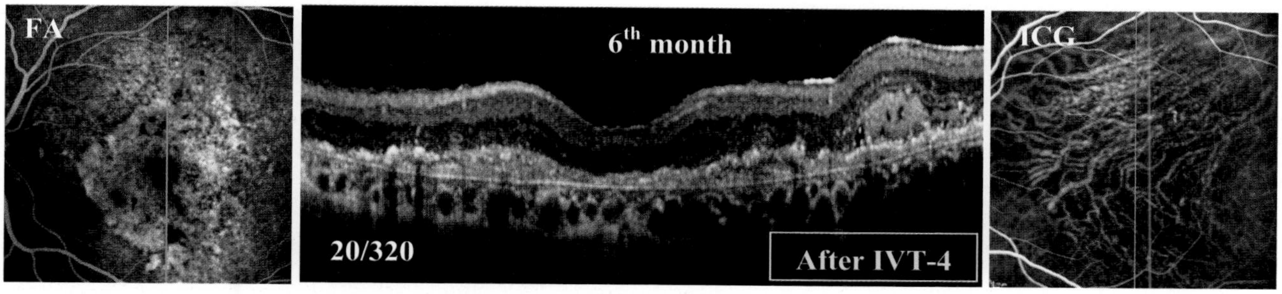

Figure 55: Old, extensive occult CNV in the process of healing and atrophy, still active in the periphery.
b): At the 6th month. VA: 20/320: flat, organized PED. Bruch's membrane remains clearly visible away from the RPE. Anterior to the RPE, the outer layers are disorganized, and the IS/OS interface is only occasionally visible. The outer nuclear layer is altered. Note the persistence of numerous bright hyper-reflective spots and a partially retracted epiretinal membrane.

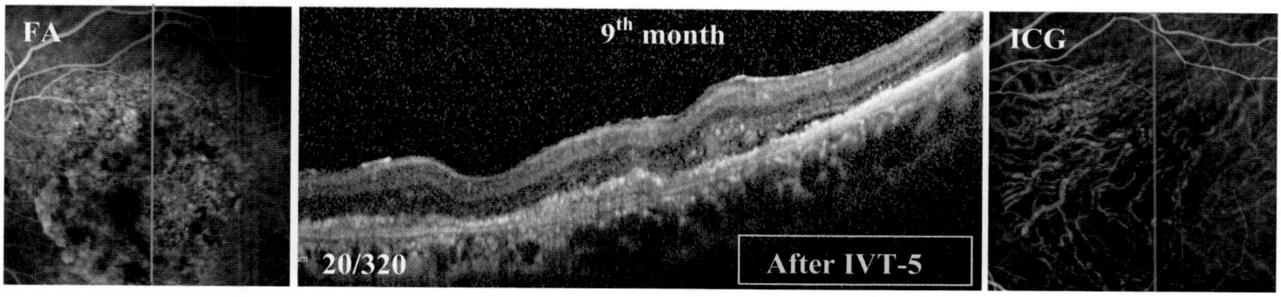

Figure 55: Old, extensive occult CNV in the process of healing and atrophy, still active in the periphery.
c): At the 9th month. VA: 20/320: decreased retinal thickness and regression of bright hyper-reflective spots.

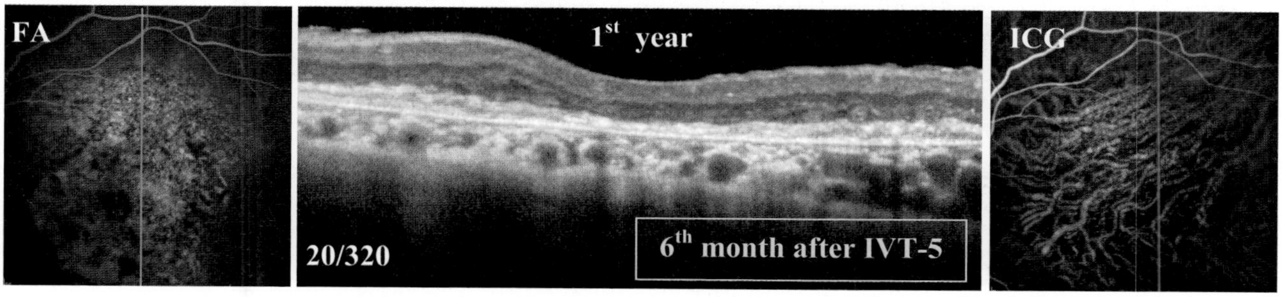

Figure 55: Old, extensive occult CNV in the process of healing and atrophy, still active in the periphery.
d): At the 12th month. VA: 20/320: the retina is thinned, especially in the foveal region, with thinning of the RPE and loss of the outer layers. The outer nuclear layer is in contact the atrophic RPE, suggesting photoreceptor atrophy.

CLINICAL CASE No. 15: ADVANCED OCCULT CNV

ENLARGED IMAGES

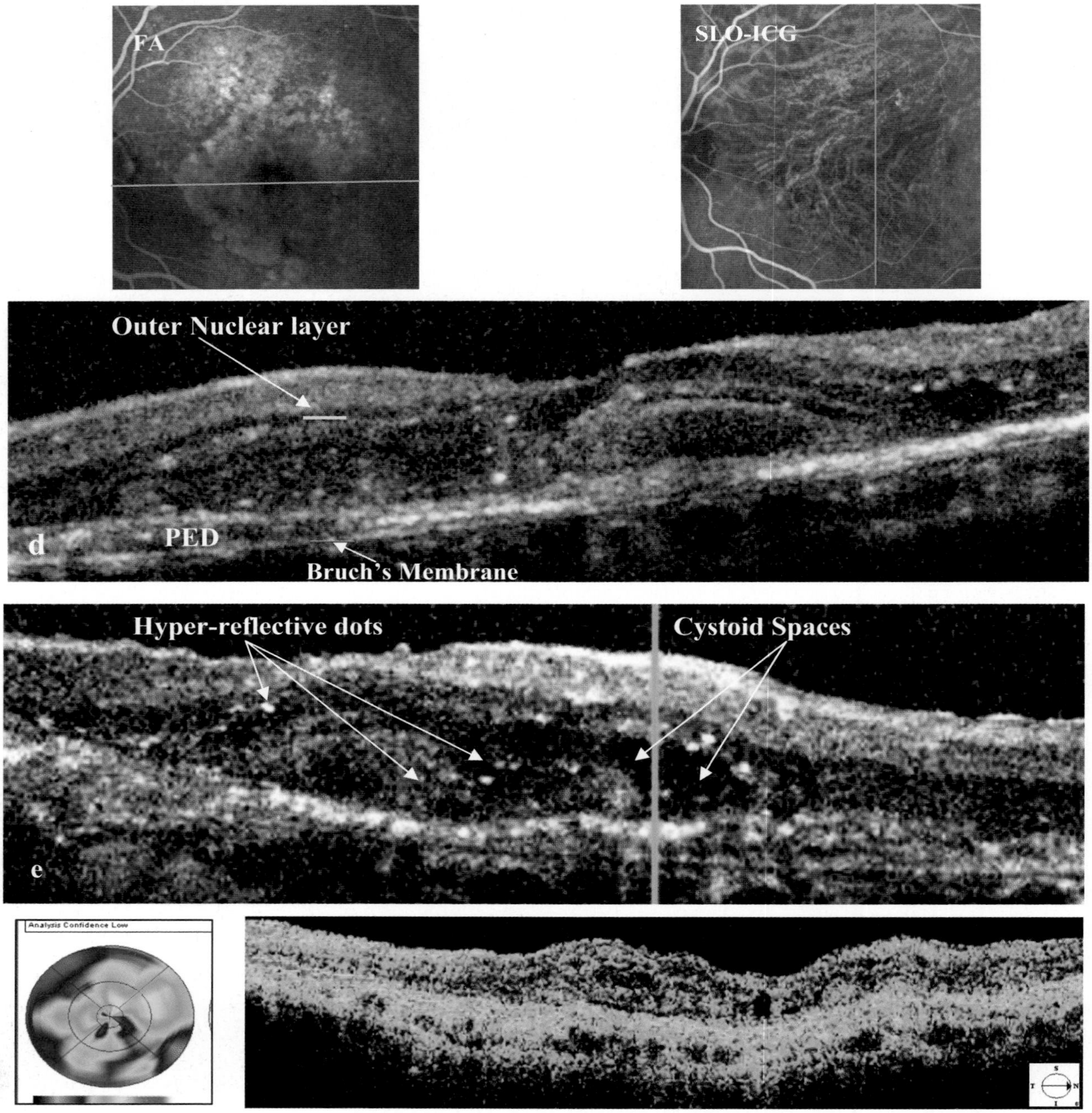

Figure 56 a): Old, extensive occult CNV in the process of healing (enlargement of Figures 54, d and e)
***Spectralis** horizontal and vertical sections.**

- *In and posterior to the RPE*: flat, organized, moderately reflective vascularized PED; irregular RPE, separated from Bruch's membrane over all of the lesion.
- *Anterior to the RPE*: the external limiting membrane and IS/OS interface are not visible. The outer nuclear layer is poorly visualized. Disorganization of the outer retinal layers: an irregular dense zone with scattered bright hyper-reflective spots, increased retinal thickness, intraretinal fluid, and retinal cysts.

***Stratus** TD-OCT section**: increased retinal thickness, cysts, and SRF are visible, but the flat vascularized PED is not visible.

CLINICAL CASE No. 15: ADVANCED OCCULT CNV

ENLARGED IMAGES

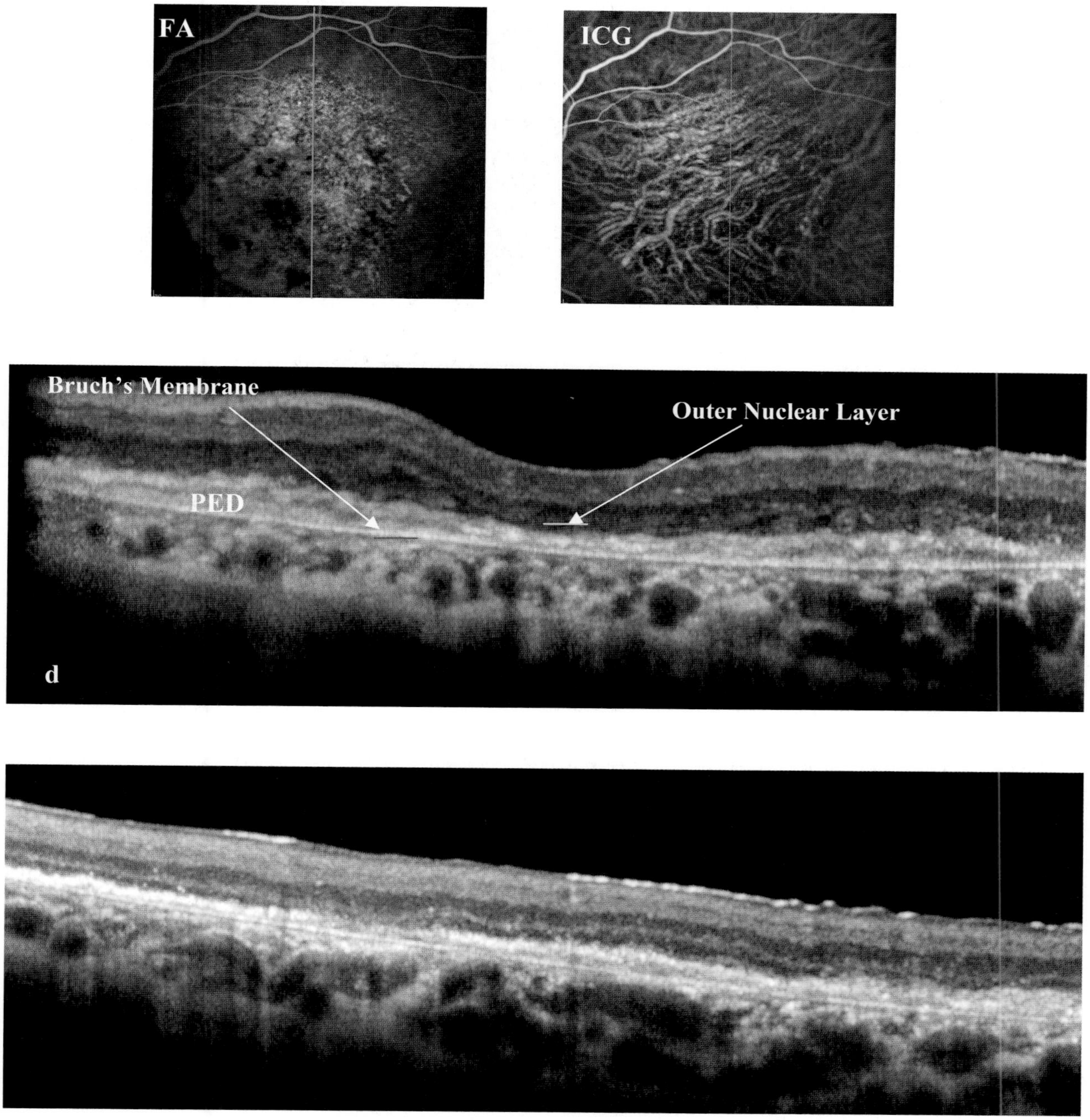

Figure 56b: Old, extensive occult CNV in the process of healing (enlargement of Figure 55d).
***Spectralis** horizontal and vertical sections.**

- *In and posterior to the RPE*: thinning and irregularities of the RPE; very flat PED with visibility of Bruch's membrane;
- *Anterior to the RPE*: thinning of the retina. Disruption of the external limiting membrane; poorly visible IS/OS interface. The outer nuclear layer is in contact with the atrophic RPE (especially in the foveal region) suggesting photoreceptor atrophy.

Conclusion

This series of clinical cases of occult CNV schematically illustrate the **polymorphic clinical features** observed in routine clinical practice.

The clinical course is usually slow but **progression** is almost inevitable, either spontaneously or despite treatment, which always requires long-term observation.

Early lesions associated with little or no symptoms can frequently be detected in the fellow eye at a stage when treatment has a better chance of preserving satisfactory vision and even maintain reading.

After the initial phase of extension of the lesions, sometimes lasting several months or several years, they can be complicated by the appearance of classic choroidal neovascularization.

Lesions are still very sensitive to treatment at this stage.

The **prognosis** is much more guarded in the presence of serous pigment epithelium detachment, which carries a risk of hemorrhage and tears These complications are serious but can still respond favorably to treatment.

Advanced lesions with mixed and/or extensive choroidal neovascularization are even more severe due to fibrosis, alterations of the RPE, and severe photoreceptor disruption. However, stabilization or even considerable improvement can be achieved in some of these cases.

At the stage of atrophy of the outer retinal layers and RPE, treatment is intended to prevent extension of the lesions or massive hemorrhage.

Early diagnosis and detection of AMD therefore improve prognosis, and close observation of the fellow eye by repeated imaging can preserve vision.

Patients are **not always aware** of the risks related to poor follow-up at this early stage.

Chorioretinal Anastomoses

Clinical Features and OCT Follow-Up after Treatment

Gabriel COSCAS
Florence COSCAS, Sabrina VISMARA,
Alain ZOURDANI, C.I. Li CALZI

(Créteil and Paris)

Chorioretinal Anastomoses

Clinical Features and OCT Follow-Up after Treatment

Described for the first time in 1994 as an active and progressive form of AMD, **chorioretinal anastomoses** (CRA), constitute a unique entity among the various clinical forms of wet AMD (*Coscas 1994, International Symposium on Fluorescein Angiography, Toronto*). Chorioretinal anastomoses are active lesions and frequently involve both eyes.

They are different from the chronic anastomoses observed at the advanced stage of disciform scars, (*Oeller, 1903*).

Even from its early stages, **CRA typically presents** with the following signs:

- Juxtafoveal **retinal hemorrhage**,
- An area of **choroidal neovascularization** (small and limited but clearly visible on fluorescein angiography and even more precisely on SLO-ICG angiography),
- located within a **pigment epithelium detachment**.

On SLO-ICG, a round Pigment Epithelium Detachment (PED) centered on the fovea can be detected in the early phases and gradually increases in size at the same rate as choroidal neovascularization and the anastomosis. The anastomosis **between CNV and a retinal arteriole or veinule** becomes increasingly visible in the late phase angiograms.

Chorioretinal anastomoses are relatively frequent, with a prevalence of 9% in our series of 200 consecutive cases of wet AMD.

Pathogenic Hypotheses

Choroidal origin

The theory that CRA originates from the choroidal circulation, originally suggested by the Créteil Group (*Kuhn, 1995*) and then by *Slakter* (1996), was also confirmed by *Gass* (2003).

Gass emphasized not only the importance of retinal hemorrhage as the first sign of this entity, but also that the origin of the choroidal neovascularization is located over a small area of atrophy of the RPE. He postulated that contact and subsequent anastomosis between CNV and retinal vessels associated with the development of a serous PED.

Gass therefore concluded that the neovascularization associated with CRA is of "***choroidal origin and subretinal localization***".

Retinal origin

A retinal origin **for the neovascular proliferation** has been suggested by other authors. The vascular proliferation, subsequently extends to the outer retina and then underneath the RPE. After it communicates with choroidal vessels, it is accompanied by a vascularized PED (*Hartnett, 1996* and *Yannuzzi, 2001*).

The success of this latter hypothesis has led to the name "*retinal angiomatous proliferation*" (RAP), which is widely used in the literature despite the unresolved controversy of its origin.

Until now, no case of early RAP followed throughout its natural history to the complete form of a vascularized PED with chorioretinal anastomosis has been well documented.

Type 3 neovascularization

The term "*type 3 neovascularization*" has been more recently proposed, indicating that the initial neovascularization may be derived from either:

- The choroid or
- Deep retinal capillaries,

with subsequent formation of anastomosis and intraretinal fluid (*Freund, 2008, Yannuzzi, 2008*).

Regardless of the *initial subclinical stage*, the **symptomatic phase** consists of:

- Choroidal neovascularization,
- Anastomoses with retinal vessels, and both
- Subretinal and intraretinal neovascular proliferation.

The clinical pattern of CRA is as follows:

- In the context of wet AMD,
- With a vascularized PED,
- Associated with high-risk soft drusen.

The lesion becomes *bilateral* and *symmetrical* in almost every case.

Clinical Features

Clinical Examination

In most cases, *biomicroscopic examination* demonstrates one or more juxtafoveal retinal hemorrhages arising at the end of a retinal vessel near the fovea.

This retinal vessel has an abnormal course and (in contrast with adjacent vessels) becomes dilated and tortuous (**Figure 1a, b, and c**). Specifically, it appears to be disrupted as it plunges **deeply** towards the choroid, next to the hemorrhage, forming a right angle or an arch.

Its course and communications are often poorly visualized by biomicroscopy.

Fluorescein Angiography

Fluorescein angiography may provide better visualization of the retinal vessels and the retino-choroidal anastomosis.

The deep neovascularization rapidly induces intense and localized leakage and hyper-fluorescence (hot spot) (**Figure 2**).

This hot spot is often initially partially masked by the retinal hemorrhage. Later, the progressive filling of the PED space with dye, does not allow visibility of the retino-choroidal anastomosis.

SLO-ICG Angiography

In contrast, SLO-ICG angiography allows precise analysis of the neovascularization and its communications with one or several retinal arterioles and/or venules (**Figure 1b and c**).

The site of the anastomosis is hyper-fluorescent and contrasts markedly against the dark background of the PED. There is no early leakage of the ICG dye and this leakage is only observed in the late phase of the angiogram (**Figure 1b and c, and Figure 2**).

Time-Domain OCT (*Stratus**)

Time-Domain OCT (*Stratus**) readily demonstrates:
- The ***PED*** (usually optically empty), and
- The intraretinal ***leakage***.

Exudative reactions are always marked with increased retinal thickness and particularly numerous and confluent cystoid spaces (**Figure 2**).

They are often present in two layers of the retina and are sometimes accompanied by subretinal fluid with sub-RPE detachment (PED) induced by the presence of deep choroidal neovascularization. In some cases, a hyper-reflective band may be observed through the PED, suggestive of a *fibrovascular tract.*

Spectral-Domain OCT (*Spectralis**)

The SD-OCT appearance of the lesion is very suggestive of the anatomical location with:
- **Localized disruption** of the RPE, and
- **Hyper-reflective tissue** derived from the choroid, bulging into the retina, which appears to correspond to the chorioretinal anastomosis.

Early stages of the disease can sometimes be detected during follow-up for the **fellow eye.** At this stage, a small and limited PED may be found. Within this PED, a localized zone of hyper-reflectivity is initially located underneath the RPE and then crosses the RPE band through a disruption. The lesion then extends towards and into the retinal tissue.

During progression, choroidal neovascularization may spread to invade the entire area of the PED (*see Clinical Cases, p. 282 to 300*).

Complications

Extensive proliferations, retraction, or progression of this neovascularization can cause further complications such as:
- RPE tears
- Macular hemorrhages
- Multiple anastomoses

Prognosis

Even without treatment the lesion may remain dormant for many months. But the natural history is always severe resulting in severe visual disability as the disease is almost always **bilateral.**

CHORIORETINAL ANASTOMOSES

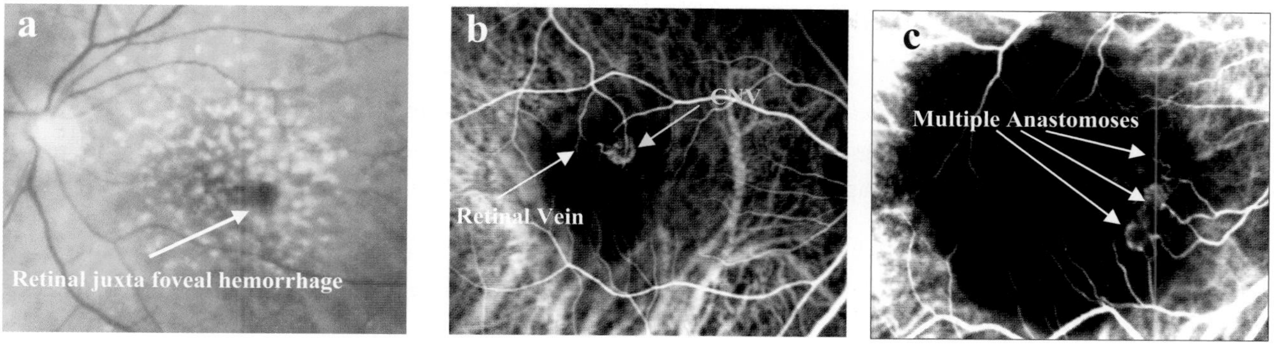

Figure 1: Typical chorioretinal anastomosis: different clinical features.
a): Color fundus photograph: numerous soft drusen and juxtafoveal hemorrhage.
b): SLO-ICG angiography: the anastomosis between two retinal vessels and choroidal neovascularization are clearly visible and contrasts against the dark PED.
c): SLO-ICG angiography: another case with multiple anastomoses.

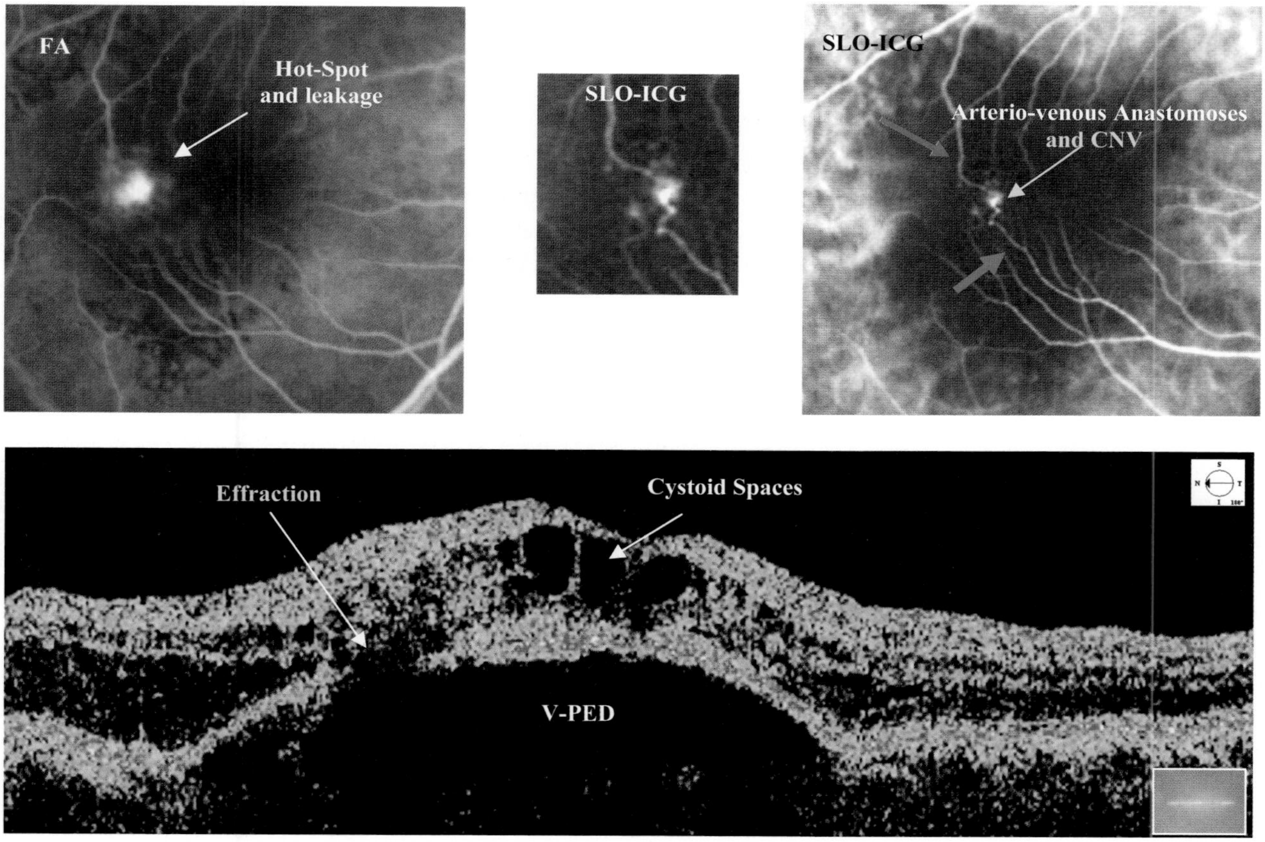

Figure 2: Typical chorioretinal anastomosis–*Stratus TD-OCT.**
Vast, prominent, homogeneous, hypo-reflective PED with moderate back-shadowing. Bruch's membrane is visible.
There is a localized disruption of the RPE band. A (moderately) reflective tract appears to protrude through this **break** towards a dense intraretinal structure that is surrounded by fairly large cysts. These cystoid spaces are almost confluent in the foveolar zone.
Note the retinal thickening with accentuated intraretinal fluid accumulation.

Treatment Modalities

Treatment Modalities

Different treatment options have been proposed, but their results have remained largely disappointing.

Laser Photocoagulation

Thermal laser photocoagulation has been almost abandoned due to the high rate of neovascular recurrence and clinical relapse.

These recurrences are sometimes very severe and accompanied with hemorrhages and RPE tears.

The only cases with a chance of success are those eyes treated at a very early stage.

However, at this initial stage of minimal lesions associated with fairly good visual acuity, the benefit of treatment must be weighed against the high risk of complications, especially when more benign treatment modalities are available.

Photodynamic Therapy

This treatment can provide improvement in some cases, usually at an early stage, but it does not appear to provide reproducible results.

Several cases of RPE tears following PDT have been reported.

Cases of delayed *treatment in advanced forms* are especially associated with a high risk of spontaneous RPE tears.

Anti-Angiogenic Therapy

Intravitreal injections of anti-VEGF appear to provide more favorable results, as demonstrated by several pilot studies.

Persistent lesions, relapses, and long-term recurrences are still frequent.

Nevertheless, these lesions appear to remain sensitive to on-going anti-VEGF injections, especially when treatment is initiated rapidly. Long-term follow up after treatment is therefore important.

Combined Therapy

PDT combined with other treatment modalities has also demonstrated useful results in CRA.

To date, only pilot studies have been reported.

These combination therapies require prolonged follow-up after treatment, and the long-term prognosis of these eyes remains guarded.

Protection of the Fellow Eye

Prevention of vision loss therefore appears to be crucial. Prolonged follow-up with repeated comprehensive imaging of the fellow eye in patients already presenting with lesions in one eye is important.

Diagnostic imaging is therefore at least as important, if not more important, in this context than in all other forms of wet AMD.

TABLE OF CONTENTS OF CLINICAL CASES

CLINICAL CASE No. 01: CHORIORETINAL ANASTOMOSIS

Recent juxtafoveal macular hemorrhage and small central PED in a patient with drusen. Follow-up by TD-OCT and SD-OCT after anti-VEGF therapy .... Page 282

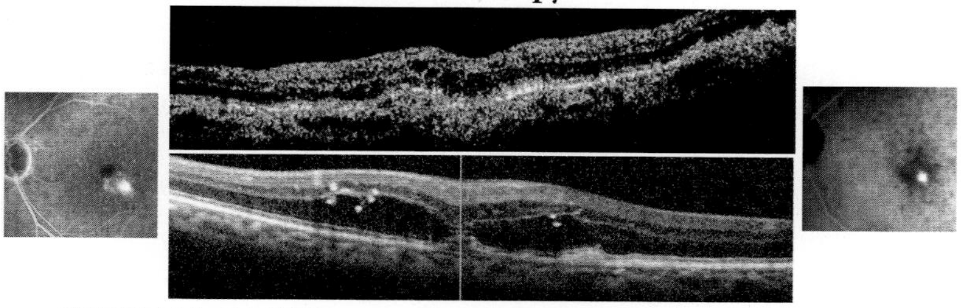

CLINICAL CASE No. 02: CHORIORETINAL ANASTOMOSIS

Juxtafoveal macular hemorrhage and small central PED. Bilateral lesion, progressing over several months. Follow-up with SD-OCT after anti-VEGF therapy .... Page 288

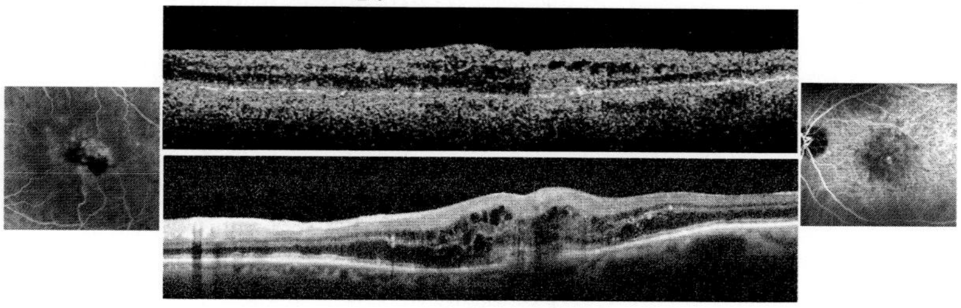

CLINICAL CASE No. 03: CHORIORETINAL ANASTOMOSIS

Vascularized PED with hot spots, macular hemorrhage, and anastomosis on SLO-ICG angiography. Follow-up by SD-OCT after anti-VEGF therapy .... Page 292

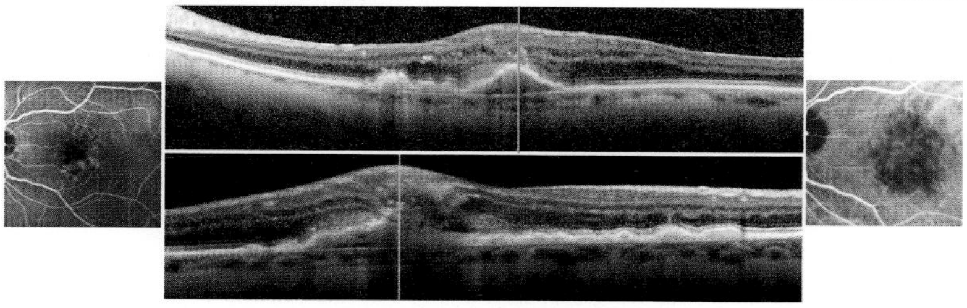

CLINICAL CASE No. 04: CHORIORETINAL ANASTOMOSIS

Juxtafoveal macular hemorrhage and small central PED in a patient with drusen. Follow-up by SD-OCT OCT after anti-VEGF therapy .... Page 296

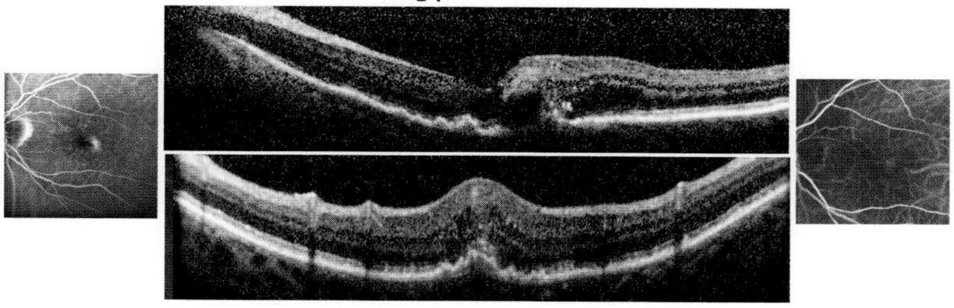

CLINICAL CASE No. 05: ADVANCED FORM OF CHORIORETINAL ANASTOMOSIS

Juxtafoveal retinal hemorrhage and vascularized PED, progressing over several years. Chronic lesion not amenable to treatment .... Page 298

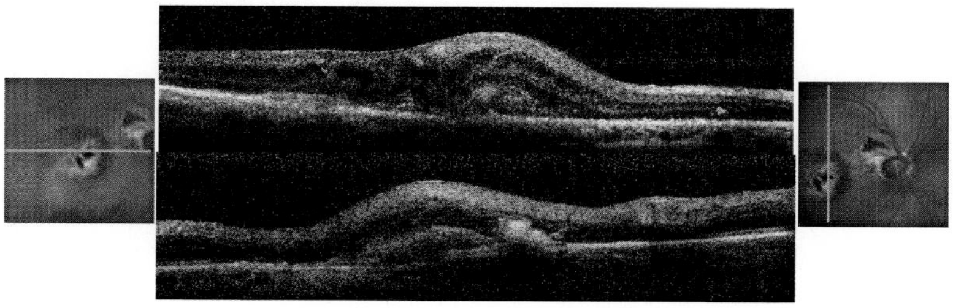

CLINICAL CASE No. 01: Chorioretinal Anastomosis

Recent juxtafoveal macular hemorrhage and small central PED in a patient with drusen. Follow-up by TD-OCT and SD-OCT after anti-VEGF therapy

An 87-year-old monocular man with a history of central retinal artery occlusion in his right eye presented with recent, moderate loss of vision in his left eye.

This patient had a history of systemic cardiovascular disease with well-controlled hypertension. Coronary, popliteal, and iliac artery bypass grafts were well-tolerated. VA: RE: LP - LE: 20/50.

Biomicroscopic Examination

Several disseminated soft drusen and a microscopic juxtafoveal hemorrhage at 5 o'clock (**Figure 3a and b**). **Autofluorescence** demonstrated a small territory of inferior temporal juxtafoveal hyper-fluorescence.

Fluorescein Angiography

- A small (200 microns) zone of early, intense hyper-fluorescence, adjacent to the hemorrhage, was detected but rapidly masked by fluorescein leakage (**Figure 3a**).
- The hyper-fluorescent area was located adjacent to the distal end of the retinal vessel, but the anastomosis was masked by fluorescein leakage.
- *Late phase*: progressive staining, close to the zone of intense fluorescein leakage, suggested progressive filling of a small PED (**Figure 3b**).

SLO-ICG Angiography

a): *Early phase*: hypo-fluorescent area suggestive of a PED. There was also a small, round, well-delineated, deep hyper-fluorescent lesion indicative of choroidal neovascularization. Retinal vessels were visualized but their terminations were fine and indistinct (**Figure 3c**).

The ***enlarged view*** clearly demonstrated the chorioretinal anastomosis with a direct communication between retinal vessels and the deeper choroidal neovascularization. There was also an end-to-end retino-retinal anastomosis between a retinal arteriole and a retinal venule (**Figure 3d**).

b): *Late phase*: the edges of the dark and hypo-fluorescent PED were well-defined with hyper-fluorescent neovascularization contrasting against this dark background.

Suggested Diagnosis:
Initial stage of chorioretinal anastomosis with a small serous PED, which had progressed over several weeks.

Contribution of OCT (*Spectralis**)

Horizontal cross-section
The RPE was raised with a moderately reflective cavity and a wavy contour, corresponding to the **initial small PED**. (**Figure 4a**).

A localized disruption of the RPE was observed adjacent to the PED, close to the center of the fovea. The CNV appeared to protrude through this **disruption in the RPE** and proliferate within the retina.
Abundant SRF was observed *anterior to the RPE band.*

Vertical cross-section
The vertical cross-section, centered directly on the angiographically hyper-fluorescent area, showed the same break in the RPE and unequivocally demonstrated protrusion of the CNV towards the retina (**Figure 4b**).
Anterior to the RPE, the cross-section showed increased retinal thickness with subretinal and intraretinal fluid. The outer retinal layers were clearly visible and only altered over the zone of protruding CNV. Numerous bright hyper-reflective spots were present.

Diagnosis
At this stage, SD-OCT demonstrated the highly suggestive and characteristic signs of CNV and their extension through the RPE. Other findings seen include a retino-retinal anastomosis, adjacent leakage, bright hyper-reflective spots, and a subfoveal and juxtafoveal PED.
All these clinical signs allowed an exact diagnosis, especially when **correlated with** angiographic findings (hot spots and anastomosis visible on the SLO-ICG angiography) and OCT images.
The combination of imaging confirmed the diagnosis. The lesions were small and localized at this stage, but too close to the center of the fovea to be treated by laser photocoagulation. These features indicated immediate *IVT injections of anti-VEGF* in an attempt to stop progression of the lesions before deterioration of VA.

CLINICAL CASE No. 01: CHORIORETINAL ANASTOMOSIS

Recent juxtafoveal macular hemorrhage and small central PED in a patient with drusen. Follow-up by TD-OCT then SD-OCT after anti-VEGF therapy.

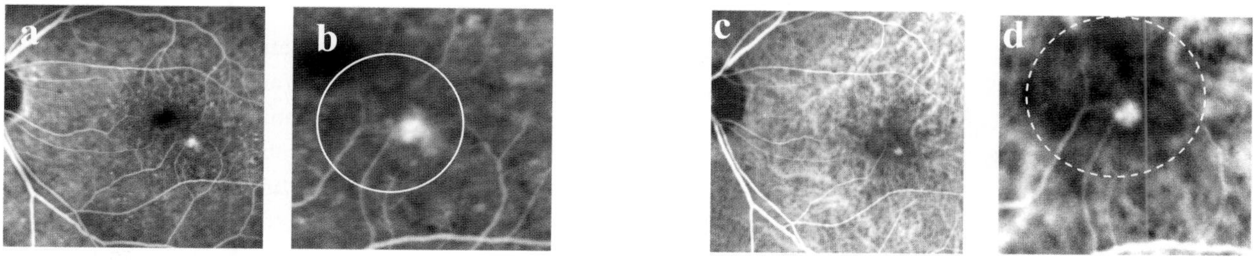

Figure 3: Chorioretinal anastomosis. VA: 20/50. (First examination).
a and b): Fluorescein angiography: small zone of hyper-fluorescence adjacent to the hemorrhage, masked by fluorescein leakage. This zone is adjacent to the termination of retinal vessels. Progressive filling of a small PED.
c and d): SLO-ICG angiography: hypo-fluorescent zone suggestive of a PED (*circle*). Small hyper-fluorescent lesion characteristic of choroidal neovascularization.
The *enlarged view* (d) clearly demonstrates the anastomosis and the direct communication between the deeper choroidal neovascularization and retino-retinal anastomosis. This is seen within the hypo-fluorescent PED (*dotted circle*).

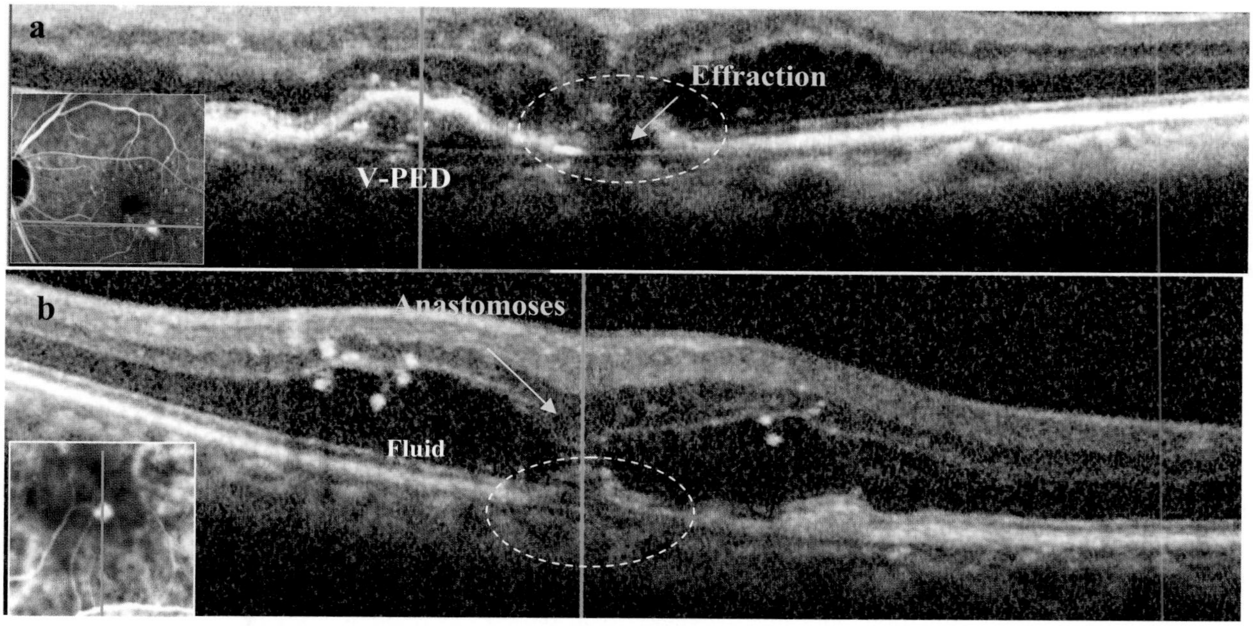

Figure 4: Chorioretinal anastomosis. VA: 20/50. (First examination).
a): *Spectralis horizontal section**: elevation of the RPE corresponding to the initial PED.
Localized disruption of the RPE, forming a discontinuity through which the CNV protrudes into the retina.
Note the SRF accumulation anterior to the RPE band.
b): *Spectralis vertical cross-section (centered on the hyper-fluorescent zone)**: protrusion of the CNV into the retina is visible with subretinal and intraretinal fluid accumulation and numerous bright hyper-reflective spots.

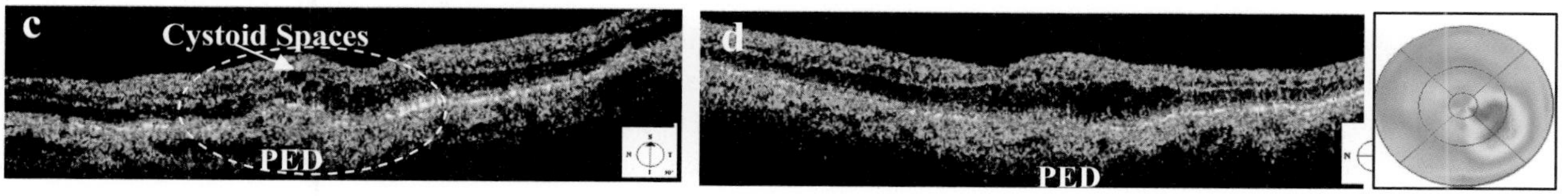

Figure 4: Chorioretinal anastomosis. VA: 20/50. (First examination).
c): *Stratus horizontal cross-section**: the abnormalities are barely visible: small PED, intraretinal abnormalities, and intraretinal fluid.
d): *Stratus vertical cross-section**: the small zone of the lesions is not visible on this cross-section.

CLINICAL CASE No. 01: Chorioretinal Anastomosis

Recent juxtafoveal macular hemorrhage and small central PED in a patient with drusen.
Follow-up by TD-OCT then SD-OCT after anti-VEGF therapy

Monthly intravitreous injections of anti-VEGF (*Lucentis**) were continued for 9 months and the response to treatment was evaluated with visual acuity, OCT, fluorescein and ICG angiography.

The patient demonstrated reliable compliance with follow-up and injections. This treatment initially achieved a good result but each attempt to defer injections was followed by recurrences of variable severity.
During these 9 months of follow-up, treatment maintained the lesions to a limited stage, and the pathology always remained sensitive to anti-VEGF therapy (**Figure 5**).

Visual acuity was relatively good, but the patient experienced changes in visual acuity after a maximum of two months between injections.

At the last follow-up, VA remained stable at 20/63, allowing satisfactory reading. Maintenance treatment with alternating ranibizumab and pegaptanib was considered.

*Spectralis** OCT

- *By the first follow-up examination*, the retinal thickness had decreased considerably to almost normal. The vertical cross-section, selected exactly over the lesion detected by fluorescein angiography, showed almost complete resolution of the intraretinal lesion (**Figure 5a**).

Only a few large bright hyper-reflective spots and disruption of the *IS/OS interface* and *external limiting membrane* were still present.

- *Two months later*, the situation appeared to have improved with VA of 20/50 and barely detectable lesions, with similar features but attenuated and more localized (**Figure 5b**).
- *Two months later*, the patient experienced a recurrence. The OCT appearance was identical to the initial findings: discontinuity of the RPE, disruption of the outer layers, intraretinal extension, fluid accumulation, and numerous bright hyper-reflective spots (**Figure 5c**).
- *After another injection*, the features improved immediately, but another recurrence was observed 2 months later with return of the same fluorescein angiography, ICG angiography, and OCT signs (**Figure 5d**).
- *The last examination* showed a satisfactory appearance.

Retinal layers were well-organized, with normal thickness and regression of the signs, even at the site of the original lesions.
Several bright hyper-reflective spots, occasionally confluent, were still visible (**Figure 5e**).

Fluorescein Angiography

The small (300 μm) hyper-fluorescent zone remained visible but became almost punctate during phases of improvement (**Figure 5a and b**).
Each relapse was marked by reappearance of fluorescein leakage but with no new hemorrhage and no change in the numerous adjacent drusen.
Dark hypo-fluorescent lipofuscin material was visualized in the foveal region.

ICG Angiography

The dark PED remained small, poorly-delineated, and with poor contrast.
Choroidal neovascularization was barely visible with no marked neovascular membrane (**Figure 5a-d**).

At this Stage

In this case of **chorioretinal anastomosis** diagnosed and treated at a very early stage, each injection was rapidly followed by resolution of exudative phenomena and the improvement in the appearance of the lesion on imaging, resulting in an almost normal appearance of the zone of neovascularization and chorioretinal anastomosis (**Figure 5**).

Combined PDT-IVT therapy was not used in this patient with monocular blindness.
These phases of improvement included not only the OCT findings but also the angiographic signs and visual acuity.
However, 3 recurrences were observed, every 2 months, suggesting that treatment only has a palliative effect and would have to be continued for many months.

CLINICAL CASE No. 01: CHORIORETINAL ANASTOMOSIS

Recent juxtafoveal macular hemorrhage and small central PED in a patient with drusen.
Follow-up by TD-OCT and SD-OCT after anti-VEGF therapy

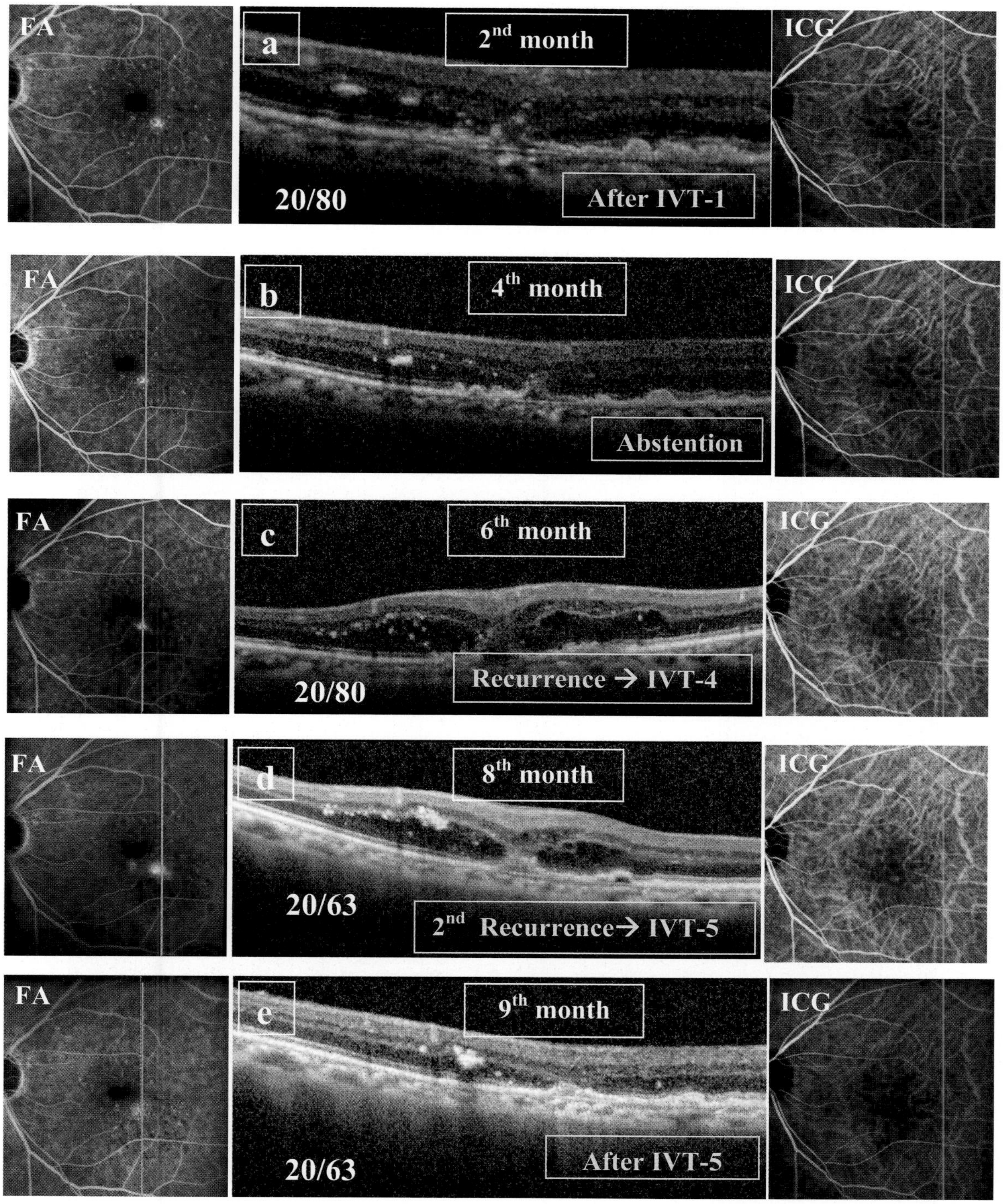

Figure 5 (a-e): Chorioretinal anastomosis: follow-up during treatment.
Each injection was rapidly followed by resolution of exudative phenomena and improvement in the appearance of the lesion, resulting in an almost normal appearance of the zone of neovascularization and chorioretinal anastomosis on SD-OCT cross-sections. There remained persistence of bright hyper-reflective spots that were occasionally confluent.
The last examination showed a satisfactory appearance with well-organized retinal layers of normal thickness and regression of the signs, even at the site of the lesions.

CLINICAL CASE No. 01: Chorioretinal Anastomosis

Recent juxtafoveal macular hemorrhage and small central PED in a patient with drusen. Follow-up by TD-OCT and SD-OCT after anti-VEGF therapy

During follow-up of this case, a calliper placed on the angiogram allowed simultaneous visualization of the corresponding lesion on the OCT cross-section together with *graphic representation of retinal thickness.*

A numerical representation of retinal thickness at the green line selected with the calliper was also displayed. **At each subsequent examination**, retinal thickness was obtained by a simple click with automatic alignment on the lesion selected at the first examination.

In this particular case, follow-up demonstrated very rapid and spectacular improvement after the first injection (green zone on the graph) (**Figure 6 a and b**).

Subsequently, at the time of recurrence, retinal thickness returned to the pretreatment value (**Figure 6c and d**).

Finally, after the 4th injection, retinal thickness returned to normal (260 µm, i.e. 166 µm less than on the initial examination).

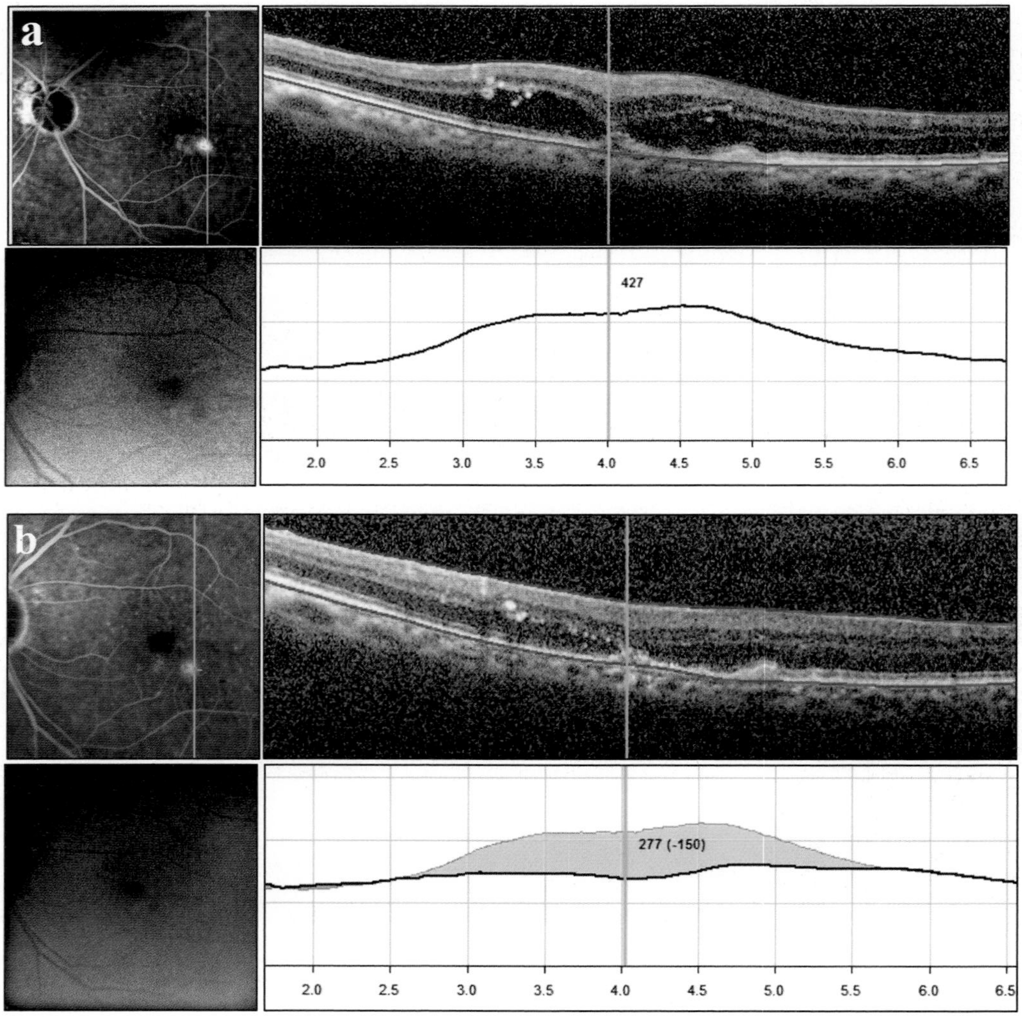

Figure 6: Automatic graphic comparison of retinal thickness at the same location as on the initial examination. a and b): *Spectralis vertical cross-sections, fluorescein angiography, and ICG angiography**: automatic graphic comparison of retinal thickness.

CLINICAL CASE No. 01: CHORIORETINAL ANASTOMOSIS

Recent juxtafoveal macular hemorrhage and small central PED in a patient with drusen. Follow-up by TD-OCT and SD-OCT after anti-VEGF therapy.

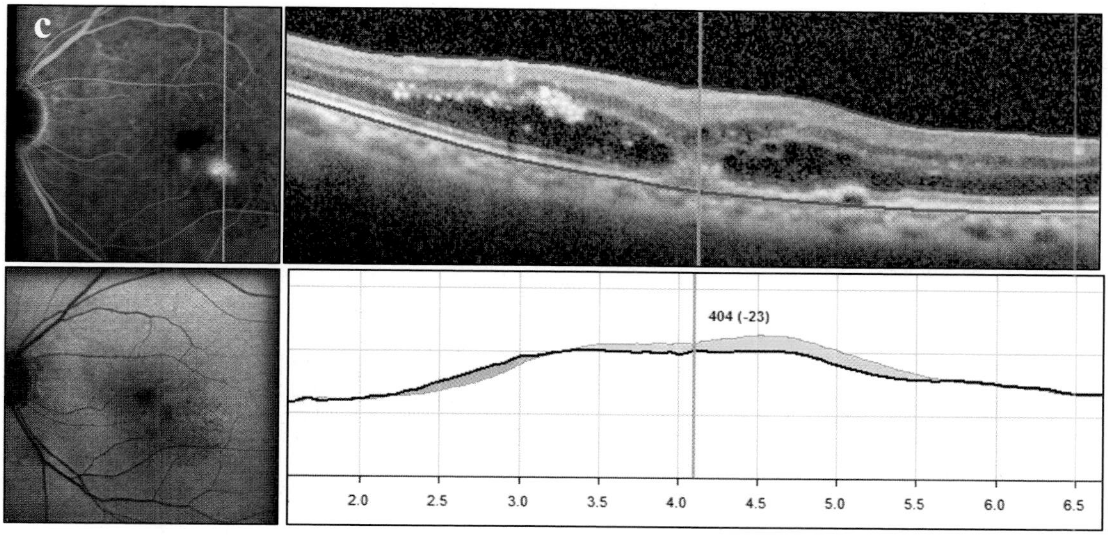

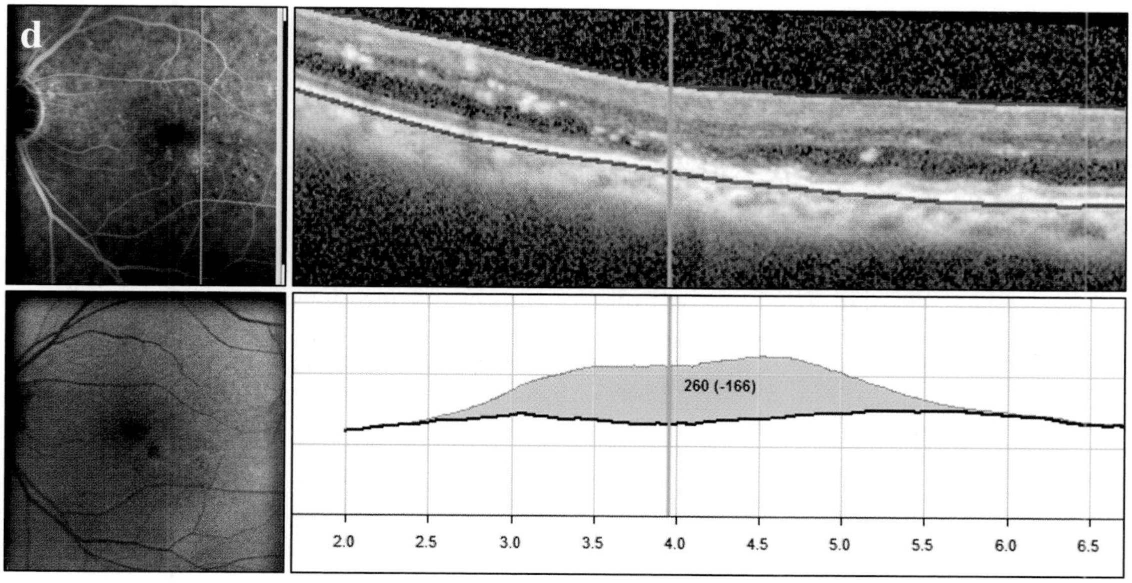

◘ Figure 6: Automatic graphic comparison of retinal thickness at the same location as on the initial examination.

c and d): ***Spectralis*** *** vertical cross-sections, fluorescein angiography, and ICG angiography**: follow-up after the second recurrence.

CLINICAL CASE No. 02: Chorioretinal Anastomosis

Juxtafoveal macular hemorrhage and small central PED. Bilateral lesion, progressing over several months. Follow-up by SD-OCT after anti-VEGF therapy

A 95-year-old woman with bilateral AMD progressing over many years and monocular blindness (due to longstanding chorioretinal anastomosis in the right eye) presented with a recent, moderate decline of visual acuity in the left eye.
VA RE: 20/320 – VA LE: 20/50.
Biomicroscopic examination revealed a few disseminated soft drusen and a highly suggestive, small juxtafoveal hemorrhage at 5 o'clock, (**Figure 8, color**).

Fluorescein Angiography

- Small zone (200 µm) of early hyper-fluorescence adjacent to the macular termination of retinal vessels with fluorescein leakages partially masked by hemorrhage (**Figure 7a**).
- In the late phase, progressive filling of a small PED and the overlying SRF with numerous cysts (**Figure 7b**).

SLO-ICG Angiography

a): *Early phase*: small, round, juxtafoveal hyper-fluorescent lesion.
The enlarged image more clearly visualized the end-to-end retino-retinal anastomosis between a retinal arteriole and a retinal venule and a direct communication between retinal vessels and a deeper, small choroidal neovascularization (**Figure 7c**).
b): *Late phase*: dark, hypo-fluorescent, low-density PED containing a zone of hyper-fluorescent choroidal neovascularization (**Figure 7d**).

Suggested Diagnosis:
Early chorioretinal anastomosis with active fluorescein leakage and a small serous PED.

Contribution of OCT (*Spectralis**)

Horizontal cross-section
Characteristic and immediately suggestive appearance:

- Discontinuity of the RPE, disruption of the external limiting membrane, alteration of the IS/OS interface,
- Presence of a pre-RPE dense zone and numerous bright hyper-reflective spots,
- Marked intraretinal fluid with numerous small cysts in two layers.

The **chorioretinal anastomosis** was visualized as a hyper-reflective zone appearing to arise from the choroid and protruding anterior to the RPE.
The **retinal hemorrhage** induced a juxtafoveal hyper-reflective zone in the inner layers with characteristic shadowing (**Figure 8a**).

The vertical cross-section centered on the hyper-fluorescent zone demonstrated the same characteristic signs: disruption of the RPE and clearly visible protrusion of CNV into the retina (**Figure 8b**).

***Stratus** TD-OCT** cross-sections showed the same lesions but with much less detail (**Figure 8c and d**).

- *Anterior to the RPE*, increased retinal thickness with subretinal and intraretinal fluid and numerous cysts.
- *The outer retinal layers* were severely altered over the zone of protrusion of the CNV with numerous bright hyper-reflective spots.

Diagnosis
The OCT appearance was therefore highly suggestive of chorioretinal anastomosis and characteristic of the presence of choroidal neovascularization protruding through the RPE.
Extension of intraretinal proliferations was reflected by the adjacent major exudative reaction, bright hyper-reflective spots on OCT, the small subfoveal and juxtafoveal PED, and numerous cysts.
All these signs were consistent with the diagnosis of chorioretinal anastomosis. The calliper allowed precise correlation between the angiographic lesion (especially on SLO-ICG) and the SD-OCT appearance, localizing the hemorrhage in the inner retinal layers.
These findings justified immediate IVT injections of anti-VEGF therapy.

CLINICAL CASE No. 02: CHORIORETINAL ANASTOMOSIS

Juxtafoveal macular hemorrhage and small central PED. Bilateral lesion, progressing over several months. Follow-up by SD-OCT after anti-VEGF therapy

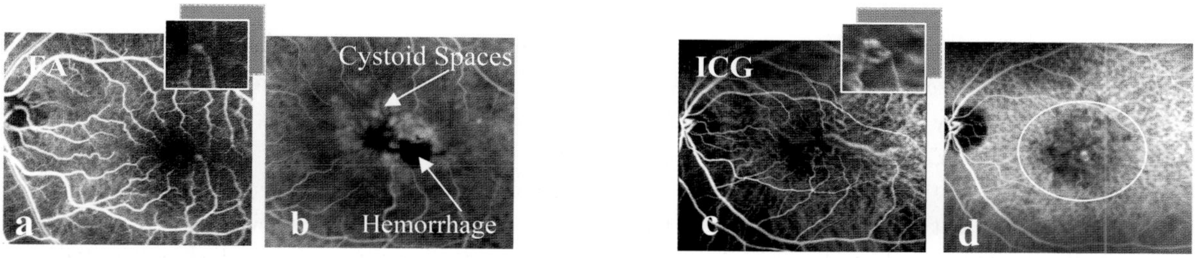

Figure 7: Chorioretinal anastomosis. VA: 20/50. First examination.
a and b): Fluorescein angiography: zone of hyper-fluorescence adjacent to the macular termination of retinal vessels with fluorescein leakage partially masked by hemorrhage. Progressive filling of a PED and SRF with cystoid spaces.
c and d): SLO-ICG angiography: small round, hyper-fluorescent, juxtafoveal lesion. The enlarged view shows the end-to-end retino-retinal anastomosis between a retinal arteriole and a retinal venule and direct communication between retinal vessels and the deeper choroidal neovascularization. The PED is dark and hypo-fluorescent.

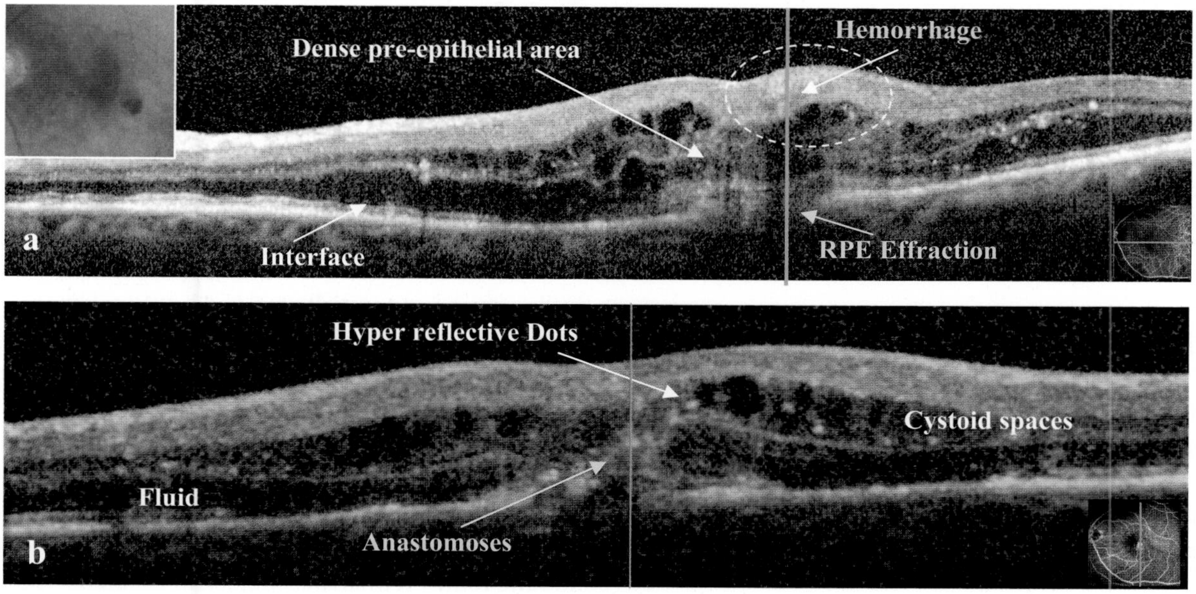

Figure 8: Chorioretinal anastomosis. VA: 20/50. First examination.
a): *Spectralis horizontal section**: discontinuity of the RPE, disruption of the external limiting membrane, alteration of the IS/OS interface, presence of a pre-RPE dense zone, and numerous bright hyper-reflective spots; abundant intraretinal fluid and a large number of cysts.
Hyper-reflective juxtafoveal zone in the inner retinal layers corresponding to the retinal hemorrhage with characteristic shadowing extending as far as the choroid.
b): *Spectralis vertical cross-section**: discontinuity of the RPE; protrusion of CNV into the retina was clearly visible.
Anterior to the RPE, increased retinal thickness with subretinal and intraretinal fluid and numerous cysts. The outer retinal layers are altered with numerous bright hyper-reflective spots.

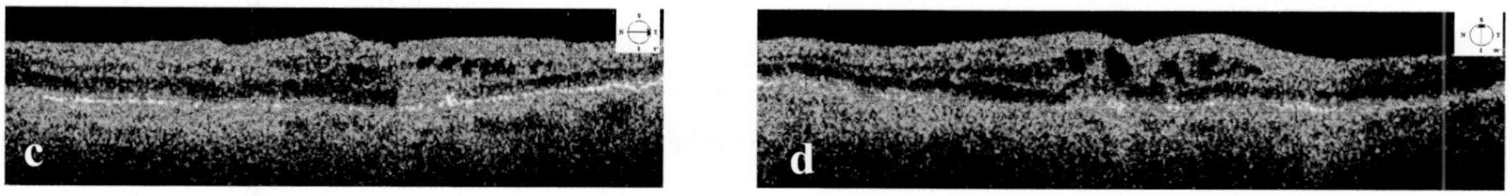

Figure 8: Chorioretinal anastomosis. VA: 20/50 VA: 20/50 First examination.
c and d): *Stratus horizontal and vertical cross-sections**: increased retinal thickness and numerous cysts.

CLINICAL CASE No. 02: Chorioretinal Anastomosis

Juxtafoveal macular hemorrhage and small central PED. Bilateral lesion, progressing over several months. Follow-up by SD-OCT after anti-VEGF therapy

A long course of intravitreous injections of anti-VEGF was planned with monthly follow-up of visual acuity, OCT, and fluorescein and ICG angiography.

However, this elderly patient elected to suspend her treatment after the third injection when she obtained subjectively satisfactory stabilization.

During these 4 months of follow-up, the various imaging modalities demonstrated partial regression of the lesions that appeared to respond to treatment without completely resolving (**Figure 9**).

This patient's visual acuity stabilized at 20/125 with subjective improvement of functional disability.

*Spectralis** OCT

By the first examination, the lesion appeared to decrease in size, although retinal thickness remained markedly increased.

Horizontal cross-section

All of the initial signs were still present but less marked: disruption of the RPE, hyper-reflective zone anterior to the RPE, numerous cysts in two layers, and multiple bright hyper-reflective spots (mainly around the zone of intraretinal fluid).

The localized zone of juxtafoveal hyper-reflectivity corresponding to hemorrhage persisted with shadowing extending throughout the choroid. All these signs were less marked than on the initial examination.

Vertical cross-section

The appearance on the vertical section was just as diagnostic with disruption of the RPE, intraretinal fluid, and juxtafoveal hemorrhage. The numerous bright hyper-reflective spots indicated that the lesion was still active despite a relative improvement (**Figure 10a and b**).

Graphic thickness representations

Comparison of the same location as on the initial examination with two graphs of the horizontal and vertical cross-sections showed a slight increase of retinal thickness despite attenuation of the patient's symptoms (**Figure 11a and b**).

Fluorescein Angiography

The neovascular membrane and anastomosis were less well perfused and initially masked by retinal hemorrhage. In the late phase, several fluorescein leakages were visible beyond the hemorrhage with almost no staining or cystoid edema (**Figure 9a and b**).

ICG Angiography

The neovascular membrane was not clearly visualized and the retino-retinal anastomosis was barely visible. The dark area, indicative of PED, remained visible but presented low contrast (**Figure 9c and d**).

At this Stage

In this typical case of bilateral CRA, the first 3 injections provided an improvement or halted progression of the lesions. Visual acuity appeared to be stabilized and, although relatively poor, was considered to be satisfactory by the patient.

However, despite persistence of the characteristic SD-OCT features, the clinical features appeared to be stabilized with no new complications, relapses, or recurrences. The patient preferred to suspend treatment in view of this functional stabilization.

This lesion can be considered to be in the process of resolution (**Figure 10**).

The prognosis remains reserved and guarded, and ideally long-term follow-up should be maintained.

CLINICAL CASE No. 02: CHORIORETINAL ANASTOMOSIS

Juxtafoveal macular hemorrhage and small central PED. Bilateral lesion, progressing over several months. Follow-up by SD-OCT after anti-VEGF therapy

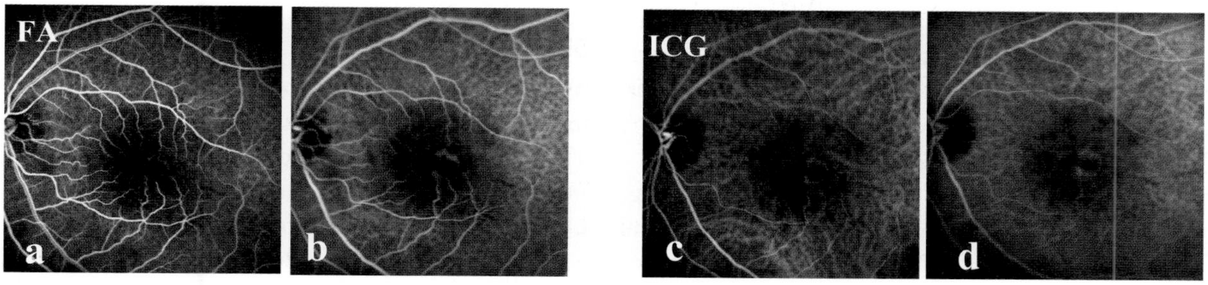

Figure 9: Chorioretinal anastomosis. VA: 20/125. After the third IVT injection.
a and b): Fluorescein angiography: neovascular membrane and less perfused anastomosis. Several fluorescein leakages.
c and d): SLO-ICG angiography: the neovascular membrane and retino-retinal anastomosis are now barely visible. The dark PED remains visible but with low contrast.

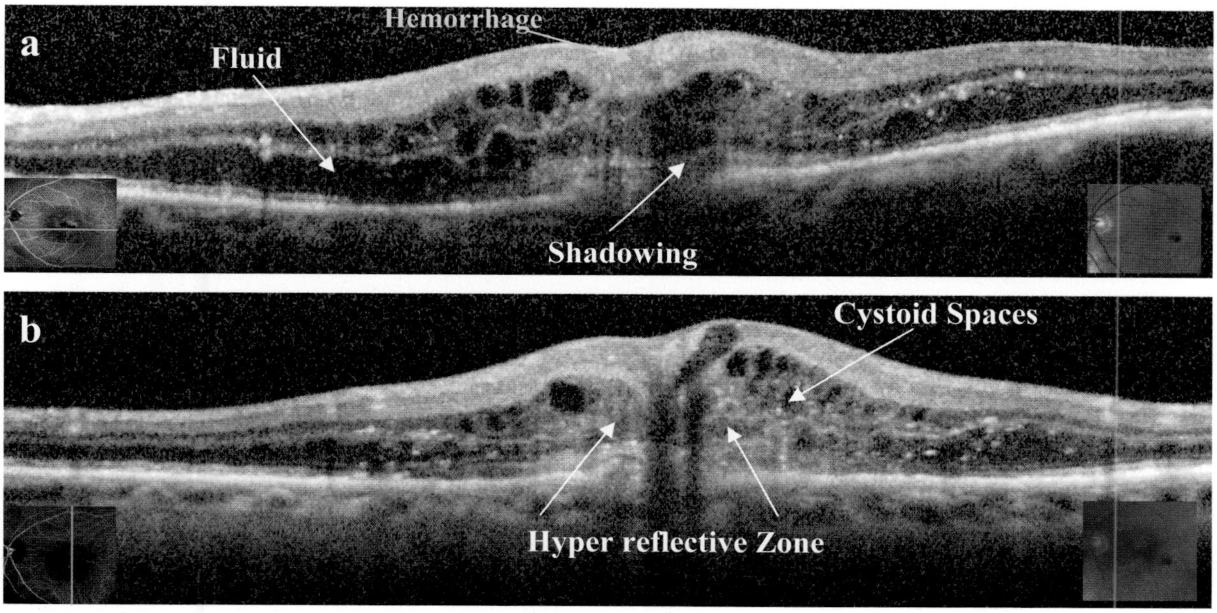

Figure 10: Chorioretinal anastomosis. VA: 20/125. After the third IVT.
a and b): *Spectralis horizontal and vertical cross-sections**: Discontinuity of the RPE, hyper-reflective zone anterior to the RPE, numerous cysts in two layers, and numerous bright hyper-reflective spots.
Localized juxtafoveal hyper-reflectivity corresponding to hemorrhage with less marked shadowing than on initial examination.

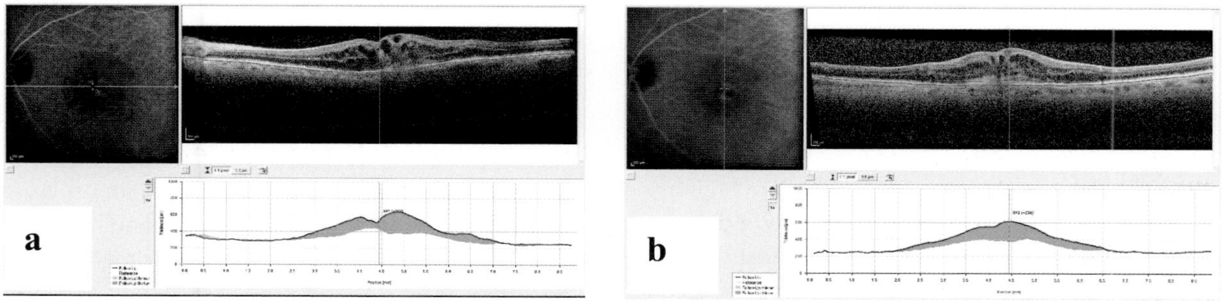

Figure 11: Automatic graphic comparison of thickness in the same location as on the initial examination.
a and b): ICG angiography, *Spectralis horizontal and vertical cross-sections.**

CLINICAL CASE No. 03: Chorioretinal Anastomosis

Vascularized PED with hot spots, macular hemorrhage, and anastomosis on SLO-ICG angiography. Follow-up by SD-OCT after anti-VEGF therapy.

An 86-year-old woman with AMD, predominantly affecting the left eye and evolving slowly for several months, presented with loss of visual acuity.
VA RE: 20/50 – VA LE: 20/160.
Biomicroscopic examination demonstrated highly suggestive pigment migrations forming a network, several perifoveal soft drusen, and most notably, a small juxtafoveal hemorrhage at 5 o'clock (**Figure 13a**, color).
On **autofluorescence**, the pigmented network was autofluorescent and xanthophyll pigment was normal.

Fluorescein Angiography

- *Early phase*, minimal hyper-fluorescent, juxtafoveal lesion at the termination of a retinal venule, which was partially masked by hemorrhage (**Figure 12a**).
- *Late phase*, the lesion was rapidly masked by staining of the material (**Figure 12b**).

SLO-ICG Angiography

a) *Early phase*: the deep, round, hyper-fluorescent, juxtafoveal neovascular membrane was immediately visible. The enlarged view clearly demonstrated that the lesion was in contact with a terminal retinal venule (**Figure 12c**).
b) *Late phase*: the initial juxtafoveal lesion was visualized within the dark, hypo-fluorescent PED with irregular margins. It was associated with a large hyper-fluorescent area that invaded almost all of the surface of the PED (**Figure 12d**).

Suggested Diagnosis:
Chorioretinal anastomosis associated with PED almost completely invaded by choroidal neovascularization, indicating a chronic lesion.

Contribution of OCT (*Spectralis**)

Horizontal cross-section
The horizontal cross-section showed the inferior part of the PED and the autofluorescent lesions.
The RPE was irregular and thickened due to deposits.
It was also elevated and separated from Bruch's membrane, demonstrating the vascularized PED.

Anterior to the RPE, OCT showed
- Disruption of the external limiting membrane,
- Alteration of the IS/OS interface,
- Presence of a pre-RPE dense zone,
- Several bright hyper-reflective spots,
- Marked intraretinal fluid, and
- Numerous, and small, tightly packed cysts.

The neurosensory retina was also globally thickened (**Figure 12a**).

Vertical cross-section
The vertical cross-section centered directly over the hemorrhage and the neovascular lesion immediately demonstrated characteristic signs: discontinuity of the RPE and clearly visible protrusion of CNV into the retina (**Figure 12b**).
Anterior to the RPE, increased retinal thickness with subretinal and intraretinal fluid and a large number of cysts. The outer retinal layers were altered over the protrusion of CNV with numerous bright hyper-reflective spots. The severely altered outer nuclear layer was no longer detectable in the central retina.
The hyper-fluorescent zone in the *inner retinal layers* was visualized simultaneously on ICG angiography and by the vertical line on OCT. The hyper-reflective zone corresponded to the juxtafoveal retinal hemorrhage with shadowing extending as far as the choroid.

Diagnosis
The OCT appearance was therefore highly indicative of chorioretinal anastomosis and characteristic of the presence of choroidal neovascularization protruding through the RPE with an intense exudative reaction. The lesion was already advanced with extension of neovascularization inside the PED, visible on ICG angiography. All of these signs, including the retinal hemorrhage in the inner layers, indicated the same diagnosis as for the first eye.
This clinical features justified immediate introduction of IVT injections of anti-VEGF therapy.

CLINICAL CASE No. 03: CHORIORETINAL ANASTOMOSIS

Vascularized PED with hot spots, macular hemorrhage, and anastomosis on SLO-ICG angiography. Follow-up by SD-OCT after anti-VEGF therapy.

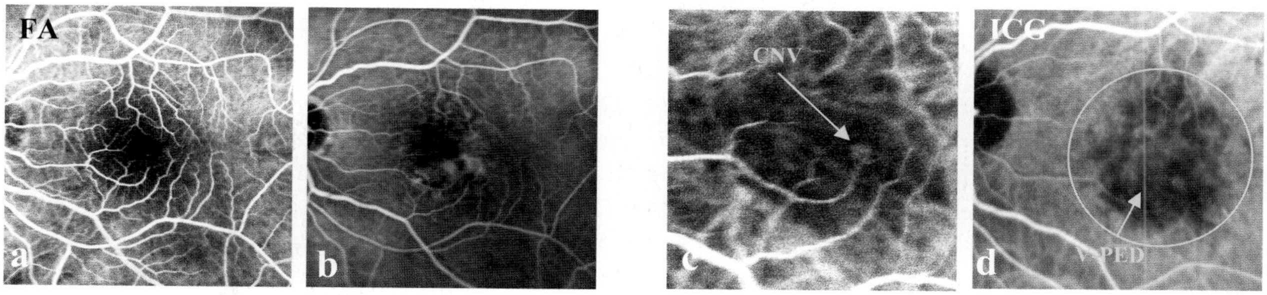

Figure 12: Chorioretinal anastomosis. VA: 20/160. Before the first IVT injection.
Fluorescein angiography
a): ***Early phase***: minimal hyper-fluorescent lesion.
b): ***Late phase:*** the lesion is rapidly masked by staining of the autofluorescent material.
SLO-ICG angiography
c): ***Early phase***: immediately visible, juxtafoveal deep neovascular lesion in contact with a terminal retinal venule.
d): ***Late phase***: large hyper-fluorescent zone inside and invading almost the entire surface of the PED.

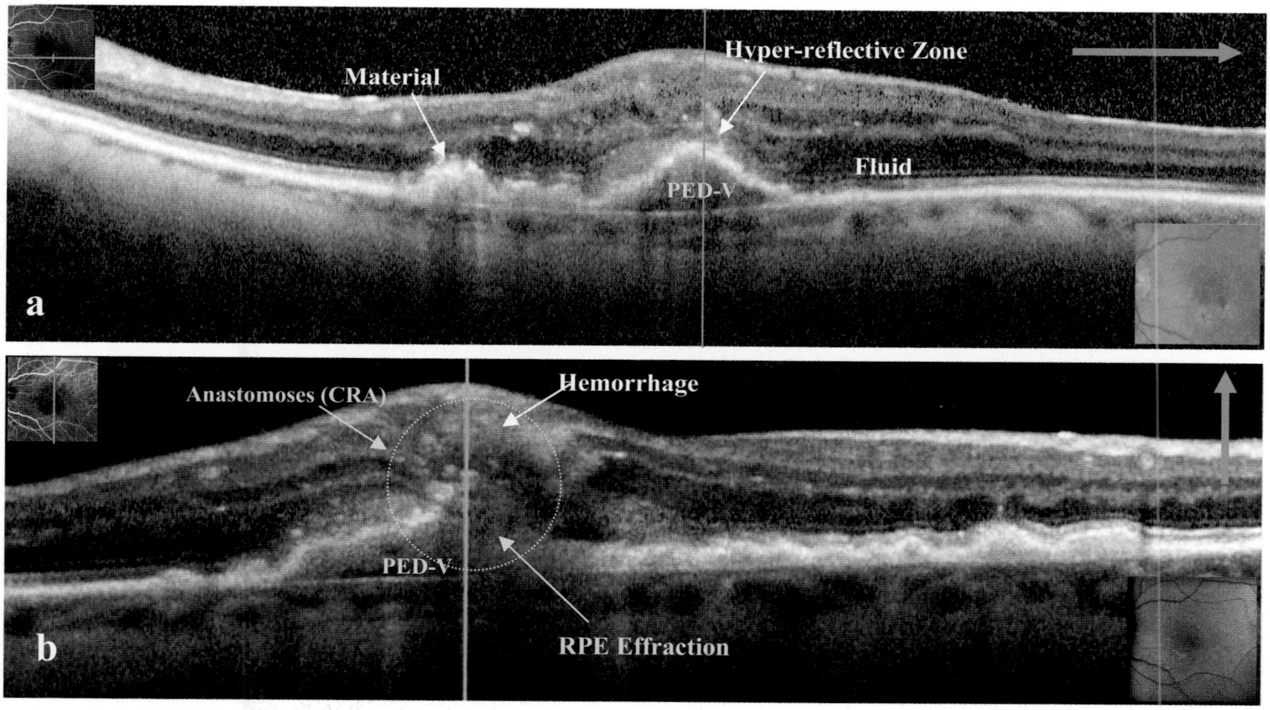

Figure 13: Chorioretinal anastomosis. VA: 20/160. Before the first IVT injection.
a): ***Spectralis**** **horizontal cross-section** through the inferior part of the PED and autofluorescent lesions (thickening corresponding to deposits): vascularized PED with elevation of the RPE.
Anterior to the RPE, disruption of the external limiting membrane, alteration of the IS/OS interface, presence of a pre-RPE dense zone, and several bright hyper-reflective spots; marked intraretinal fluid; numerous cysts.
b): ***Spectralis**** **vertical cross-section** centered on the lesion and the hemorrhage, showing characteristic signs: discontinuity of the RPE and very clearly visible protrusion of the CNV into the retina. *Anterior to the RPE*, increased retinal thickness and subretinal and intraretinal fluid and numerous cysts. The outer layers are altered over the zone of protrusion of the CNV with numerous bright hyper-reflective spots. The outer nuclear layer is severely altered.

CLINICAL CASE No. 03: Chorioretinal Anastomosis

Vascularized PED with hot spots, macular hemorrhage, and anastomosis on SLO-ICG angiography. Follow-up by SD-OCT after anti-VEGF therapy.

This patient was followed for a period of 3 months during which she received 2 intravitreous injections of anti-VEGF (*Lucentis**) with routine monthly observation by visual acuity, OCT, fluorescein angiography, and ICG angiography.

During these 3 months of follow-up, the various imaging modalities demonstrated satisfactory regression of morphological lesions, which, although already longstanding, showed a remarkable response to treatment. This was demonstrated by retinal thickness measurements with automated comparison to initial measurements on successive graphs (**Figure 14**).

However, **visual function** was barely improved, as only subjective symptoms regressed but visual acuity remained relatively low at 20/125 on the last examination.

*Spectralis** OCT

- **By the first follow-up examination**, all of the retinal architecture had almost returned to normal.

On the ***horizontal cross-section***, the foveal depression regained a normal structure. The inner retinal layers were well-organized and the outer nuclear layer had a normal appearance.

Only multiple localized elevations of the RPE were observed, corresponding to multiple soft drusen.

The external limiting membrane and IS/OS interface were almost intact, except in the juxtafoveal and inferior temporal region, where the RPE was slightly raised (**Figure 13a**).

On the ***vertical cross-section,*** the RPE also had numerous elevations corresponding to drusen with minimal alterations of the outer layers over the dome of the drusen.

In the inferior part of the scan, the neurosensory retina was still abnormally thickened with several cysts. The foveal depression had a normal profile (**Figure 13b**).

- **At the third examination and after 2 intravitreous injections**, the normal appearance of the horizontal cross-section was confirmed with a normal foveal depression and well-organized retinal layers.

Only a small juxtafoveal and temporal PED persisted with adjacent alterations of the external limiting membrane and especially the outer nuclear layer, as well as several bright hyper-reflective spots (**Figure 13c**).

Due to a moderate adverse drug reaction limited to a rash and at the patient's request, follow-up angiography was not performed.

At this Stage

In this case of advanced CRA, the first 2 injections clearly induced an improvement, at least morphological, with control of exudation and resorption of subretinal and intraretinal fluid (**Figure 14**).

In view of the good visual acuity in the other eye, the patient considered the result to be fairly satisfactory. Functional and imaging observation was maintained, and the patient was warned about the risk of recurrence over the months to come.

In contrast with the cases described above, presenting the earliest possible lesions, functional improvement appeared to be more difficult to achieve in this case treated after several months of progression to these more advanced lesions.

Rigorous long-term observation is essential to guide subsequent treatment.

CLINICAL CASE No. 03: CHORIORETINAL ANASTOMOSIS

Vascularized PED with hot spots, macular hemorrhage, and anastomosis on SLO-ICG angiography. Follow-up by SD-OCT after anti-VEGF therapy.

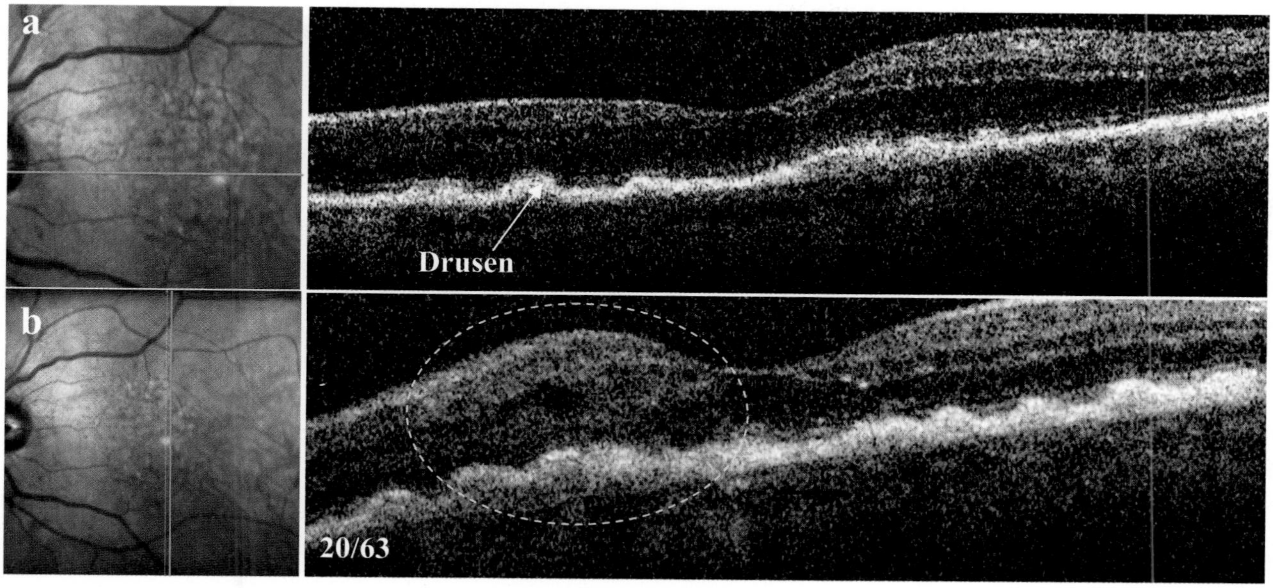

Figure 13: Chorioretinal anastomosis. VA: 20/63. After the first IVT injection.
a): *Spectralis horizontal cross-section**: normal foveal depression, well-organized inner layers and normal outer nuclear layer. Multiple localized elevations of the RPE corresponding to soft drusen. The external limiting membrane and IS/OS interface are intact except in the juxtafoveal and inferior temporal region where the RPE is slightly raised.
b): *Spectralis vertical** cross-**section**: Numerous elevations of the RPE corresponding to drusen with minimal alterations of the outer layers. Several cystoid spaces in the inferior part of the scan.

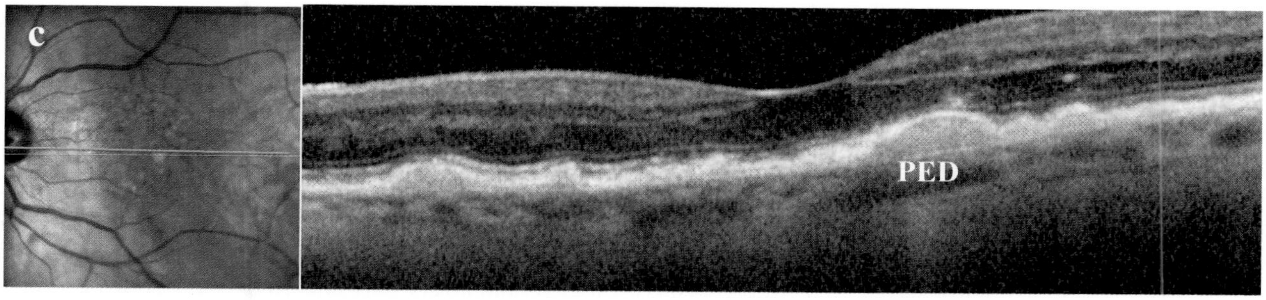

Figure 13: Chorioretinal anastomosis. VA: 20/125. After the 2nd IVT injection.
c): *Spectralis horizontal cross-section**: normal foveal depression and well organized retinal layers.
Persistence of a small temporal juxtafoveal PED with several bright hyper-reflective spots and alteration of the external limiting membrane and especially the outer nuclear layer.

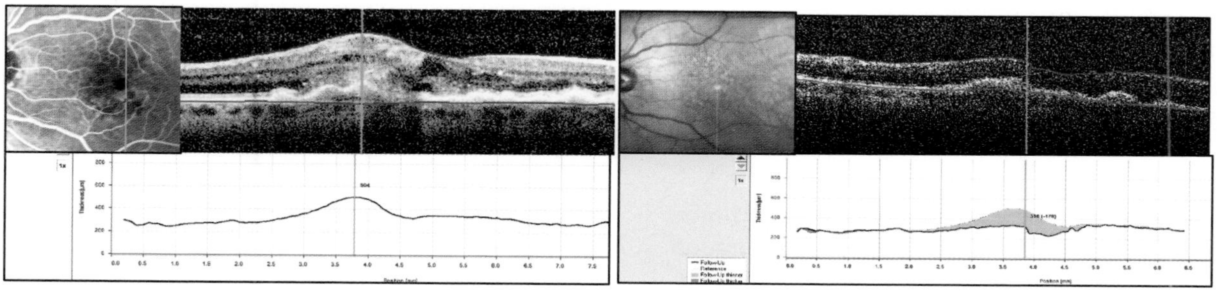

Figure 14: Automatic retinal thickness comparison graph:
Comparison with the same location as on the initial examination demonstrates improvement in terms of retinal thickness.

CLINICAL CASE No. 04: Chorioretinal Anastomosis

Juxtafoveal macular hemorrhage and small central PED in a patient with drusen. Follow-up by SD-OCT OCT after anti-VEGF therapy.

An 87-year-old woman with *bilateral lesions* progressing over many years and *monocular blindness* presented with recent, moderate loss of visual acuity in the left eye.
VA RE: LP - VA LE: 20/32.

Biomicroscopic Examination

Fairly numerous, non-confluent perifoveal soft drusen and a highly suggestive juxtafoveal hemorrhage, 1/3 DD in diameter, at 5 o'clock (**Figure 15a**).

Autofluorescence

No changes of the central zone, but presence of granular, perimacular hyper-fluorescence mainly in the inferior 2/3 of the macular region (**Figure 15b**).

9

Fluorescein Angiography

A localized zone (measuring about 300 μm) of early, progressive hyper-fluorescence adjacent to the termination of an inferior retinal vein with fluorescein leakages partially masked by hemorrhage (**Figure 15c, d, and e – enlarged images**).

SLO-ICG Angiography

Barely visible, small, juxtafoveal hyper-fluorescent lesion (**Figure 15f and g**).

Enlarged image: end-to-end retino-retinal anastomosis between a retinal arteriole and a retinal venule with communication between retinal vessels and the deeper choroidal neovascularization (**Figure 15h**).

Suggested Diagnosis:
Juxtafoveal retinal hemorrhage, suggesting on early chorioretinal anastomosis with active fluorescein leakage.

Contribution of OCT (*Spectralis**)

Horizontal cross-section

The OCT features were characteristic and diagnostic: discontinuity of the RPE, disruption of the external limiting membrane, alteration of the IS/OS interface, presence of a pre-RPE dense zone, numerous bright hyper-reflective spots, abundant intraretinal fluid, and numerous small cysts.
The juxtafoveal hyper-reflective zone in the inner retinal layers, corresponding to the **retinal hemorrhage**, showed characteristic posterior shadowing as far as the choroid (**Figure 16a**).

Vertical cross-section

The cross-section centered on the hyper-fluorescent zone showed the same characteristic signs: discontinuity of the RPE; clearly visible protrusion of the CNV into the retina that appeared to be derived from the choroids, and bulging anterior to the RPE, indicating a chorioretinal anastomosis (**Figure 16b**).
Anterior to the RPE, increased retinal thickness with subretinal and intraretinal fluid and numerous cysts. The outer retinal layers were altered over the zone of protruding CNV. These signs were associated with numerous bright hyper-reflective spots.

At this Stage

This clinical case illustrates the typical appearance of retinal hemorrhage, often the first sign of chorioretinal anastomosis. Angiography and enlarged views also clearly visualized the features of chorioretinal anastomosis.
The OCT appearance was highly suggestive of choroidal neovascularization and protrusion of CNV through the RPE, as well as the presence of an anastomosis with an intense adjacent exudative reaction. This appearance was accompanied by numerous bright hyper-reflective spots, a small subfoveal and juxtafoveal PED, and numerous cysts. The retinal hemorrhage caused a hyper-reflective zone in the inner layers with marked shadowing.
All of these features led to a clinical diagnosis, which was confirmed with angiography and OCT.
The lesions were too close to the center of the retina to consider laser photocoagulation. The clinical picture indicated immediate treatment with IVT injections of anti-VEGF therapy in an attempt to halt progression of the disease before loss of visual acuity.

CLINICAL CASE No. 04: CHORIORETINAL ANASTOMOSIS

Juxtafoveal macular hemorrhage and small central PED in a patient with drusen. Follow-up by SD-OCT OCT after anti-VEGF therapy.

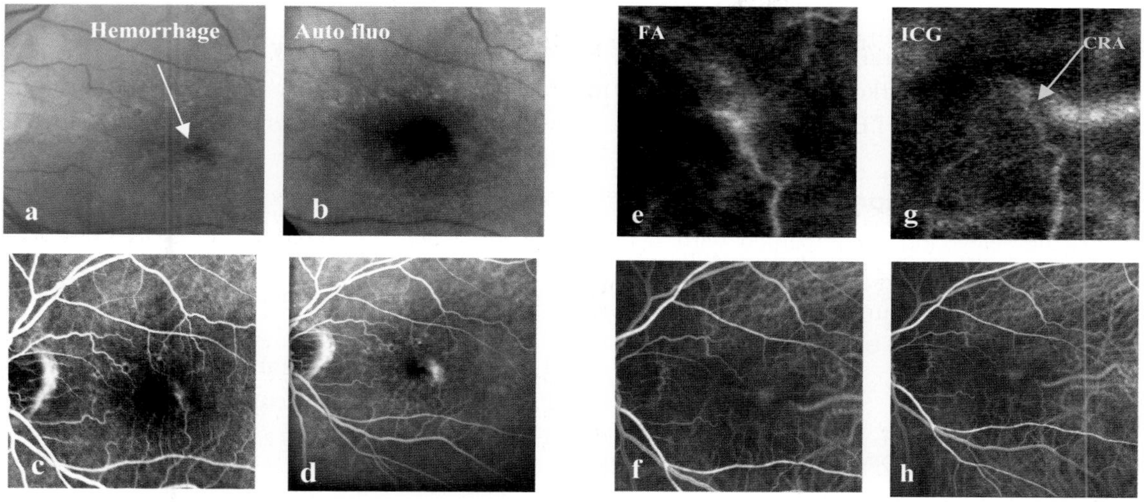

Figure 15: Chorioretinal anastomosis. VA: 20/32. First examination.
a): Color fundus photograph: juxtafoveal retinal hemorrhage and drusen.
b): Autofluorescence: perifoveal and inferior abnormalities.
c, d, and e): Fluorescein angiography: localized hyper-fluorescence at the termination of a retinal vein.
f, g, and h): SLO-ICG angiography: choroidal neovascularization at the extremity of a retino-retinal anastomosis, more clearly visible on the enlarged image (g).

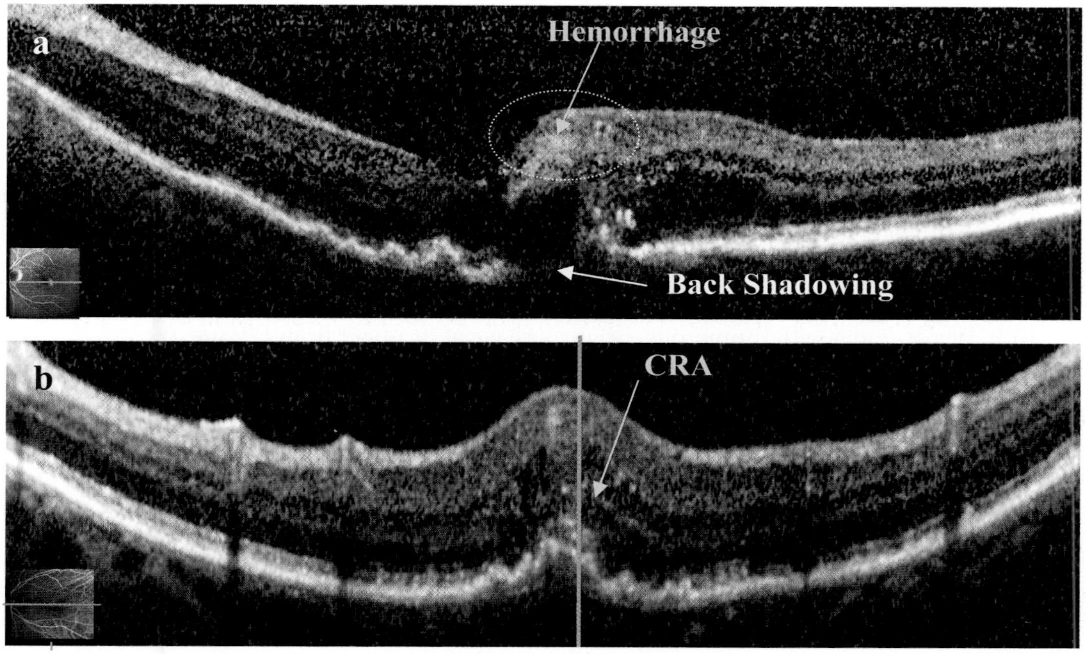

Figure 16: Chorioretinal anastomosis. VA: 20/32. First examination.
a): *Spectralis horizontal cross-section through the zone of hyper-fluorescence**: discontinuity of the RPE and clearly visible protrusion of the CNV into the retina. Increased retinal thickness, subretinal and intraretinal fluid, and numerous cysts. Note the hemorrhage and posterior shadowing (back-shadowing).
Anterior to the RPE, disruption of the external limiting membrane, alteration of the IS/OS interface, presence of a pre-RPE dense zone and several bright hyper-reflective spots.
b): *Spectralis vertical cross-section centered on the lesion and the hemorrhage**, showing the same characteristic signs and the vascularized PED with elevation of the RPE.

CLINICAL CASE No. 05: Advanced Form of Chorioretinal Anastomosis

Juxtafoveal retinal hemorrhage and vascularized PED, progressing over several years. Chronic lesion not amenable to treatment.

A 91-year-old man with bilateral lesions progressing over many years presented with marked loss of visual acuity in both eyes. VA RE: 20/400.-VA LE: 20/160.

Biomicroscopic Examination

Moderate macular elevation accompanied with several juxtafoveal hemorrhages and a fine crown of lipid exudates. A juxtapapillary lesion surrounded by exudates was also observed (**Figure 17a and b**).

Autofluorescence

Several perifoveal changes, especially in the peripapillary region (**Figure 17c**).

Fluorescein Angiography

Juxtafoveal and subfoveal zone of hyper-fluorescence predominantly inferior nasal with intense fluorescein leakage, partially masked by hemorrhage (**Figure 17d**).

SLO-ICG Angiography

Vast oval-shaped, inferior nasal neovascular membrane with a clearly visible peripheral arcade surrounded by hemorrhage.

An inferior nasal retinal vein changed direction at its termination and descended towards the center of the deep choroidal neovascular membrane.

The neovascular membrane was visible against the dark PED which was almost entirely invaded by CNV (**Figure 17e**).

Suggested Diagnosis:

Vascularized PED with advanced chorioretinal anastomosis communicating with a vast deep neovascular membrane.

Contribution of OCT (*Spectralis**)

Horizontal cross-section

OCT demonstrated a large subfoveal and juxtafoveal fibrovascular lesion with large cysts and features suggestive of CRA: localized discontinuity of the RPE, disruption of the external limiting membrane and IS/OS interface, pre-RPE dense zone with numerous bright hyper-reflective spots, marked intraretinal fluid, and numerous cysts.

A juxtafoveal hyper-reflective zone in the inner layers corresponded to the **retinal hemorrhage** with characteristic shadowing (**Figure 18a**).

Vertical cross-section

The cross-section *centered on the hyper-fluorescent zone* demonstrated the same characteristic signs: disruption of the RPE and a hyper-reflective lesion anterior to the RPE with a zone of hyper-reflectivity related to deep hemorrhage at its upper limit (**Figure 18b**).

Anterior to the RPE, increased retinal thickness with intraretinal fluid. The outer layers were altered with a dense area over the zone of protruding CNV with several bright hyper-reflective spots.

At this Stage

The angiographic signs and the discontinuity of the RPE visualized on OCT allowed a retrospective diagnosis of very advanced chorioretinal anastomosis.
This chronic lesion in the right eye was known to be present for several years, leaving little hope for any functional improvement after treatment.

However, the lesion was still active, which lead the ophthalmologist to offer IVT injections. The 91-year-old patient refused any treatment for his right eye and preferred to focus treatment on his left eye. He wanted to take care of the eye with more recent changes, which had the potential of functional improvement.

CLINICAL CASE No. 05: ADVANCED CHORIORETINAL ANASTOMOSIS

Juxtafoveal retinal hemorrhage and vascularized PED, progressing over several years. Chronic lesion not amenable to treatment

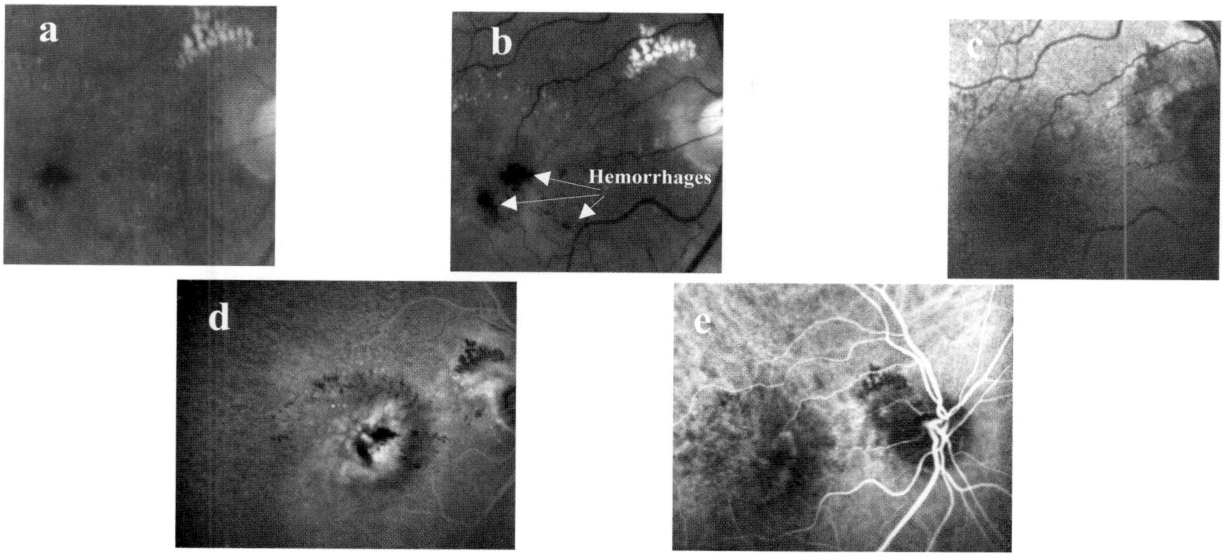

Figure 17. Advanced form of chorioretinal anastomosis. VA: 20/320. First examination.

a and b): Color and red-free fundus photographs: juxtafoveal retinal hemorrhages.
c): Autofluorescence: perifoveal and peripapillary abnormalities.
d): Fluorescein angiography: 2 DD hyper-fluorescent zone with fluorescein leakage, partially masked by hemorrhage.
e): SLO-ICG angiography: vast deep neovascular membrane communicating with retinal vessels.

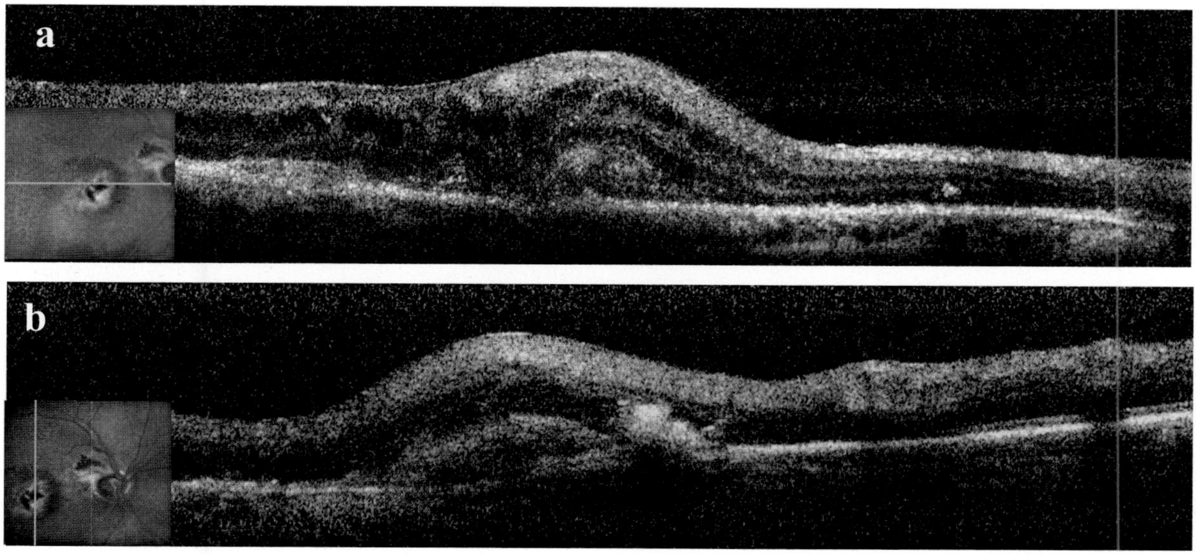

Figure 18. Advanced form of chorioretinal anastomosis. VA: 20/320. First examination.

a): *Spectralis horizontal cross-section**: large subfoveal and juxtafoveal fibrovascular lesion with large cysts.
b): *Spectralis vertical cross-section**: discontinuity of the RPE. Hyper-reflective lesion anterior to the RPE with a zone of hyper-reflectivity related to deep hemorrhage at its upper limit.

Conclusion

The **early stages** of typical chorioretinal anastomosis have a characteristic appearance: juxtafoveal retinal hemorrhage, angiographic hyper-fluorescence at the macular termination of retinal vessels, and retino-retinal anastomosis communicating with a small choroidal neovascularization.

The **SD-OCT image** (*Spectralis**) is characteristic with disruption of the RPE, protrusion of the neovascularization, an intense exudative reaction, and bright hyper-reflective spots.

At this early stage, **treatment** provides rapid and dramatic improvement (despite persistence of localized alterations of the outer layers and discontinuity of the RPE). However, the effect of treatment appears to be limited, as it usually lasts barely more than 2 months after each injection.

Combination therapy does not appear to be initially indicated at the present time, but long-term follow-up is essential.

Polypoidal Choroidal Vasculopathy

Clinical Features and OCT Follow-Up after Treatment

Gabriel COSCAS

Florence COSCAS, Sabrina VISMARA,
Alain ZOURDANI, C.I. Li CALZI

(Créteil and Paris)

Polypoidal Choroidal Vasculopathy

Polypoidal choroidal vasculopathy does not constitute part of the classical definition of AMD, but these two entities have a number of features in common.

This entity was initially described as "*multiple, recurrent serosanguinous pigment epithelium detachments,*" but the most widely accepted term is now idiopathic **polypoidal choroidal vasculopathy** (PCV) (*Yannuzzi 1997*).

SLO-ICG angiography identify and localize these abnormalities in the peripapillary region and also more peripherally. When located in the **macular region**, they can cause more serious functional impairment.

Clinical Features

Polypoidal Formations

The name of this disease refers to the presence of choroidal vascular branches with dilated, aneurismal, or polypoidal terminations often grouped like bunches of grapes.

These **polypoidal formations** can cause leakage and/or hemorrhage, accounting for the associated multiple, serous, and/or hemorrhagic pigment epithelium detachments.

Polypoidal lesions show delayed filling on angiography with pooling of dye and they remain very hyper-fluorescent in the late phases.

These **polyps** are polymorphous, ranging from small and/or solitary to multiple and grouped in various formations.

During the course of the disease, with successive acute exudative or hemorrhagic episodes, the polyps may be relatively difficult to detect in the context of multiple elevations of the retina and retinal pigment epithelium.

Abnormal Choroidal Vessels

The polyps are associated with abnormal choroidal vessels, usually grouped in localized areas, presenting with dilatations and circulatory abnormalities.

These choroidal vascular abnormalities are most clearly visualized on early and intermediate phases of SLO-ICG angiography, which remains the best diagnostic imaging modality.

Two types of abnormal choroidal vessels can be distinguished:

- A branching network with terminal polyps, or
- Disseminated polypoidal dilatations on capillaries or relatively fine vessel branches.

The abnormal choroidal vascular network is visible on early and intermediate phases of SLO-ICG. It is usually *peripapillary* (**Figure 1**), but can also be observed in the posterior pole and in the *macula*.

Some polypoidal dilatations appear to be attenuated at the end of the angiographic sequence, while others become increasingly hyper-fluorescent with fluorescein leakage. These latter forms appear to be more frequently complicated by hemorrhage.

Hyper-Fluorescent Plaque

A polypoidal hyper-fluorescent plaque is frequently observed in the late phases of the SLO-ICG angiography sequence. This plaque, often extensive, is not always correlated with the normal choroidal vasculature. Intensely hyper-fluorescent zones corresponding to ectasias can be observed in this plaque.

Choroidal Neovascularization

During the long course of this disease, polypoidal choroidal vasculopathy can be accompanied by true choroidal neovascularization, making its diagnosis even more challenging.

Polypoidal choroidal vasculopathy is observed at a relatively young age, usually without drusen. Lesions are not confined to the macula and choroidal neovascularization remains a relatively rare complication.

These features clearly distinguish PCV from the usual form of AMD.

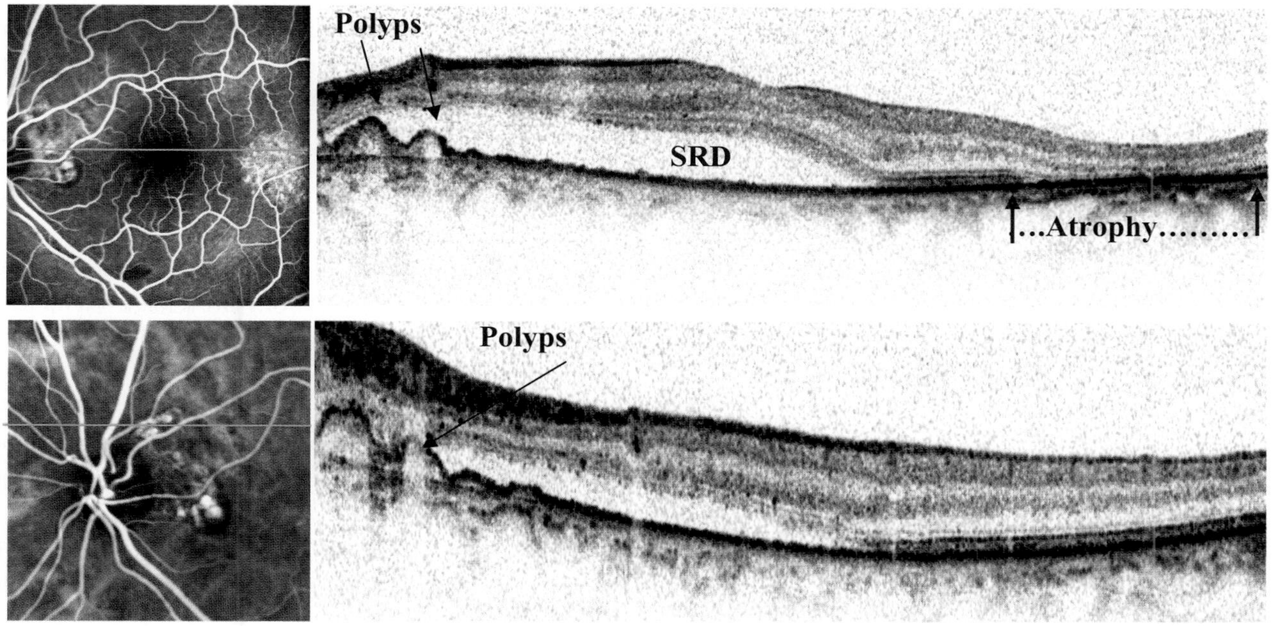

Figure 1: Polypoidal choroidal vasculopathy, predominantly peripapillary. VA: 20/63.
a): Fluorescein angiography correlated with a *Spectralis horizontal section** showing an intense exudative reaction.
b): SLO-ICG angiography correlated with a *Spectralis horizontal section** showing a cluster of small polyps.

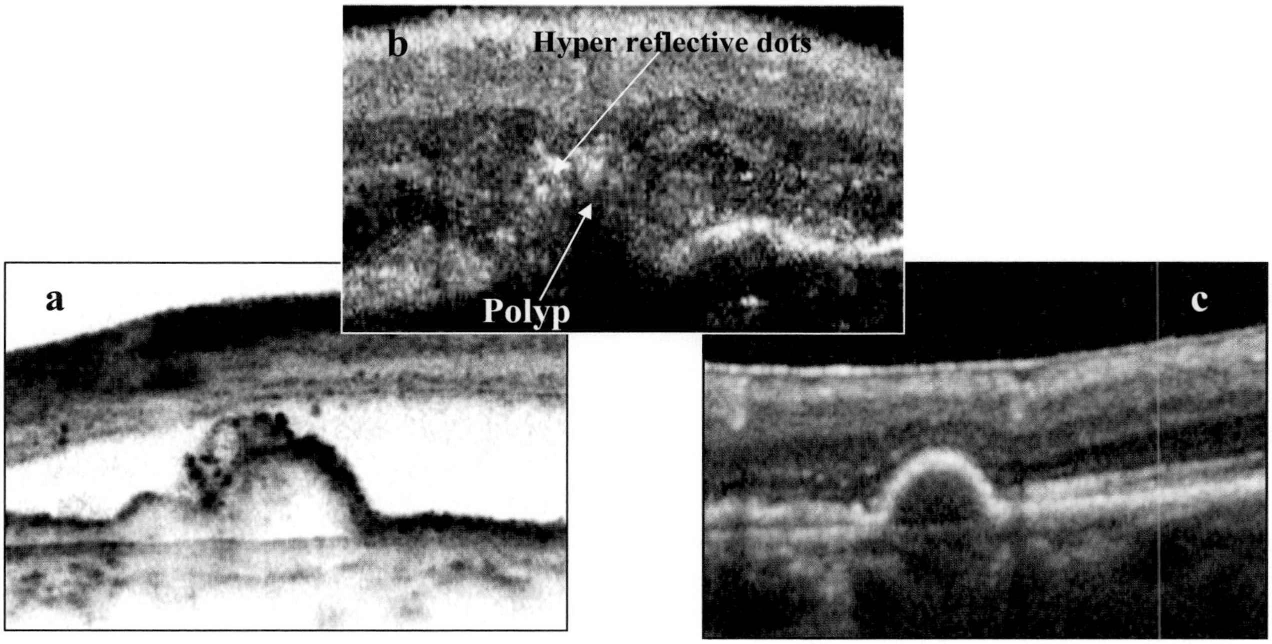

Figure 2: Several appearances of polyps:
a): Juxtapapillary polyp with RPE proliferation and marked SRF.
b): Prominent polyp with protrusion into the inner retinal layers, bright hyper-reflective spots, and dense zones.
c): Residual polyp after treatment with no adjacent reaction.

The **incidence of PCV** appears to be higher in some countries, For example in Japan it appears to account for more than 40% cases of macular hemorrhage in the elderly.
Genetic correlation studies demonstrate a relationship with true AMD (*Goth 2008, Lee 2008*).
In our series of 200 consecutive patients, the incidence of polypoidal choroidal vasculopathy (PCV) was relatively high at 8%.

Contribution of OCT

Time-Domain OCT (*Stratus**) clearly demonstrates alterations of the RPE band related to protrusion of *polypoidal ectasias*.

These ectasias induce localized, steeply sloped elevation of the retinal pigment epithelium, in contrast with a serous PED, which is usually gently sloped and relatively flat.

The *PED cavity* is generally optically empty, revealing Bruch's membrane away from the RPE, but the cavity may also have a heterogeneous appearance.

More marked *shadowing* in the choroid may be observed in the case of concomitant active neovascularization.

The *size of the polyps* may be limited to that of drusen or, on the contrary, can be large and severely deform the RPE band. Polyps may be observed either within a zone of serous or serosanguinous PED or, more often, at the edge of the PED.

SD-OCT sections (*Spectralis**) provide more detailed visualization of polyps that can be seen as relatively prominent, isolated, or multiple and clustered in groups (**Figure 1**).

Actively evolving polyps are associated with an *exudative reaction* that can become intense and sometimes create large cysts.

A large number of bright hyper-reflective spots adjacent to polyps are often observed in the **outer retinal layers** and even deeper (**Figure 2a and b**).

The outer retinal layers can be severely altered over the protruding polyps, with displacement of the outer nuclear layer, which is thinned and fragmented. The external limiting membrane and IS/OS interface can be lost and often replaced by a more or less extensive hyper-reflective dense zone (**Figure 2b**).

Spectral-Domain OCT provides an important advantage over TD-OCT by allowing the acquisition of 3D volume images and **dense serial sections**. This allows systematic examination of the entire macular region and the detection of even small polyps.

Natural History

The typical natural history of PCV has not been clearly elucidated. PCV has been known to remain asymptomatic or to extend with multiplication of the lesions and progression of the late plaque.

Particularly interesting **transitional forms**, which are between small polyps and occult CNV, have been observed.

The development of exudative and hemorrhagic complications and choroidal neovascularization is particularly important when they involve the macular region.

Treatment

The treatment of PCV has not been clearly defined, and the course of PCV in response to treatment is variable.

Laser photocoagulation can be used to destroy extrafoveal polypoidal formations and/or photocoagulate feeder vessels in the abnormal vascular network.

However, this treatment modality is not satisfactory due to the subsequent development of new channels, alterations of the choroidal vascular network, and recurrences of polypoidal formations.

Clinical trials of **photodynamic therapy** have demonstrated fairly good efficacy, particularly in patients who have already developed exudative and hemorrhagic complications.

Intravitreous injections of **anti-angiogenic therapy** have been used in many cases when these vasculopathies are associated with occult CNV (**Figure 2c**).

Despite a definite improvement, recurrences and active progression with **fibrosis** appear to be relatively frequent and may justify combination therapy.

Combined treatments must only be considered when the patient's vision is at stake, such as in the case of progressive leakage or hemorrhage. Long-term observation is necessary in every case.

TABLE OF CLINICAL CASES

CLINICAL CASE No. 01: POLYPOIDAL CHOROIDAL VASCULOPATHY
Macular lesion with an extensive serosanguinous PED and polypoidal choroidal vasculopathy, progressing over several years.
Follow-up by TD-OCT and SD-OCT after anti-VEGF therapy................................. Page 306

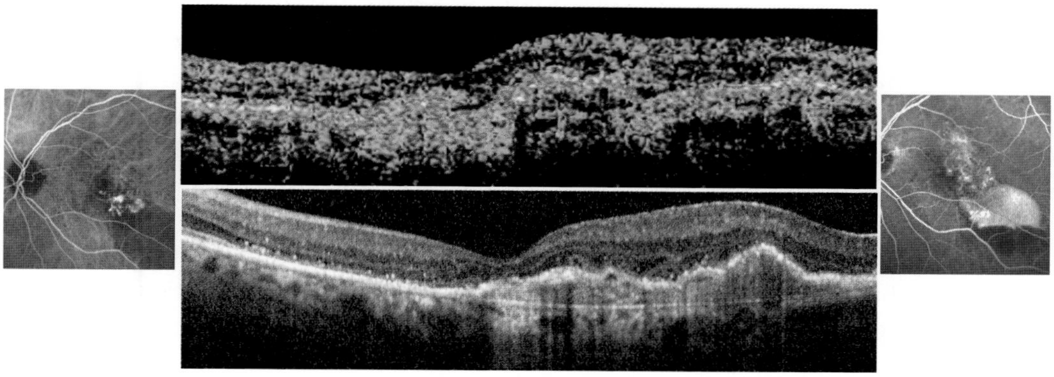

CLINICAL CASE No. 02: POLYPOIDAL CHOROIDAL VASCULOPATHY
Macular lesion with drusen and a vascularized PED, progressing over several years.
Follow-up by SD-OCT after anti-VEGF therapy .... Page 314

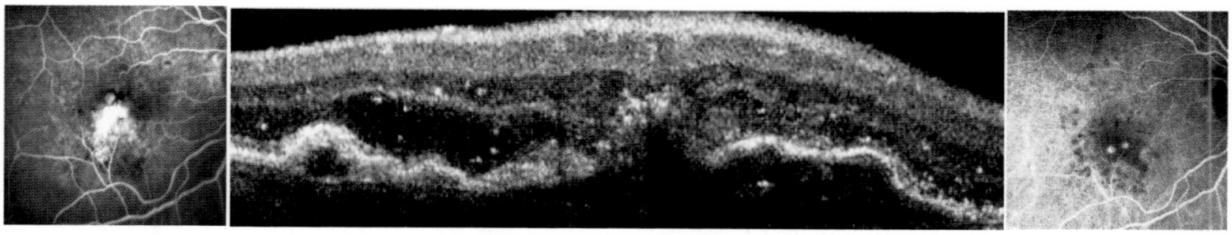

CLINICAL CASE No. 03: POLYPOIDAL CHOROIDAL VASCULOPATHY
Extensive, exudative macular lesion with several drusen, progressing over several years.
Follow-up by SD-OCT after anti-VEGF therapy .... Page 318

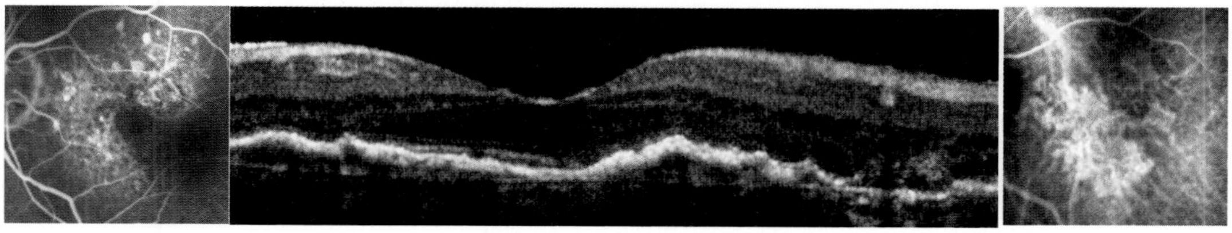

CLINICAL CASE No. 01: Polypoidal Choroidal Vasculopathy

Macular lesion with extensive serosanguinous PED and polypoidal choroidal vasculopathy, progressing over several years. Follow-up by TD-OCT and SD-OCT after anti-VEGF therapy.

A 73-year-old man presented with slowly progressive decline of visual acuity in his left eye, which interfered with his daily activities. He had a central scotoma in his other eye, existing for several years.
VA RE: 20/400 - VA LE: 20/50.

Biomicroscopic Examination

Central macular discoloration and inferior temporal bullous detachment extending well into the periphery; no lipid exudates (**Figure 3a and b**).

Autofluorescence

A vast hyper-fluorescent halo is visible in the macular region and spreading inferiorly and beyond the temporal vessels. The central zone and xanthophyll pigment were spared (**Figure 3c**).

Fluorescein Angiography

- **In the superior half**, a zone of irregular hyper-fluorescence suggestive of alteration of the RPE, with no fluorescein leakage. A series of small, rounded, foveal and temporal lesions that became hyper-fluorescent at the late phases.
- **In the inferior half**, progressive filling of the well-demarcated bullous PED with pooling of dye, except in the inferior sector, which remained hypo-fluorescent with a horizontal limit. This suggested a blood-filled fluid level (**Figure 3e and f**).

SLO-ICG Angiography

a): *Early phase*: fine, abnormal, juxtafoveal and inferior temporal network at the superior edge of the dark, hypo-fluorescent zone corresponding to the inferior PED.

b): *Late phase*: progressive and increasingly dense filling of a series of polypoidal formations, forming a group, like a bunch of grapes.

These high-contrast polyps were clearly visible adjacent to the well-demarcated, dark PED (**Figure 3g and h**).

Suggested Diagnosis:
Macular polypoidal choroidal vasculopathy with extensive serosanguinous PED, progressing over several years.

Contribution of OCT (*Stratus**)

Horizontal section

In the **center of the fovea**, *anterior to the RPE*, a localized zone of hyper-reflectivity suggested moderate fibrosis.

Immediately adjacent to this lesion, the RPE was elevated with a moderately reflective cavity and a wavy contour, corresponding to the polypoidal formations.

Slight shadowing was observed with no increase in retinal thickness (**Figure 4**).

Vertical section

Multiple irregularities of thickness and reflectivity were observed in the RPE with slight elevation in the central zone.

Anterior to the RPE, increased retinal thickness and diffuse intraretinal fluid with a few cysts (**Figure 4**).

Diagnosis

OCT examination alone could not provide a diagnosis at this stage, but it did confirm the presence of a ***moderately reflective PED*** with a minor intraretinal exudative reaction.
Correlation with angiographies confirmed the diagnosis of a lesion comprising:

- An atrophic zone in the superior and foveal part, and
- A vast, inferiorly eccentric serosanguinous PED.

The diagnosis was affirmed by the presence of ***polypoidal formations*** in the superior part of this PED.
The existence of an exudative and serosanguinous reaction with recent decline of VA justified immediate treatment.

Although treatment of this disease has not been clearly established, therapy by ***intravitreous injections of anti-VEGF*** was offered.

CLINICAL CASE No. 01: POLYPOIDAL CHOROIDAL VASCULOPATHY
Follow-up by TD-OCT and SD-OCT after anti-VEGF therapy.

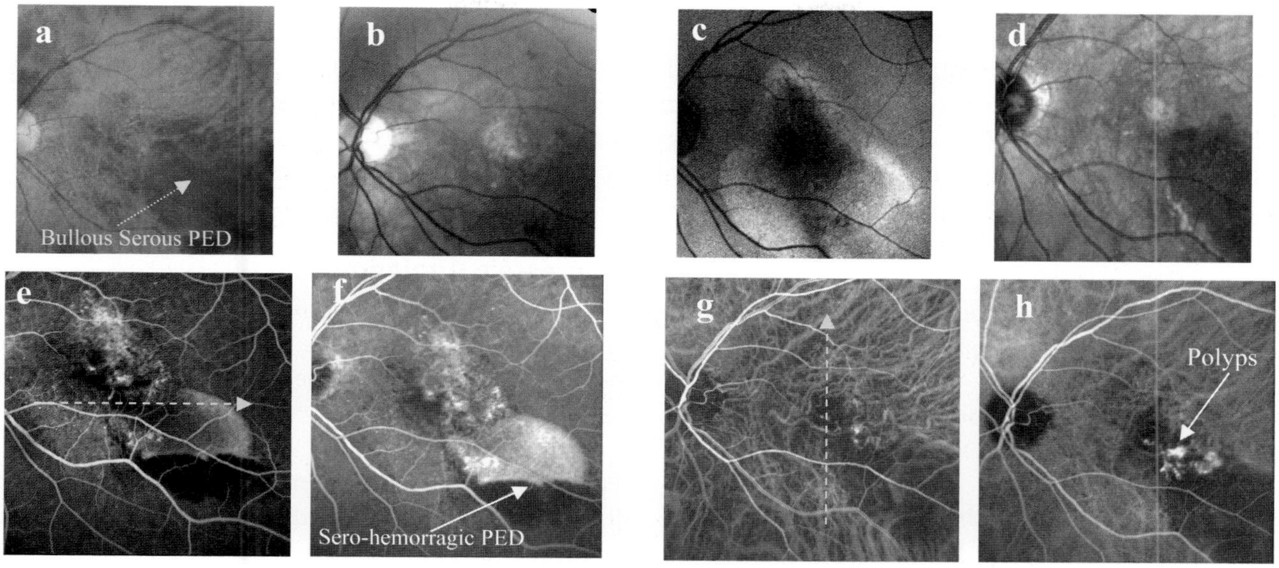

Figure 3: Polypoidal choroidal vasculopathy with serosanguinous PED. VA: 20/50.
a): Color fundus photograph. b): Monochromatic red-free fundus photograph. c): Autofluorescence. d): Infrared.
e and f): Fluorescein angiography. g and h): SLO-ICG angiography.

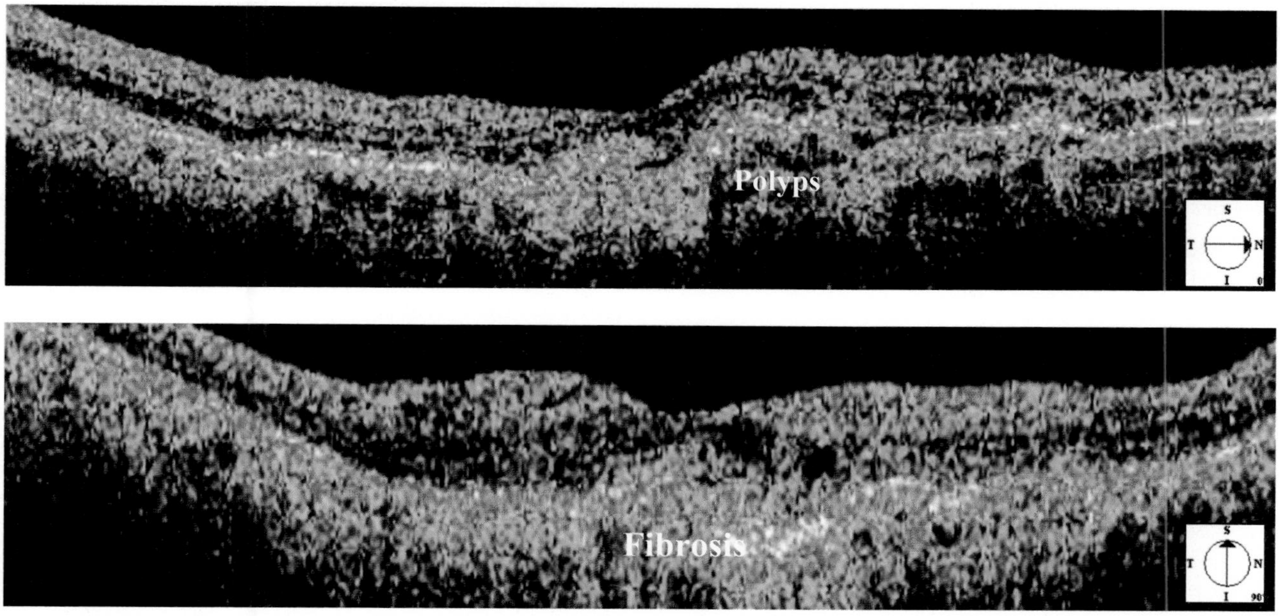

Figure 4: Polypoidal choroidal vasculopathy with serosanguinous PED. VA: 20/50.
***Stratus** horizontal and vertical sections.**
The ***horizontal section*** in the center of the fovea, anterior to the RPE, reveals a localized zone of hyper-reflectivity suggestive of moderate fibrosis. Adjacent to this lesion, elevation of the RPE with a moderately reflective cavity and a wavy contour corresponded to the polypoidal formations.
The ***vertical section*** shows multiple irregularities of thickness and reflectivity of the RPE. Anterior to the RPE, increased retinal thickness with several small cysts.

CLINICAL CASE No. 01: Polypoidal Choroidal Vasculopathy

Follow-up by TD-OCT and SD-OCT after anti-VEGF therapy.

Treatment by monthly intravitreous injections of anti-VEGF (*Lucentis**) was continued for more than 2 years with follow-up by visual acuity, OCT, fluorescein angiography, and ICG angiography. The response to treatment was favorable but often incomplete and marked by several recurrences.

During the first year, the patient was followed by conventional *Stratus** TD-OCT (**Figure 5**).

During the second year, follow-up was based on simultaneous angiography and SD-OCT (*Spectralis**) (**Figure 5**).

Analysis of the course over the first year

Visual acuity slowly improved, providing the patient with more comfortable vision, although it remained at a relatively low level after each injection. Visual acuity stabilized at 20/100 or 20/63 throughout this period.

OCT

On the first follow-up examination, retinal thickness gradually decreased. Intraretinal fluid resolved, and the foveal depression became more clearly visible (**Figure 5a**).

IVT injections were regularly repeated due to persistence of the angiographic signs and development of progressive macular fibrosis. This justified combined IVT and *photodynamic therapy* (**Figure 5b**).

After the 6th injection, a recurrence was observed with return and extension of a serosanguinous detachment, structural changes of the polyps, and formation of cystoid macular edema (**Figure 5c**).

After the 8th injection, the OCT horizontal section showed a satisfactory appearance of the fovea with restoration of a normal profile and resolution of edema. This was accompanied with a gain in visual acuity.

Fluorescein Angiography

All of the abnormal choroidal vascular network persisted with changes in the structure and number of polyps but with no increase in the surface area of the lesion.

Fluorescein angiography demonstrated alteration of the RPE in the foveal region and persistence of the pigment epithelium detachment (**Figure 5a-d**).

ICG Angiography

The choroidal vascular network and the polyps were clearly visualized, allowing analysis of morphological changes as well as extension and recurrence of the serosanguinous PED (**Figures 5, 6, and 7**).

During the second year

The lesions gradually healed: the PED became flattened and organized, bright hyper-reflective spots decreased, and the outer nuclear layer became more clearly visible.

However, the foveal zone presented features of RPE atrophy and a small band of **fibrosis** (**Figure 7**).

At the end of the second year, this patient developed exudative phenomena with degenerative cystoid edema and an epiretinal membrane (**Figure 8**).

At this Stage

Lasting stabilization of the lesion with limited improvement but acceptable visual acuity justified suspension of IVT injections (**Figure 5**). This improvement was slow and only partial, marked by an episode of recurrence that responded to treatment.

Persistence of the choroidal vascular abnormalities, polyps, fibrosis, cystoid edema, and extrafoveal PED justified continued follow-up throughout the second year with a poor long-term prognosis (**Figures 7, 8, and 9**).

CLINICAL CASE No. 01: POLYPOIDAL CHOROIDAL VASCULOPATHY
Follow-up by TD-OCT and SD-OCT after anti-VEGF therapy.

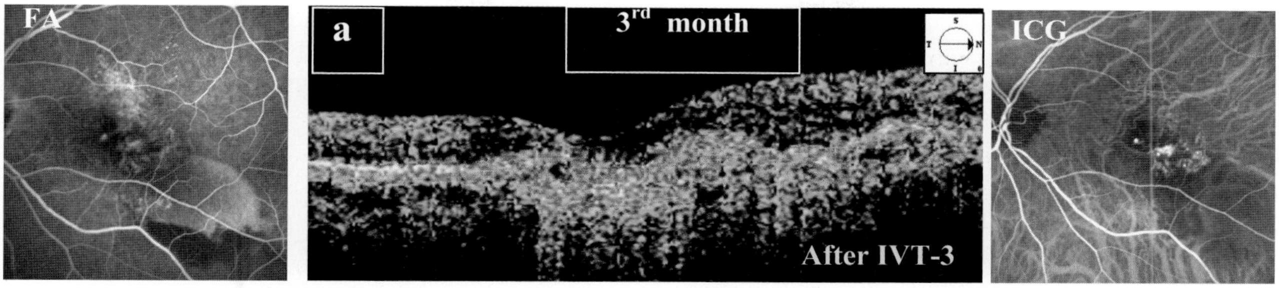

Figure 5: Polypoidal choroidal vasculopathy with serosanguinous PED. VA: 1.5/10.
a): After the 3rd IVT injection: stabilization of the lesions, decreased exudation, persistence of the polyps, and serosanguinous PED.

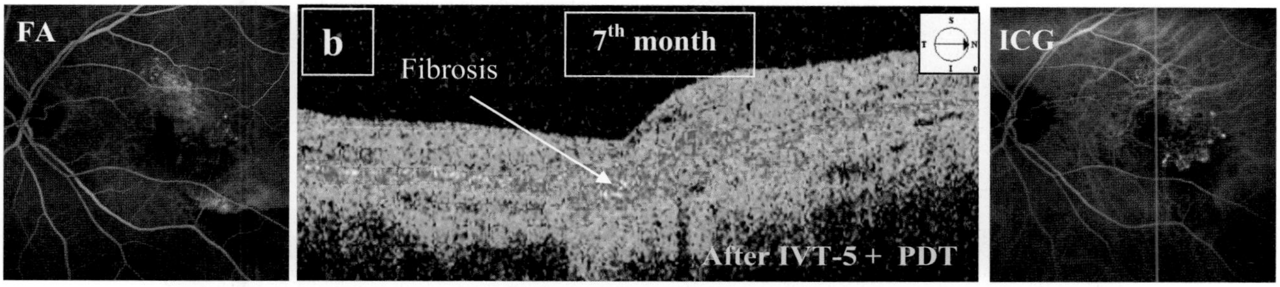

Figure 5: Polypoidal choroidal vasculopathy with serosanguinous PED. VA: 1.5/10.
b): After the 5th IVT injection: retinal reattachment but subfoveal fibrosis and persistence of the polyps.

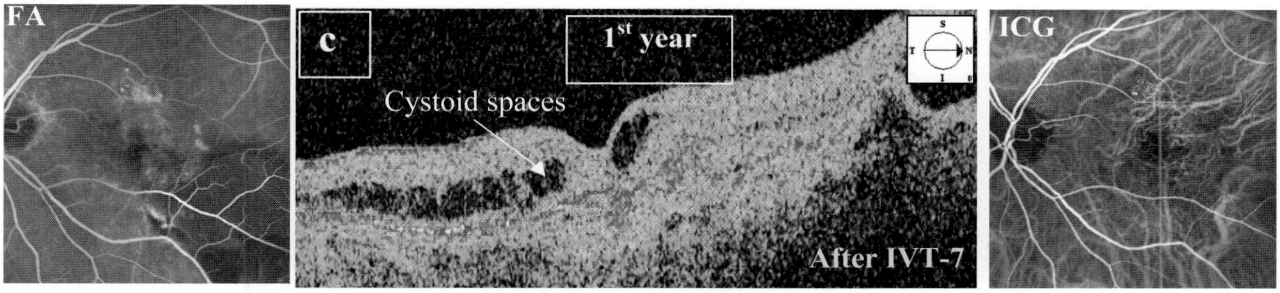

Figure 5: Polypoidal choroidal vasculopathy with serosanguinous PED. VA: 2/10.
c): After the 7th IVT injection: slight functional improvement despite the development of cystoid macular edema.

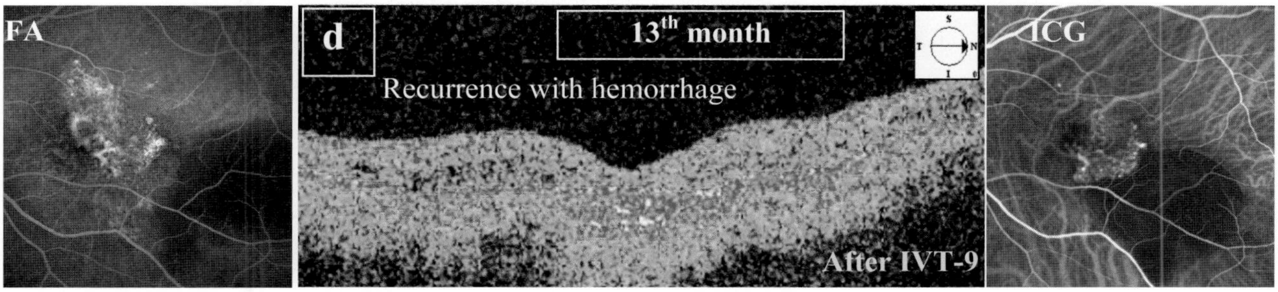

Figure 5: Polypoidal choroidal vasculopathy with serosanguinous PED. VA: 3/10.
d): After the 9th IVT injection: improvement of VA with retinal reattachment despite a recurrent hemorrhagic PED.

CLINICAL CASE No. 01: POLYPOIDAL CHOROIDAL VASCULOPATHY
Follow-up by TD-OCT and SD-OCT after anti-VEGF therapy.

ENLARGED IMAGES

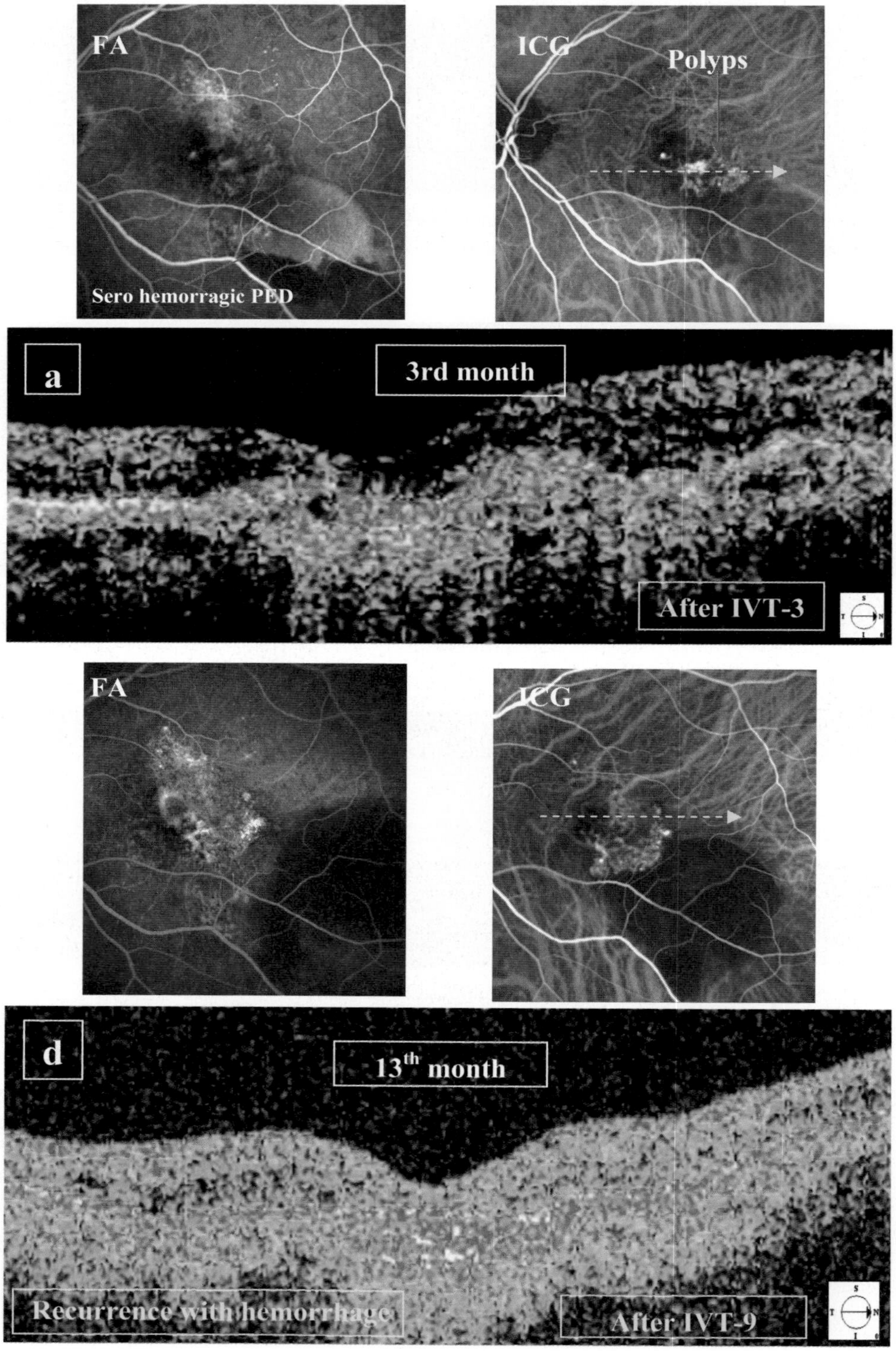

Figure 6: Polypoidal choroidal vasculopathy with serosanguinous PED.
Enlarged views of Figures 5a and d.

CLINICAL CASE No. 01: POLYPOIDAL CHOROIDAL VASCULOPATHY FOLLOW-UP AFTER TREATMENT

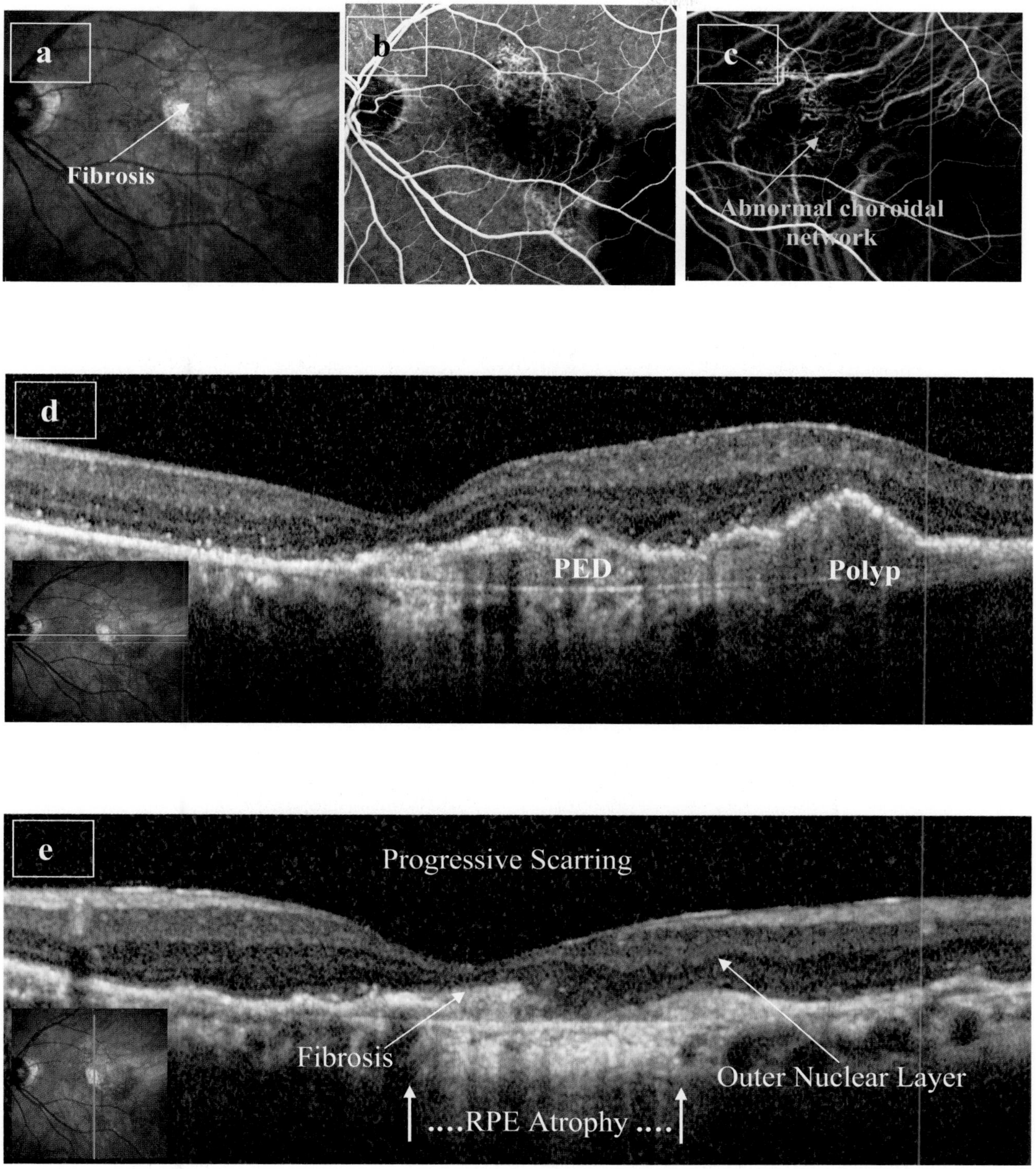

Figure 7: Polypoidal choroidal vasculopathy with serosanguinous PED. VA: 3/10.

a-e): During the first year: progressive healing: atrophy of the RPE, fibrosis and organization of the PED. Marked alterations of the outer nuclear layer, external limiting membrane, and IS/OS interface.

CLINICAL CASE No. 01: POLYPOIDAL CHOROIDAL VASCULOPATHY FOLLOW-UP AFTER TREATMENT

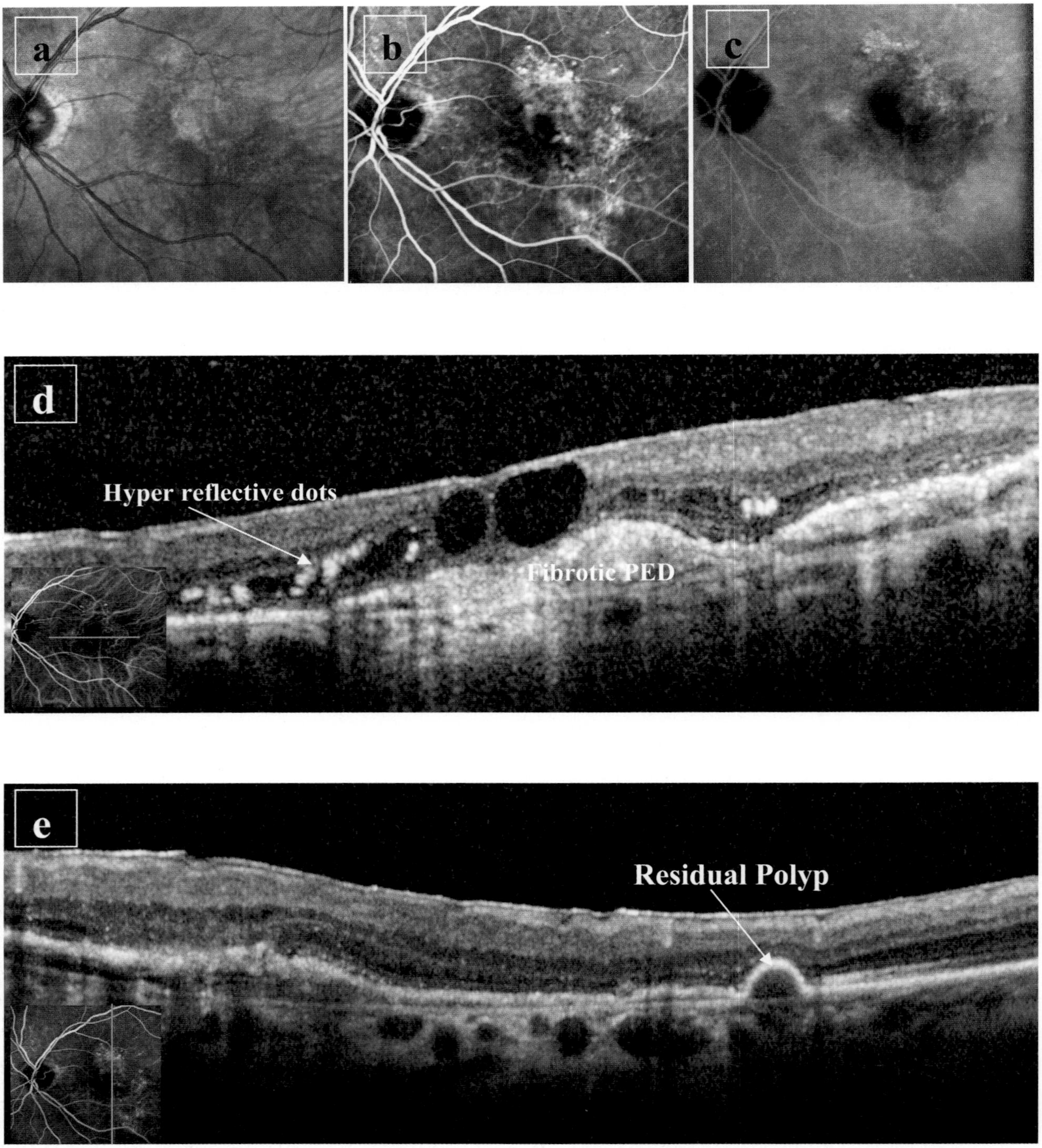

Figure 8: Polypoidal choroidal vasculopathy with serosanguinous PED. VA: 3/10.
a-e): At the end of the second year: recurrence and deterioration of the SD-OCT signs:
- Flat but hyper-reflective PED suggesting fibrosis;
- Intraretinal fluid with cysts and bright hyper-reflective spots;
- Central atrophy and loss of the outer nuclear layer in the foveal zone;
- A residual polyp in the superior macula.

CLINICAL CASE No. 01: POLYPOIDAL CHOROIDAL VASCULOPATHY FOLLOW-UP AFTER TREATMENT

a

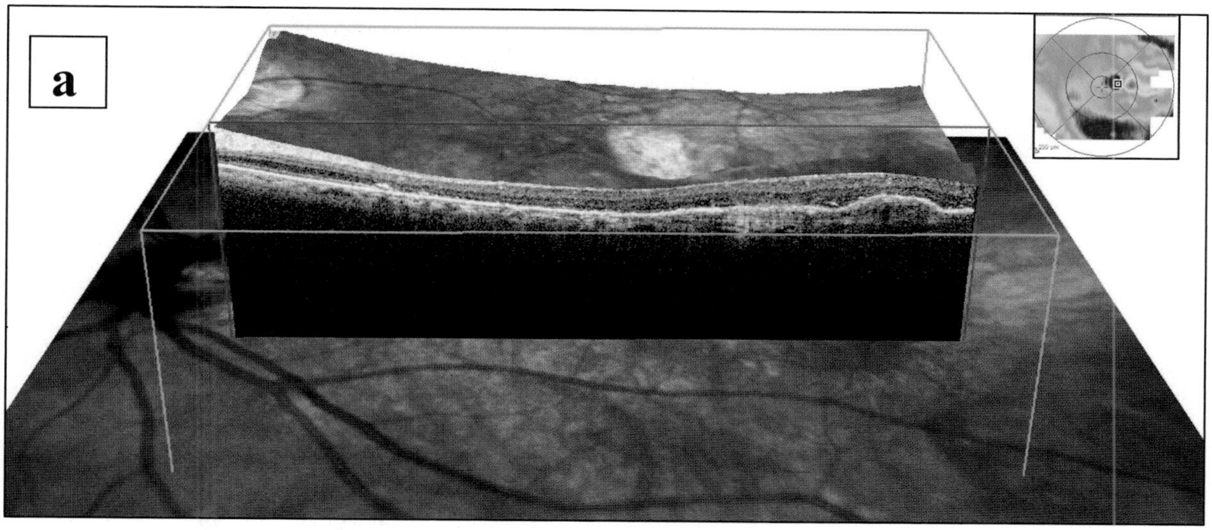

b

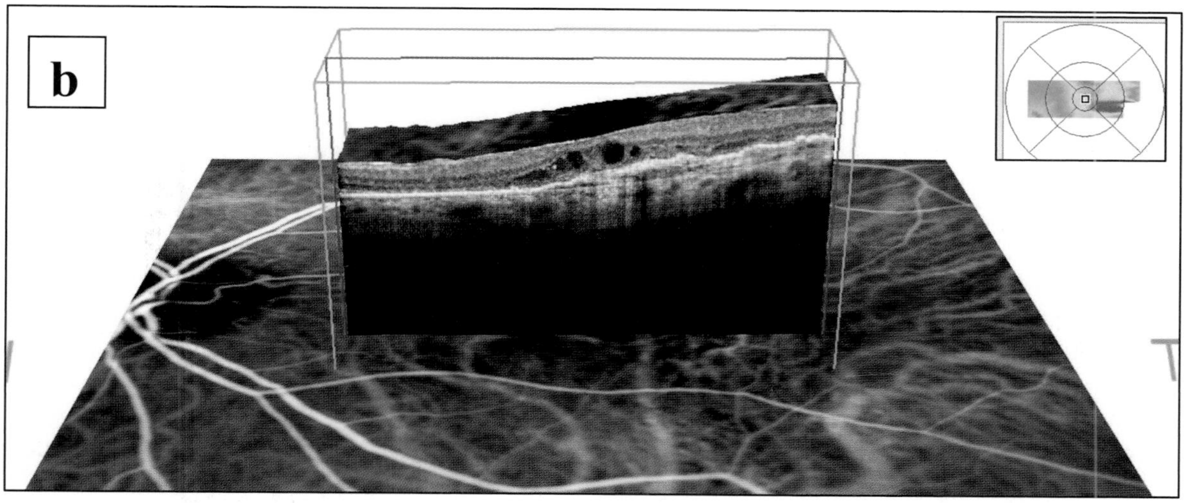

Figure 9: Polypoidal choroidal vasculopathy with serosanguinous PED. VA: 3/10

3D images for comparison of the changes:

a): At the end of the 1st year: stabilization after treatment.

b): At the end of the 2nd year: recurrence and alteration of the abnormal choroidal vascular structures.

CLINICAL CASE No. 02: Polypoidal Choroidal Vasculopathy

Macular lesion with drusen and vascularized PED, progressing over several years.
Follow-up by SD-OCT after anti-VEGF therapy.

An 84-year-old man presented with slowly progressive decline of visual acuity in the right eye, discovered in the context of a routine examination for numerous bilateral soft drusen.

VA RE: 20/100 - VA LE: 20/63.

Biomicroscopic Examination

Numerous soft drusen, predominantly in the temporal and inferior macula, with several calcified drusen.

The inferior macular region was raised with a grayish color but without signs of hemorrhage (**Figure 10a and b**).

On autofluorescence, reticular drusen were clearly visible in the region of the superior temporal arcade.

The zone of xanthophyll pigment was altered and irregular. Intense and irregular autofluorescence was observed all around the inferior macular elevation (**Figure 10c**).

Fluorescein Angiography

- Heterogeneous hyper-fluorescence of all the raised region with progressive staining in certain areas.
- Pooling of fluorescein in the juxtafoveal zone.
- Cystoid spaces were stained in the late phases (**Figure 10d and e**).

SLO-ICG Angiography

a): *Early phase*, a small territory of hypo-fluorescence, with two small hot spots.
b): *Late phase*: the small PED was clearly visible and well-demarcated, but the contours were irregular with a crown of soft drusen.
The two hot spots in the PED were increasingly visible (**Figure 10f and g**).

> **Suggested Diagnosis:**
> *Small polypoidal formations associated with a PED and no detectable neovascular membrane.*

Contribution of OCT (*Spectralis**)

Horizontal section

The RPE was irregular with several small thinned and thickened zones.
The RPE was separated from Bruch's membrane with anterior protrusions corresponding to the two *polypoidal formations*.
Posterior to the RPE, almost all of the heterogeneous PED cavity was optically empty.
Anterior to the RPE, an intense exudative reaction was observed with markedly increased retinal thickness and fluid infiltration between the outer retinal layers. A serous retinal detachment was demonstrated in the inferior and temporal macular region.
A large number of bright hyper-reflective spots were observed around the zones of intraretinal fluid and adjacent to the polyps. The outer retinal layers and outer nuclear layer were no longer visible and were invaded by dense zones, bright hyper-reflective spots, and protruding polyps (**Figure 11**).

Vertical section

The vertical section through the largest polyp demonstrated similar features, with steeply sloped edges. Intraretinal fluid was increased with large central cysts and multiple cysts in the outer plexiform layer.

The polyp protruded as far as the outer plexiform layer. The outer nuclear layer was disorganized, irregular, and poorly-defined (**Figure 11**).

> **Diagnosis**
> The **SD-OCT examination** provided a wealth of diagnostic information by clearly demonstrating three key signs: the *PED*, *polypoidal formations*, and *intraretinal fluid* with bright hyper-reflective spots and dense zones.
>
> Comparison with angiographies confirmed and refined the diagnosis of a complex lesion, comprised of multiple soft drusen, a vascularized PED with intraretinal fluid, and **polypoidal formations complicating AMD.**

CLINICAL CASE No. 02: POLYPOIDAL CHOROIDAL VASCULOPATHY
Macular lesion with drusen and vascularized PED, progressing over several years

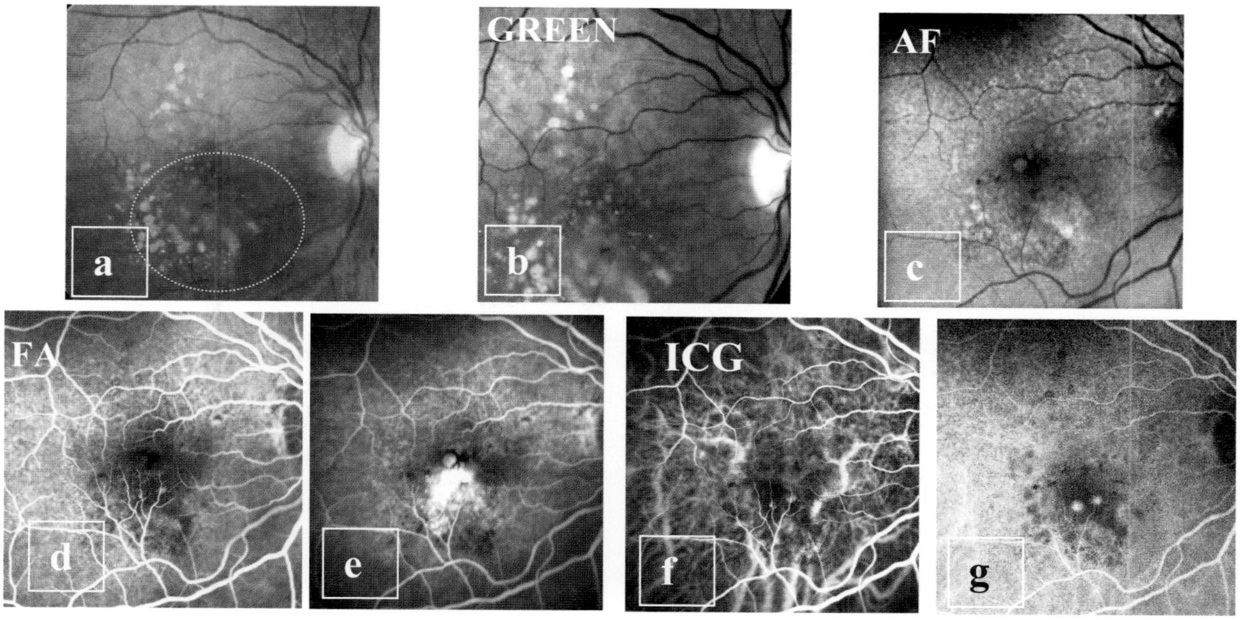

Figure 10: Polypoidal choroidal vasculopathy with serosanguinous PED. VA: 20/100.
a): Color fundus photograph. b): Red-free fundus photograph. c): Autofluorescence. d and e): Fluorescein angiography. f and g): SLO-ICG angiography.

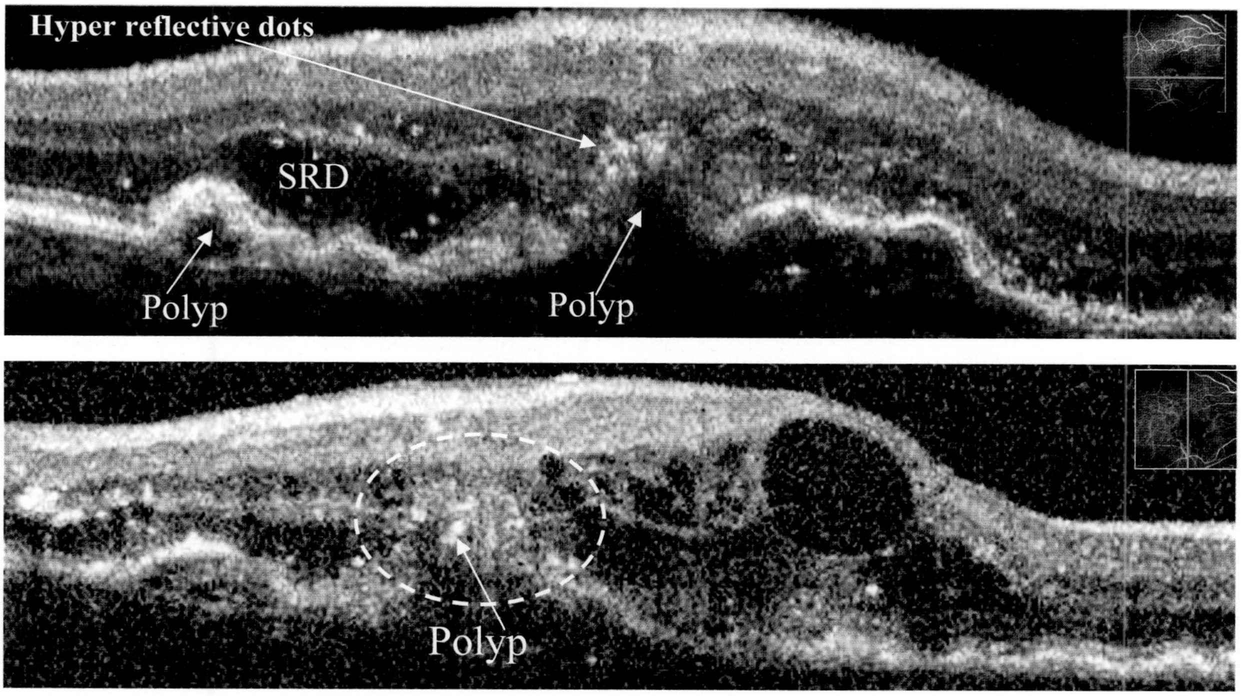

Figure 11: Polypoidal choroidal vasculopathy with serosanguinous PED. VA: 20/100.
***Spectralis** horizontal section**: irregular PED with anterior protrusions corresponding to two polypoidal formations. SRF and intraretinal fluid.
Vertical section: Large central cysts and multiple cysts in the outer plexiform layer.
The polyp protrudes as far as the outer plexiform layer. The outer nuclear layer is disorganized, irregular, and poorly visible.

CLINICAL CASE No. 02: Polypoidal Choroidal Vasculopathy

Follow-up by SD-OCT after anti-VEGF therapy.

Treatment by monthly intravitreous injections of anti-VEGF (*Lucentis**) was continued for one year with follow-up by visual acuity, OCT, fluorescein angiography, and ICG angiography.
The response to treatment was encouraging although incomplete, and no recurrence was observed.
Visual acuity remained stable and relatively low at 20/160, despite improvement in subjective symptoms throughout follow-up.

OCT

- ***By the first follow-up examination***, retinal thickness had considerably decreased, intraretinal fluid had almost completely disappeared, and the foveal depression was clearly visible.

The outer plexiform layer was visible with normal thickness. Multiple small cysts and especially the large central cysts resolved over a period of several weeks.
The outer nuclear layer and external limiting membrane were again visible with only a small number of bright hyper-reflective spots.

Protrusion of the polyp was much less marked, although a persistent dense zone was present (**Figure 12**).

- ***After the third injection***, improvement continued with a normal appearance of all the retinal layers.

However, a small SRF with several dense spots on its edge and a localized hyper-reflective zone corresponding to the polyp anterior to the RPE were still present (**Figure 12b**).

- ***After the fourth injection***, the horizontal OCT section of the fovea showed a satisfactory appearance with a normal profile and resolution of the edema. There was a persistent subfoveal hyper-reflective zone, suggestive of fibrosis.

The *vertical section* confirmed almost complete resolution of the polyps and absence of intraretinal fluid with persistence of the juxtafoveal dense zone and localized loss of the external limiting membrane and IS/OS interface (**Figure 13**).

Visual acuity did not improve.

Fluorescein Angiography

The abnormal choroidal vascular network present on the first examination gradually decreased in terms of both surface area and perfusion.

This vascular network was virtually no longer visible on the last examination (**Figures 12 and 13**).

ICG Angiography

The choroidal vascular network, the polyps, and the PED progressively resolved with each successive examination and were no longer visible on the last examination (**Figures 12 and 13**).

At this Stage

This case of *polypoidal formations associated with occult neovascular membrane* (**transitional form or active complications**) was improved with treatment.

The polyps and the exudative and inflammatory reactions (intraretinal dense spots and zones) were rapidly and dramatically ameliorated.

This improvement was clearly demonstrated by *Spectralis** OCT, particularly in the outer retinal layers.

The persistence and progression of limited but subfoveal fibrosis explained the absence of functional improvement with only stabilization of visual acuity.

The rapid resolution of the choroidal vascular abnormalities, polyps, and PED reflect the efficacy of treatment.

Long-term observation must be maintained as these lesions often recur.

CLINICAL CASE No. 02: POLYPOIDAL CHOROIDAL VASCULOPATHY
Follow-up by SD-OCT after anti-VEGF therapy.

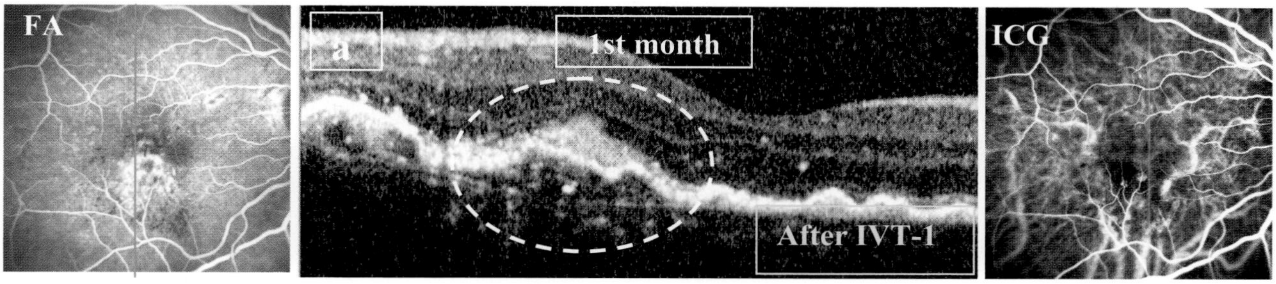

Figure 12: Polypoidal choroidal vasculopathy with serosanguinous PED. VA: 20/125.
a): After the first IVT injection: dramatic improvement: resolution of the cysts and regression of the polyp and bright hyper-reflective spots.

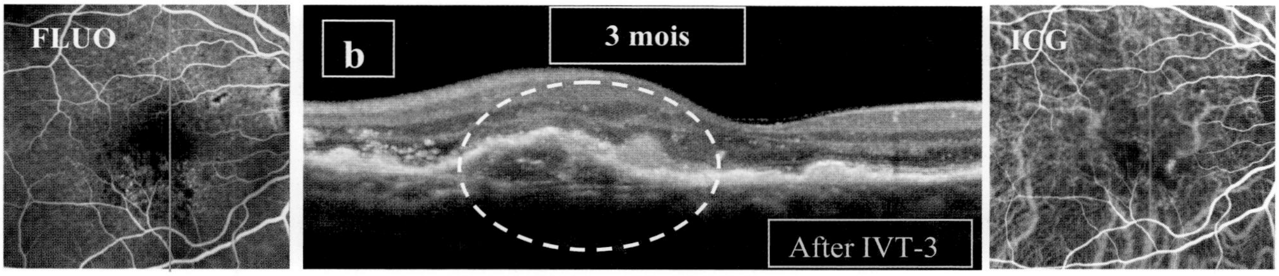

Figure 12: Polypoidal choroidal vasculopathy with serosanguinous PED. VA: 20/160.
b): After the third IVT injection: normal appearance of all layers; persistence of a small SRF, several dense points on the edges of the PED, and a localized hyper-reflective zone corresponding to the polyp, anterior to the RPE.

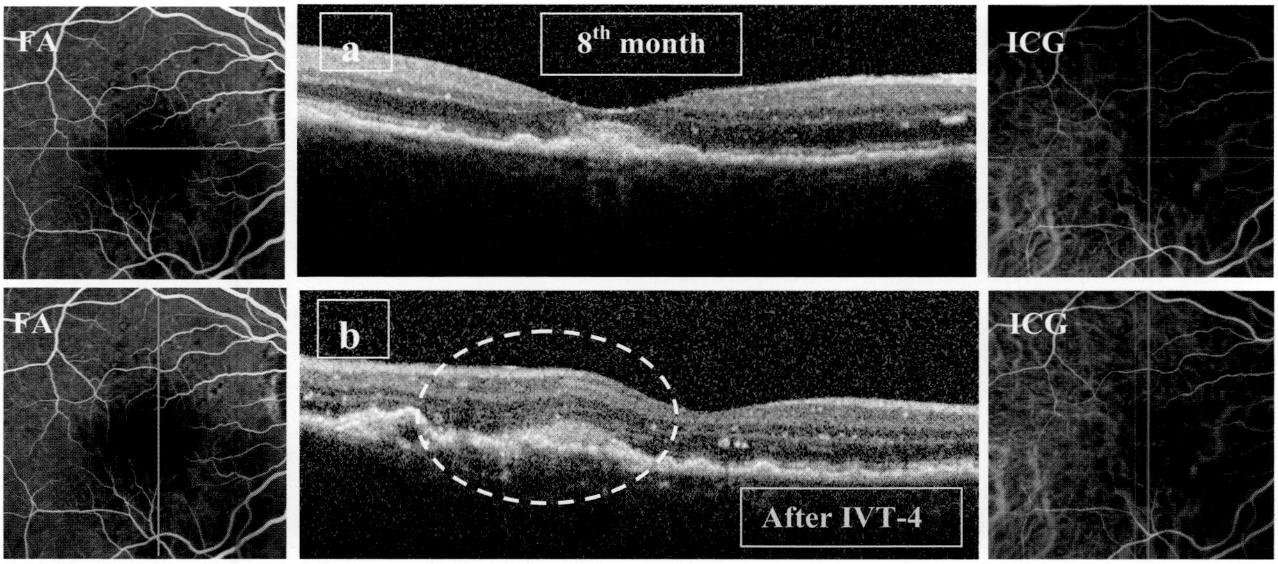

Figure 13: Polypoidal choroidal vasculopathy with serosanguinous PED. VA: 20/160.
a and b): After the fourth IVT injection: horizontal and vertical sections: normal profile and resolution of edema; persistence of a subfoveal hyper-reflective zone, suggestive of fibrosis; almost complete resolution of the polyps; no intraretinal fluid. Persistence of a juxtafoveal dense zone and localized loss of the external limiting membrane and IS/OS interface.

CLINICAL CASE No. 03: Polypoidal Choroidal Vasculopathy

Extensive, exudative macular lesion with several drusen, progressing over several years. Follow-up by SD-OCT after anti-VEGF therapy.

An 84-year-old man presented with progressive decline of visual acuity in the *left eye*, which was particularly worrying because it was his better eye. He had a central scotoma in the right eye for several years due to an extensive atrophic lesion.
VA RE: 20/80 - VA LE: 20/40.

Biomicroscopic examination and autofluorescence demonstrated minor abnormalities with a few perifoveal soft drusen. Note a slight retinal elevation, predominantly in the superior macular sector. No hemorrhage or lipid exudates (**Figure 14a and b**).
On autofluorescence, the central zone was surrounded by a large band of hyper-fluorescence surrounding the central zone, predominantly in the superior temporal sector (**Figure 14c**).

Fluorescein Angiography

Early hyper-fluorescence of the entire posterior pole with a false image of central sparing (due to xanthophyll pigment). This irregular hyper-fluorescence was composed of numerous, small zones of intense hyper-fluorescence, without fluorescein leakage.
At the late phase, fairly numerous punctate lesions were observed, suggesting small polyps (**Figure 14d and e**).

SLO-ICG Angiography

a): *Early phase*: rapid filling of an abnormal network, initially in the superior nasal sector and then extending inferiorly.
b): *Late phase*: partial emptying of the superior part of the network, while the inferior part became increasingly visible and well-contrasted. This initially suggested occult choroidal neovascularization, but there was no leakage phenomenon (**Figure 14f and g**).

Suggested Diagnosis:
Vast abnormal choroidal network and numerous polyps with a slowly progressive course causing limited leakage. No detectable choroidal neovascularization.

Contribution of OCT (*Spectralis**)

Vertical section

The vast macular lesion detected on angiography was responsible for few signs on SD-OCT, essentially a moderate and flat PED, involving almost all of the fovea.

The RPE, separated from Bruch's membrane except in the foveolar region, was irregular with thinner and thicker zones and numerous hyper-reflective dense spots. Numerous small prominences were also observed, probably corresponding to small polyps.

The outer retinal layers were altered: the IS/OS interface was thickened in the center and fragmented and was only partially visible.

The outer nuclear layer was severely altered with thinned zones and denser zones, mainly in the superior part, over a small zone of RPE atrophy.

Minimal intraretinal fluid was observed in the central region (**Figure 15**).

Diagnosis

The **clinical features and angiographic signs** could have initially suggested a diagnosis of extensive choroidal neovascularization.
However, the slow course, relative central sparing, presence of several polyps, and especially the absence of fluorescein leakage supported slowly progressive polypoidal choroidal vasculopathy.

The **SD-OCT examination** was compatible with this diagnosis by showing multiple small polyps with a moderate exudative reaction and an extensive PED (with progression to atrophy in the superior part). Analysis of the **outer retinal layers** demonstrated the presence of alterations with bright hyper-reflective spots and dense zones.

CLINICAL CASE No. 03: POLYPOIDAL CHOROIDAL VASCULOPATHY

Extensive, exudative macular lesion with several drusen, progressing over several years. Follow-up by SD-OCT after anti-VEGF therapy.

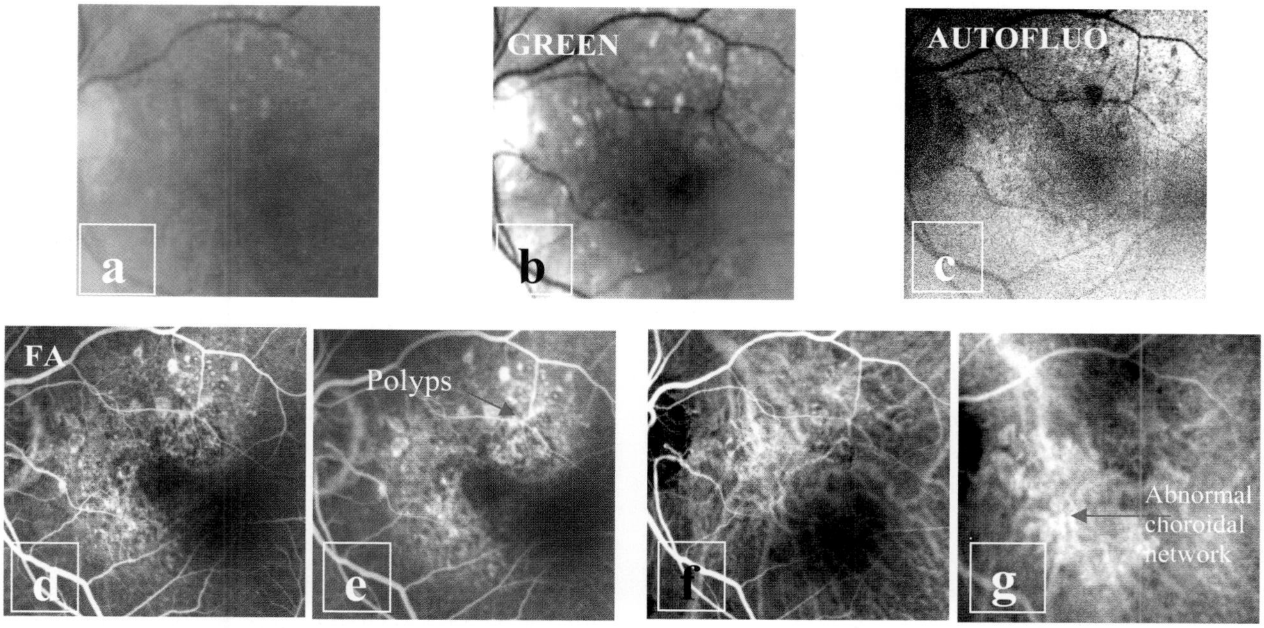

Figure 14: Polypoidal choroidal vasculopathy. VA: 20/40.
a): Color fundus photograph.
b): Red-free fundus photograph: minor abnormalities: several perifoveal soft drusen. Slight superior macular elevation.
c): Autofluorescence: vast band of hyper-fluorescence, predominantly in the superior temporal sector.
d and e): Fluorescein angiography: early, irregular hyper-fluorescence of the posterior pole with many small zones of hyper-fluorescence without fluorescein leakage, suggestive of small polyps in the superior temporal sector.
f and g): SLO-ICG angiography: rapid filling of an abnormal network, initially superior nasal and then extending inferiorly. Partial emptying of the superior part of the network, while the inferior part becomes increasingly visible and well-contrasted.

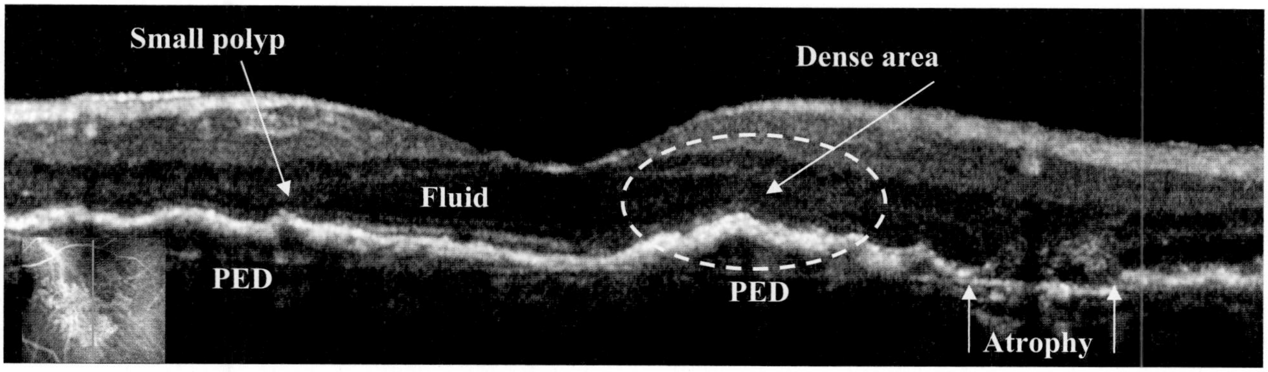

Figure 15: Polypoidal choroidal vasculopathy. VA: 20/40.
Spectralis* vertical section: the vast juxtafoveal and interpapillomacular abnormal choroidal network causes limited signs on SD-OCT. Multiple irregularities of the RPE and irregularities and fragmentation of the IS/OS interface and external limiting membrane (which are only clearly visible in the foveal region).
Multiple alterations of the outer nuclear layer with dense zones, particularly in the superior part. Presence of a flat, very extensive (3 to 4 DD) pigment epithelium detachment, mainly in the superior sectors, over the most severely elevated zone with only minimal intraretinal fluid in the central region.

CLINICAL CASE No. 03: Polypoidal Choroidal Vasculopathy

Extensive, exudative macular lesion with several drusen, progressing over several years. Follow-up by SD-OCT after anti-VEGF therapy.

Treatment by monthly intravitreous injections of anti-VEGF (*Lucentis**) was continued for 6 months with follow-up by visual acuity, OCT, fluorescein angiography, and ICG angiography.

Visual acuity improved to 20/32 after the first injection, then remained stable throughout follow-up with no subsequent improvement.

OCT

On the first follow-up examination
Retinal thickness was considerably decreased. Intraretinal fluid was decreased but was still present, and the foveal depression remained clearly visible.

Abnormalities of the outer layers had barely changed with persistence of the irregularities and minimal prominences of the RPE (**Figure 16a**).

After the second injection
Improvement continued with flattening of the PED and visibility of the external limiting membrane (**Figure 16b**).

After the third injection
The retinal profile became almost normal on the horizontal and vertical sections (**Figure 16c and d**).

The PED persisted over its entire surface, but was flat and barely visible, essentially marked by persistence of several small polyps. The external limiting membrane and IS/OS interface were clearly visualized.

Several persistent zones of thinning and hyper-reflectivity were observed in the outer nuclear layer over the residual polyps.

The inner retinal layers had a normal, well-organized appearance.

However, thickening of the inner limiting membrane was observed in the superior temporal sector, corresponding to relative RPE atrophy (**Figure 16c**).

Fluorescein Angiography

All of the abnormal vascular network remained visible with the same topography. The small polyps also remained visible, but their density and staining were markedly decreased.

No fluorescein leakage was observed (**Figure 16**).

ICG Angiography

Only the abnormal choroidal network remained visible, although the branches appear to be fewer and smaller with lower contrast, even in the late phase (**Figure 16**).

At this Stage

A relatively favorable response to treatment was observed in this case, comprising numerous small polyps (especially in the superior temporal sector) and a vast, juxtafoveal and interpapillomacular abnormal choroidal network.

The polyps and exudative and inflammatory reactions (intraretinal dense spots and zones) resolved rapidly. Polyps were barely detectable following treatment. Intraretinal fluid was no longer visible, and the PED had almost completely resolved.

These results justified suspension of treatment after the third injection.

However, the abnormal choroidal network still persisted, with a superior temporal zone of thinning and atrophy of the RPE.

The prognosis remained fairly reserved due to the persistence of this abnormal choroidal network, justifying 6-month or annual follow-up due to the risk of recurrence.

CLINICAL CASE No. 03: POLYPOIDAL CHOROIDAL VASCULOPATHY

Extensive, exudative macular lesion with several drusen, progressing over several years.
Follow-up by SD-OCT after anti-VEGF therapy.

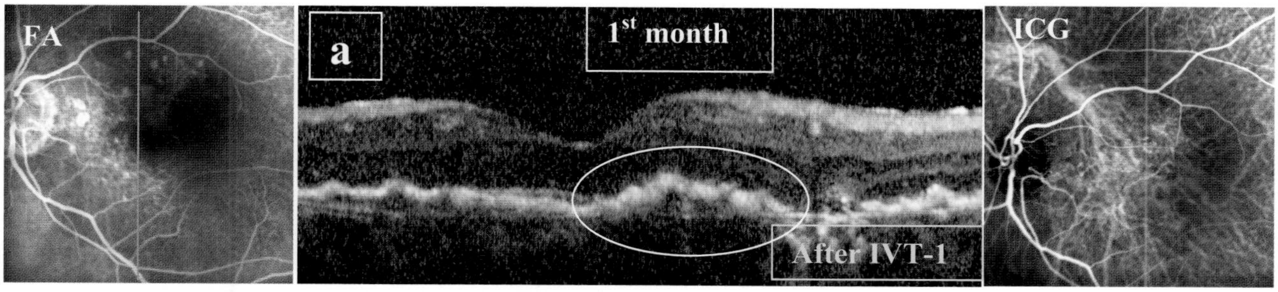

Figure 16: Polypoidal choroidal vasculopathy. VA: 20/40.
a): After the first IVT injection: immediate improvement. Reduction of retinal thickness and intraretinal fluid. The foveal depression remains clearly visible. Persistence of abnormalities of the outer retinal layers and irregularities of the RPE.

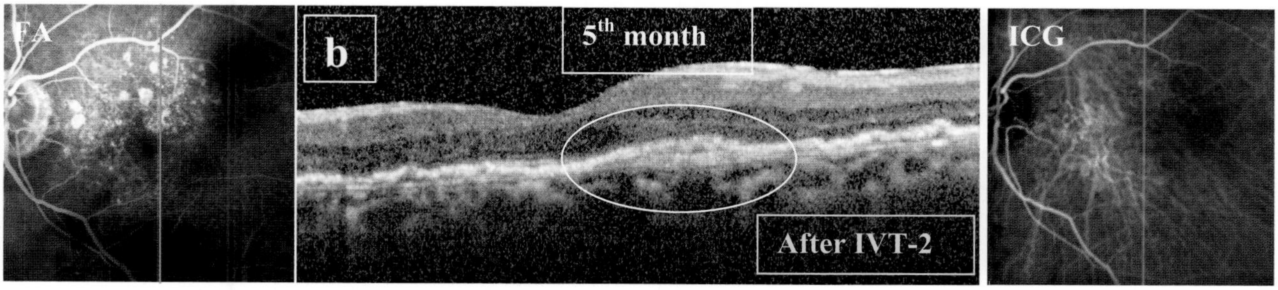

Figure 16 polypoidal choroidal vasculopathy. VA: 20/40.
b): After the second IVT injection: the PED has become flat. The external limiting membrane is now visible. All of the abnormal vascular network persists.

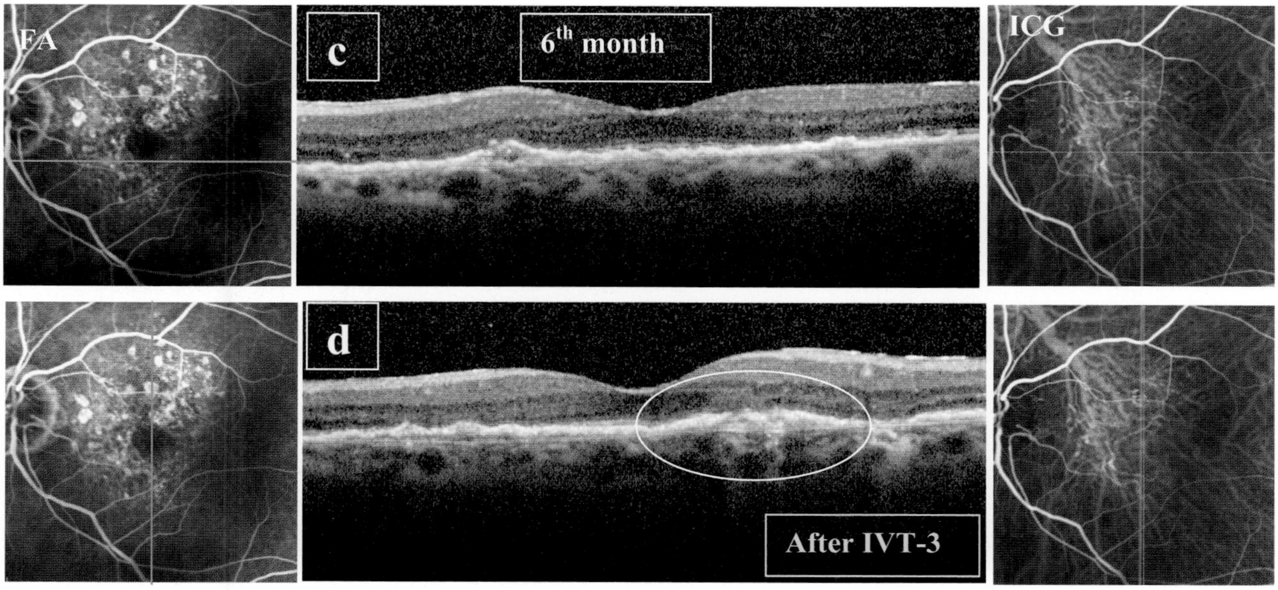

Figure 16c and d: Polypoidal choroidal vasculopathy. VA: 20/160.
c and d): After the third IVT injection: the retinal profile is almost normal on both the horizontal section and the vertical section. Several zones of thinning of the outer nuclear layer with dense zones over the residual polyps. Thickening of the inner limiting membrane in the superior temporal sector.

Conclusion

Idiopathic polypoidal choroidal vasculopathy, or PCV, is a particular entity, distinct from the usual definition of AMD.

Polypoidal choroidal vasculopathy can be clearly **distinguished from AMD** by its polymorphic clinical features, the presence of extramacular lesions, onset at a younger age, and the absence of the usual precursor signs of AMD.

However, these two diseases share many features in common.

The presence of multiple, recurrent serosanguinous pigment epithelium detachments is suggestive of AMD.

The typical form of an **abnormal branching choroidal** network with polypoidal formations at the terminations of these vessels appears to constitute a distinct entity.

As illustrated by this **series of clinical cases**, polypoidal ectasias can also be observed within very small choroidal vessels, almost at the level of capillaries. Polypoidal dilatations can also be observed in advanced forms of AMD.

Transitional forms between initial PCV and subsequent development of occult choroidal neovascularization with hemorrhagic complications can also be observed.

It is still unclear at the present time whether these lesions are related or different manifestations of the same disease.

The frequency of these forms in Asian countries raises the question of a **genetic predisposition**. Recent genetic correlation studies advocate for a common genetic background.

Classic Choroidal Neovascularization

Clinical Features and OCT Follow-Up after Treatment

Gabriel COSCAS

Florence COSCAS, Sabrina VISMARA,
Alain ZOURDANI, C.I. Li CALZI

(Créteil and Paris)

contrast, are extremely suggestive and characteristic, OCT is able to provide additional information:

- By evaluating the presence of an exudative (and/or hemorrhagic) reaction by means of indirect signs, such as intraretinal fluid, even initially limited.
- By demonstrating the presence of the hyper-reflective, subretinal complex anterior to the RPE, typical of classic CNV.
- By demonstrating in many opportunities, the presence of a PED, indicating the concomitant presence of poorly-defined occult CNV that may be missed on fluorescein angiography.

Comparison of fluorescein angiography and SLO-ICG angiography findings with OCT images validates interpretation of the direct and indirect signs observed on OCT, confirms the diagnosis of classic CNV, and helps to guide treatment.

Imaging Modalities

TD-OCT visualizes indirect signs and direct signs.

Indirect signs:
Indirect signs are related to abnormal leakage with subretinal and intraretinal fluid accumulation.

The *serous detachment of the neurosensory retina* is usually moderate, essentially visible at the edge of the hyper-reflective zone. It may sometimes be more extensive.

Accentuation of vascular leakage results in *intraretinal fluid*, either diffuse with increased **retinal thickness**, or collected in the cystoid spaces of inner retinal layers (**Figure 1**).

During the progression of disease, cysts can become numerous, larger, spread to multiple layers, or travel towards the center of the fovea.

Intraretinal fluid and the presence of a hyper-reflective complex and their associated inflammatory reaction induce progressive loss of the **foveal depression**, which is sometimes replaced by a marked elevation.

A zone of **posterior shadowing** is another fairly specific indirect sign of hyper-reflective classic CNV that limits passage of light towards the posterior pole.

Finally, OCT demonstrates irregularities or thickening of the RPE band and sometimes even localized disruption, suggesting protrusion of neovascularization.

Direct signs:
The essential direct sign indicating the presence of classic CNV is a fairly intense **zone of hyper-reflectivity** anterior to the RPE (**Figure 1**).

This hyper-reflective complex is usually spindle-shaped, sometimes distinct from the RPE or, on the contrary, adherent and even fused with the RPE. It is outlined by a zone of posterior shadowing. The exact nature of this poorly-demarcated hyper-reflective zone is difficult to determine on TD-OCT.

SD-OCT

Indirect signs of intraretinal fluid and *direct signs* of hyper-reflectivity are also seen, but even more information can be learned from analysis of the retinal layers and their abnormalities.

The RPE (although attenuated by shadowing due to the neovascular lesion) remains clearly visible and is ***not detached from Bruch's membrane.***

Analysis of serial (*raster*) sections often reveals one or several disruptions in the RPE allowing passage of classic CNV.

Anterior to the RPE, a **SRF** is almost always present (often with shifting fluid), and its internal and external margins are often highlighted by **bright hyper-reflective spots**.

The neovascular membrane is visualized by **a zone of hyper-reflectivity**, whose contours appear to be continuous with a thickened and hyper-reflective *IS/OS interface*. The *external limiting membrane* is displaced and often disrupted over the neovascularization.

The hyper-reflective zone corresponding to classic CNV comprises a denser zone (with scattered bright hyper-reflective spots) that invades or displaces the outer nuclear layer. As a consequence, the outer nuclear layer becomes poorly visualized.

Diffuse intraretinal fluid and cysts induce major changes of the middle and inner retinal layers. The hyper-reflective lesion and intraretinal fluid induce loss of the **foveal depression** and a marked increase in central retinal thickness.

Vitreomacular adhesions often persist.

RECENT ONSET CLASSIC CHOROIDAL NEOVASCULARIZATION

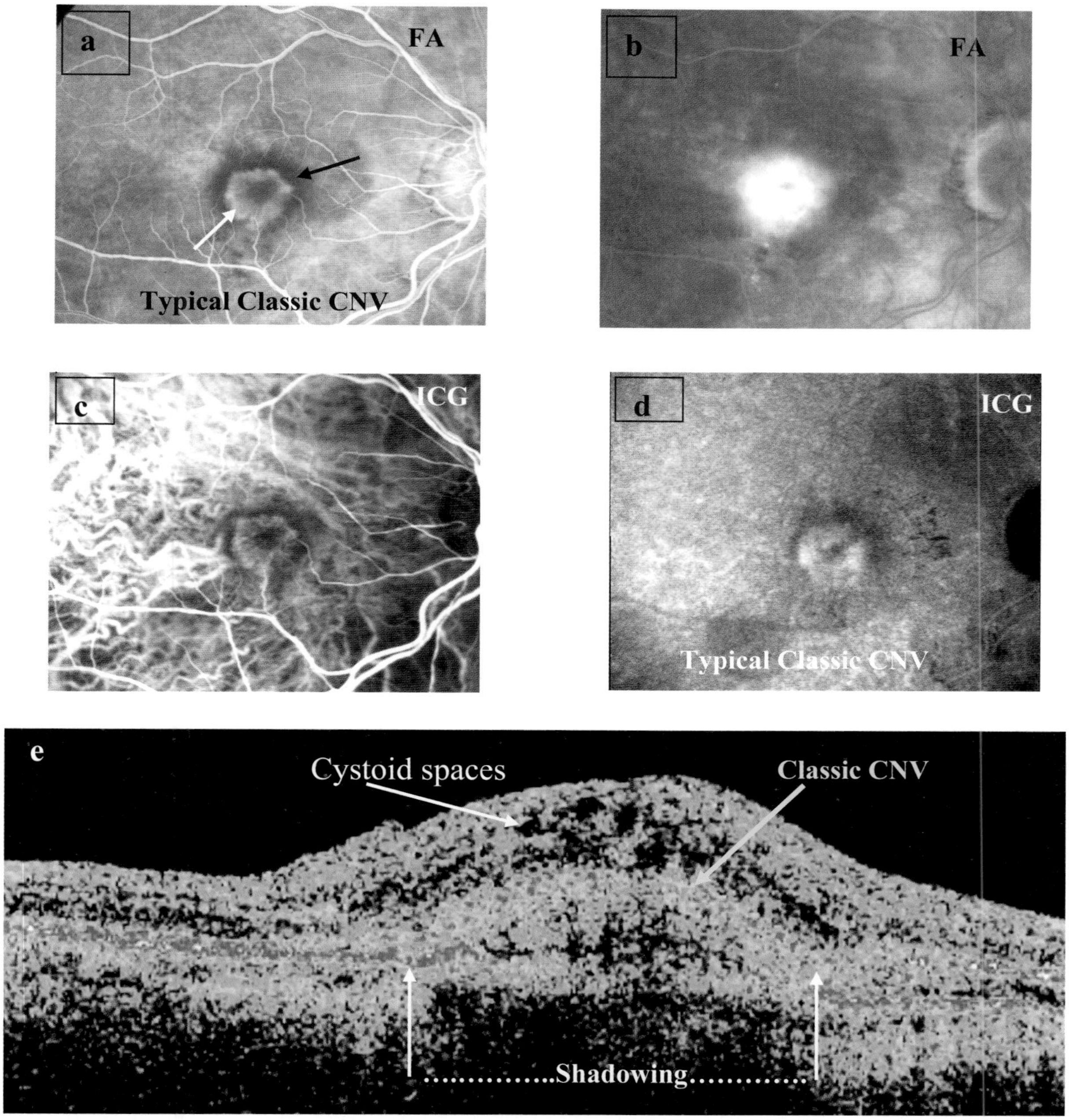

Figure 1: Recent-onset classic choroidal neovascularization: a typical case.

a and b): Fluorescein angiography: 1 DD hyper-fluorescent bicycle wheel (*white arrow*) with late fluorescein leakage (b) masking the peripheral pigment ring (*black arrow*).

c and d): SLO-ICG angiography: rapid perfusion of the neovascular membrane with late staining of other structures. Similar appearance on fluorescein angiography but with minimal leakage. The choroidal arteries are clearly visualized.

e): TD-OCT (*Stratus)**: intraretinal fluid and several cysts (*white arrow*) in the neurosensory retina.
Classic CNV is visualized as a hyper-reflective band anterior to the retinal pigment epithelium (*yellow arrow*) but separated by a less reflective band and inducing relatively marked posterior shadowing in the zone between the arrows.

CLINICAL CASE No. 01: Small Classic CNV

Follow-up by SD-OCT after anti-VEGF therapy.

Monthly intravitreous injections of anti-VEGF (*Ranibizumab**) were continued for 6 months with follow-up by visual acuity, OCT, fluorescein angiography, and ICG angiography.

Immediately satisfactory results were obtained with rapid stabilization.

Visual acuity was markedly improved by the first examination, increasing to 20/40 and then stabilizing at 20/32 with resolution of metamorphopsias.

SD-OCT

By the first follow-up examination
Intraretinal fluid decreased considerably with resolution of cysts and a marked decrease in retinal thickness (429 μm).

The *hyper-reflective lesion* remained unchanged, but the outer retinal layers were more clearly visible: the IS/OS interface remained thickened and the external limiting membrane was visible with several bright hyper-reflective spots.

The *dense zone of hemorrhage* was markedly decreased and the outer nuclear layer regained a regular appearance (**Figure 3a**).

After the second injection
Improvement continued with resolution of intraretinal fluid and bright hyper-reflective spots. Outer retinal layers were almost normal.

At the third month
Recurrence of a small SRF and several bright hyper-reflective spots, justifying a third injection.

At the sixth month
No signs of leakage were present and the outer retinal layers were clearly visible and well-organized. However, the fovea remained elevated by the well-delineated, dense, pre-RPE hyper-reflective complex, suggestive of progressive fibrosis of classic CNV.

Fluorescein Angiography

The neovascular membrane rapidly decreased in size and became retracted with no fluorescein leakage. Only a limited zone of late staining with a small peripheral residual hemorrhage was still visible (**Figure 3a-d**).

ICG Angiography

Rapid regression of the membrane was seen and it was no longer visible after the second month (**Figure 3a-d**).

At this Stage

This case of **isolated classic CNV** associated with macular hemorrhage immediately showed a favorable response to treatment.

Pre-treatment SD-OCT demonstrated a pre-RPE hyper-reflective complex with leakage and disorganization of the outer retinal layers.

Intraretinal fluid **resolved rapidly** with improvement of visual acuity, a normal appearance to the outer retinal layers, and resolution of inflammatory signs.

No marked relapse was observed during 6 months of follow-up, but a 3rd injection was helpful.

Even still, the pre-RPE hyper-reflective complex persisted, suggesting **progressive fibrosis**.

It was denser than at the beginning but was well-tolerated with no major reactive signs.

Treatment was suspended in view of the rapid stabilization of the lesion with satisfactory visual acuity.

The persistence of fibrosis anterior to the RPE justified continuing observation.

A close and prolonged observation remained necessary, particularly due to the fact of the irreversible loss of vision in the fellow eye.

CLINICAL CASE No. 01: SMALL CLASSIC CNV

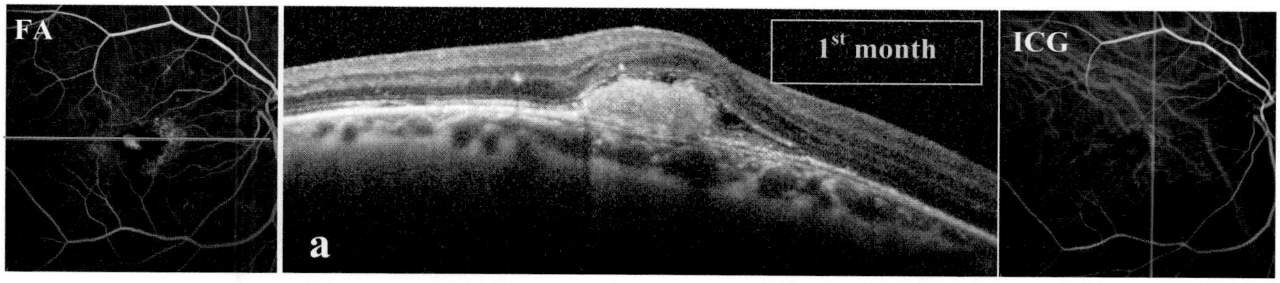

Figure 3: Small classic CNV. VA: 20/40. Thickness: 429 μm.
a): After the 1st IVT injection: resolution of intraretinal fluid and cysts and decreased retinal thickness, but the hyper-reflective lesion remained unchanged. The outer retinal layers were visible, the IS/OS interface was thickened, and the external limiting membrane was visible with several bright hyper-reflective spots. The dense zone of hemorrhage was in the process of resolving. The outer nuclear layer was more clearly visualized.

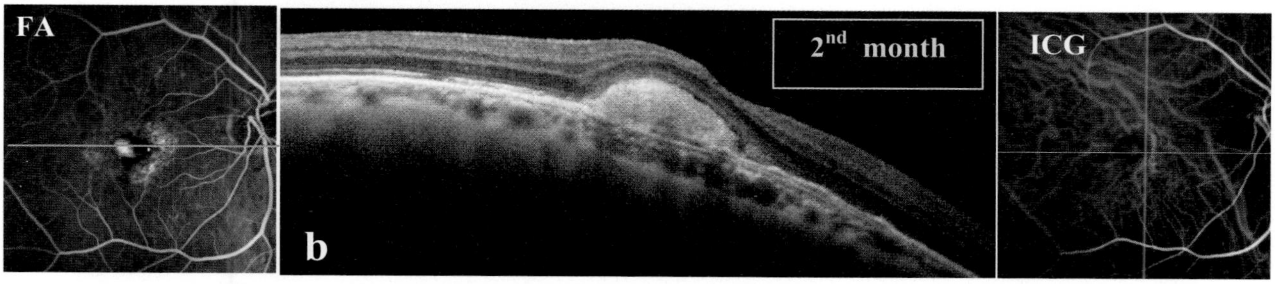

Figure 3: Small classic CNV. VA: 20/32. Thickness: 359 μm.
b): After the 2nd IVT injection: resolution of intraretinal fluid and bright hyper-reflective spots. Almost normal appearance of the outer retinal layers.

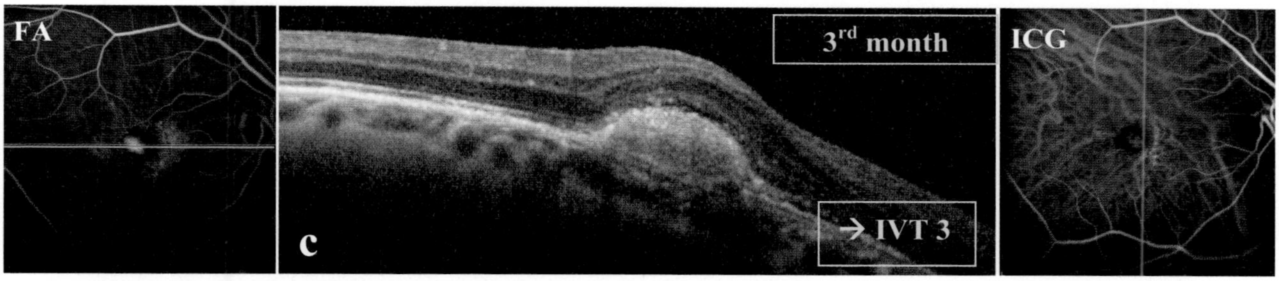

Figure 3: Small classic CNV. VA: 20/32. Thickness: 359 μm.
c): Before the 3rd IVT injection: recurrence of a small SRF and several bright hyper-reflective spots.

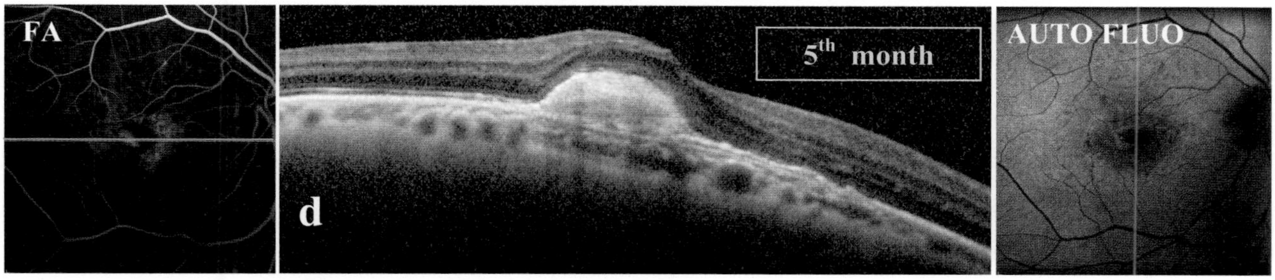

Figure 3: Small classic CNV. VA: 20/40. Thickness (Spectralis*): 351 μm.
d): At the 5th month: no exudative signs. The outer retinal layers were well visualized and well organized.
The fovea remained elevated by the hyper-reflective lesion, suggesting progressive fibrosis of the classic CNV.

CLINICAL CASE No. 01: SMALL CLASSIC CNV

ENLARGED IMAGES

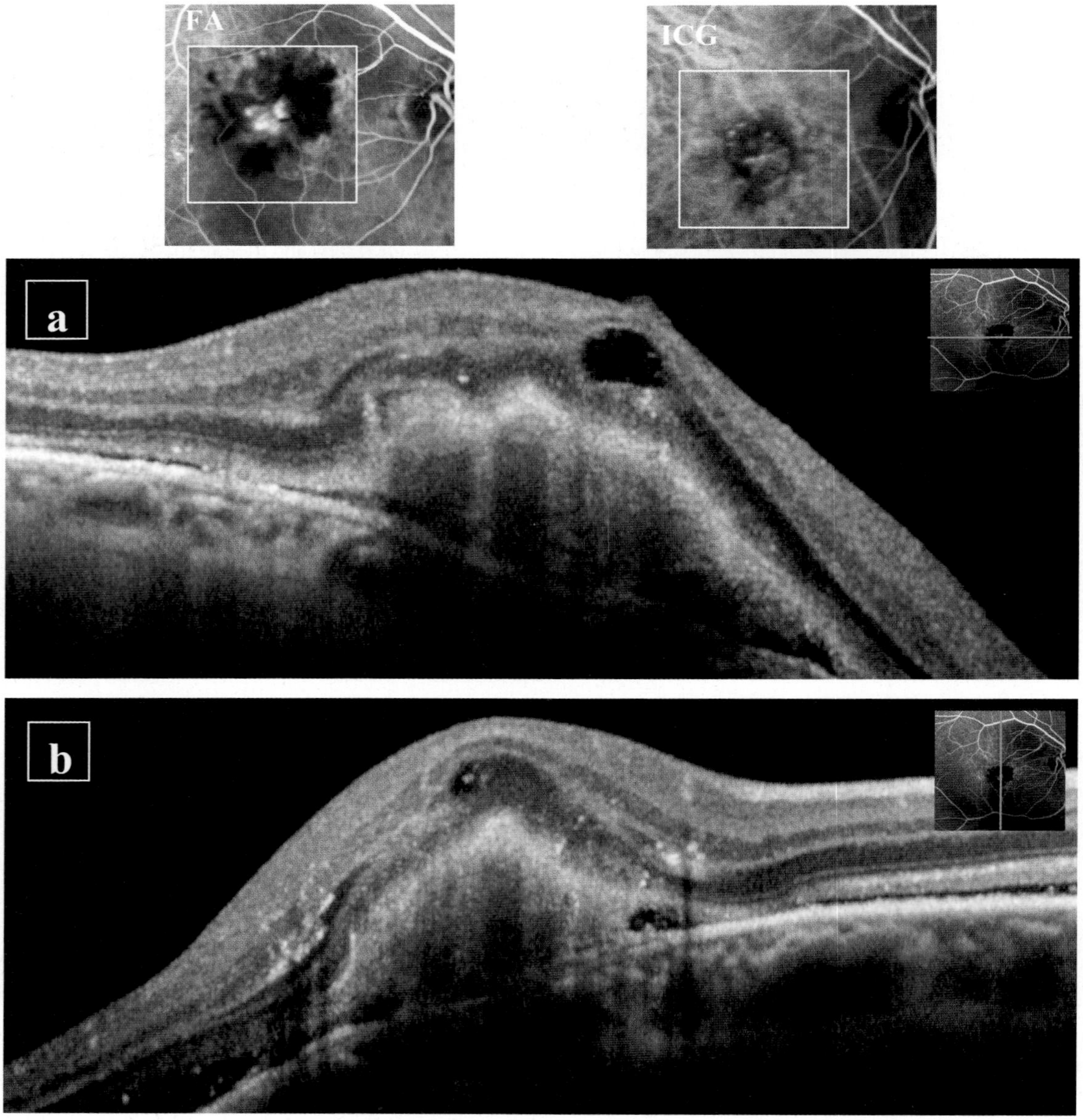

Figure 4: Small classic CNV (enlarged view of Figure 2).
a and b): *Spectralis horizontal and vertical sections.**

- Within and posterior to the RPE:
  The RPE was not detached or separated from Bruch's membrane.
  The RPE was partially masked by shadowing due to the pre-RPE hyper-reflective lesion.
- Anterior to the RPE:
  The IS/OS interface was gradually thickened, delineating a hyper-reflective complex anterior to the RPE.
  The outer nuclear layer was visible and invaded by a more reflective zone, related to hemorrhage.
  Increased retinal thickness (687 µm), intraretinal fluid, and cysts.

CLINICAL CASE No. 01: SMALL CLASSIC CNV

ENLARGED IMAGES

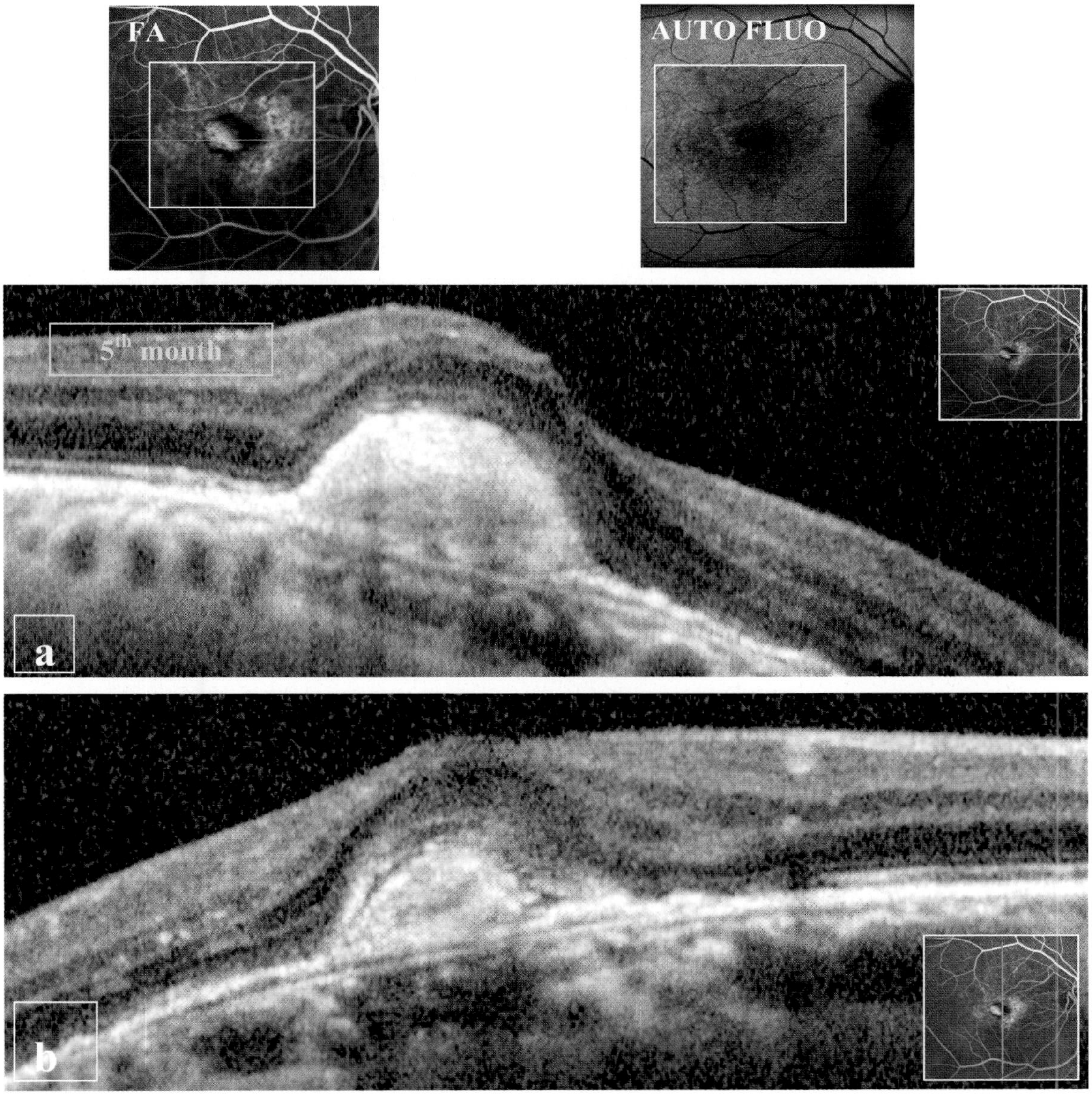

▪ Figure 5: Small classic CNV (enlarged view of Figure 3c)
a and b): *Spectralis horizontal and vertical sections.**

- Within and posterior to the RPE:
  The RPE was partially masked.
  The hyper-reflective lesion was denser and more fibrotic.
- Anterior to the RPE:
  No exudative signs.
  The outer retinal layers were well-visualized and well-organized.
  The IS/OS interface remained thickened. The subfoveal outer nuclear layer was well-visualized. Thickness (*Spectralis**): 351 µm.
  The fovea remained elevated by the hyper-reflective lesion, suggesting progressive fibrosis of the classic CNV.

CLINICAL CASE No. 02: Large Classic CNV

Classic choroidal neovascularization, progressing over many months, with moderate symptoms. Follow-up by TD-OCT and SD-OCT after anti-VEGF therapy.

Clinical Signs

An 83-year-old monocular woman due to longstanding AMD presented with recent, progressive decline of visual acuity in the right eye with metamorphopsias, which interfered with reading.
VA RE: 20/63 - VA LE: 20/200.

Biomicroscopic Examination

Vast, heterogeneous, grayish lesion of the posterior pole, 3 DD in diameter, located subfoveally but extending as far as the optic disc without hemorrhage.

Autofluorescence

An elongated, interpapillomacular, heterogeneous, hypofluorescent area with an irregular crown of hyper-fluorescence (**Figure 6a, b, and c**).

Fluorescein Angiography (Figure 6d)

Early and intense hyper-fluorescence of the entire well-defined and well-delineated interpapillomacular lesion with a network of **radial neovascularization** and a **peripheral anastomotic arcade**. These encroached onto the fovea and caused intense fluorescein leakage.

SLO-ICG Angiography (Figure 16e)

The neovascular membrane rapidly filled and was drained by several large vessels in the region between the optic nerve and macula. The network was composed of thin but dense vessels, which occupied all of the foveal region.

Suggested Diagnosis:

Large subfoveal classic CNV extending to the optic disc. It arose in the region between the optic disc and the macula with no detectable occult CNV associated with it.

Contribution of OCT (*Stratus**)

Horizontal section

The RPE was clearly visible and appeared to be thickened in the foveal region and as far as the optic disc, with a **hyper-reflective band** just anterior to and almost fused with the RPE.

Anterior to the RPE, a small amount of intraretinal fluid with increased retinal thickness, displacement of the central retina, and loss of the foveal depression (**Figure 7a**).

Vertical section

The hyper-reflective band anterior to the RPE was more clearly visualized in the foveal region with a moderate increase of retinal thickness and diffuse intraretinal fluid.

The hyper-reflective **classic CNV** displaced the neurosensory retina anteriorly with slight attenuation of the foveal depression (**Figure 7b**).

Diagnosis

The OCT examination demonstrated a spindle-shaped zone of **intense hyper-reflectivity** anterior to and in contact with the RPE (from which it was occasionally separated), suggestive of a large (3 DD) classic CNV.
The *leakage* was limited with diffuse intraretinal fluid and loss of the foveal depression but without any disorganization of the retinal tissue. Central retinal thickness (*Stratus**): 267 µm
Angiography confirmed the presence of an isolated, large, subfoveal, and interpapillomacular classic choroidal neovascular membrane with moderate fluorescein leakage and no hemorrhage.
This recently enlarging lesion, causing severe symptoms, justified immediate anti-VEGF therapy.

CLINICAL CASE No. 02: LARGE CLASSIC CNV

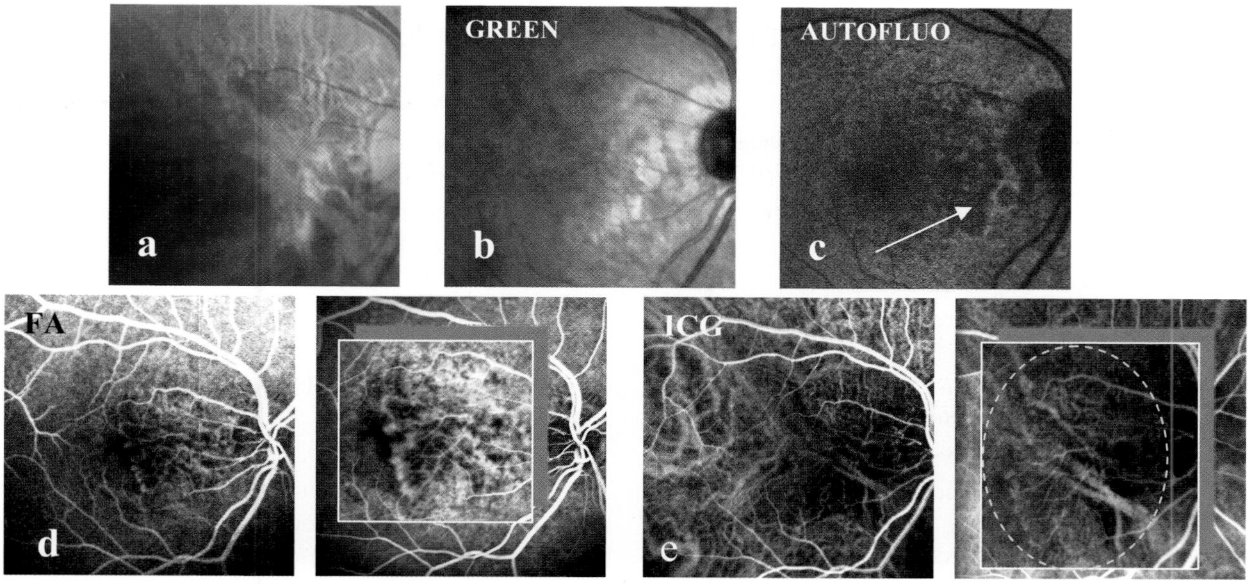

Figure 6: Large classic CNV. VA: 20/63.
a): Color. b): Red-free. c): Autofluorescence.
d): Fluorescein angiography: early and intense interpapillomacular hyper-fluorescence with a network of radial neovascularization and a peripheral anastomotic arcade, encroaching into the central zone and causing intense fluorescein leakage.
e): SLO-ICG angiography: the neovascular membrane was rapidly filled and drained by several large vessels situated in the region between the optic disc and the macula. The network appears to be composed of small but dense vessels, which occupied all of the foveal region.

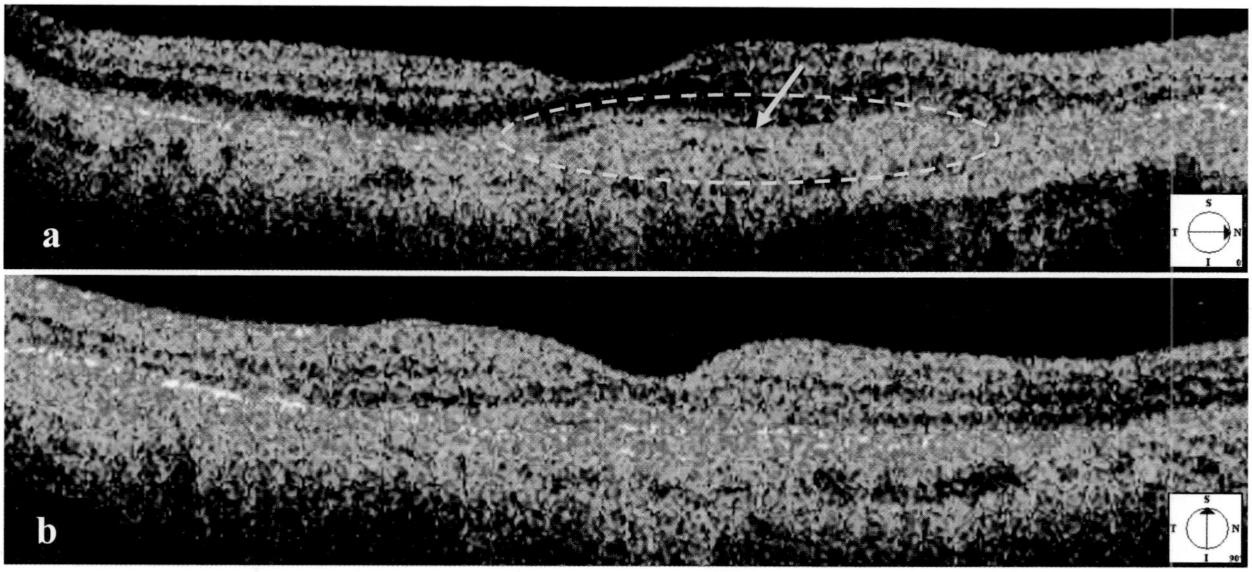

Figure 7: Large classic CNV. VA: 20/63.
*Stratus** TD-OCT.
a): Horizontal section: thickening of the RPE, with a hyper-reflective band, just anterior to and almost fused with the RPE (*yellow arrow*). Anterior to the RPE, a small amount of intraretinal fluid, increased retinal thickness, displacement of the central retina, and loss of the foveal depression.
b): Vertical section: moderate increase of retinal thickness with diffuse intraretinal fluid.
The hyper-reflective material of classic CNV displaced the neurosensory retina anteriorly with slight attenuation of the foveal depression.

CLINICAL CASE No. 02: Large Classic CNV

Monthly intravitreous injections of anti-VEGF therapy were continued for 1 year with follow-up by visual acuity, OCT, fluorescein angiography, and SLO-ICG angiography. The response to treatment was initially satisfactory but was followed by gradual deterioration of visual function over the last months of follow-up.

Visual acuity initially improved to 20/40 after the first 3 injections, then gradually decreased to 20/80.

TD-OCT

On the first follow-up examination
Regression of intraretinal fluid and reduction of retinal thickness (206 µm), but the pre-RPE hyper-reflective band became more clearly visible and denser (false white color) (**Figure 8a**).

At the third month
The appearance was similar, but the increased thickness of the hyper-reflective zone justified a third intravitreous injection, which was followed by functional improvement (**Figure 8b**).

SD-OCT

At the ninth month
The SD-OCT signs showed partial improvement, especially in the foveal region. However, despite quarterly maintenance IVT injections, examination of layers demonstrated the presence of a fine hyper-reflective band just anterior to the RPE, suggestive of **fibrosis** of the neovascular membrane.
The IS/OS interface was visible and thickened with alteration of the nuclear layer in the central region (**Figure 8c**). Most importantly, signs of complete *atrophy of the outer retinal layers* were observed with loss of the outer nuclear layer in the region between the optic disc and the macula.

On the last examination
One year after onset of the disorders, atrophy of the outer retinal layers in the region between the optic disc and the macula was confirmed.

The external limiting membrane and IS/OS interface were visible in the foveal zone and a fine hyper-reflective band was still present anterior to the RPE (**Figure 8d**).

Fluorescein Angiography

The neovascular membrane and fluorescein leakage regressed and then completely resolved by the third month. However, atrophy of the RPE gradually spread to involve the entire macular region as far as the optic disc.
This atrophy was confirmed on autofluorescence by extension of hypo-fluorescent spots throughout this region (**Figure 8a-d**).

ICG Angiography

Rapid regression of the membrane, which became undetectable by the second month (**Figure 8a-d**).

At this Stage

This case of large, isolated classic CNV was demonstrated on OCT as hyper-reflective material, which displaced the neurosensory retina anteriorly, with slight attenuation of the foveal depression.
These signs were suggestive of a well-delineated, large, subfoveal **classic CNV membrane** extending as far as the optic disc and without any associated occult neovascularization.
The response to treatment was immediately favorable with regression of the small amount of intraretinal fluid and fluorescein leakage (but without major alteration of the outer retinal layers).

A **minor recurrence** justified a 3rd injection followed by maintenance therapy every 3 months.

After one year of follow-up, 3 months after the last treatment, improvement was maintained. However, persistence of a fine hyper-reflective band just anterior to the RPE, (suggestive of **fibrosis**) with thickening of the IS/OS interface and alteration of the nuclear layer was demonstrated by SD-OCT.

Stabilization of the lesion with useful VA justified suspension of IVT injections but with prolonged and close follow-up.

11

CLINICAL CASE No. 02: LARGE CLASSIC CNV

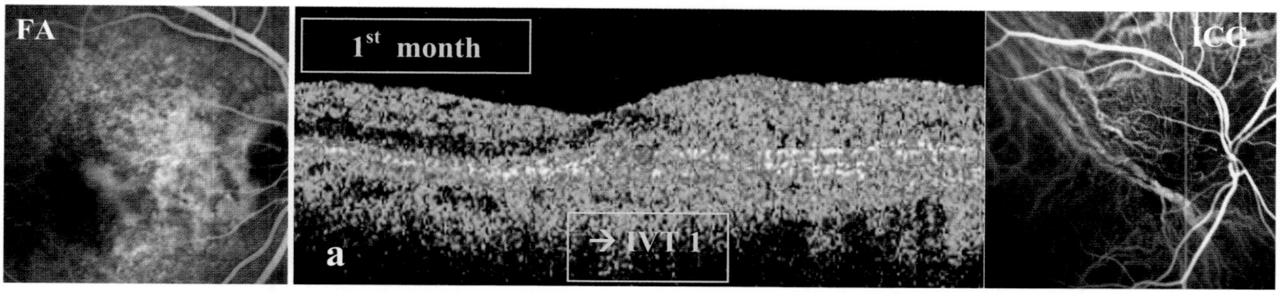

Figure 8: Large classic CNV. VA: 20/63. Central retinal thickness: 206 µm.
a): After the 1st IVT injection: resolution of intraretinal fluid and reduction of retinal thickness. The pre-RPE hyper-reflective band became more clearly visible and denser (false white color).

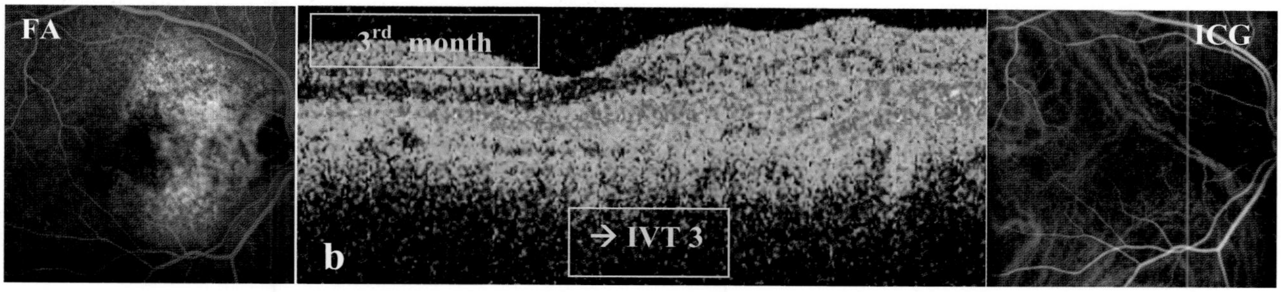

Figure 8: Large classic CNV. VA: 20/63. Central retinal thickness: 188 µm.
b): After the 3rd IVT injection: increased thickness of the hyper-reflective zone.

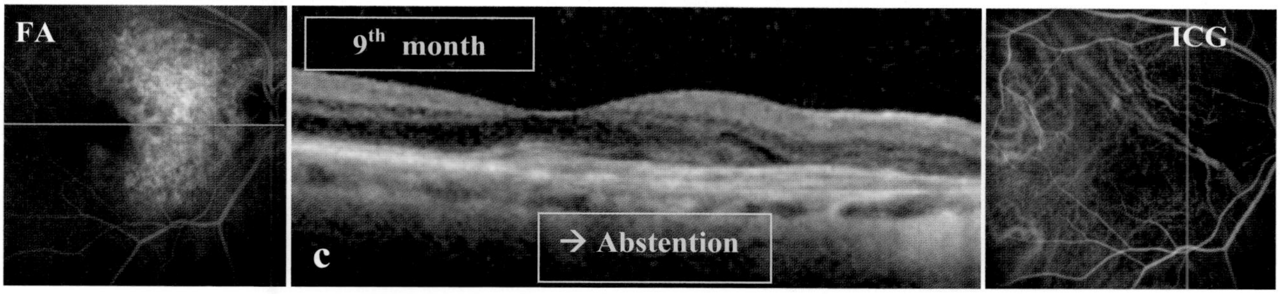

Figure 8: Large classic CNV. VA: 20/63. Thickness (*Spectralis**): 307 µm.
c): After the 5th IVT injection: fine hyper-reflective band just anterior to the RPE, suggestive of fibrosis of the neovascular membrane. The IS/OS interface was visible and thickened. Alteration of the nuclear layer in the central region.
Note a localized area of complete atrophy of the outer retinal layers and loss of the outer nuclear layer in the region between the optic disc and the macula.

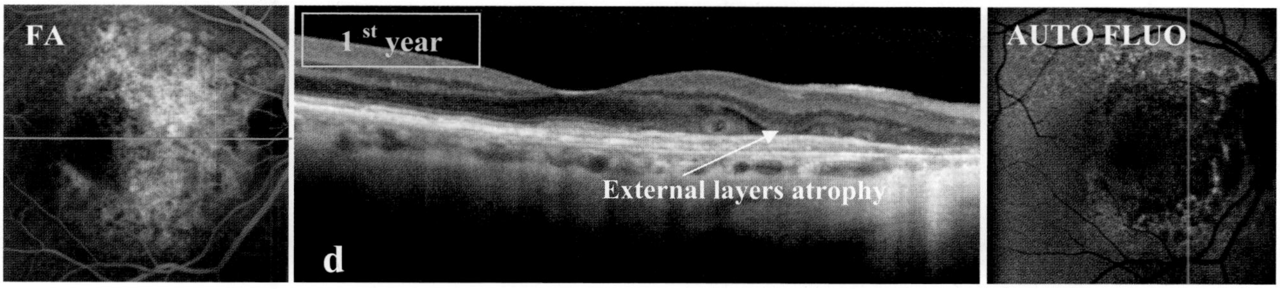

Figure 8: Large classic CNV. VA: 20/63. Thickness (*Spectralis**): 232 µm.
d): Three months after stopping treatment: atrophy of outer retinal layers in the zone between the optic disc and the macula (*arrow*). The external limiting membrane and IS/OS interface were visible in the foveal zone. A fine hyper-reflective band was still present anterior to the RPE.

CLINICAL CASE No. 02: LARGE CLASSIC CNV

ENLARGED IMAGES

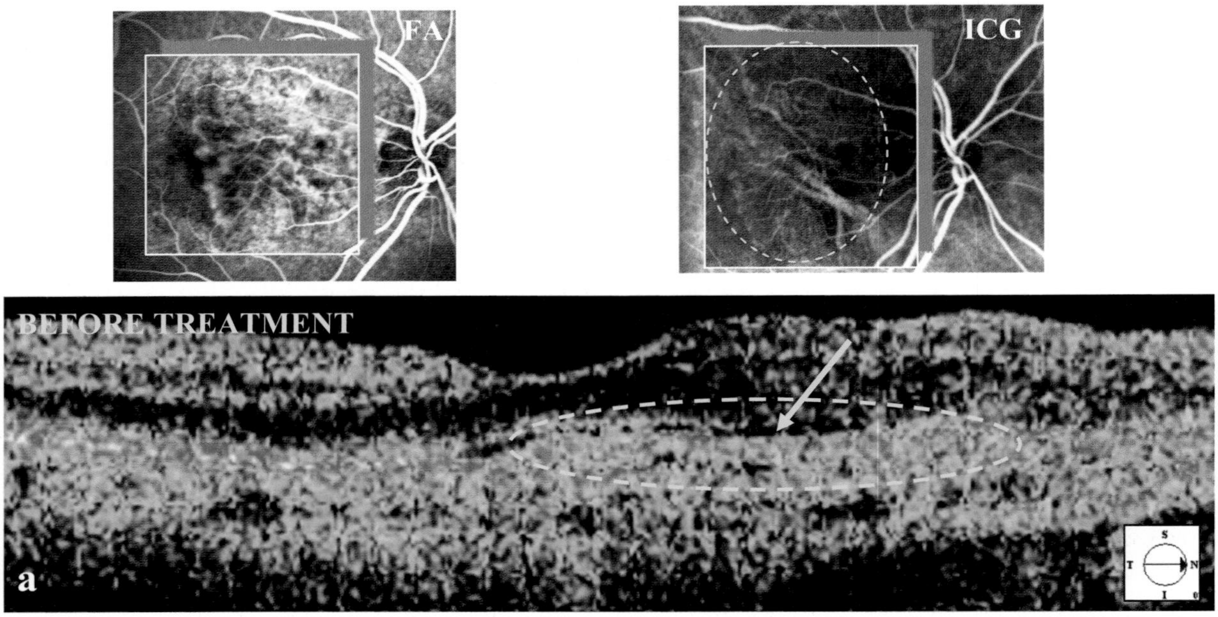

Figure 9: Large classic CNV (enlarged view of Figure 7).
***Stratus** horizontal section: first examination.**
Presence of subfoveal hyper-reflective material anterior to the RPE, extending to the optic disc and distinct from the RPE (*oval and arrow*). Diffuse intraretinal fluid with increased retinal thickness, confirming the angiography findings.

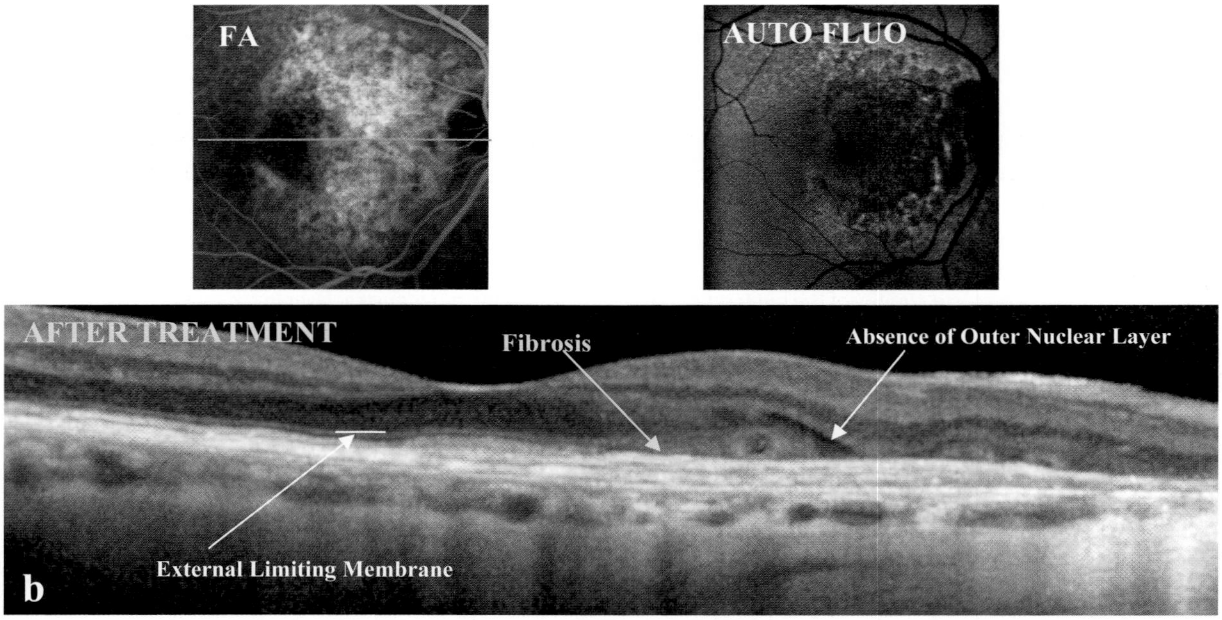

Figure 10: Large classic CNV (enlarged view of Figure 8d).
***Spectralis** horizontal section: last examination.**
Regression of intraretinal fluid. The external limiting membrane was visible except in the region between the optic disc and the macula, where all of the outer retinal layers had completely disappeared, particularly the outer nuclear layer (*arrow*).
Presence of a residual, linear, hyper-reflective band anterior to the RPE, suggestive of fibrosis of the classic CNV.

Conclusion

- **Fluorescein angiography** provides major, easy to interpret, and a recognized source of information for the diagnosis of ***classic choroidal neovascularization.***

It demonstrates the neovascular membrane, its afferent and efferent branches, its anastomotic arcade, and the characteristic *fluorescein leakage* (when at least one early frame and one late frame are available).

Fluorescein angiography has therefore become the "gold standard" for the diagnosis and localization of classic choroidal neovascularization.

- **Time-Domain OCT** has rapidly acquired an important role, as it is easy to perform and allows almost intuitive interpretation of the main findings.

Classic CNV is usually visualized as a spindle-shaped hyper-reflective subretinal band anterior to and in contact with the RPE (**Figure 9**).

This band is accompanied by an *exudative reaction*, easily identified as a subretinal optically empty zone associated with diffuse intraretinal fluid and cysts that can become large.

Variations of intraretinal fluid can be easily compared by following retinal thickness (central or in various sectors in the macular region).

TD-OCT has therefore become a first-line test to evaluate response to treatment.

- However, TD-OCT findings must be confirmed by angiograph–not only in unclear and difficult cases–but also for decision making.

This is particularly helpful when deciding whether to continue intravitreous injections, the intervals between injections, and when treatment should be stopped.

Other imaging modalities also provide complementary data that are useful to establish a precise diagnosis, and to more accurately follow the natural history or the response to treatment.

These other imaging modalities can also help identify those cases with a good prognosis ("*good responders*") and those more difficult cases requiring more complex treatments.

- **SLO-ICG angiography** therefore appears to be essential to determine whether classic CNV is isolated or associated with occult CNV, either at presentation or subsequently.

ICG angiography is also important to identify polypoidal formations and its accompanying abnormal choroidal vascular membrane.

Another use of ICG angiography is in the detection of chorioretinal anastomosis within a hot spot and with intense leakage.

- The more recently available **SD-OCT imaging** provides more information for the demonstration of classic choroidal neovascularization.

SD-OCT confirms the typical features of CNV such as:
- The absence of a PED,
- The pre-RPE site of classic CNV, and
- Intraretinal leakage.

SD-OCT also allows visualization of the outer retinal layers and can therefore detect alterations of photoreceptors (inner segments/outer segments) and the outer nuclear layer (**Figure 10**).

These structures are profoundly altered by proliferation of classic CNV, but their presence or reappearance are excellent **markers of a favorable outcome.**

Complete resolution of hyper-reflective classic CNV or, on the contrary, persistence of more or less intense subretinal fibrosis are usually well-correlated with visual acuity.

- SD-OCT, when **correlated** with the various imaging modalities, is particularly useful in classic choroidal neovascularization to:
  - Confirm whether classic CNV is isolated or associated with occult CNV,
  - Monitor the response to treatment, and
  - Determine the frequency and duration of IVT injections.

Atrophic Forms (Dry AMD)

Clinical Features and OCT Follow-Up

Gabriel COSCAS
Florence COSCAS, Sabrina VISMARA,
Alain ZOURDANI, C.I. Li CALZI

(Créteil and Paris)

Atrophic Forms (Dry AMD)

Clinical Features and OCT Follow-Up

Introduction

Definitions

Atrophic form or "Dry AMD" is defined by areas of RPE atrophy, often resulting from regression of confluent soft drusen.

These **areas of atrophy**, usually perifoveal, gradually spread to become confluent, forming a partial, then complete ring, and finally involving the center of the macula.

At this stage, the visual symptoms, initially moderate and related to a paracentral scotoma, suddenly deteriorate with marked loss of visual acuity because the fovea is no longer spared.

The **primary RPE lesion** is associated with alteration, then obliteration of the underlying choriocapillaris, and death of photoreceptors in the zones of RPE atrophy.

These **areas of atrophy** generally present with clearly demarcated, irregularly shaped margins ("geographic atrophy"). They are frequently highlighted by a hyperpigmented border in the junctional zone. Accumulation of lipofuscin in this area results in accentuated autofluorescence.

Histologically, RPE atrophy is accompanied by a loss of the outer nuclear layer, and the outer plexiform layer becomes in direct contact with *basal laminar deposits.*

Complications

Atrophy therefore constitutes one of the major complications of age-related maculopathy (ARM or precursor stage) which progresses to age-related macular degeneration.

Dry AMD is characterized by the absence of an exudative reaction.

However, **choroidal neovascularization** can occur at any time during the course, usually on the foveal margin of an area of atrophy.

Deterioration of visual impairment therefore may not only be directly correlated with extension of atrophy but also to CNV proliferation.

This justifies a complete imaging assessment whenever a patient with already diagnosed dry AMD experiences a deterioration of visual acuity.

There are several possible causes of atrophy.

- **Geographic atrophy** is the most common form. This term refers to all types of RPE atrophy, which extend and progressively coalesce and cause degeneration of overlying photoreceptors.

These lesions are well-delineated and sometimes present with irregular "geographical" contours.

Atrophic areas, derived from degeneration of **drusen,** are initially isolated and perifoveal. They then gradually enlarge to form areas measuring 1/4 to 1/2 DD with retinal pigment migrations.

Areas of atrophy slowly become organized all around the fovea, initially with **central sparing.** Slow involvement of the central fovea follows, which results in severe loss of visual acuity. These lesions are often *bilateral* and *symmetrical* but not necessarily simultaneous.

- **RPE tears** can lead to the formation of an atrophic area in the zone exposed by retraction of the retinal pigment epithelium.
- **Loss of vitelliform material**, replaced by a zone of macular atrophy, is another way dry AMD may develop. There is sometimes residual vitelliform material around the edges associated with this type of atrophy.

Frequency

The frequency of dry AMD is much higher than suggested by the first studies, which were conducted in tertiary care centers.
General population studies tend to show that dry AMD is just as frequent as wet AMD.

The incidence of dry AMD with **severe loss of visual acuity** is poorly-defined, but appears to be at least half as frequent as severe forms of wet AMD.

Biomicroscopy

Biomicroscopic examination can visualize the first stages of RPE depigmentation.

The extent and location of typical areas of atrophy, which may be associated with retinal pigment migration and drusen, can be easily identified (**Figures 1a, b, and c**).

Fluorescein Angiography

Atrophic areas induce progressive **hyper-fluorescence** due to well-demarcated transmission defects that persist in the late phases but remain without fluorescein leakage.

A pigmented border is often visible and a few large choroidal vessels may sometimes be seen on the late phases.

The RPE surrounding the lesions is altered with irregular hyper-fluorescence and retinal pigment migrations (**Figures 1d and e**).

Indocyanine Green Angiography

The screen formed by the normal RPE is attenuated in infrared light. However, loss of RPE allows visualization of the rare, but persistently perfused choroidal vessels that may cross beneath these areas.

In the late phases, RPE atrophy is characterized by slight hypo-fluorescence (**Figures 1f and g**).

The course of dry AMD may be complicated by choroidal neovascularization, particularly at the foveal margins. CNV is clearly visible on SLO-ICG angiography.

Contribution of OCT

OCT constitutes an easy-to-use imaging modality for follow-up and detection of complications of dry AMD that must subsequently be confirmed by angiography.

Time-Domain OCT

The intense **back-shadowing** in zones of atrophy, extending well into the choroid, is the defining sign of atrophy. This is easily demonstrated on multiple TD-OCT sections. This shadowing usually masks the thinning and/or loss of the RPE.

- The second diagnostic sign is **thinning of the neurosensory retina** over zones of atrophy, which is particularly serious when it involves the central zone.

Thinning of the central retina correlates well with loss of central visual acuity.

On closer examination, loss of the hypo-reflective layer corresponding to the outer nuclear layer can be seen.

- The third important feature is the **absence of exudative signs.**

Any increase in retinal thickness at the edge of a zone of atrophy must raise the suspicion of a neovascular complication.

Spectral-Domain OCT

The signs described above are easily demonstrated on SD-OCT. In addition, the following attributes can be seen:

- Thinning and loss of the RPE are clearly visualized, but maintenance of the straight line representing Bruch's membrane is an important sign.
- The *external limiting membrane* and *IS/OS interface* are severely altered and/or no longer visible and become disrupted early.
- In the most severe forms, the *outer nuclear layer* is no longer visible in the zones of atrophy.
- The *outer plexiform layer* comes directly in contact with Bruch's membrane. This accounts for thinning of the neurosensory retina, while the inner retinal layers may remain relatively unchanged.

Prognosis

RPE atrophy is irreversible and causes death of almost all **photoreceptors** in the atrophic area, resulting in a corresponding scotoma.

Due to the current absence of effective treatment, dry AMD has a poor prognosis despite the hopes raised by a recent clinical trial (AREDS study), which demonstrated the benefits of antioxidants, vitamin A, and vitamin C supplements.

Future research includes ongoing studies on micro-nutrition and as well as RPE transplantation procedures.

DRY AGE-RELATED MACULAR DEGENERATION SPARING THE FOVEA

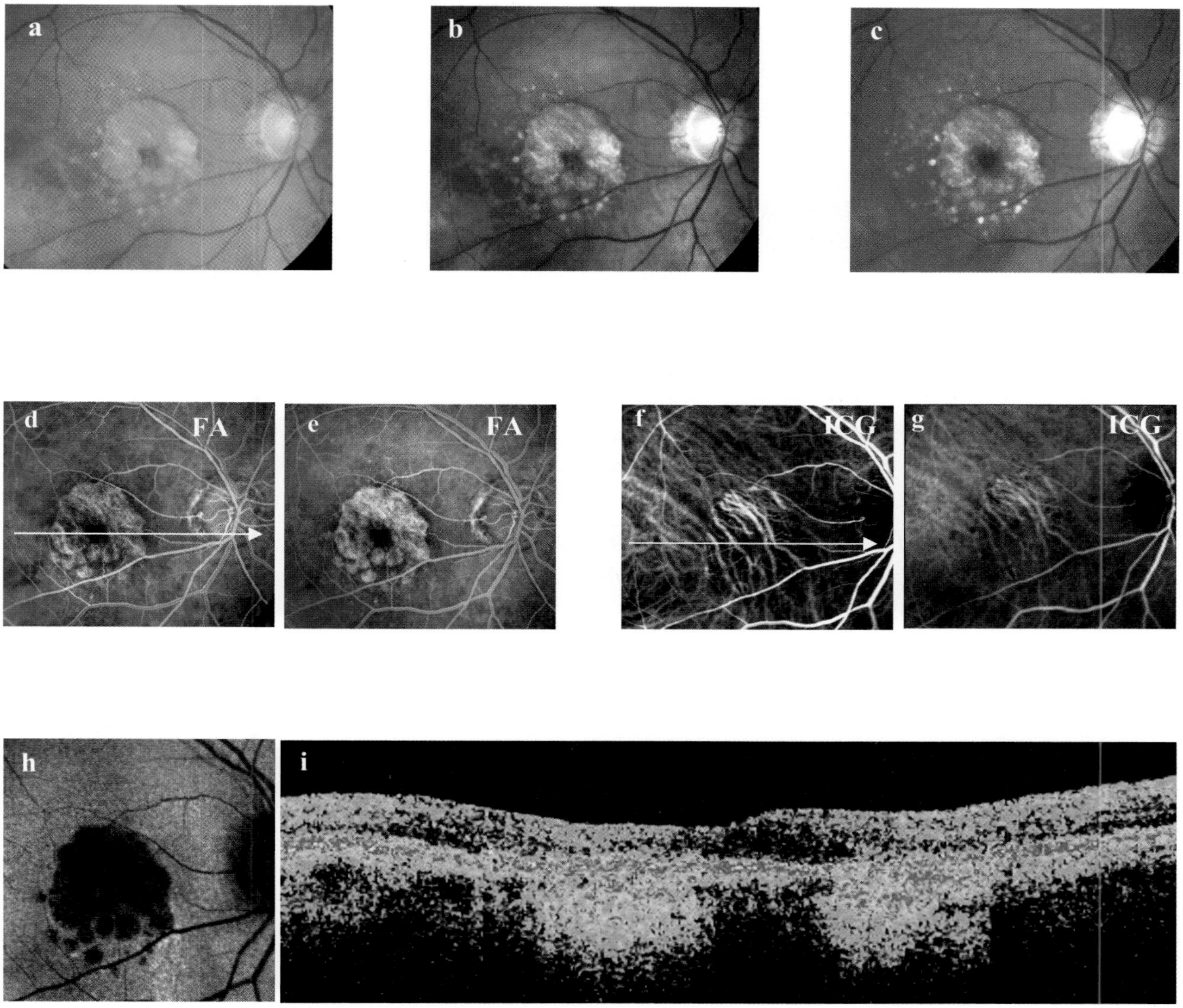

Figure 1: Dry age-related macular degeneration sparing the fovea.

a, b, and c): Color, red-free, and blue: rounded, slightly irregular, de-pigmented area with well-defined margins. In the center can be seen a small, darker central zone in which xanthophyll pigment is preserved.

d and e): Fluorescein angiography: progressive hyper-fluorescence due to a transmission defect and central sparing. Note a few soft drusen in the inferior part.

f and g): SLO-ICG angiography: note the more marked visibility of choroidal vessels in the zone of atrophy.

h): Autofluorescence: marked hypo-fluorescence in the entire zone of atrophy and atrophic drusen in inferior sectors. No zones of hyper-autofluorescence.

i): OCT: marked hyper-reflectivity extending posteriorly to the choroid with retinal thinning in the entire zone of atrophy. There is a central zone which spares the RPE and xanthophyll pigment with shadowing.

CLINICAL CASES OF DRY AMD

CLINICAL CASE No. 01: DRY AMD: INITIAL STAGE

Area of juxtafoveal atrophy with progressive extension and increasing functional repercussions.

Follow-up by SD-OCT .... Page 348

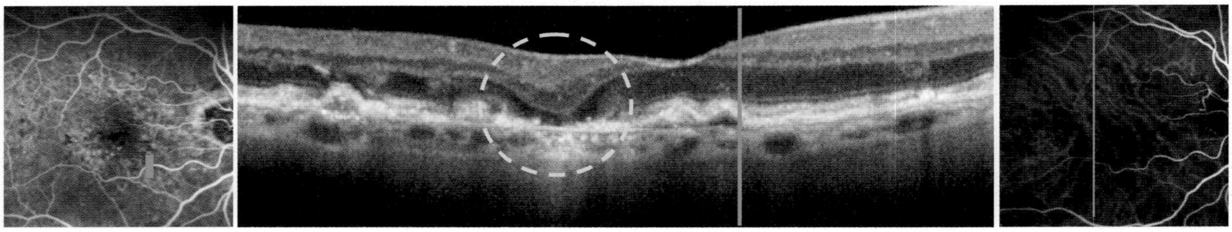

CLINICAL CASE No. 02: DRY AMD: EARLY EXTRAFOVEAL FORM

Areas of localized and nonconfluent juxtafoveal atrophy.

Spectral-Domain OCT examination .... Page 352

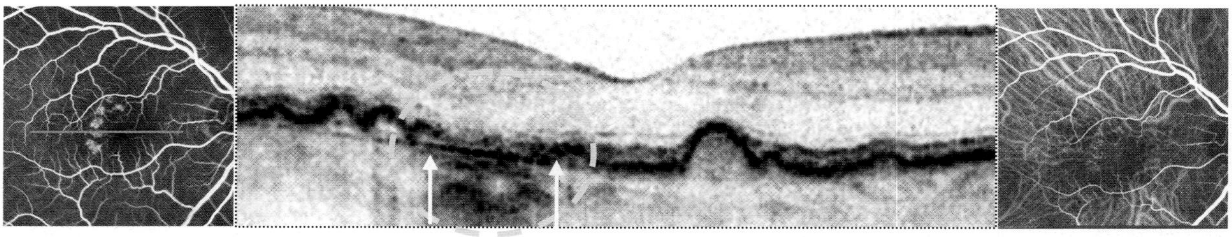

CLINICAL CASE No. 03: DRY AMD: ADVANCED PERIFOVEAL AND SUBFOVEAL FORM

Extensive and almost confluent areas of perifoveal and subfoveal atrophy.

Spectral-Domain OCT examination .... Page 354

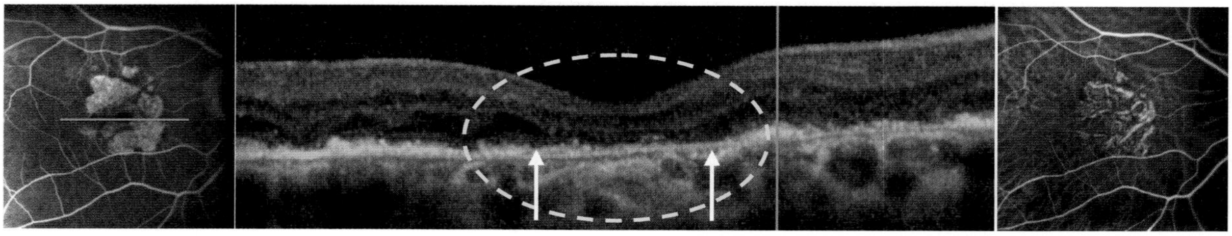

CLINICAL CASES OF DRY AMD

CLINICAL CASE No. 04: MACULAR ATROPHY FOLLOWING RPE TEAR

Vascularized pigment epithelium detachment with an old large tear and atrophy in the zone of RPE retraction.

TD-OCT and SD-OCT examination .... Page 356

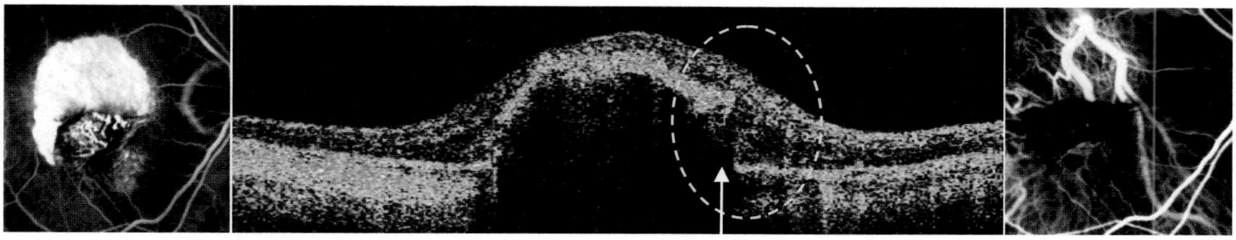

CLINICAL CASE No. 05: MACULAR ATROPHY DUE TO VITELLIFORM MACULAR DYSTROPHY

Bilateral, asymmetrical adult-onset vitelliform macular dystrophy progressing to atrophy

TD-OCT and SD-OCT examination .... Page 360

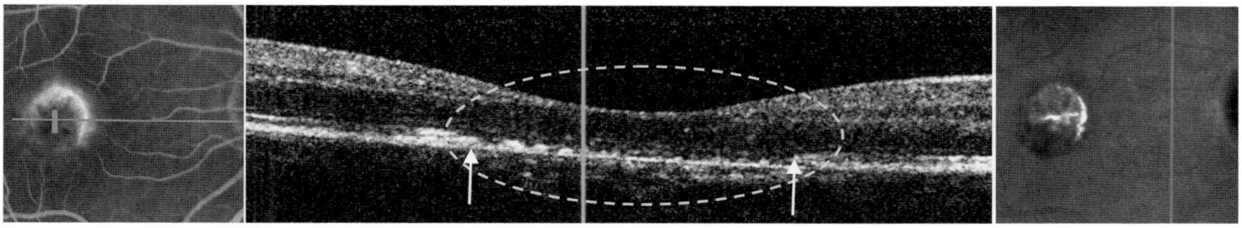

CLINICAL CASE No. 06: MACULAR ATROPHY DUE TO VITELLIFORM MACULAR DYSTROPHY

Bilateral, asymmetrical adult-onset vitelliform macular dystrophy progressing to atrophy

SD-OCT examination .... Page 362

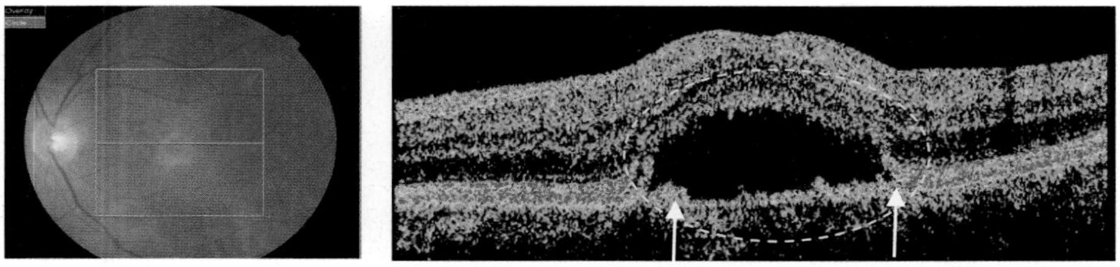

CLINICAL CASE No. 01: Dry AMD: Initial Stage

Area of juxtafoveal atrophy with progressive extension and increasing functional repercussions. Follow-up by SD-OCT.

Clinical Signs

An 89-year-old woman with precursor signs of AMD had been regularly followed for 3 years with a moderate decline in visual acuity. She did not have any metamorphopsias, but her vision was consistently deteriorating, and she was having difficult with reading.
VA RE: 20/80 - VA LE: 20/80.

Biomicroscopic Examination

Fairly numerous disseminated drusen of various sizes located away from the center. A depigmented grayish 1/3 DD area with a dark peripheral border was observed in the paracentral and inferior juxtafoveal region.

Autofluorescence

Numerous, irregularly shaped bright hyper-fluorescent spots, forming several parts of a network, especially in the region between the optic disk and the macula (**Figures 2a and b**).

Fluorescein Angiography (Figures 2c and d)

Several soft drusen, which slowly stained. The juxtafoveal area presented slight late hyper-fluorescence without fluorescein leakage.

SLO-ICG Angiography (Figures 2e and f)

Few abnormalities in the central macular region apart from several disseminated soft drusen.

Visualization of choroidal vessels in the central region, which were crossed by large veins. The small choroidal vessels were only visible in the superior temporal sector.

Suggested Diagnosis:

Poorly contrasted, poorly-delineated area of initial RPE atrophy, possibly related to regression of a group of drusen.

Contribution of OCT (*Spectralis**)

Horizontal section

The section, slightly off-centered inferiorly, demonstrated a normal retinal profile with decreased thickness of 218 µm (*Spectralis**).

The RPE also showed numerous irregularities with small drusen.

In particular, highly suggestive, but diffuse and non-localized thinning of the RPE was observed in the central and paracentral zone.

Vertical section

The off-centered section visualized the atrophic zone (detected by biomicroscopy and monochromatic films). The external limiting membrane was readily visible almost everywhere on this section and was raised by numerous drusen.
In the de-pigmented area (marked by the calliper), the IS/OS interface and external limiting membrane were no longer visible. They were replaced by a moderately dense zone masking the outer nuclear layer which was otherwise normal (*circle*).

Diagnosis

The OCT examination demonstrated minor changes at this stage, with moderate thinning of the retina, relative thinning of the RPE, and localized damage to the IS/OS interface and external limiting membrane.
These changes were localized to the small area of RPE depigmentation, more clearly visible on biomicroscopy and monochromatic films than on angiography.
These alterations, associated with reduction in the density of centrally located drusen, suggested the presence of early RPE. In the absence of any exudative signs, it was decided to regularly follow-up the patient, who was offered continued use of AREDS formulated supplements.
SD-OCT demonstrated thinning then atrophy of the RPE, localized disappearance of the IS/OS interface and *external limiting membrane*, followed by loss of the *outer nuclear layer*. This brought the outer plexiform layer directly in contact with Bruch's membrane, with localized loss of photoreceptors.

CLINICAL CASE No. 01: DRY AMD: INITIAL STAGE

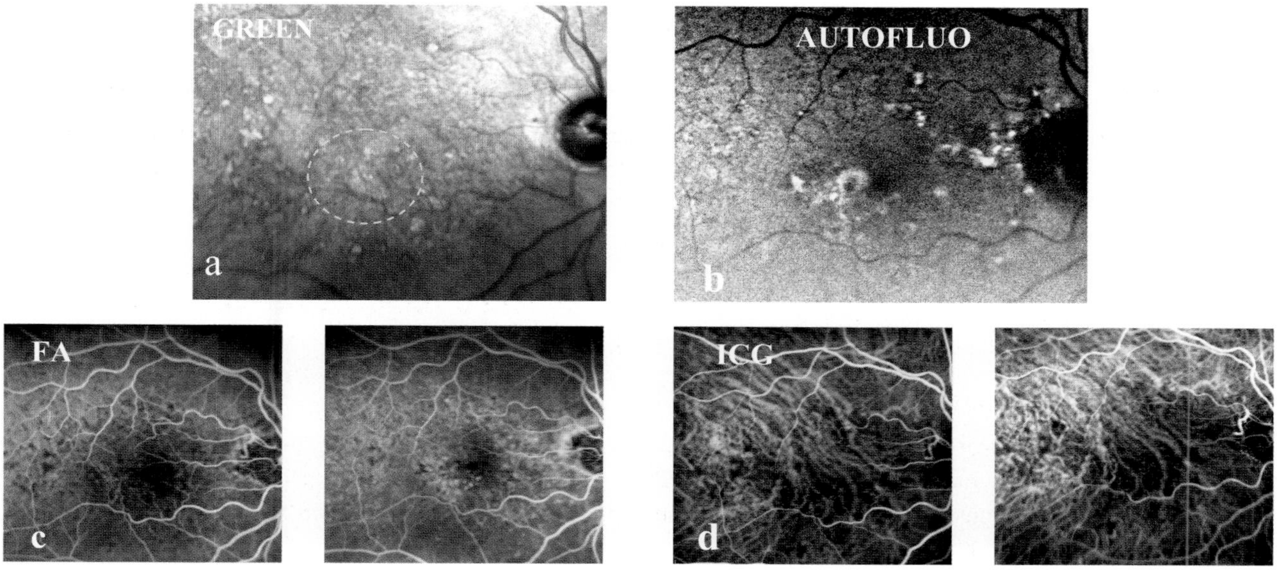

Figure 2: Dry AMD: initial stage. VA: 20/80.
a and b): Red-free and autofluorescence: disseminated drusen of various sizes located away from the center. A de-pigmented grayish 1/3 DD area with a dark peripheral border can be seen in the paracentral and inferior juxtafoveal region (*circle*).
Autofluorescence: numerous, irregularly disposed hyper-fluorescent spots in the region between the optic disc and the macula.
c): Fluorescein angiography: juxtafoveal area with slight late hyper-fluorescence without fluorescein leakage.
d): SLO-ICG angiography: disseminated soft drusen. Reduction of choroidal vessels in the central region, which was only crossed by large veins with no smaller choroidal vessels.

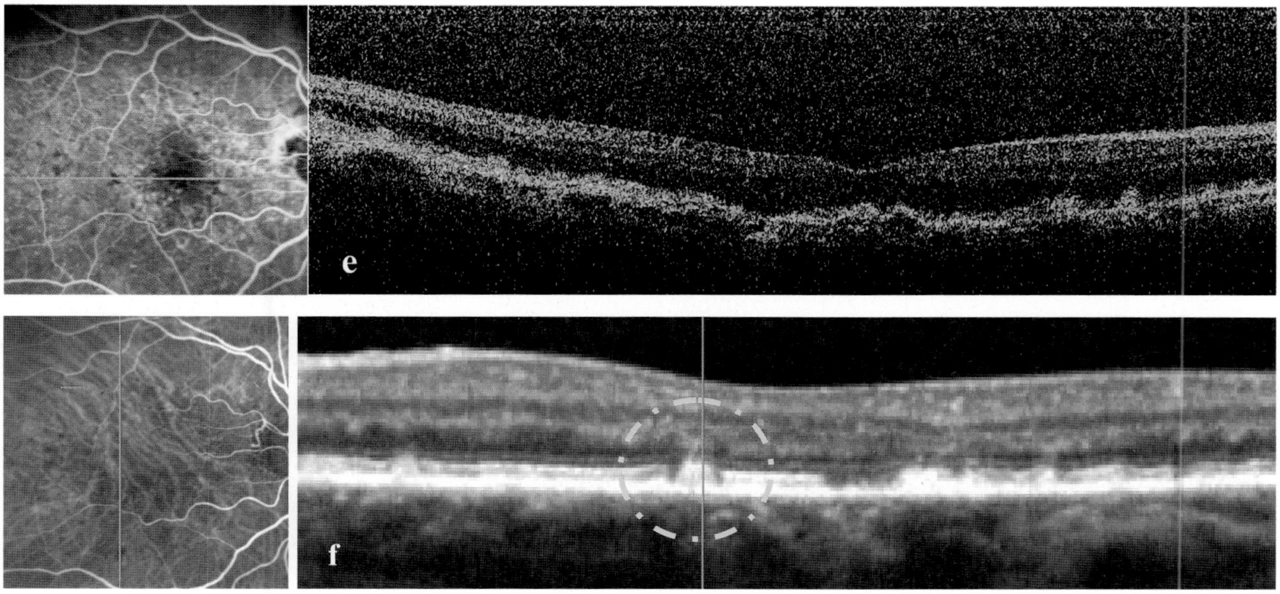

Figure 2: Dry AMD: initial stage. VA: 20/80 (same patient).
e): Horizontal section: normal retinal profile but with decreased thickness. The RPE presented numerous irregularities with small drusen. Highly suggestive, but diffuse and non-localized thinning of the RPE in the central and paracentral zone. Central retinal thickness: 218 μm.
f): Vertical section: The external limiting membrane was readily visible almost everywhere and was raised by numerous drusen. In the de-pigmented area (marked by the calliper), the IS/OS interface and external limiting membrane were no longer visible and were replaced by a moderately dense zone masking the outer nuclear layer, which was otherwise normal (*circle*).

CLINICAL CASE No. 01: DRY AMD: INITIAL STAGE

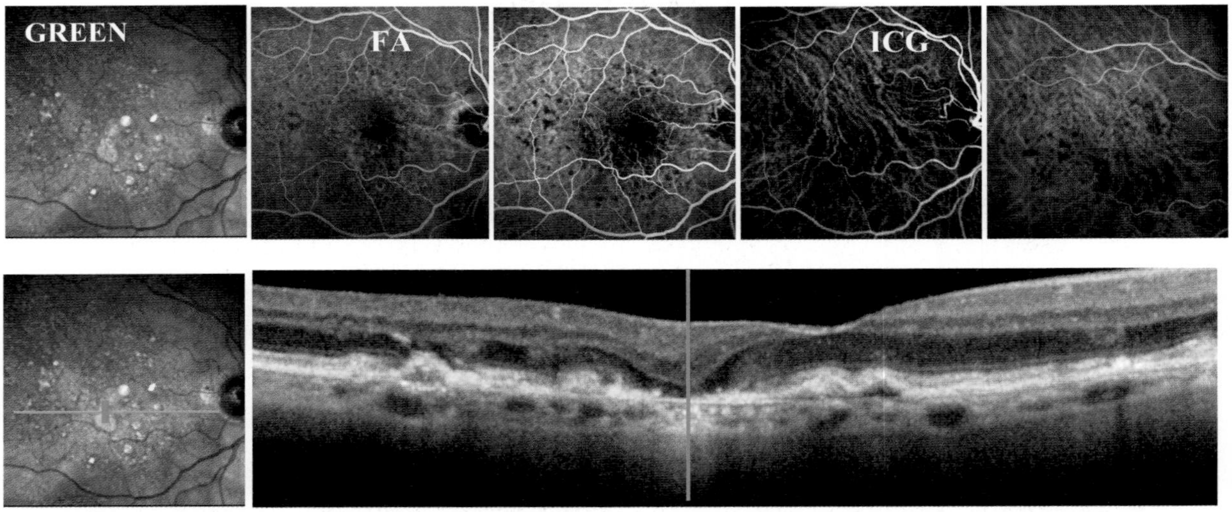

Figure 3: Dry AMD: six months later (same patient as in Figure 1). VA: 20/100.

***Spectralis** horizontal section**: localized juxtafoveal atrophy in the de-pigmented area of the RPE, which was now clearly visible. In this zone, the outer retinal layers were no longer visible, apart from the outer nuclear layer.
Note the hypertrophy of the RPE at the edges of the atrophy and the alterations of the outer retinal layers over each large drusen.

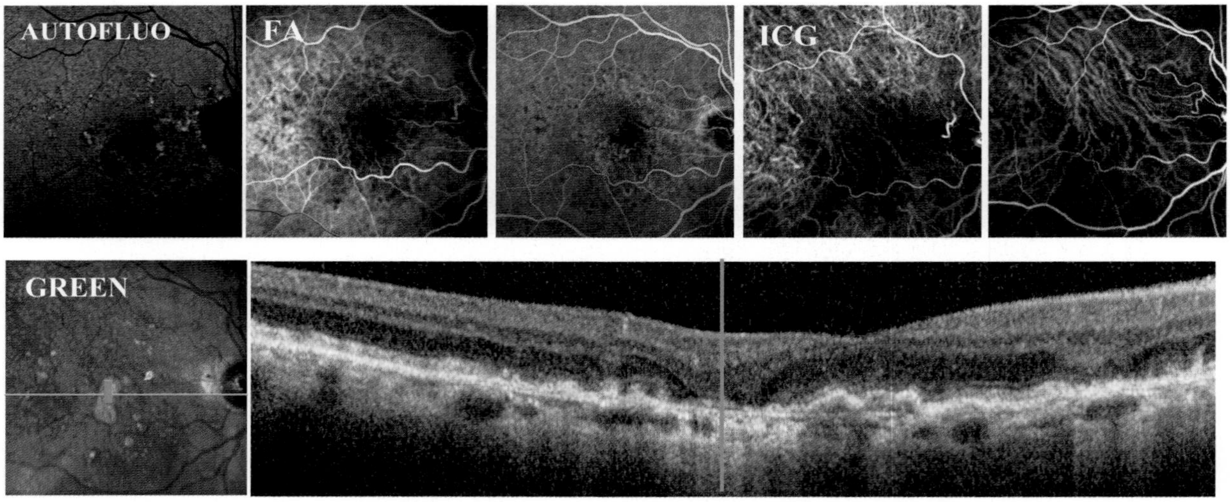

Figure 4: Dry AMD: one year later (same patient as in Figure 1). VA: 20/100.

***Spectralis** horizontal section**: the area of atrophy was slightly larger and the outer nuclear layer had completely disappeared in this zone, which induced a juxtafoveal scotoma that interfered with reading.

CLINICAL CASE No. 01: DRY AMD: INITIAL STAGE

ENLARGED IMAGES

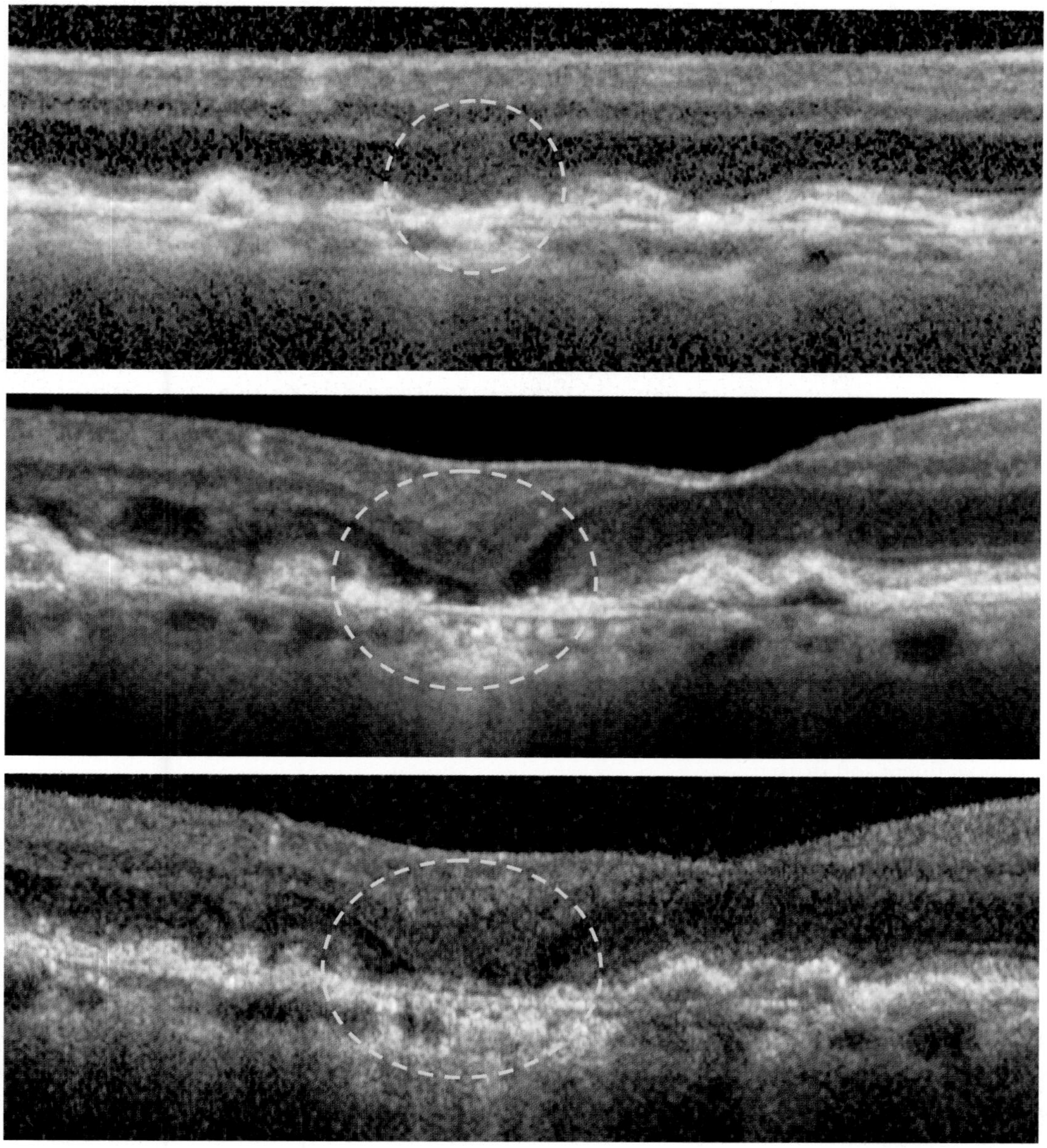

Figure 5: Dry AMD: Enlarged images of Figures 2, 3, and 4 (same patient).

At this Stage

Comparison of images on 3 successive examinations over a period of 1 year clearly demonstrated the causes of decreased visual acuity and difficulty with reading: appearance of a small area of **juxtafoveal atrophy** was barely visible on biomicroscopy but was detected by autofluorescence.

CLINICAL CASE No. 02: Dry AMD: Early Extrafoveal Form

Areas of localized and nonconfluent juxtafoveal atrophy.
Spectral-Domain OCT examination.

Clinical Signs

An 82-year-old woman, regularly followed for AMD for 3 years, presented for a check-up due to a moderate decline in visual acuity without metamorphopsias.

VA RE: 20/40 - VA LE: 20/40.

Biomicroscopic Examination

Five round, irregular, whitish, nonconfluent 1/5 DD spots without a peripheral border were observed in the paracentral and temporal extrafoveal region. Fairly numerous hard drusen were observed further away from the center.

Autofluorescence

The same dark spots were surrounded by a large number of autofluorescent spots (**Figures 6a and b**).

Fluorescein Angiography

Progressive hyper-fluorescence of each of the atrophic spots due to abnormal transmission without fluorescein leakage (**Figure 6c**).

SLO-ICG Angiography

The same spots were observed on SLO-ICG angiography together with subfoveal hyper-fluorescence, reflecting extension of the lesions towards the central region (**Figure 6d**).

Suggested Diagnosis:
Nonconfluent areas of extrafoveal RPE atrophy, apparently isolated and without an exudative reaction.

12

Contribution of OCT (*Spectralis**)

Horizontal section

The RPE was clearly visible with normal thickness on either side of the fovea. Multiple peaks corresponded to the presence of nonconfluent soft drusen.

In the zone corresponding to the small and *de-pigmented areas*, the RPE was atrophic and no longer visible. Only the straight line of Bruch's membrane was observed with *hyper-reflectivity* extending a long way posteriorly, only in the extrafoveal area.

Anterior to the RPE, the external limiting membrane and the IS/OS interface were initially clearly visible, but were disrupted over the area of atrophy, where the outer nuclear layer also disappeared.

This brought the outer plexiform layer in contact with Bruch's membrane and confirmed the localized atrophy of the RPE and photoreceptors in this zone (**Figure 7a**).

The signs of damage to the outer retinal layers extended as far as the subfoveal region, but were less marked and spared the outer nuclear layer.

These alterations of the subfoveal region were well correlated with the ICG angiography findings.

Oblique section (Figure 7b)

This section also clearly demonstrated the same features of atrophic zones with an only slightly altered juxtafoveal region.

Conclusion

SD-OCT examination of this clinical case presented multiple, small, and nonconfluent **areas of extrafoveal atrophy**, which confirmed the findings of the other imaging modalities (monochromatic, autofluorescence).
SD-OCT confirmed the presence of a small number of soft drusen, poorly visible on fundus examination. They were adjacent to areas of atrophy (probably related to regression of pre-existing drusen).

SD-OCT allowed detailed analysis of the degree of alteration of the outer layers. Changes in the foveal region accounted for the progressive decline in central visual acuity. Finally, SD-OCT confirmed the absence of a PED and other signs of exudation.

CLINICAL CASE No. 02: DRY AMD: EARLY EXTRAFOVEAL FORM

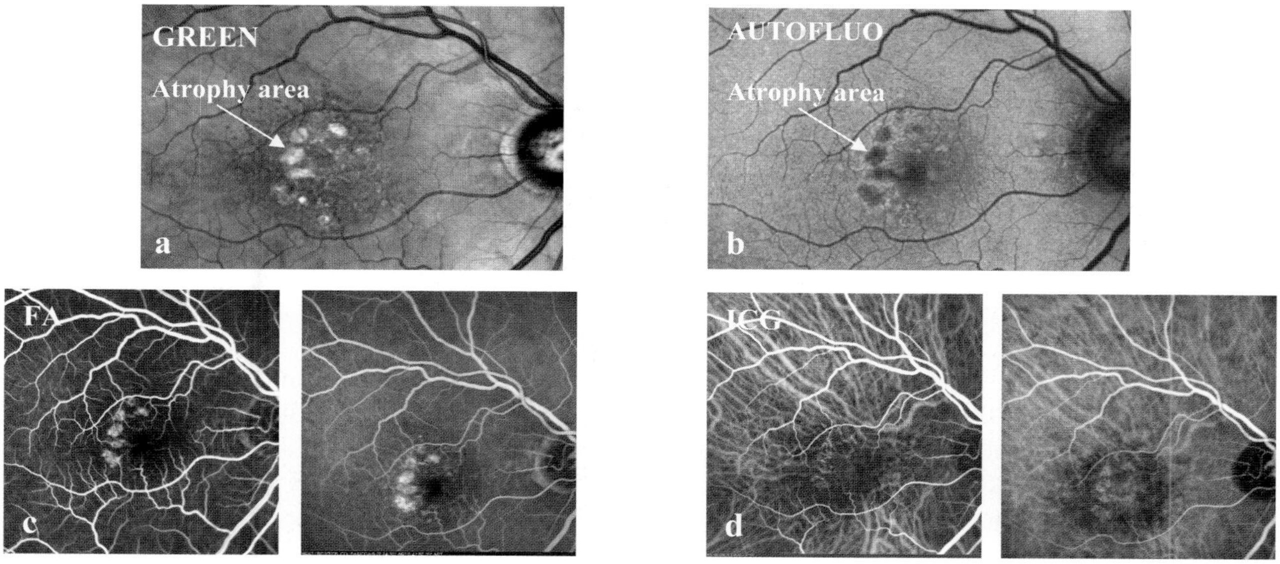

Figure 6: Early extrafoveal dry AMD. VA: 20/40.
a and b): Red-free and autofluorescence: five, round, irregular, whitish, nonconfluent spots. On autofluorescence, the same dark, hypo-fluorescent spots were surrounded by a large number of autofluorescent spots.
c): Fluorescein angiography: hyper-fluorescence of each of the spots due to abnormal transmission with no fluorescein leakage.
d): SLO-ICG angiography: the same spots were observed, together with subfoveal hyper-fluorescence, which reflected extension of the lesions towards the central region.

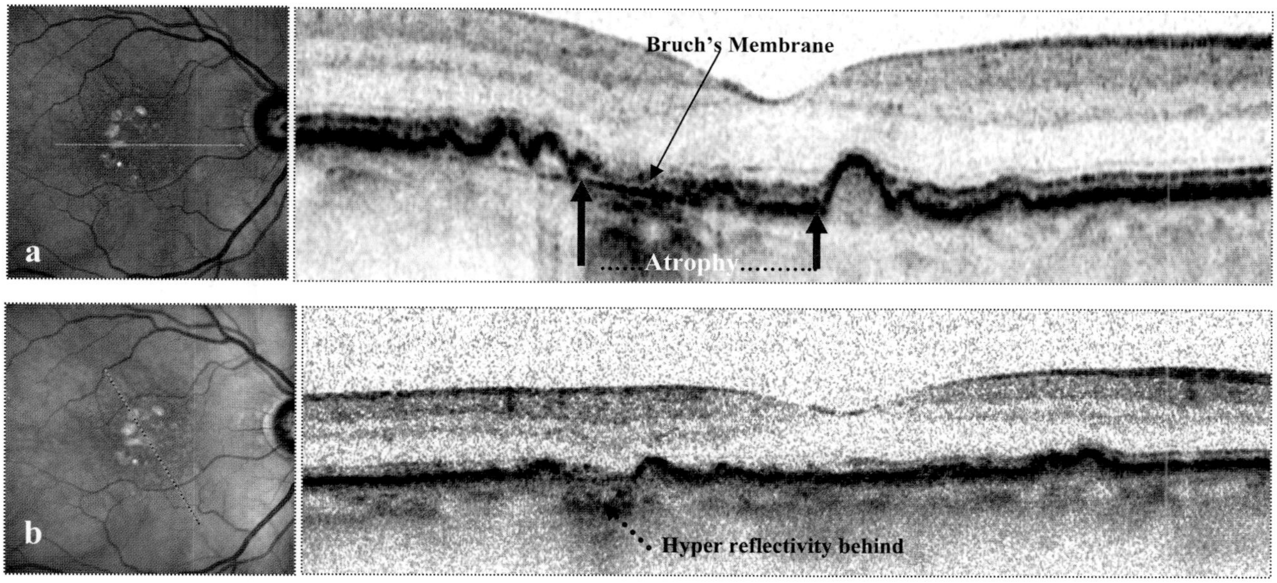

Figure 7: Early extrafoveal dry AMD. VA: 20/40.
a): Horizontal section: the RPE was clearly visible with numerous drusen. Atrophy of the RPE over the hyper-fluorescent spots and visibility of the straight line of Bruch's membrane with marked back-shadowing.
Anterior to the RPE, the external limiting membrane and IS/OS interface were clearly visible and were disrupted over the area of atrophy. Disruption of the external limiting membrane and IS/OS interface and especially loss of the outer nuclear layer. The outer plexiform layer was in contact with Bruch's membrane. Note that signs of outer layer damage extended as far as the subfoveal region.
b): Vertical section: demonstration of one of the atrophic zones. The juxtafoveal region was only slightly altered.

CLINICAL CASE No. 03: Dry AMD: Advanced Perifoveal and Subfoveal Form

Extensive and almost confluent areas of perifoveal and subfoveal atrophy.
Spectral-Domain OCT examination.

Clinical Signs

An 80-year-old man presented with slowly progressive bilateral decline of visual acuity over many months. Symptoms predominantly affected his right eye with no metamorphopsias, but there were multiple central microscotomas which interfered with reading.
VA RE: 20/200 - VA LE: 20/125.

Biomicroscopic Examination

Multiple, round, but irregular and almost confluent whitish areas, measuring 1/3 DD, with a slightly darker peripheral border forming an incomplete ring and a juxtafoveolar central spot in the macular region. A few shiny hard drusen were also observed.

Autofluorescence

The same spots were dark, hypo-fluorescent, and surrounded by several fine autofluorescent spots (**Figures 8a and b**).

Fluorescein Angiography

Fluorescein angiography showed progressive hyper-fluorescence of each of the atrophic spots due to abnormal transmission without fluorescein leakage. Persistence of residual xanthophyll pigment in the central region (**Figure 8c**).

ICG Angiography

The same spots were observed on SLO-ICG angiography with abnormal visibility of the large choroidal vessels. Spots appeared to be larger and almost confluent, suggesting that the more or less intense lesions occupied almost all of the macular zone (**Figure 8d**).

Suggested Diagnosis:
Almost confluent areas of perifoveal RPE atrophy with minimal foveal sparing but apparently isolated with no exudative reaction.

12

Contribution of OCT (*Spectralis**)

Horizontal section

The RPE was irregular, with small localized zones of proliferation, and areas in which the RPE was no longer visible. This was particularly apparent in the foveal region where only Bruch's membrane remained clearly visible.

This subfoveal area was associated with marked **backshadowing**.

Anterior to the RPE, the *IS/OS interface* was not visualized, and the *external limiting membrane* (occasionally visible) was absent over the area of atrophy.

Anterior to the RPE, the outer nuclear layer was also absent, bringing the outer plexiform layer in contact with Bruch's membrane and confirming localized atrophy of RPE and photoreceptors in this zone (**Figures 9a and b**).

Signs of outer retinal layer damage extending beyond the central zone with numerous irregularities and jagged portions in the outer nuclear layer. These various alterations of the subfoveal region were well-correlated with ICG angiography findings. Central retinal thickness was 160 μm (**Figures 9a and b**).

Conclusion

This case presented multiple areas of fairly extensive and almost confluent **subfoveal atrophy**.

The SD-OCT examination confirmed the findings of the other imaging modalities (monochromatic, autofluorescence, and angiography) and demonstrated the presence of several residual hard drusen.

SD-OCT provided detailed analysis of the degree of alteration of outer retinal layers, not only on areas of atrophy, but also in the foveal region.

These alterations accounted for the progressive and marked loss of central visual acuity. Finally, SD-OCT confirmed the absence of an exudative reaction or PED.

CLINICAL CASE No. 03: DRY AMD: ADVANCED PERIFOVEAL AND SUBFOVEAL FORM

Extensive and almost confluent areas of perifoveal and subfoveal atrophy.
Spectral-Domain OCT examination.

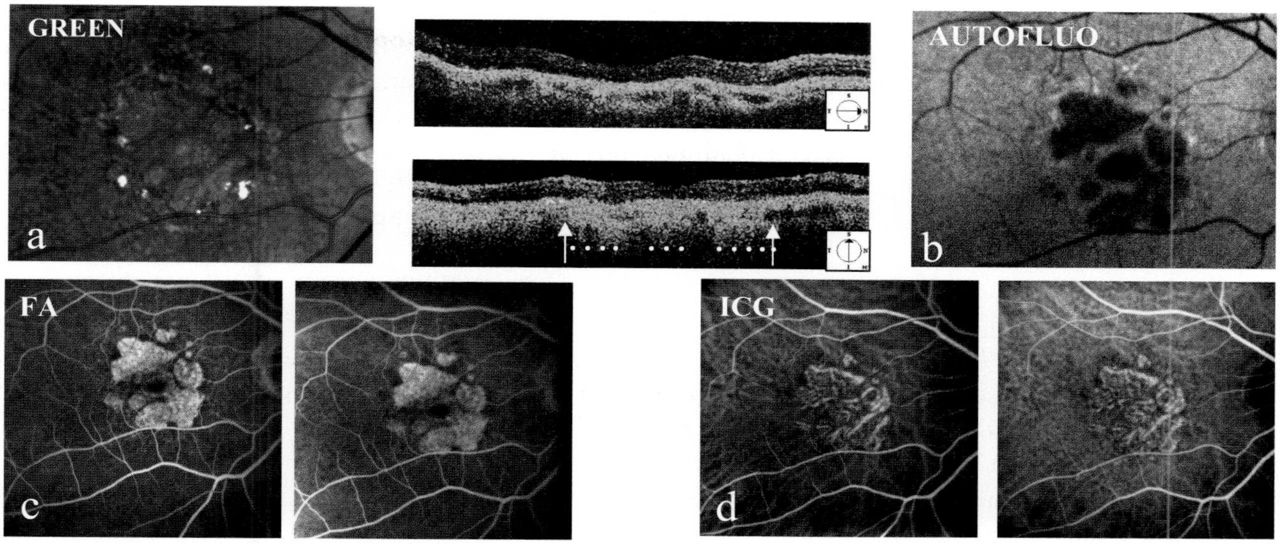

Figure 8: Dry AMD: advanced perifoveal and subfoveal form. VA: 20/200.
a and b): Red-free and autofluorescence: multiple, round, but irregular and almost confluent whitish areas formed an incomplete ring and a juxtafoveolar central spot. A few shiny hard drusen were present all around these lesions.
On autofluorescence, the same spots were dark and hypo-fluorescent with several fine autofluorescent spots.
c): Fluorescein angiography: progressive hyper-fluorescence of each of the spots due to abnormal transmission.
d): SLO-ICG angiography: spots appear larger and almost confluent, suggesting that the more or less intense lesions occupy almost the entire macular zone.

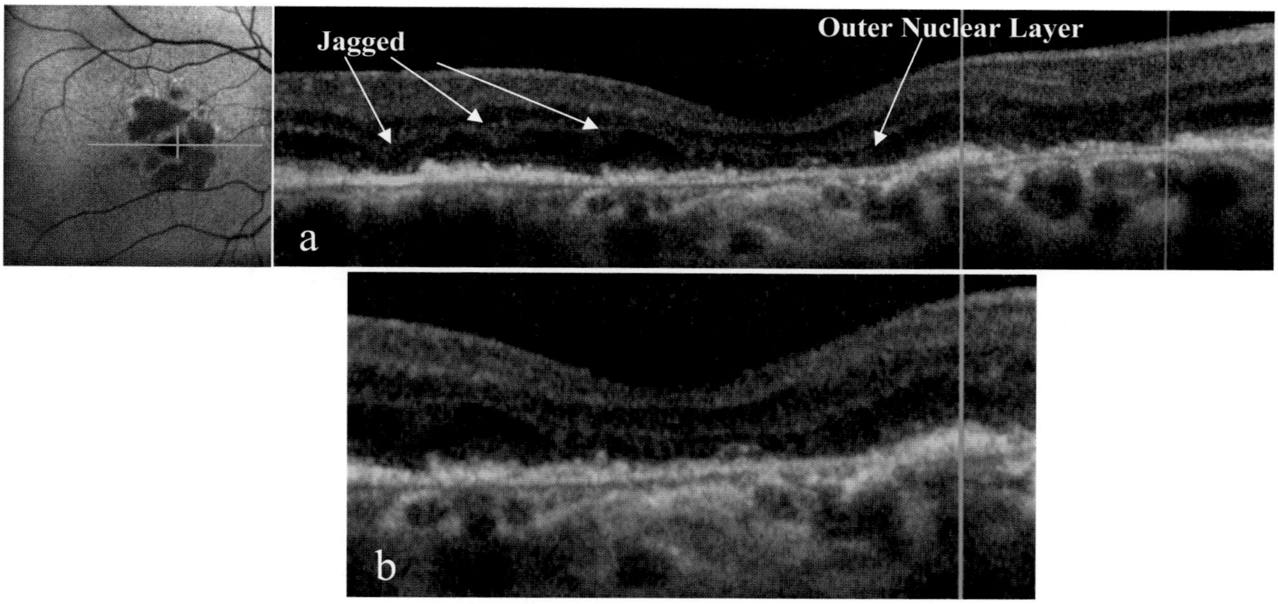

Figure 9: Dry AMD: advanced perifoveal and subfoveal form. VA: 20/200.
a): SD-OCT horizontal section: irregular RPE, no longer visible in the foveal region, where only Bruch's membrane remained clearly visible with marked back-shadowing.
b): Enlarged images: anterior to the RPE, the IS/OS interface and external limiting membrane were no longer visible over the zone of atrophy. The outer nuclear layer was also lost, bringing the outer plexiform layer in contact with Bruch's membrane, which confirmed the localized atrophy of the RPE and photoreceptors in this zone.

CLINICAL CASE No. 04: Macular Atrophy Following RPE Tear

Vascularized pigment epithelium detachment with an old large tear and atrophy in the zone of RPE retraction. TD-OCT and SD-OCT examination.

Clinical Signs

An 81-year-old woman, followed for AMD for 3 years, initially presented with sudden loss of visual acuity in her right eye. The fellow eye had several soft drusen and nonconfluent areas of atrophy.
VA RE: 20/800 - VA LE: 20/125.

Biomicroscopic Examination

Highly suggestive, large round lesion in the fundus with a de-pigmented and atrophic zone in the superior 2/3. There were several large choroidal vessels visualized in this area.

Autofluorescence

The zone was black and dense on autofluorescence.
In contrast, the inferior 1/3 was hyper-pigmented with scattered autofluorescent spots (**Figures 10a, b, and c**).

Fluorescein Angiography

Fluorescein angiography showed progressive hyper-fluorescence due to staining of the entire superior atrophic zone.

Small fluorescent spots were observed in the inferior zone due to abnormal transmission through the altered RPE (**Figure 10d**).

SLO-ICG Angiography

Abnormal visibility of several large choroidal vessels in the area of the RPE tear.

In the inferior part, the retracted RPE was hyper-pigmented, dense, and masked the choroid (**Figure 10e**).

Suggested Diagnosis:

Large, old tear in 2/3 of the circumference of a vascularized PED. The inferior part of the lesion corresponded to the prominence of the retracted RPE and the fibrovascular scar tissue.

Contribution of OCT (*Stratus**)

Vertical section

The RPE was visualized from below upwards. It was initially normal and then formed a dome-shaped detachment from the choroid and was completely absent in the atrophic zone.

In the elevated zone, the RPE was irregular, partially retracted, and rolled onto itself.

The hyper-pigmentation caused intense back-shadowing, which completely masked the choroid.

Beyond this dome, the RPE was no longer visible and the choroid was directly in contact with the retina (which was thinned at this level). This thinning and absence of the RPE accounted for the intense posterior shadowing.

Oblique section

The section started at the superior part and showed retinal thinning and loss of the RPE in the area of the tear. The section then showed the rest of the retracted fibrovascular PED and finally the normal peripheral territory (**Figures 11a and b**).

Conclusion

The TD-OCT examination clearly demonstrated the exposed area of an old vascularized PED (with atrophy of the choriocapillaris in the zone of RPE retraction) and the hyper-pigmented residual inferior fibrovascular detachment.
There were no signs of SRF or intraretinal fluid. The neurosensory retina was thinned in the area of the tear and the outer retinal layers and outer nuclear layer were no longer visible.

This lesion appeared to be chronic and stabilized without preservation of useful central vision, even in the zone of the fovea that was still lined by RPE. There was no indication for treatment in the absence of an exudative reaction.

CLINICAL CASE No. 04: MACULAR ATROPHY FOLLOWING AN RPE TEAR

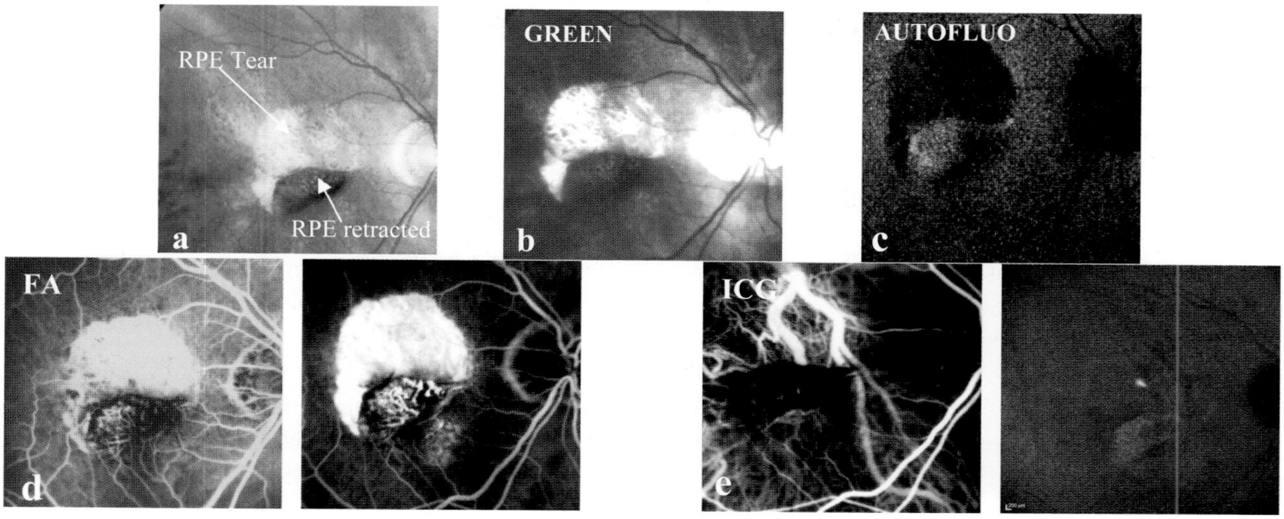

Figure 10: Dry AMD: macular atrophy following an RPE tear. VA: 20/800.
a, b, and c): Color, red-free, and autofluorescence: large rounded lesion with a de-pigmented and atrophic zone in the superior 2/3 that appears black on autofluorescence. The inferior third was hyper-pigmented with scattered autofluorescent spots.
d): Fluorescein angiography: progressive hyper-fluorescence due to staining of the entire superior atrophic zone. Small fluorescent spots were observed in the inferior zone due to abnormal transmission through the altered RPE.
e): SLO-ICG angiography: abnormal visibility of several large choroidal vessels in the area of the tear. In the inferior part, the retracted RPE was hyper-pigmented, dense and masked the choroid.

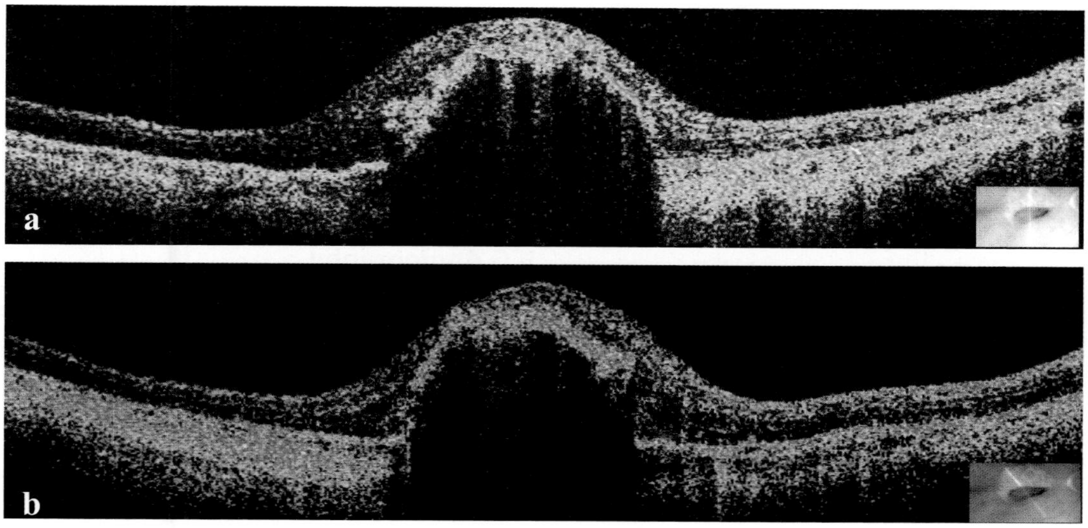

Figure 11: Dry AMD: macular atrophy following RPE tear. VA: 20/800.
a): *Stratus horizontal section**: the RPE was initially normal and then formed a dome-shaped detachment from the choroid and was completely absent in the atrophic zone.
In the elevated zone, the RPE was irregular, partially retracted, and rolled onto itself with intense back-shadowing due to hyper-pigmentation of the RPE. Beyond this dome, the RPE was no longer visible and the choroid was in contact with the thinned retina (loss of the outer nuclear layer).
b): *Stratus oblique section**: retinal thinning and absence of the RPE in the area of the tear. Retracted remnant of the fibrovascular PED and then normal peripheral area.

CLINICAL CASE No. 04: Macular Atrophy Following RPE Tear

Vascularized pigment epithelium detachment with an old large tear and atrophy in the zone of RPE retraction. TD-OCT and SD-OCT examination

The patient agreed to close follow-up for 3 years due to the severity of the lesions in the right eye, and the risk for the fellow eye. During the first year, this observation was performed by conventional imaging and TD-OCT (*Stratus**) (**Figure 12**).
During the second year, observation was based on simultaneous angiography and SD-OCT (*Spectralis**) imaging (**Figure 13**).

At the end of the first year

Central visual acuity remained low (20/800), but without metamorphopsias.

*Stratus** TD-OCT, vertical section

The neurosensory retina was elevated with loss of the foveal depression due to the central lesion, but there was no SRF.
The RPE presented a persistent dome-shaped detachment from the choroid, but this was slightly less prominent than before. Beyond this residual PED, the RPE was completely absent in the superior atrophic zone.

In the elevated zone, the RPE was irregular, retracted, and rolled up without signs of CNV proliferation. This thickening and hyper-pigmentation caused complete back-shadowing as far as the choroid.
Beyond this dome, the RPE was no longer visible and the choroid was in direct contact with the retina, which was thinned at this level.
Thinning and loss of the RPE were responsible for intense back-shadowing (**Figure 12**).

At the end of the second year

Central visual acuity remained unchanged (20/800).

*Spectralis** SD-OCT vertical section

In the elevated zone, the RPE was irregular and rolled up with marked hyper-reflectivity and thickening, which indicated reactive proliferation of the RPE that had invaded all of the outer retinal layers. Beyond this dome, the RPE was no longer visible, confirming the tear and retraction of the RPE with atrophy of the underlying layers.

Anterior to the RPE, in the residual PED, the IS/OS interface and external limiting membrane remained occasionally visible but were not clearly identified. The outer nuclear layer was invaded by a hyper-reflective extension of the RPE, sometimes extending as far as the inner limiting membrane.
In the atrophic zone, the IS/OS interface, external limiting membrane, and outer nuclear layer were absent, which brought the outer plexiform layer in contact with Bruch's membrane and confirmed photoreceptor atrophy (**Figure 13**).

Fluorescein Angiography

Fluorescein angiography showed persistent zone of progressive hyper-fluorescence due to staining of all of the superior atrophic area. Numerous spots were visible in the inferior zone due to abnormal transmission through the RPE (**Figures 12 and 13**).

ICG Angiography

Abnormal visibility of several large choroidal vessels in the area of the tear. In the inferior part, the hyper-pigmented and retracted RPE was dense and masked the choroid (**Figures 12 and 13**).

At this Stage

This tear of the superior 2/3 of a vascularized PED remained stable throughout follow-up with no new proliferation of CNV.
In the zone of atrophy following retraction of the RPE, the neurosensory retina was thinned. The outer plexiform layer was directly in contact with the hyper-reflective choroid with a fibrotic appearance, crossed by only a few rare choroidal vessels.
In the zone of the residual detachment, the RPE was markedly thickened and hyper-reflective with a hyper- pigmented and proliferating appearance.
The central macular zone was not spared by retraction of the RPE and visual acuity remained poor at 20/800.
There was no indication for treatment in the absence of an exudative reaction, but annual review was recommended.

CLINICAL CASE No. 04: MACULAR ATROPHY FOLLOWING RPE TEAR

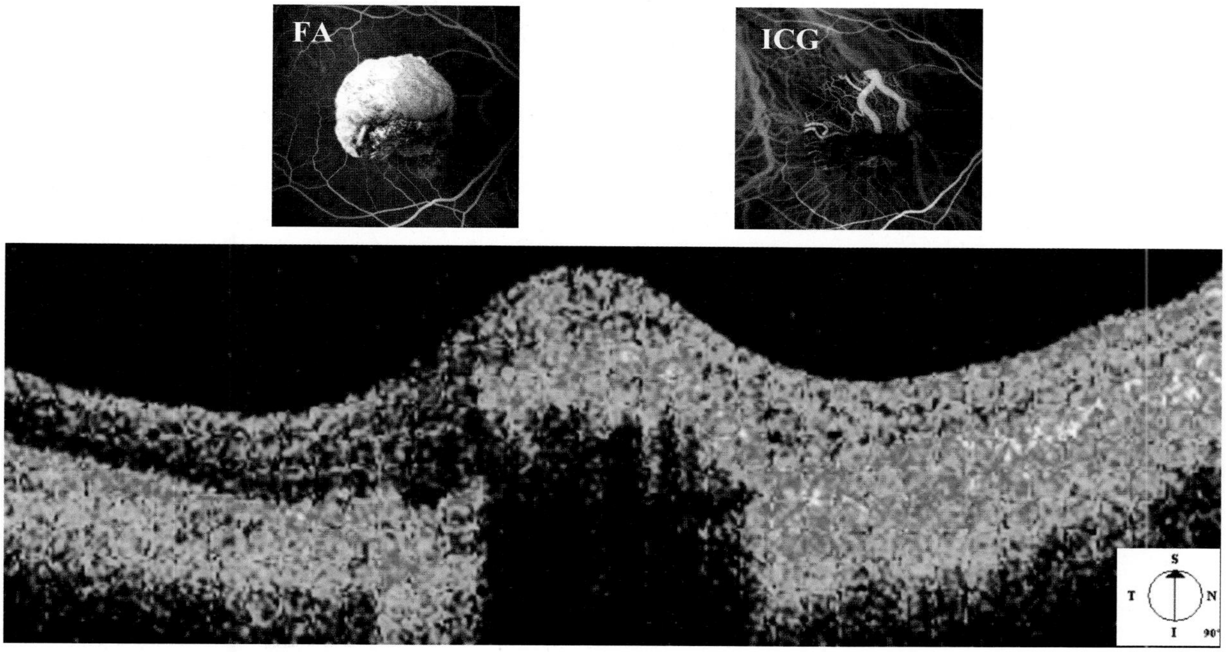

Figure 12: Macular atrophy following an RPE tear: advanced perifoveal and subfoveal form. VA: 20/800.
***Stratus** vertical section**: the residual, dome-shaped PED had become less prominent, raising the retina, but without SRF. Within this PED, the RPE was irregular, retracted, and rolled up with signs of proliferation. Complete back-shadowing as far as the choroid. Beyond the PED, the RPE was completely absent from the superior atrophic zone. The choroid was directly in contact with the thinned retina, accounting for the intense back-shadowing.

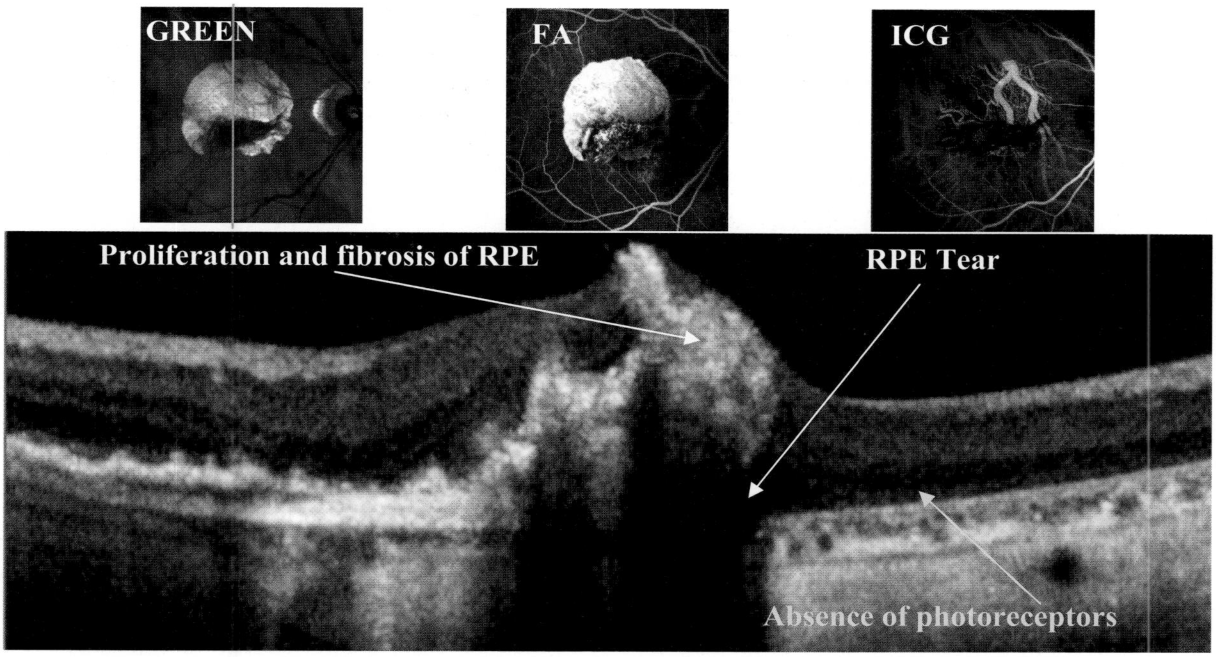

Figure 13: Macular atrophy following RPE tear: advanced perifoveal and subfoveal form. VA: 20/800.
***Spectralis** vertical section**: in the elevated zone, the RPE was irregular, rolled up, and hyper-reflective (reactive proliferation of the RPE that invaded all of the outer retinal layers). The IS/OS interface and external limiting membrane were occasionally visible but not clearly identified. The outer nuclear layer was invaded by the RPE, sometimes extending as far as the inner limiting membrane. In the atrophic zone, the outer retinal layers were absent, bringing the outer plexiform layer in contact with Bruch's membrane and confirming photoreceptor atrophy.

CLINICAL CASE No. 05: Macular Atrophy due to Vitelliform Macular Dystrophy

Bilateral, asymmetrical adult-onset vitelliform macular dystrophy progressing to atrophy. TD-OCT and SD-OCT examination.

Clinical Signs

A 63-year-old woman, who had been followed for bilateral, asymmetrical macular lesions for more than two years, presented with progressive decline of visual acuity in her right eye for several months.

VA RE: 20/80 - VA LE: 20/40.

Biomicroscopic Examination

Biomicroscopic examination showed a central, oval lesion with a fairly well-delineated de-pigmented and atrophic superior portion and a darker, brownish inferior semicircle (**Figure 14a**).

Autofluorescence

The two parts were clearly distinguished: the inferior part was intensely fluorescent, while the superior part was globally, but not homogeneously, hypo-fluorescent (**Figure 14b**).

Fluorescein Angiography

Almost all of the lesion was hypo-fluorescent, masking the hyper-fluorescent fundus. This hyper-fluorescence was especially visible in the periphery and superior part of the lesion and corresponded to abnormal transmission of fundus hyper-fluorescence due to alteration of the RPE without fluorescein leakage (**Figures 14c and d**).

ICG Angiography

The lesion was composed of hypo-fluorescent material, dense in the inferior half and in the superior periphery, with several fine extensions. This material was more rare and almost absent in the superior part, revealing the hyper-fluorescent fundus crossed by several large choroidal vessels but with no fluorescein leakage (**Figures 14e and f**).

Suggested Diagnosis:
Vitelliform macular dystrophy with regression and atrophy of the material in more than half of the superior lesion.

Contribution of OCT (*Spectralis**)

Horizontal section

The RPE was almost completely absent in the central subfoveal zone with persistence of several scattered hyper-reflective islands anterior to Bruch's membrane.

The *IS/OS interface* was completely absent in the same zone, while the *external limiting membrane* was still visible. The hypo-reflective *outer nuclear layer* presented normal thickness.

Vertical section

The RPE in the inferior zone of the lesion was preserved with accumulation of fairly dense hyper-reflective material.

This material appeared to proliferate anteriorly in a localized zone of the outer nuclear layer at the center of the section. The other retinal layers were normal (**Figures 15a and b**).

Conclusion

SD-OCT examination clearly demonstrated the presence of **accumulated vitelliform material** in the inferior part of the lesion, which was visible anterior to the RPE. In contrast, the superior part of the lesion had absent RPE and only a few islands of hyper-reflective material that persisted with marked alteration of the IS/OS interface. The external limiting membrane and outer nuclear layer remained intact.

All these findings were *confirmed* by fluorescein and ICG angiography, which clearly demonstrated the oval macular lesion, persistence of hypo-fluorescent material in the inferior part, and regression in the superior part with RPE atrophy.
The absence of any visible lesions in the external limiting membrane and outer nuclear layer explained the relative sparing of VA of 20/80. There **was no indication for treatment** in the absence of an exudative reaction.

CLINICAL CASE No. 05: MACULAR ATROPHY DUE TO VITELLIFORM MACULAR DYSTROPHY

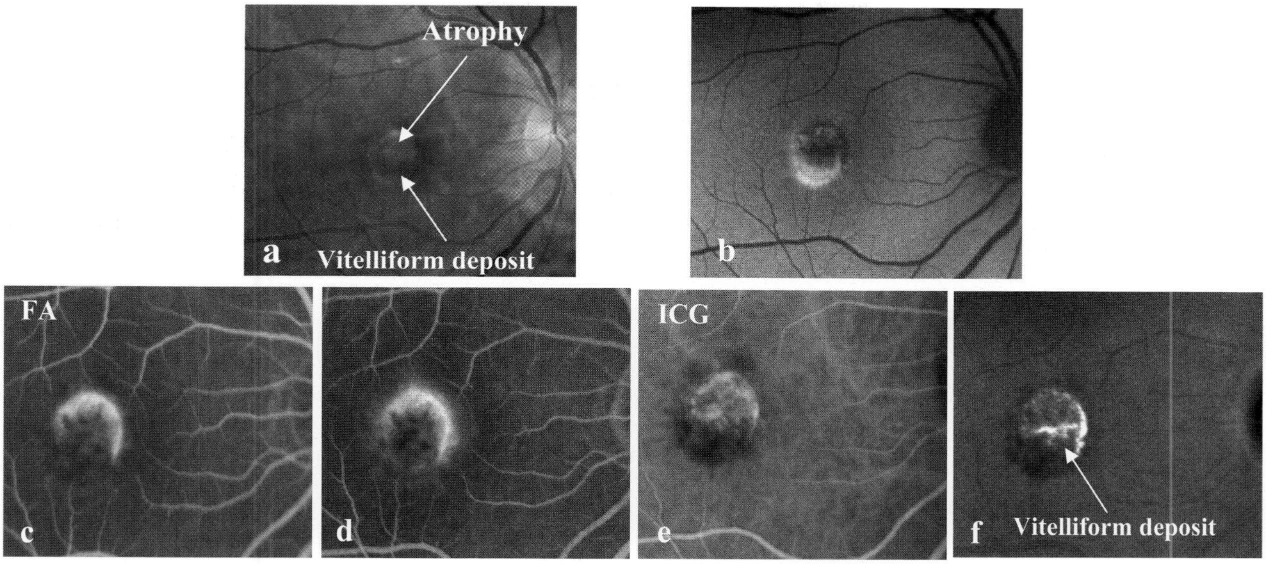

Figure 14: Macular atrophy due to vitelliform macular dystrophy VA: 20/80.
a and b): Color and autofluorescence: the superior part of the central oval lesion was de-pigmented and atrophic. The inferior semi-circle was darker with a brownish color. On autofluorescence, the two parts were clearly distinguished: the inferior part was intensely fluorescent and the superior part was hypo-fluorescent but not homogeneous.
c and d): Fluorescein angiography: hyper-fluorescence of the periphery and superior part of the lesion due to abnormal transmission related to alteration of the RPE without fluorescein leakage. Non-homogeneous masking in the inferior half.
e and f): SLO-ICG angiography: the material was hypo-fluorescent and dense in the inferior half with irregular margins and several fine extensions. This material was rare and almost absent in the superior part, which revealed the hyper-fluorescent fundus.

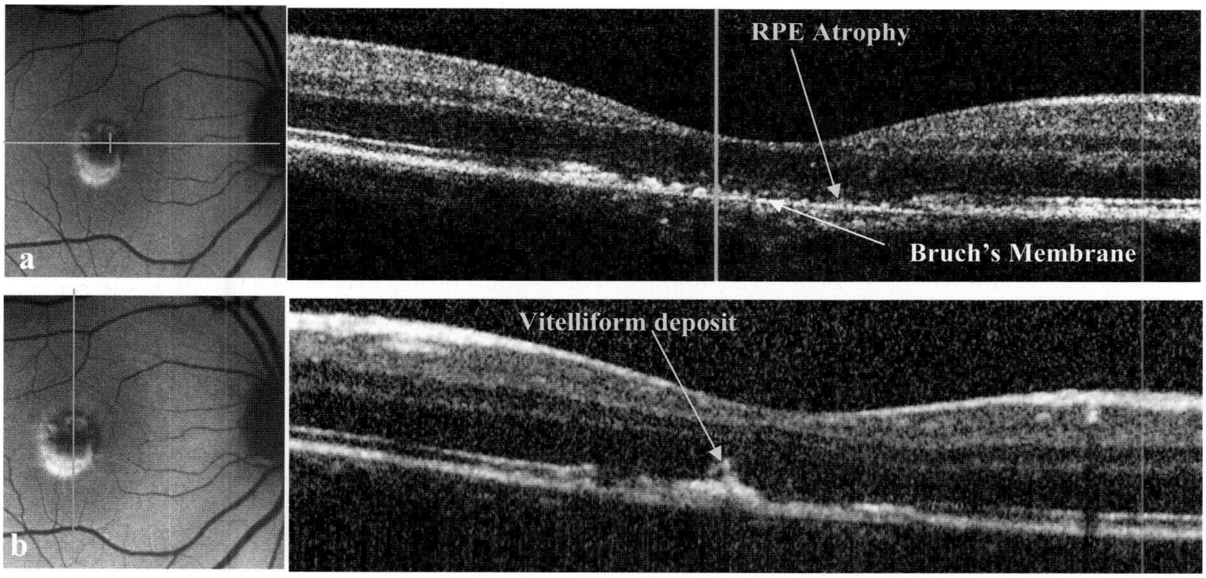

Figure 15: Macular atrophy due to vitelliform macular dystrophy VA: 20/80.
a): *Spectralis horizontal section**: almost complete disappearance of the RPE in the central subfoveal zone. Persistence of several scattered hyper-reflective islands anterior to Bruch's membrane. Loss of the IS/OS interface. The external limiting membrane and outer nuclear layer were normal.
b): *Spectralis vertical section**: the RPE was preserved but with accumulation of fairly dense hyper-reflective material that appeared to proliferate anteriorly in the outer nuclear layer.

CLINICAL CASE No. 06: Macular Atrophy due to Vitelliform Macular Dystrophy

Bilateral, asymmetrical adult-onset vitelliform macular dystrophy progressing to atrophy. TD-OCT and SD-OCT examination.

Clinical Signs

An 82-year-old woman had been followed with bilateral, asymmetrical macular lesions for several years. She presented with progressive decline of visual acuity in the left eye over several months.
VA RE: 20/63 - VA LE: 20/200.

Biomicroscopic Examination

Slightly prominent, rounded, irregular, de-pigmented lesion with jagged and slightly pigmented edges without hemorrhage.
On red-free images, the lesion had poorly-defined margins and appeared to be de-pigmented, as on the red light image (**Figures 16a, b, and c**).

Fluorescein Angiography

The lesion became rapidly hypo-fluorescent with progressive staining, particularly intense in the inferior and nasal sectors. Its surface area did not increase and no fluorescein leakage was observed (**Figure 16d**).

Suggested Diagnosis:

Vitelliform macular dystrophy with accumulation of material, which induced slight elevation in the inferior and nasal macula.

Contribution of OCT (*Topcon** 3D OCT-1000)

Horizontal section

The RPE was suddenly disrupted and was almost completely absent in the central subfoveal zone. Bruch's membrane was clearly visible with several areas of hyperreflective material. An almost optically empty hypo-reflective space was observed anterior to Bruch's membrane with marked elevation of the neurosensory retina.

The external limiting membrane was clearly visible over its entire course and outlined the elevation of the neurosensory retina. The most lateral limit of the retina over the elevation was irregular.

Anterior to the hypo-reflective zone and external limiting membrane, the outer nuclear layer was thinned, as if displaced by a zone of increased density. No cystoid spaces were observed (**Figure 17a**).

3D Examinations

The 3D image clearly visualized the regular, dome-shaped elevation of the macular surface.

The corresponding section revealed the main findings visible on the high-definition section:

- RPE atrophy,
- Hypo-reflective space,
- Elevation of outer retinal layers,
- Thinning of the outer nuclear layer, which was displaced by denser material (**Figure 17b**).

The 3D image with segmentation allowed even clearer distinction of the structures situated anterior and posterior to the RPE.
The anteroposterior section can also be located in relation to the fundus image (**Figure 17c**).

Conclusion

The SD-OCT examination (*Topcon** 3D OCT-1000) clearly visualized the zone of RPE atrophy with only a few remnants of vitelliform material visible anterior to Bruch's membrane and the intensely hypo-reflective, almost optically empty zone.
This localized zone anterior to Bruch's membrane was accompanied by elevation of the neurosensory retina.
Outer retinal layers were altered and irregular, with thinning of the outer nuclear layer, but no disorganization of the retina and no cystoid spaces.
This intensely hypo-reflective zone seemed to be related to regression of vitelliform material, with no signs of associated choroidal neovascularization.
The risk of subsequent CNV development justified prolonged observation.

CLINICAL CASE No. 06: MACULAR ATROPHY DUE TO VITELLIFORM MACULAR DYSTROPHY

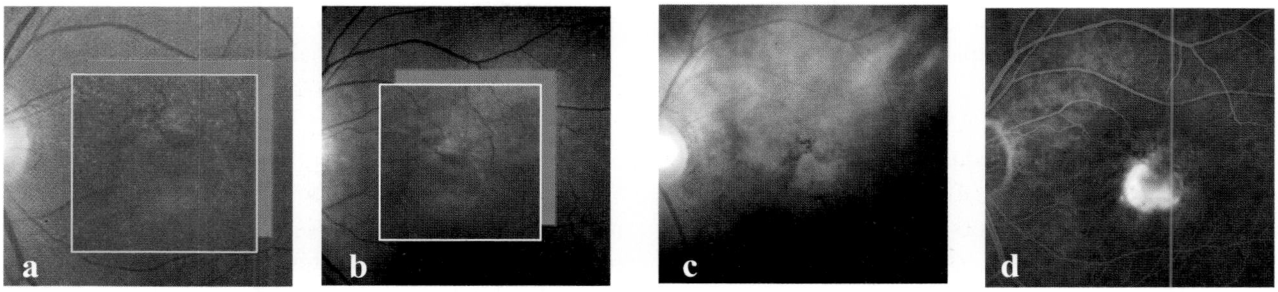

Figure 16: Macular atrophy due to vitelliform macular dystrophy. VA: 20/63.
a, b, and c): Color, autofluorescence, red-free: rounded, irregular, de-pigmented, slightly prominent lesion with jagged and slightly pigmented margins, without hemorrhage. On red-free images, the lesion had poorly-defined margins and appeared to be de-pigmented, as on the red light image.
d): Fluorescein angiography: rapidly hyper-fluorescent lesion with progressive staining, particularly intense in the inferior and nasal sectors. No fluorescein leakage.

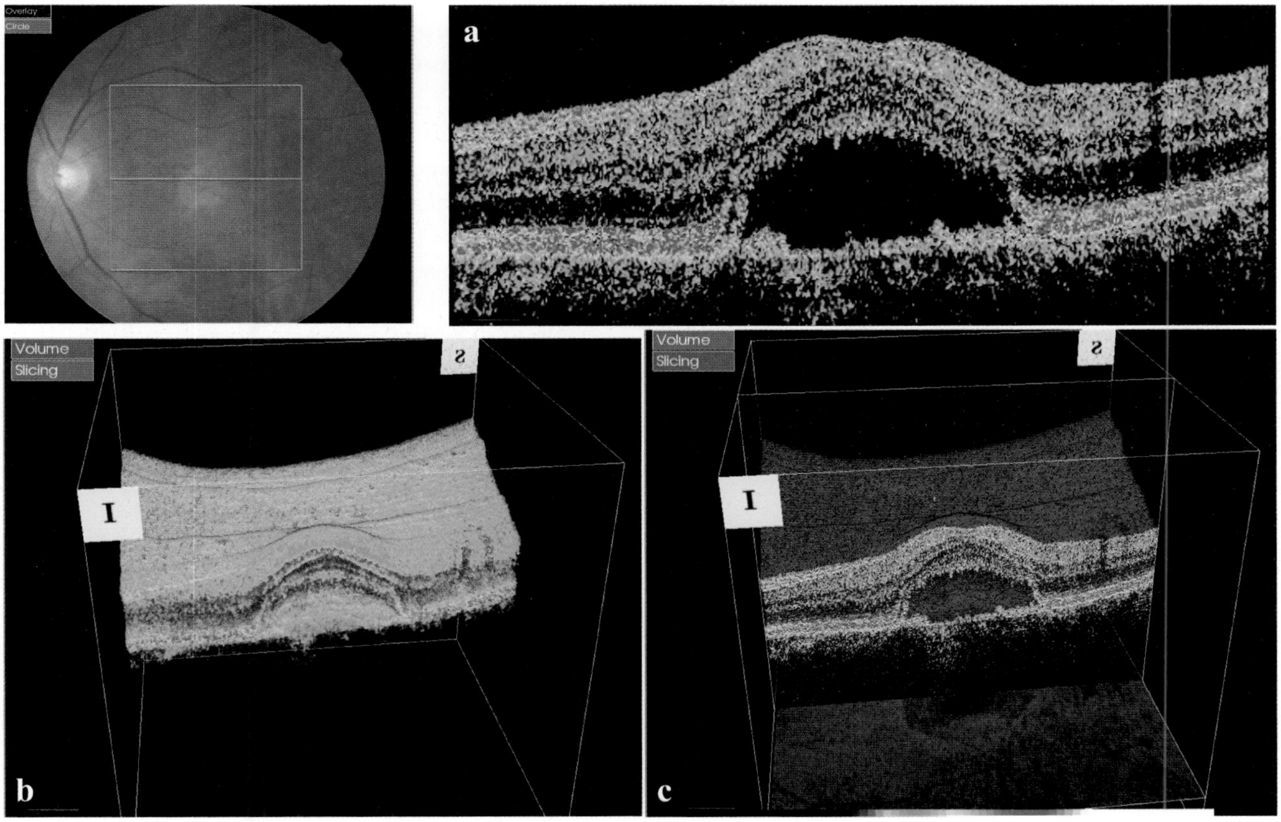

Figure 17: Macular atrophy due to vitelliform macular dystrophy. VA: 20/63.
a): *Topcon 2D horizontal section**: the RPE was almost completely absent in the central subfoveal zone. Bruch's membrane was clearly visible with several remnants of hyper-reflective material.
A marked elevation of the neurosensory retina with an almost optically empty hypo-reflective space anterior to Bruch's membrane. The external limiting membrane was clearly visible over its entire course, but the most lateral limit of the retina over the elevation was irregular and poorly-defined with variable reflectivity. The outer nuclear layer was thinned.
b): Volume 3D *Topcon (horizontal section) Cropping**: regular, dome-shaped elevation of the macular surface.
The corresponding section revealed the main findings visible on the high-definition section.
c): Volume 3D *Topcon (horizontal section) Cropping Slicing Projection**: the 3D image with segmentation allowed even clearer distinction of the structures situated anterior and posterior to the RPE (*images courtesy of Dr. Sam Razavi*).

OCT and Dry AMD

Dry AMD therefore is comprised of multiple characteristics, which must be distinguished from classic precursor signs (or age-related maculopathy).

The **common feature** of dry AMD is the presence of areas of RPE atrophy, which subsequently induces severe alteration of the choriocapillaris. The outer retinal layers and particularly the photoreceptors are affected secondarily.

This *slowly progressive* course causes functional impairment and severe loss of visual acuity, which is difficult to treat at the present time.

Several **therapeutic approaches** have been proposed, not only to treat neovascular complications, but also to prevent and halt the progression of atrophy. There are even attempts to replace atrophic zones with RPE transplantation.

Regardless of the treatment modality, it is essential to recognize the **first stages** of atrophy and follow their deterioration and/or **extension,** particularly towards the center of the fovea and the **fixation point**.

12

Various imaging modalities can achieve this objective.

- **Red light monochromatic** images often demonstrate areas of atrophy, even at an early stage when these areas are not clearly visible on biomicroscopy or red-free monochromatic images.

- Areas of atrophy are easily detected on **fluorescein and ICG angiography**, creating a window defect through which choroidal vessels of variable atrophy are clearly visible.

- **Autofluorescence** examinations, easy to perform and without the need for an IV injection, rapidly demonstrate the presence of lipofuscin-rich material. Progressive regression of this material (accompanying RPE atrophy) results in a zone of marked hypofluorescence.

Time-Domain OCT

TD-OCT provides even more precise information that is as easy to obtain as autofluorescence.

- Partial or complete atrophy of the RPE with persistence of Bruch's membrane is a very characteristic sign.
- The presence of islands of material or material accumulated in the junctional zone is also easy to recognize and can be used to follow the patient's course.

Spectral-Domain OCT

SD-OCT, especially with the *Spectralis** machine, allows much more precise analysis of alterations of the outer retinal layers and constitutes a remarkable progress in ophthalmology.

- **Various degrees of severity** of the lesion can be identified by studying visibility of the IS/OS interface and the external limiting membrane.

At a later stage, loss of the outer nuclear layer reflects not only RPE atrophy but also complete and irreversible damage to **photoreceptors**.

- The diagnosis is confirmed by thinning of the neurosensory retina, which is easily quantifiable. Separate measurement of the various retinal layers and RPE, which will be possible in the near future, will facilitate follow-up and assessment of the response to treatment.

- **3D SD-OCT studies** can also demonstrate zones of atrophy of the RPE and outer retinal layers and measure the **surface area** involved.

Progression of atrophy must be evaluated not only by measuring the surface and peripheral extension, but more importantly, its relation to the fixation point. The presence of a zone of central sparing is very important for the patient's quality of life.

Automatic eye-tracking systems allow accurate follow-up comparisons.

OCT therefore provides a major contribution, even in dry AMD, which is poorly amenable to treatment.

However, in the case of deterioration and when there is a doubt about its cause, **comparison of the various imaging modalities** can specify the diagnosis, confirm the various prognostic factors, and guide treatment.

The Contribution of Optical Coherence Tomography (OCT)

Gabriel COSCAS

(Créteil and Paris)

The Contribution of OCT

New and extremely valuable information is now provided with **Spectral Domain OCT** (SD-OCT) due to the more rapid data acquisition.

In Recent Years

The essential contribution of *Conventional Time Domain OCT* (TD-OCT, *Stratus**, Carl Zeiss Meditec, Inc.), in age-related macular degeneration (AMD) has been its ability to detect intraretinal and subretinal *fluid accumulation.*

More specifically, measurement of increased ***retinal thickness*** induced by the fluid accumulation and evaluation of response to treatment is very useful and has become part of routine clinical practice.

However, this information could be too limited and over simplistic and requires *additional detailed analysis.*

Development of Spectral Domain OCT

Technological advances leading to the development of Spectral-Domain OCT enables further examination of all *outer layers and photoreceptors*.

13

Recent Advances

The ***resolution*** of anteroposterior cross-sectional imaging has been considerably improved, allowing analysis and definition of the borders of each of the retinal layers that compare to histology.

This allows the transition between angiographic data and histological data (which remain rare).

Angiography visualizes normal and abnormal blood vessels and/or neovascularisation and detects abnormal permeability shown by dye leakage.

OCT allows detailed analysis of the different retinal layers: the spaces within or under the retina, intraretinal fluid accumulation, scarring, fibrosis, and atrophy.

Correlations with Fundus Imaging

A fundus image (color picture or angiography) can be obtained ***simultaneously*** with an OCT examination. The location of the scan can be observed directly on the fundus image. A landmark (digital *calliper)* placed on the examined area enables an immediate and automated view of this area on the OCT (and vice versa).

The ability to localize a lesion on an OCT scan and the fundus simultaneously is particularly useful for exact interpretation of the lesion.

Controversies on the Different Imaging Modalities

There are still some controversies concerning the usefulness and efficacy in comparing the main three ocular imaging modalities (fluorescein angiography, SLO-ICG angiography, and OCT).

- The controversy surrounds two issues:
  - Some authors postulate that only **OCT** should be used, replacing the other two modalities.
  - Others suggest that **combined analysis** using all three diagnostic techniques is helpful (particularly in cases which are not straightforward).
- *Fluorescein angiography* is unanimously considered to be the "gold standard" for fundus examinations. Fluorescein leakage is an extremely valuable sign. Moreover, in the era of intravitreous injections, an intravenous injection is relatively harmless.
- *Indocyanine green (ICG)* angiography performed with a scanning laser ophthalmoscope (SLO) provides detailed information on choroidal vasculature and choroidal neovascularization, which is so often occult or ill-defined on fluorescein angiography. SLO-ICG angiography can also detect and analyze lesions which are missed because of their small size (anastomoses and polyps).
- OCT performed alone (and especially when the OCT-scan cannot be precisely correlated with a fundus image) may be poorly informative, providing only indirect signs.

Related to involuntary patient eye movements, TD-OCT can give incomplete or erroneous results with a risk of errors and *artifacts.*

Thickness measurements remain imprecise. (Variations become significant only when they exceed 50 to 70 µm.) The *reproducibility* of successive examinations is not reliable, especially when the patient has poor fixation. Correlations with the fundus image remain approximate and dependent on the ophthalmologist's skill and experience. These **limitations** however are resolved by Spectral Domain-OCT.

Comparison of Fluorescein Angiography, ICG Angiography, and OCT

Several studies designed to determine the reciprocal advantages and limitations of fluorescein angiography compared with OCT have been published in the literature.

- These **pilot studies** demonstrated:
  - The advantage of fluorescein angiography in providing a precise diagnosis.
  - The value of OCT, in monitoring the course of the disease, by detecting and measuring variations in retinal thickness and intraretinal fluid accumulation.

- A **masked, prospectively controlled study** was designed in order to provide objective and statistically significant results.

This study comprised independent and masked review of fluorescein angiography, SLO-ICG angiography, and OCT data in a series of 200 patients.

It was designed to assess the importance of each of these imaging tools in the **decision to treat, re-treat,** or discontinue anti-VEGF therapy, either for

- The initial diagnosis and treatment decision, or
- During post-treatment follow-up.

The various examinations were reviewed according to **reading grids**.

Each examiner received a series of documents in random order and had to read and interpret *either OCT alone* or each of the two types of angiography separately.

Then afterwards, the examiner repeated the analysis by comparing two and three of these imaging modalities.

- **The objective of this study** was to determine which imaging modality or which combination of modalities was the most reliable for diagnosis and treatment decision.

Statistical analysis of the final results is currently underway, and the results will be published in the near future.

Preliminary results

The *preliminary results* appear to confirm the initial hypothesis that the combination of fluorescein angiography and OCT is the best combination and the most reliable at all stages of the disease.

SLO-ICG angiography provides essential data for the diagnosis of *chorioretinal anastomosis* and *polypoidal choroidal vasculopathy*, accounting for 10% to 12% of cases each.

ICG angiography is also essential to demonstrate or exclude the presence of *occult* choroidal neovascularization associated with minimally classic choroidal neovascularization.

- In all cases of advanced, extensive, complex, or treatment-refractory disease, the combination of the three imaging modalities is the most informative and constitutes the best means of diagnosis.

Therefore, the combination of SD-OCT with fundus imaging, and particularly with simultaneous fluorescein and ICG angiographies, could be the best approach to patient care. The *Spectralis** (Heidelberg Engineering, Inc.) can also combine these images with a reference autofluorecence picture.

Contribution of Time-Domain OCT

Time-Domain OCT (TD-OCT) using the *Stratus** apparatus is now part of most routine ophthalmological practice, especially in the care of patients with AMD.

The most **important results** obtained with TD-OCT are well-established:

- Detection and evaluation of vascularized retinal pigment epithelium detachment (V-PED), and
- Detection and quantification of intraretinal and subretinal fluid accumulation.

1. Different Types of Choroidal Neovascularization

Most CNV can be classified into three main categories: occult, classic, and/or mixed; they may also be recognized as:

- Type 1: **Pre-epithelial**,
- Type 2: **Sub-epithelial** (sub-RPE), and/or
- **Mixed.**

Occult or sub-RPE CNV actually comprises all forms of vascularized retinal pigment epithelium detachment (V-PED) observed during AMD.

OCT examinations showed that occult CNV develops underneath the RPE and induces separation of the RPE layer from the hyper-reflective line of Bruch's membrane (BM).

Vascularized retinal pigment epithelium detachment can be small and limited or progressively large and extensive. They may be comprised of:

- Either a *predominantly serous exudative* reaction, or on the contrary,
- A *fibrovascular* component.

The PED cavity may subsequently become organized with the formation of sub-RPE fibrosis and progressive scarring.

Mixed CNV

In cases of *active growth*, occult CNV can be transformed into mixed CNV, with more or less extensive classic CNV proliferating above the RPE.

On Time-Domain OCT, the classic CNV component presents as a localized hyper-reflective area situated above the PED and underneath the neurosensory retina.

According to the relative extent of occult and classic components, these cases of mixed CNV can be termed "*minimally classic*" or "*predominantly classic*" CNV.

The features of these (mixed) CNV are indistinct as the TD-OCT cross-section of the retinal layers becomes disorganized. In this case, angiography is useful, if not essential, for the diagnosis.

Other Clinical Forms of CNV

The other clinical forms of CNV (easily detected and analyzed by fluorescein angiography and/or ICG angiography) are not clearly identified by using TD-OCT alone:

- **Classic CNV with no occult CNV** component (whose incidence is relatively low), are associated with acute clinical symptoms including exudative reaction and hemorrhages.

Therefore, they need immediate and complete imaging assessment.

- **Chorioretinal anastomoses**, (relatively more frequent) are difficult to recognize with TD-OCT, but their occurrence may be suggested by the combination of PED with accentuated intraretinal leakage and numerous, large, and confluent cysts.
- **Polypoidal choroidal vasculopathy** is usually difficult to recognize with fluorescein angiography and needs additional information obtained with SLO-ICG.

OCT will detect and show the localized, steep elevation of the polyps (single or multiple) within or away from a sero-hemorrhagic V-PED.

The OCT examination must comprise multiple **"raster" scans** to avoid missing the lesion, which is often small and juxtafoveal.

2. Fluid Accumulation

The evidence of fluid accumulation within the retina is the second important contribution of OCT.

Fluid accumulation can be observed in the potential spaces between the RPE and Bruch's membrane (PED) and also between the RPE and the neurosensory retina.

Fluid can accumulate within the retinal tissue itself, inducing *increased macular thickness*. This presents as either diffuse or with cystoid cavities of variable size and confluence.

This exudative reaction with fluid accumulation is especially marked over the zone of neovascularization. It tends to gravitate inferiorly.

This reaction is related to the abnormal permeability of "active" choroidal neovascularization and a local increase in VEGF.

3. Demonstration of Retinal Fluid

Demonstration of retinal fluid is important as:

- Fluid accumulation has been shown to *correlate* with declining visual acuity.
- The *initial and main effect* of anti-VEGF therapy is reduction and resorption of fluid or leakage, which is followed by rapid functional improvement.

TD-OCT examination therefore shows an **indirect sign**, leakage, which by simple measurement of central retinal thickness, indicates:

- The presence or absence of active CNV,
- The initial efficacy of treatment.

4. Criteria of Stabilization or Scarring

Despite remarkable progress, current treatments rarely achieve a complete cure, but more frequently achieve short or long-lasting **stabilization** of the lesions, which may be diagnosed at an advanced stage.

Healing and scarring of these advanced forms comprises either *fibrosis* (with clearly visible hyper-reflectivity on OCT) or, more rarely, *atrophy* of the outer layers.

Fibrosis

The fibrosis is visualized as a *hyper-reflective band* of variable thickness and extent. This fibrosis can progressively regress, either spontaneously or in response to treatment.

It may also deteriorate and be associated with neurosensory retinal degeneration with the formation of persistent cystoid macular edema (CME).

The development of dense, hyper-reflective subretinal fibrosis located between the RPE and the neurosensory retina appears to have severe functional consequences. Fibrosis located beneath the RPE layer (fibrovascular PED), appears to be relatively well-tolerated offering a better visual prognosis.

Atrophy of the Outer Layers

This atrophy is easily recognized *on OCT as:*

- Hyper-reflectivity extending backwards towards the choroid,
- Localized loss of the RPE band,
- Decreased thickness of the neurosensory retina.
- In early changes, the outer nuclear layer becomes thinner and no longer detectable.

Final visual acuity depends on the extension and severity of these atrophic changes.

5. Limitations of TD-OCT

- Causes of error are related to the relative slowness of the Time-Domain OCT acquisition process, accounting for **motion artifacts** and poor localization. The lack of precision and the poor reproducibility of successive examinations during follow-up are well-known.
- Changes of the **outer retinal layers** are rarely and only poorly visualized by Time-Domain OCT. "Pixelized" information only suggests the hyper-reflective line of the IS/OS interface, which rapidly becomes non-interpretable during the course of the disease. The same applies to alterations of the outer nuclear layer.
- **Discordances** between TD-OCT data and visual acuity measurements are frequently observed. There is not always a concordance between the presence (or absence) of residual fluid, persistence of the neovascular network, and visual acuity.
- **Small lesions** or lesions situated away from the center of the macula can be easily missed, leading to erroneous conclusions or delayed diagnosis.
- Any hyper-reflective zone visible on TD-OCT can be due to **multiple causes** (neovascularization, fibrosis, lipofuscin deposits, hemorrhage, pigment, inflammatory reaction, etc.). These hyper-reflective zones should be interpreted by comparing them with other imaging modalities.
- **Progressive disease** with signs of new leakage should be examined by angiography.

This will allow the detection of new or extensive choroidal neovascularization and its complications.

Finally, not only OCT signs but also information from angiographic imaging should be gathered in order to make a precise diagnosis, treatment decision, and for follow-up. TD-OCT alone is not sufficient.

The Contribution of Spectral Domain OCT

Development and utilization of a new imaging technique called **Spectral or Fourier Domain OCT** has enabled us to overcome some limitations of TD-OCT.

Spectral Domain technology constitutes a major advancement by allowing *high-speed, high-resolution examinations* and even *3D reconstructions.*

> The advantages of Spectral Domain OCT are maximized when the three imaging modalities and reference images, as well as automated comparison of changes over time, are obtained **simultaneously**.

1. Technological Progress

Axial Resolution

In SD-OCT the interference signal is a function of the optical wavelength *simultaneously* measuring all echoes of light from different layers.

This instantaneous analysis of a light spectrum for each A-scan increases the number of points analyzed, resulting in an **axial resolution** of 4 to 6 microns (versus 8 to 10 microns for Time-Domain OCT).

Faster Imaging

A-scans can be obtained at high speed (between 15,000 and 40,000 A-scans per second), which eliminates risks of error related to involuntary patient eye movements.

Acquisition of a B-scan is 50 to 100 times faster than with TD-OCT.

This more **rapid image acquisition** and improved axial resolution allow visualization of smaller structures.

Analysis of the **outer retinal layers** and evaluation of alterations of photoreceptor layer is improved.

Reference Images

The higher image acquisition rate and the greater scan density allows co-registration of B-scans with simultaneously obtained **fundus images**, such as color, red free, infrared photography, fluorescein or SLO-ICG angiography (by using a second laser source).

Volume

Improved resolution and scan speed gives **3-dimensional (3D)** information. Video examination of OCT scans allows separate analysis of successive scans of the retina and analysis of a single cross-sectional image.

This is particularly useful for detecting small focal pathologies.

3D images can be mobilized in all directions and/or sectioned in any plane, offering a *comprehensive view of the entire foveal area* and allowing virtual "anatomical dissection."

Software is being developed to acquire precise volumetric measurements and to follow the course of certain structures, such as SRF, PED, intraretinal cystic spaces, and drusen.

These volumetric examinations require a relatively long acquisition time and usually result in reduced transverse 3D resolution at high speeds.

However, high-resolution 3D images can be obtained when the patient has good fixation and when a sufficiently long acquisition time is used.

Signal-to-Noise-Ratio

The increased background noise related to the higher sensitivity of Spectral-Domain OCT can be reduced by averaging several images (which are virtually identical due to the high-speed image acquisition).

This system can be improved by "**eye-tracking***" technology, allowing averaging of images all acquired at exactly the same place.

2. Clinical Applications

In clinical practice, SD-OCT datasets allow comparison of the various fundus imaging modalities with **precise point-by-point correlations**.

These correlations can be studied, not only during the same examination, but also during follow-up examinations to analyze the results of treatment.

Registration

Various reference images indicating the scan line can be obtained. Some machines use a scanning laser ophthalmoscope with excellent fundus image quality, providing color or infrared images.

Some equipment simultaneously allows fluorescein or indocyanine angiography or autofluorescence images, while others use a non-mydriatic fundus camera.

Measuring and Mapping Thickness

Detection and follow up of variations in retinal thickness are important. They can be represented graphically according to several modalities:

- Either overlaid on a fundus photograph, or
- A graph reproducing the B-scan profile.

An eye-tracking system can ensure that these thickness measurements are reliably reproducible on successive examinations and are performed exactly in the same location.

- The boundaries of retinal thickness measurements are different from those of TD-OCT. SD-OCT incorporates the thickness of the RPE (and could extend as far as the line representing Bruch's membrane) with only slight differences from one tool to another.

Retinal thickness measurements with SD-OCT are on average 40 to 80 micrometers larger than those measured with the *Stratus**.

However, retinal thickness measurement algorithms vary between the various currently available machines. Several detection errors can still occur, but these mistakes can be manually corrected.

Segmentation

Some SD-OCT tools provide automated segmentation of 3D images to delineate two or three layers of hyper-reflectivity.

Thickness variations in 3D can be demonstrated at the level of the internal limiting membrane (and possible vitreoretinal adhesions), RPE, or anywhere in-between.

3. Outer Retinal Layers

The **essential advantage** of the improved image quality of Spectral-Domain OCT in AMD is the increasingly precise analysis of the different intraretinal layers, especially the outer retinal layers.

- **Three hyper-reflective structures** of the outer layers of the retina are clearly defined:
  - The external limiting membrane (**ELM**),
  - The interface between inner and outer segments of the photoreceptor layer (**IS/OS interface**), and
  - The retinal pigment epithelium (**RPE**).

These structures delineate hypo-reflective spaces occupied by the outer nuclear layer and by the inner and outer segments of the photoreceptor layer.

- **The outer nuclear layer (ONL)** is dark, hypo-reflective, and normally relatively large.

Various changes may be observed during the course of AMD. This layer can be thinned or invaded by denser zones (irregular, serrated, or extensive) or they may even partially disappear. These subtle changes have major prognostic significance.

- The **external limiting membrane (ELM)** is linear, relatively thin, clearly visible, and well-delineates the outer nuclear layer.

- **The IS/OS interface** is a hyper-reflective structure, thicker than the external limiting membrane.

It can have a fragmented or irregular appearance, or may be thicker and clearly visible over a zone of neovascularization.

Thickness variations of the IS/OS interface are correlated with the activity of CNV and are often reversible with treatment.

- **Photoreceptors** are therefore situated in two well-delineated hypo-reflective spaces corresponding to:
  - **Inner segment** between the external limiting membrane and the IS/OS interface,
  - **Outer segment** between the IS/OS interface and the retinal pigment epithelium.

The hypo-reflective zone corresponding to photoreceptors and outer segments is normally larger in the center of the fovea.

> Analysis of these outer layers and particularly any alterations of the outer nuclear layer and the two hyper-reflective lines can demonstrate **photoreceptor damage**. This should be followed during the course of the disease.

4. Neovascularization

Occult CNV and V-PED

The presence and proliferation of occult CNV (sub-RPE CNV) and the accompanying exudative reactions result in detachment of the RPE (PED) from Bruch's membrane, which becomes visible.

Pigment epithelial detachment occurs gradually and is either *fibrovascular* or *predominantly serous.*

The **OCT-profile** of this detachment reflects the different phases of its development. The PED may be initially relatively *flat with a low dome* and may progressively become more elevated and *bullous.*

In late stages, it may be irregular and *undulated* with one or more elevations and wavy edges.

Fluid Accumulation

The presence of choroidal neovascularization (CNV) is *not directly visible* on OCT, as it is on angiographic images. However, the abnormal permeability of these new vessels is reflected by *fluid accumulation* (better seen on SD-OCT than on Time-Domain OCT).

Fluid accumulates not only underneath the RPE (PED), but also underneath the neurosensory retina, or it may infiltrate the retinal tissue itself (edema). The latter can present either diffusely (increased thickness) or as intraretinal cysts (CME).

These cystic spaces are usually larger in the center where they can become confluent. They may extend over one or two layers but predominate within the plexiform layers.

This fluid infiltration induces loss of the foveal depression and disorganization of the retinal layers including the inner layers.

5. Inflammatory Reactions

The presence of **actively growing CNV** is often accompanied by inflammatory reactions (best seen with the *Spectralis** SD-OCT). These reactions include numerous bright **hyper-reflective spots** and denser zones of variable size.

Bright hyper-reflective spots, which may correspond to protein precipitates, are mainly observed at the edges of subretinal fluid or around cystic spaces.

They are predominantly observed in the outer retinal layers above neovascularization but can extend into the inner retinal layers.

- **Denser zones** are ill-defined areas of moderate reflectivity observed over a fibrovascular PED or around subretinal classic CNV.

The IS/OS interface often appears to merge in these denser zones associated with bright hyper-reflective spots (or deposits), which can also displace or extend into the outer nuclear layer and beyond.

All of these signs appear to be **reversible** after treatment and seem to be correlated with visual acuity changes.

The objective of treatment is to restore the normal structure and appearance of the inner and outer retinal layers.

6. Scarring, Fibrosis, and Atrophy

In the advanced forms of AMD, such as CNV treated late and/or CNV that is refractory to treatment, SD-OCT demonstrates different amounts of hyper-reflective zones.

This hyper-reflectivity is usually **fusiform in shape**, suggesting the presence of fibrosis. The location of this fibrosis depends on the type of CNV, its proliferation, and the duration of the lesion.

- **Subretinal fibrosis**, following classic or mixed subretinal CNV, is located between the RPE and the neurosensory retina and is usually associated with a *poor visual prognosis.*

- **Sub-RPE fibrosis**, following occult or minimally classic sub-RPE CNV, develops within the fibrovascular PED, which gradually but not completely collapses.

The PED cavity becomes organized with a heterogeneous, highly reflective appearance, suggesting varying amounts of fibrosis.

This sub-RPE fibrosis is usually persistent and severe. However, it can be compatible with *preservation of use-*

ful visual acuity, especially in the absence of permanent damage to the outer retinal layers.

Macular Atrophy

Unfortunately, CNV regression can be accompanied by severe alterations of the outer retinal layers.

These changes include atrophy, not only of the RPE but also localized **loss of outer retinal layers** (IS/OS interface, external limiting membrane, and even the outer nuclear layer).

This atrophy brings outer plexiform layers in contact with Bruch's membrane.

Atrophy and loss of photoreceptors are accompanied by a **decrease in central retinal thickness** and irreversible loss of central visual acuity.

7. Correlations

With the development of Spectral Domain-OCT technology and the availability of the *Spectralis** (Heidelberg Inc.), we have initiated a *study on morphological and functional correlations in exudative AMD.*

This study was designed to systematically analyze the outer retinal layers and their variations since the initial presentation and on successive examinations during the first year.

Several **preliminary results** are already available (prior to publication of the statistical results).

The essential *objective* was:

- To assess the diagnostic and prognostic value of Spectral-Domain OCT examination of the outer retinal layers, and
- To determine correlations between baseline visual acuity, the types of lesions observed, and the extent and duration of CNV.

This *prospective study* consisted of 134 patients with exudative AMD who were followed during their treatment by color, red-free, and autofluorescence fundus photography, fluorescein and SLO-ICG angiography, and Spectral-Domain OCT using the *Spectralis* (Heidelberg Inc.)*, which allowed simultaneous imaging.

Patients in this study were divided into 4 groups according to baseline visual acuity (Group 1:≥ 20/32. Group 2: from 20/63 to 20/40. Group 3: from 20/100 to 20/80. Group 4: < 20/100).

In each group, CNV were classified into 5 categories: (1) Sub-RPE occult CNV. (2) Sub-retinal classic CNV. (3) Mixed CNV (occult + classic CNV). (4) Chorioretinal Anastomoses (CRA). (5) Polypoidal choroidal vasculopathy (PCV).

All patients were treated by intravitreous injections of anti-VEGF.

Each reinjection was decided on the basis of complete follow-up and imaging examinations. Fundus imaging was analyzed at baseline, after the first injection, after the third injection, and at one year of follow-up.

Detailed analysis of *outer retinal layers* as well as *fluid accumulation* (SRF and intraretinal cysts) and *inflammatory signs* (*highly reflective points* and *denser areas* with relative hyper-reflectivity) was performed for correlation studies.

This study addressed **three main questions**:

- In how many cases do the hyper-reflective lines of the outer retinal layers have either a normal or altered appearance or are associated with complete disorganization of the retinal layers at the baseline examination?
- How many cases presented an improvement, stabilization, or deterioration of the visibility of the outer retinal layers? These data were analyzed after the first injection, then after the third injection. and at the 1-year follow-up visit.
- What are the correlations between these various groups?

The preliminary results appear to indicate:

- A close correlation between early CNV, minimal or moderate lesions of the outer retinal layers, and good (functional) visual acuity recovery.
- The presence of fibrosis (accentuated or preventing clear depiction of the outer layers) is associated with moderate to severe loss of visual acuity.

Conclusion

As a result of current technological progress and preliminary experimental studies, **functional imaging** will soon be added to morphological and **structural imaging** in clinical practice.

Doppler blood flow measurements, *oximetry*, and studies of retinal activity in response to light stimulation are already underway.

Comparisons with *autofluorescence* data should allow analysis of alterations in the RPE.

Genotype-phenotype correlations will help to explain and possibly predict the natural history of the disease and its response to treatment.

Angiography visualizes CNV, and OCT demonstrated the exudative and inflammatory reactions associated with CNV.

The **advantage of Spectral-Domain OCT,** due to its high resolution, is to allow recognition of the outer retinal layers and photoreceptors.

Spectral-Domain OCT scans of the outer retinal layers provides new morphological, qualitative, and quantitative data that are valuable for diagnosis, developing the best treatment strategy, and to monitor treatment follow-up.

Tissue visualization is almost at the point which allows histological and cellular detail, constituting "**non-invasive eye biopsies.**" This level of information may finally be achieved by Adaptive Optics OCT.

Spectral-Domain OCT has already proven to be invaluable, and it should be part of our equipment in the same way as biomicroscopes and angiography instruments.

The essential challenge remains the interpretation of each image, facilitated by enlarged images and correlations with other imaging modalities, to ensure that OCT has the place it deserves in the assessment of macular diseases.

Interpretation of OCT Examinations

- OCT examinations can be interpreted rapidly and almost intuitively.

Fluid accumulation, increased thickness, and large intraretinal cysts can be easily indentified.

These findings *suggest CNV*, in the same way as an area of hyper-fluorescence with intense leakage on angiography does.

- However, a *more rational and precise analytical approach*, evaluating each structure point by point, is better.

- **The first step** is:
  - To identify the RPE band, and
  - To carefully examine this band looking for irregularities, thickening, fragmentation, displacement, or shadowing.

The presence of a visible and distinct separation of the RPE from the Bruch's membrane must also be assessed.

- **The second step** consists of examination of structures located posterior to the RPE band, looking for:

  - Hyper-reflectivity extending posteriorly, which suggests atrophy.

  - Hypo-reflectivity, which suggests shadowing in underlying structures or from structures above (ie, hard exudates, pigment, or hemorrhages).

- **The third step** consists of examination of structures situated anterior to the RPE band, including:
  - The thickness of the retina itself,
  - The presence of cavities or deposits,
  - The various retinal layers,
  - The vitreous and vitreoretinal adhesions.

- Examination of the outer retinal layers of the retina has been dramatically changed by Spectral-Domain OCT, which can visualize:

  - The three main landmarks of the outer retinal layers:

    - *Outer nuclear layer (ONL),*

    - *External limiting membrane (ELM),*

    - *Interface between inner and outer segments of the photoreceptor layer (IS/OS).*

  - The presence of fluid accumulation is evaluated in relation to these landmarks, either underneath the RPE (PED), underneath the neurosensory retina, or infiltrating the retina itself (with or without intraretinal cysts).

- The SD-OCT scan is then examined for:

  - Signs suggestive of the presence of choroidal neovascularization, either underneath the RPE, above the RPE, or both.

  - Surrounding reactive signs suggestive of associated inflammation:

    - Bright **hyper-reflective spots,**

    - **Denser** and relatively hyper-reflective **areas,**

    - Scarring, fibrosis, or atrophy.

- The examination is completed by studying:

  - *Inner retinal layers,*

  - *Foveal depression,*

  - *Vitreoretinal adhesions.*

A READING CHART can facilitate detection of these various signs, leading to a diagnosis in the majority of cases.

This diagnosis is then immediately or subsequently **confirmed** with angiographic findings and clinical features (see READING CHART, P 377).

This point-by-point analysis of ocular structures and their changes observed on an OCT scan remains schematic.

Lesions involving only one layer or only one tissue type are extremely rare and interpretation of localized lesions must *take all adjacent changes into account.*

OCT Reading Grid / Chart of Exudative AMD

Date	Name Age		Initial diagnosis	Comments
Vitreous	❑ Normal	❑ Detached	❑ Adhesions	
Inner retinal layers	❑ Normal	❑ Altered	❑ Disorganized	
Foveal depression	❑ Normal	❑ Flattened	❑ Inverted/lost	
Outer nuclear layer	❑ Normal	❑ Thinned	❑ Absent	
External limiting membrane	❑ Normal	❑ Altered	❑ Absent	
IS/OS interface	❑ Normal	❑ Altered	❑ Absent	
RPE	❑ Normal	❑ Altered	❑ Absent	
PED	❑ Absent	❑ Optically empty/ serous	❑ Fibrovascular	
Bruch's membrane	❑ Normal	❑ Visible	❑ Altered	
Intraretinal cysts	❑ Absent	❑ Few	❑ Confluent	
SRF	❑ Slight	❑ Moderate	❑ Large	
Thickness	❑ Normal	❑ Increased	❑ Decreased	
Highly reflective points	❑ Absent	❑ Numerous	❑ Disseminated	
Dense zones/deposits	❑ Absent	❑ Moderate	❑ Extensive	

Appendix

Commercially Available Spectral-Domain OCT Equipment

Since the initial development of Spectral-Domain OCT, a number of companies now manufacture equipment based on this technology for use by ophthalmologists: clinicians and scientists.

Each of these machines offers all of the advantages of Spectral-Domain OCT: rapid acquisition, high resolution, capability of 3D reconstruction.

Point-to-point correlations can also be established with fundus photography, fluorescein angiography, and ICG angiography images. However, each machine has its own specific characteristics.

The following pages were written with the help of manufacturers to more clearly define the advantages and disadvantages of each machine.

SanoTek

Spectralis™ HRA-OCT
Heidelberg Engineering / SanoTek

HEIDELBERG ENGINEERING

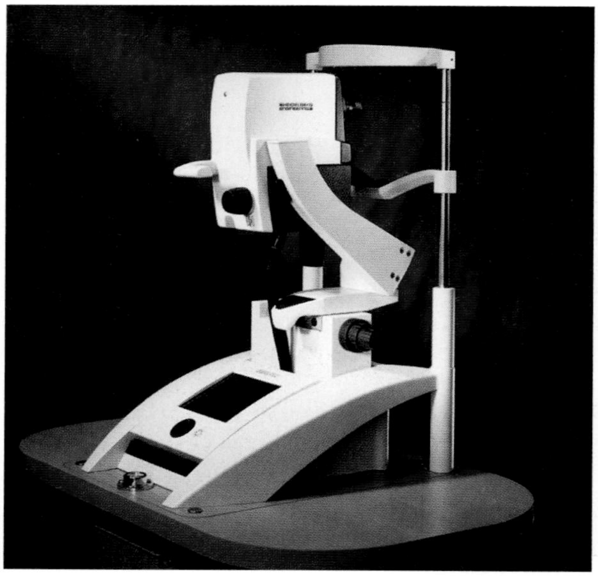

- **Scan speed:** 40,000 A-scans/second.
- **Minimum pupil diameter:** 2 mm.
- **Internal and external fixation targets.**
- **Focus Range: -24.00 to +40.00 D.**
- **Scanning field:** 30° for OCT - 57° for angiography.

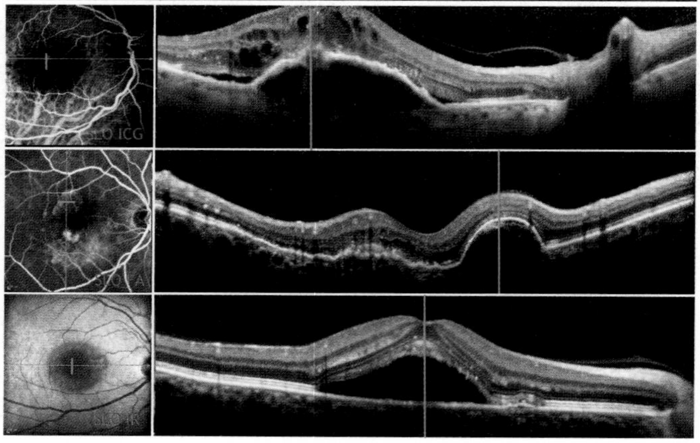

Main technical characteristics of OCT and HRA-OCT

4 light sources:

Use	Type of laser	Wavelength
Fluorescein angiography and Red-free	Sapphire laser	488nm (blue)
SLO-ICG angiography	Laser diode	785nm (near infrared)
Infrared	Laser diode	820nm (infrared)
OCT	Superluminescent diode	880nm (infrared)
OCT resolution	**Axial**	**Transverse**
	3.8 μ	14 μ

Unique functions:

- **High acquisition speed:** 40,000 scans/second.
  Avoids artifacts from microsaccades and increases image definition.
- **Noise reduction technology** (*Heidelberg Noise Reduction Technology™*).
  Allows visualization of fine structures.
- **Automatic real-time image averaging system** (*ART or Automatic Real Time*).
- **Eye-tracking** (*TruTrack™ Technology and Tracking Laser Tomography™*):
  Tracks eye movements,
  Maintains scan position on the retina during the examination,
  Automatically repositions scan at the same location as a previous examination.
- **Reference image:** Infrared, high quality angiography (SLO), autofluorescence.
- **Composite image:** real-time and automated.

Retina

- **Retinal thickness mapping** (maps, color scales, ETDRS target, segmentation)
- **3D modeling:** various sections, multiframe movie, single frame.

Disc region

- Optic disc ring analysis program (ultrarapid circular scans).
- Comparison to a normative database.
- Analysis of asymmetry between the two eyes.

Upgradeable

- Glaucoma module in the final stages of development.

Spectralis™ HRA-OCT
Heidelberg Engineering / SanoTek

Color-coded retinal thickness mapping

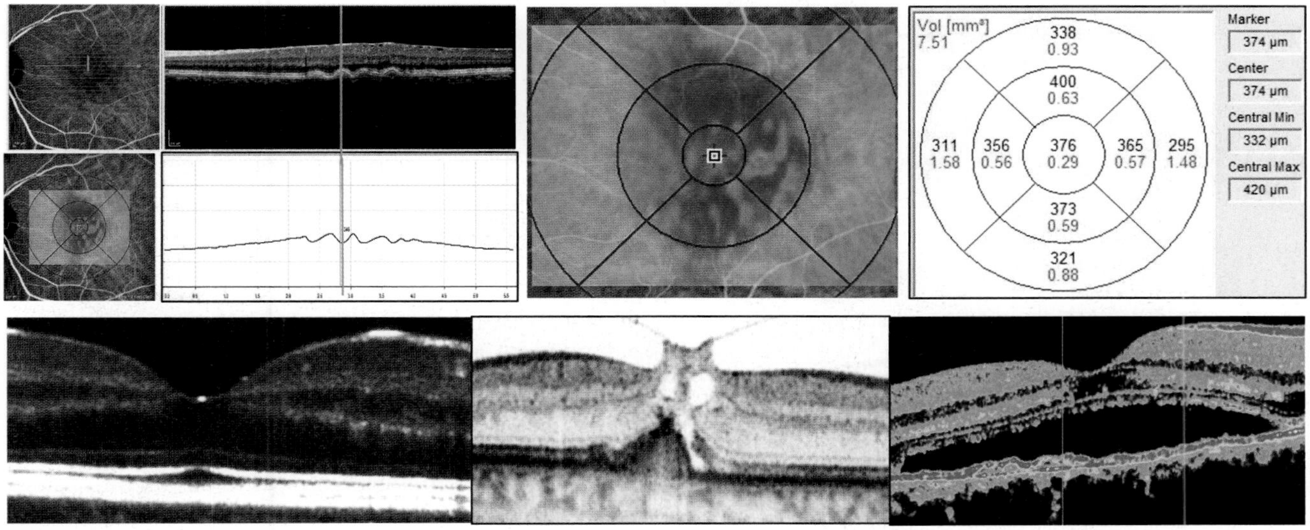

Follow-up of response to treatment and enlarged images

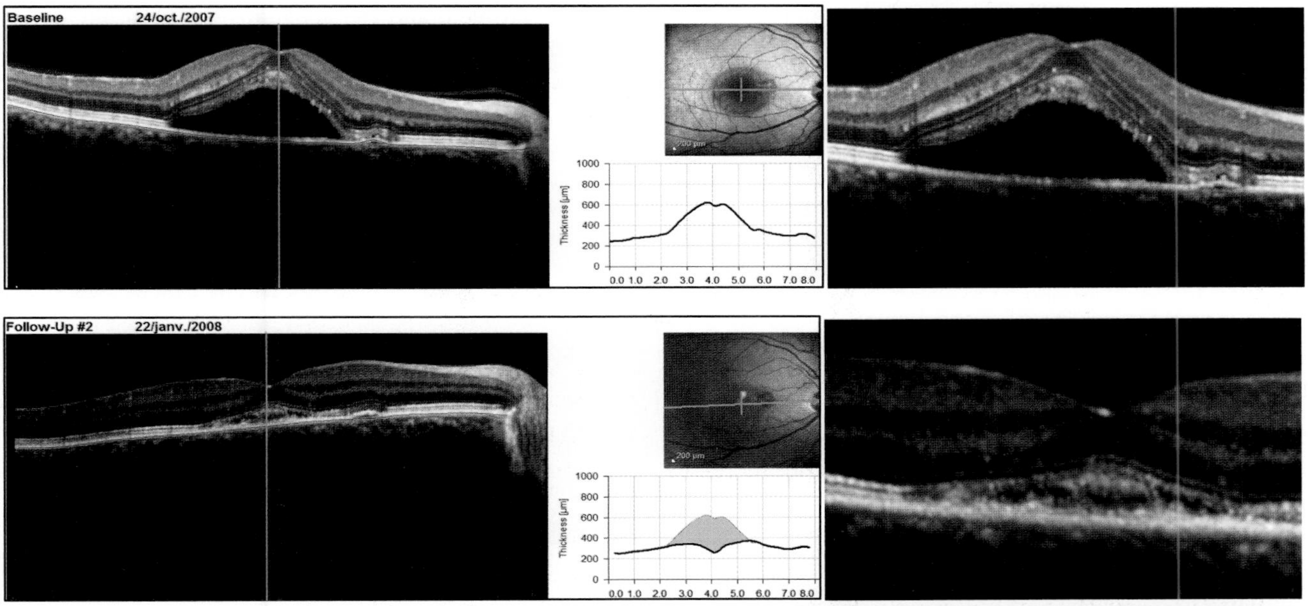

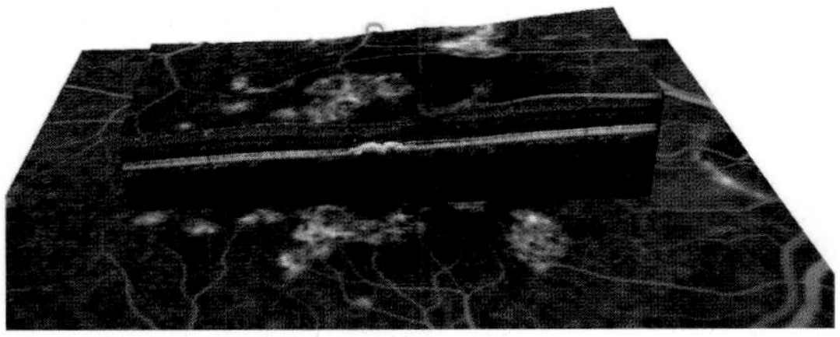

3D modeling, multiframe movie, single frame

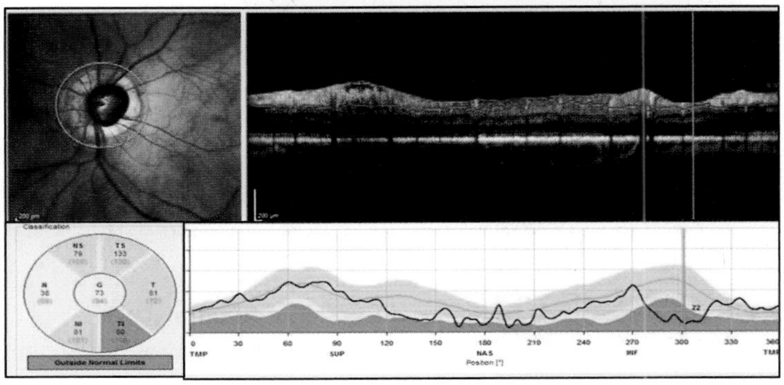

Glaucoma module (in final stages of development)

CONNECTING VISIONS

TOPCON

TOPCON 3D OCT

3D OCT-1000

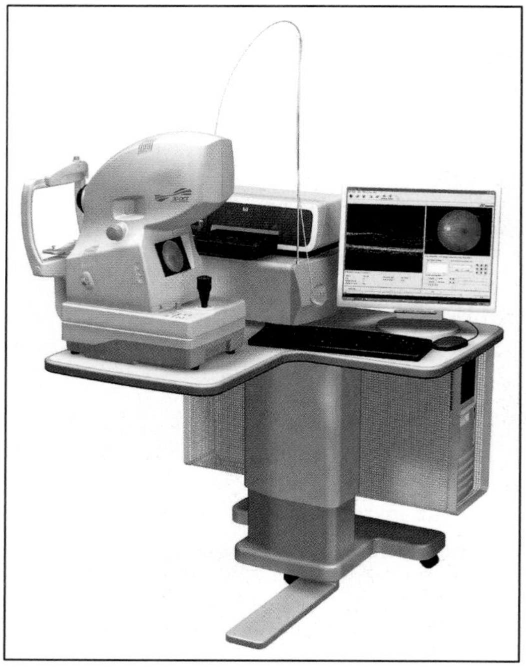

- <u>Optical Coherence Tomography (OCT)</u>, using a Spectral or Fourier domain system connected, for the first time, to a non-mydriatic fundus camera.
- <u>Simple and rapid acquisition</u>, both for patients side and photographers, allowing the ophthalmologist to capture and analyze a selection of OCT sections and merge them with the color fundus image.
- <u>Characteristics:</u>
  Wavelength: 840 nm
  Horizontal resolution: ≤ 20 µm
  Longitudinal resolution: 5 µm
- <u>Patient positioning:</u>
  The patient is positioned on a motorized chinrest and looks at a target that can be adjusted according to the level of the patient's vision.
- <u>Photographer manipulations</u>
  They are simple, either manual or automatic depending on the setting. In automatic mode, once the patient has been installed, an AUTO Z key is activated, and the apparatus automatically detects the position of the OCT section. A quality score from 0 to 100 is displayed.

<u>Quantification and thickness measurements:</u>

After scanning the retinal zone, the software calculates the thicknesses of the OCT zone and displays them as a chart or EDTRS scale, providing *pachymetric quantification* of the various layers of the retina, including optical fibers. This information can be compared with the normative database.

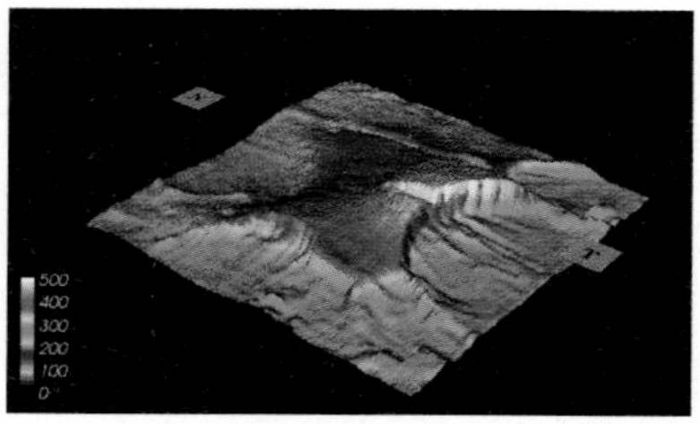

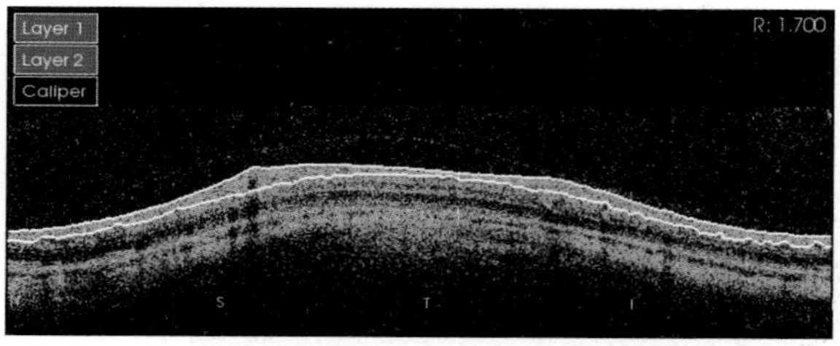

- The color image remains the reference image to compare examinations taken at different times. The B-Scan is always **positioned on the same location** as the color image and is independent of the patient's fixation point.
- The color image can be replaced by another image (fluorescein angiography, ICG angiography, etc.)
- A database network can be created with multiple viewing stations to allow analysis at other locations.

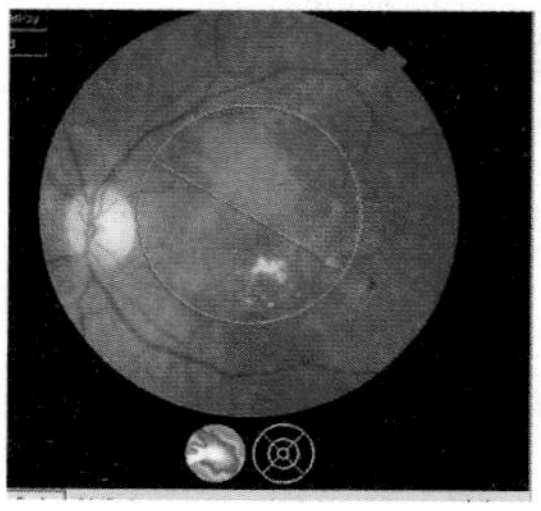

<u>Color images:</u>

- This color image is obtained with a set of alignment targets and automatic flash.
- With an angle of 45° through a 4 mm pupil, it covers the posterior pole, optic disc, and macula.
- Various imaging enhancements can be done, such as separation of green, red and blue light, area measurements, and enlarged views.

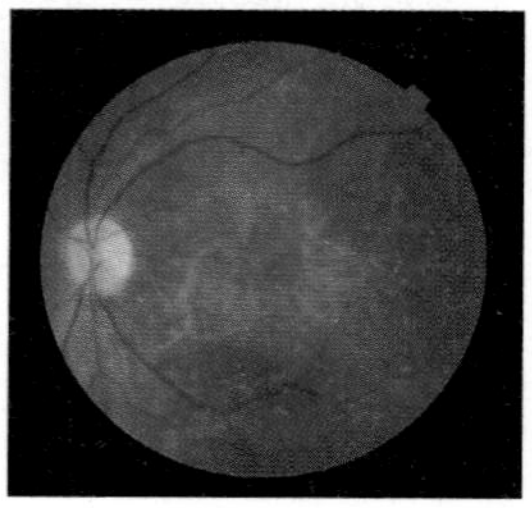

TOPCON 3D OCT

TOPCON

CONNECTING VISIONS

OCT SCANS

- OCT scans are acquired before acquisition of color fundus images.
- The software provides a large choice of *scan areas* (3 mm x 3 mm - 4.5 mm x 4.5 mm - 6 mm x 6 mm - 8.2 mm x 3 mm), *scan number* (1 to 128), *scan resolution* (512 points to 4,096 points), scan interval, and allows overlapping of the same scan (2 – 16 passages).

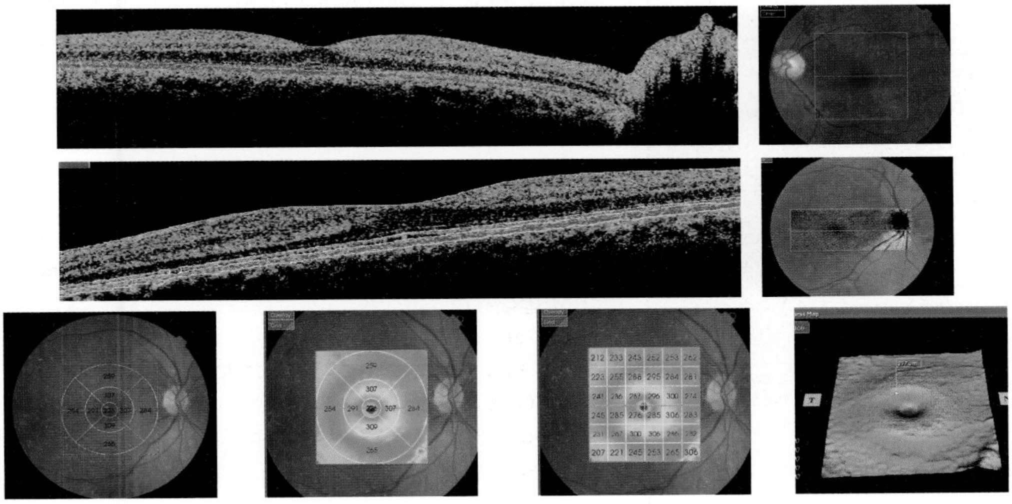

3D IMAGING

- A **3D image** can be obtained by reconstituting the series of scans over a zone of 6 mm x 6 mm or a zone of 8.2 mm x 3 mm. Horizontal, vertical, or oblique examinations are all possible in this 3D image.
- The **various layers** can be easily studied. They are pre-identified with computer analysis (nerve fiber layer - pigment epithelium).
- The **3D reconstitution** of all B-scans allows various applications, such as examination of the vitreoretinal interface and ensuring that the intended area is visualized.
- This technique avoids the need for the patient to be present once the examination has been completed.
- **Searching capabilities:**
  Once the examination has been completed, the user can, with the on-screen display, review the automatic analyses (registration – thickness measurements, etc.)
  Previous examinations are accessible in the patient list as images, allowing a rapid overview of all examinations: 3D - RASTER, etc.
- Able to export movies for 3D presentations.

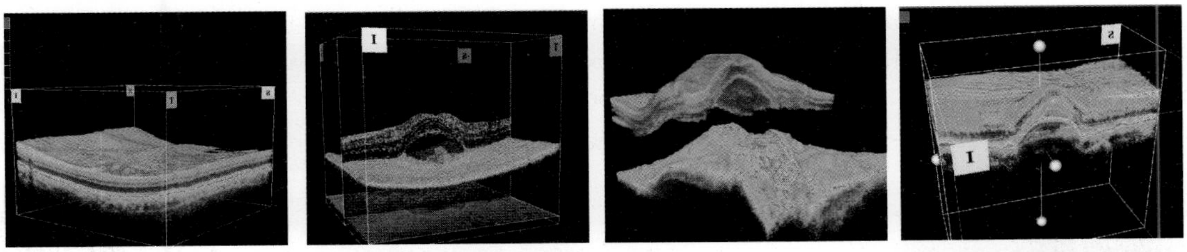

- **Glaucoma**

Color image of the optic disc

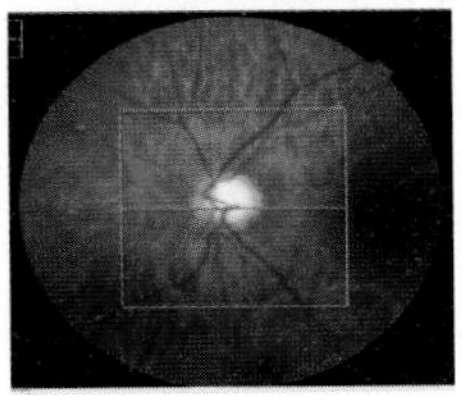

OCT scan of the optic disc

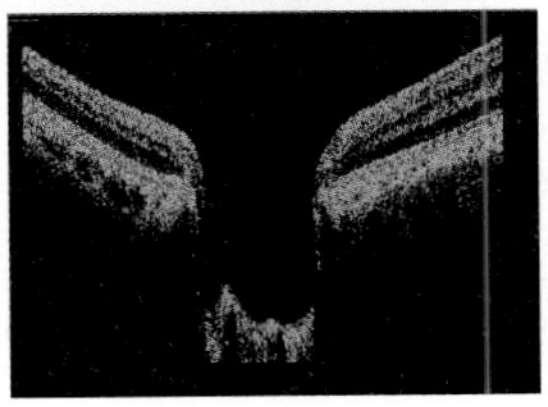

RTVue
FOURIER DOMAIN OCT
in-vivo histology

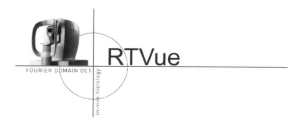

The Most Comprehensive OCT

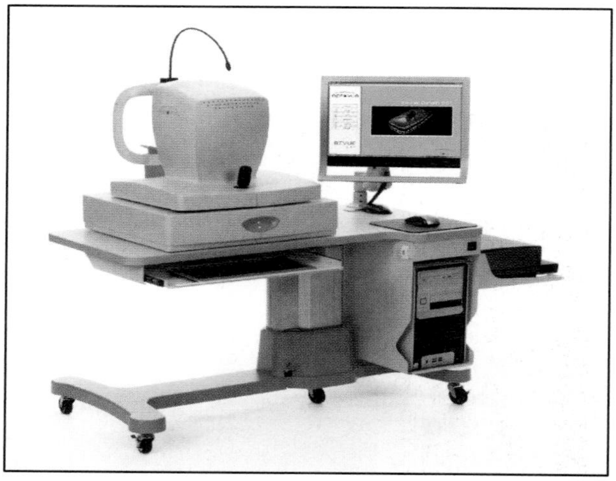

- The RTVue provides high-resolution imaging of the retina layers, with detail and precision.
- A range of scan patterns is available to fit the imaging needs of a retina practice.
- These patterns are designed to take advantage of the speed and resolution offered by Fourier-domain OCT technology.

Technical specifications

Scanner	
OCT image	26,000 A-scan/second
Frame rate	256 to 4096 A-scan/frame
Depth resolution (in tissue)	5.0 µm
Transverse resolution	15 µm
Scan range	Depth: 2- 2.3 mm Transverse: 2 mm to 12 mm
Wavelength	840 ± 10 nm
Exposure power	750 µm
Fundus imager	
Field of view	32° (H) x 23° (V)
Illumination	Near IR
Type of camera	IR
Minimum pupil diameter	2.0 mm
Patient interface	
Working distance	22 mm
Motorized focus range	-15 to +12 D

- The **Line, Cross Line, and Grid Line** scans a high detailed slice through the targeted area of the fundus.
- The averaging function provides noise reduction to enhance the overall image and increase detail.
- All scan presentations are user selectable for Grayscale or Color, either as the default or at any time during viewing.

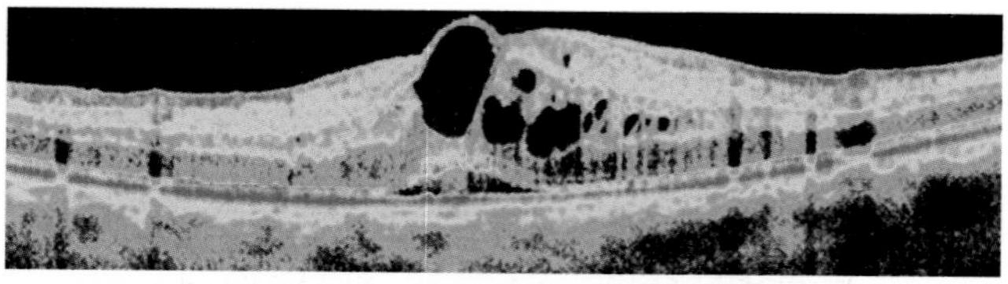

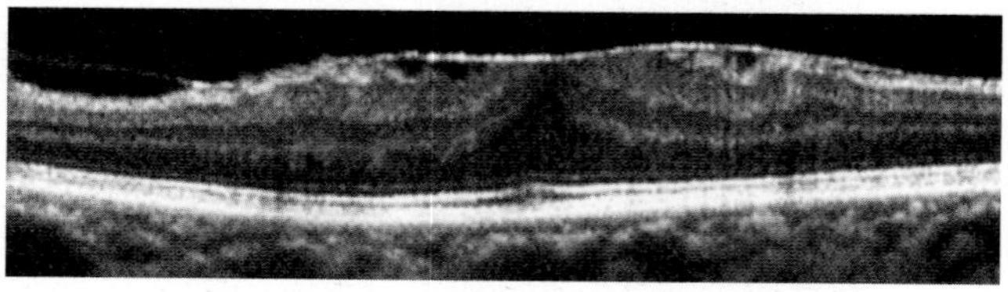

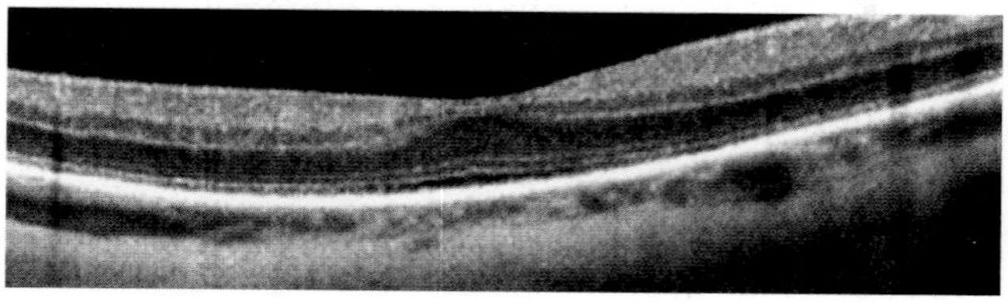

RTVue
FOURIER DOMAIN OCT
in-vivo histology

The Most Comprehensive OCT

EMM5 scan (5 mm Macular Map)

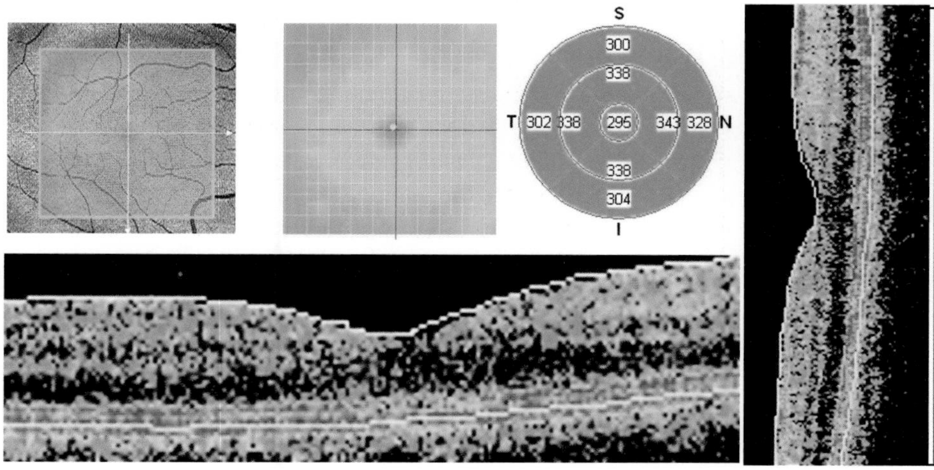

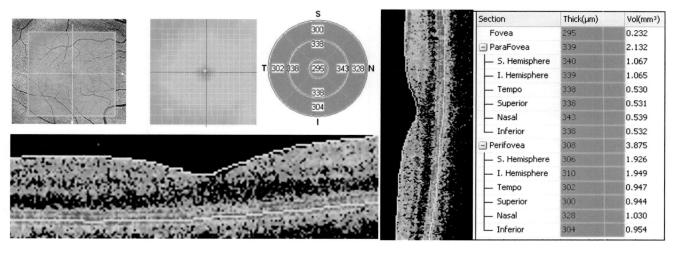

Section	Thick(µm)	Vol(mm³)
Fovea	295	0.232
ParaFovea	339	2.132
S. Hemisphere	340	1.067
I. Hemisphere	339	1.065
Tempo	338	0.530
Superior	338	0.531
Nasal	343	0.539
Inferior	338	0.532
Perifovea	308	3.875
S. Hemisphere	306	1.926
I. Hemisphere	310	1.949
Tempo	302	0.947
Superior	300	0.944
Nasal	328	1.030
Inferior	304	0.954

- **Detailed retinal mapping** (23,768 data points) in a 5 mm x 5 mm area of the macula. A dense grid of 42 scans allows reconstruction of the map.
- **Thickness topographies** available for the total retina, inner retina, outer retina, and also for an retinal pigment epithelium detachment.
- **Averages** per quadrant, thicknesses and volumes for each retinal layer. Localization of the lesion is facilitated by the high-contrast SLO reconstruction.
- For more reliable **comparison of examinations** over time, the measuring algorithm identifies blood vessels to register examinations from one visit to the next.

3D Macular scan

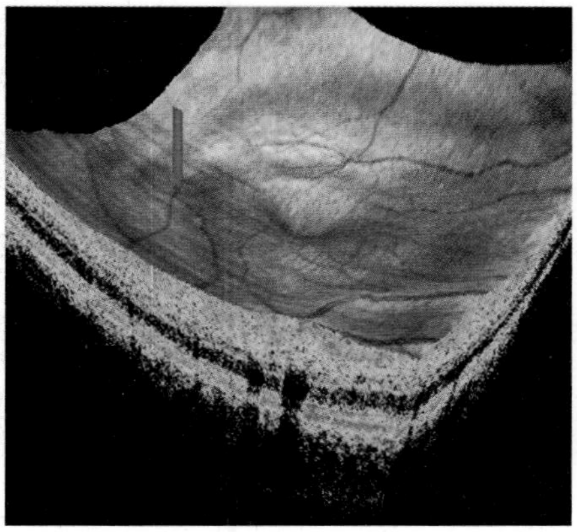

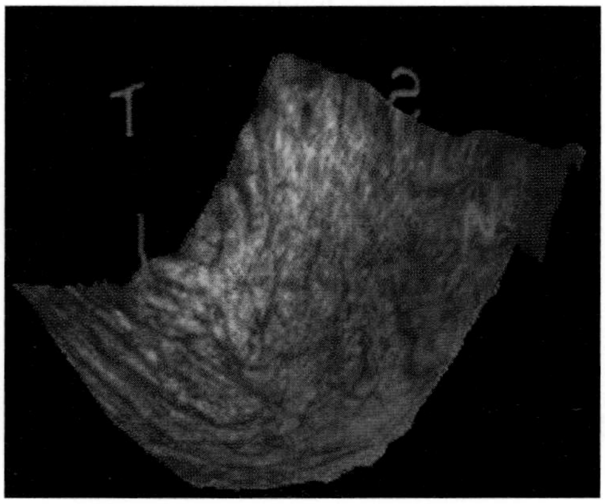

- More than 54,000 A-scans are used for the **3D display** and high-contrast SLO reconstruction.
- Overview of the 3D image and viewing from **multiple angles** provide a maximum of options that can be customized.
- The creation of short full-screen **video** sequences provides a teaching tool for patient information.
- The **3D C-scan option** using summation of C-scans allows visualization of the deep layers of the retina and choroid.

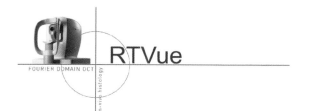

OPKO/OTI INSTRUMENTATION
A Division of OPKO Health, Inc.

Spectral OCT/SLO –
Ophthalmic Technologies, Inc.
(OTI, Toronto, ON, CANADA)

HAAG-STREIT FRANCE

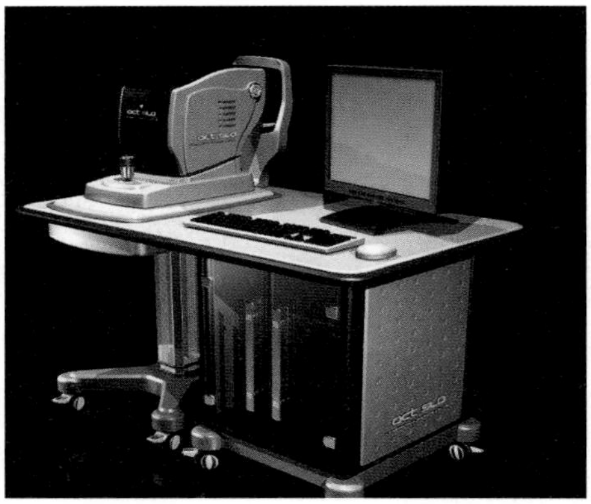

OCT/SLO Imaging

Spectral OCT/SLO is an imaging system which combines:
- **Optical Coherence Tomography**
- and **Scanning Laser Ophthalmoscope (SLO)**,

designed to:
- image the retina, *choroidal,* and the vitreo-retinal interface
- provide a *confocal fundus image*, which is linked to the OCT B-Scan image of the retina.

Spectral OCT/SLO is a versatile system which can be used in a wide range of clinical applications.

RETINA

Retinal imaging

Due to utilization of spectral technology, the OTI system generates high-resolution images in a fraction of the time required by temporal-domain systems.
Imaging with the Spectral OCT/SLO generates an image of such high resolution that the different layers of the inner retina are clearly seen. Subtle abnormalities may be detected sooner, allowing earlier intervention.

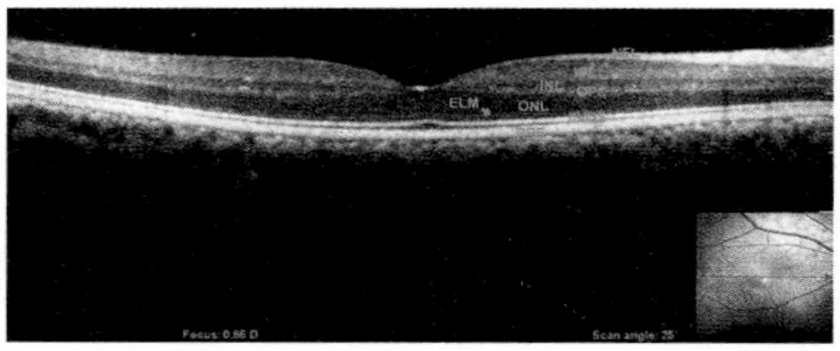

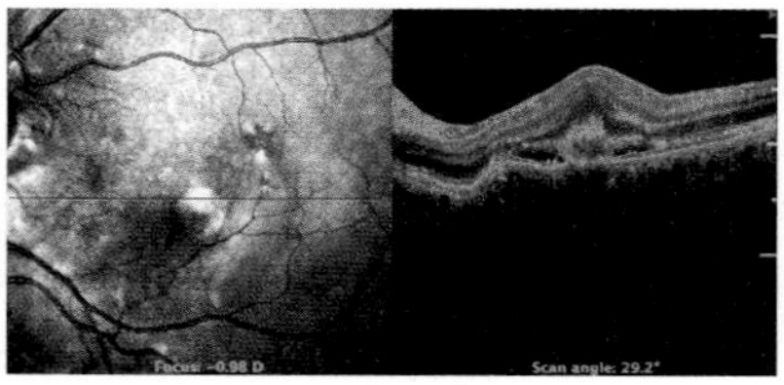

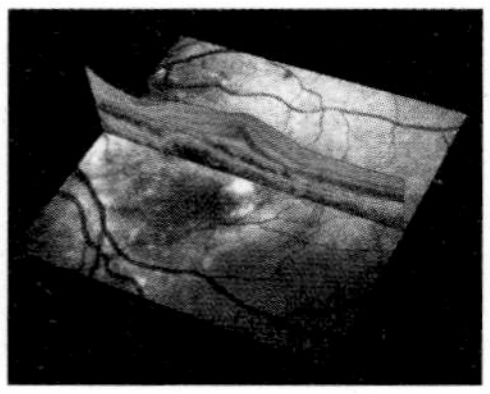

The OTI Spectral OCT/SLO provides an **axial resolution of 4-6 µm** with a scan rate of up to *27,000 A-scans per second*. The shorter examination time reduces patient movement artifacts and makes the examination much easier for the patient and the operator, especially in patients with low vision, small pupils, and opaque media.
The OTI system provides a **wide range of B-scan options:** linear scan, radial scan, retinal scanning, graphic retinal thickness mapping, and various visualization modes such as grayscale, color, side-by-side visualization with the SLO image, and vitreous enhancement.

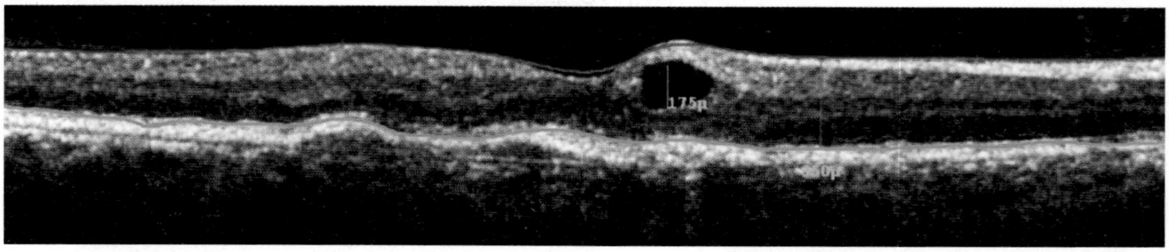

REAL-TIME REGISTRATION

Spectral OCT/SLO acquires OCT and SLO images **simultaneously** through a single optical system using the same light source.
This allows **direct correlation** between the characteristics of the retinal surface on the SLO image and the internal characteristics of the retina visualized on the OCT image, providing precise *real-time registration and orientation.*

OPKO/OTI INSTRUMENTATION
A Division of OPKO Health, Inc.

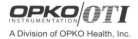

Spectral OCT/SLO – Ophthalmic Technologies, Inc. (OTI, Toronto, ON, CANADA)

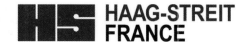

HAAG-STREIT FRANCE

3D TOMOGRAPHY

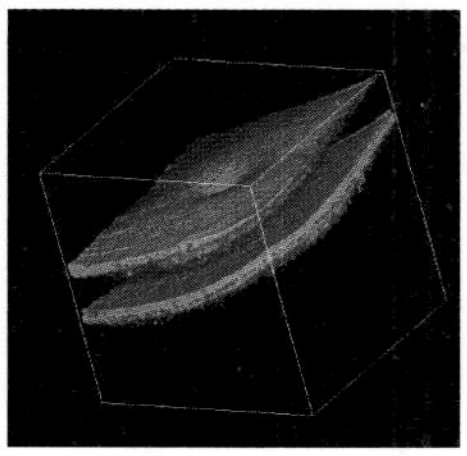
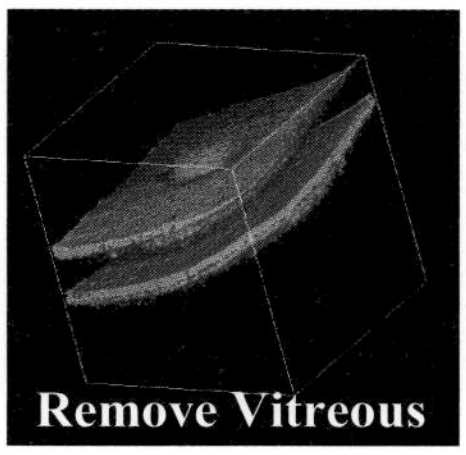 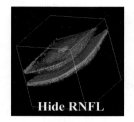

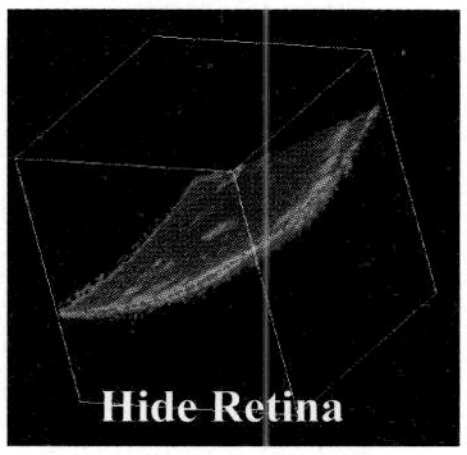

3D TOMOGRAPHY

SLO allows exact localization of the OCT topographic mapping by using a vascular pattern.

Retinal thickness is visualized in the form of a 8 x 8 grid, a 5 x 5 grid or in as zones. With SLO, the exact localization of the topographic mapping is determined by using information contained in the patient's vascular pattern.

Topographic mapping is obtained from a sequence of parallel B-scans, captured in TV scanning mode in 1 or 2 seconds. Sections can be extracted to demonstrate internal structures under the surface of the map.

Topographic maps can be visualized in the form 3D topography or 3D tomography.

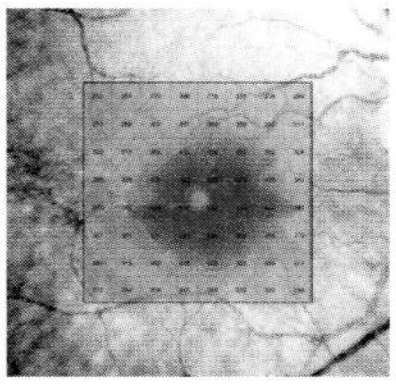
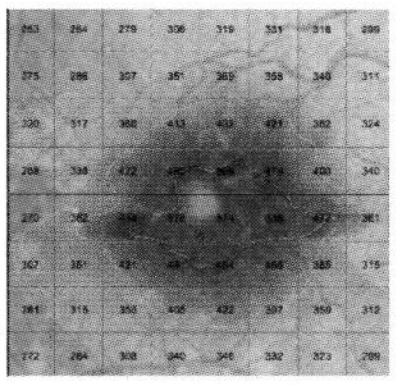
 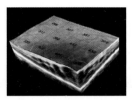

Comparison and topography subtraction

Microperimetry on the OTI Spectral OCT/SLO

- **The SLO module** of the OTI apparatus allows integration of **microperimetry** in the Spectral OCT/SLO. This capacity to perform a functional examination of the retina is specific and unique to the OTI Spectral OCT/SLO.
- **The results** are mapped on the SLO image of the fundus and can also be overlaid onto the retinal thickness map to establish the link between *retinal function* and *thickness* in specific points of the retina.
- If the patient uses eccentric fixation, the system tracks the position of fixation, allowing continuation of the examination rather than useless repetition of stimuli when the patient's eye moves.

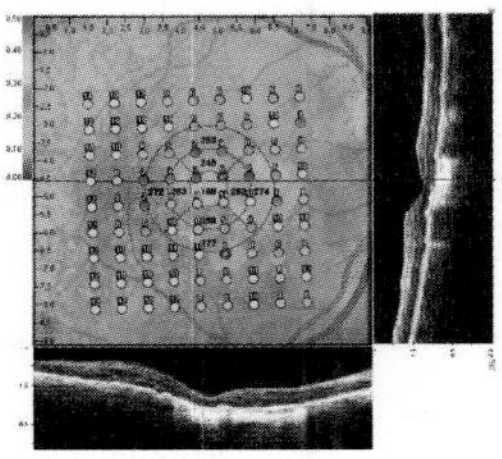
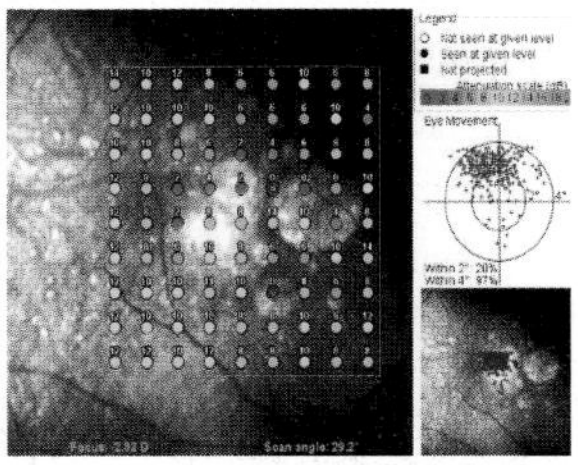
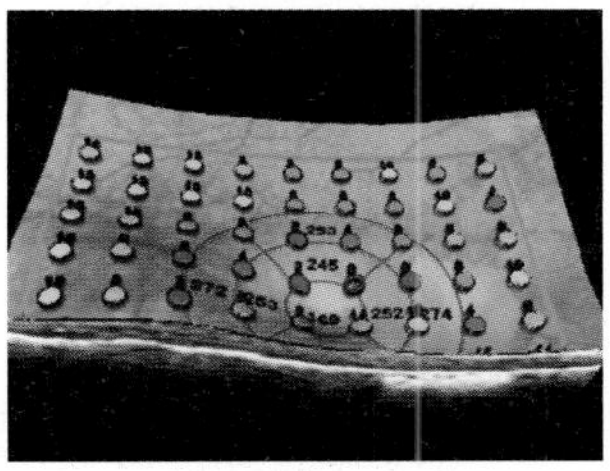

GLAUCOMA

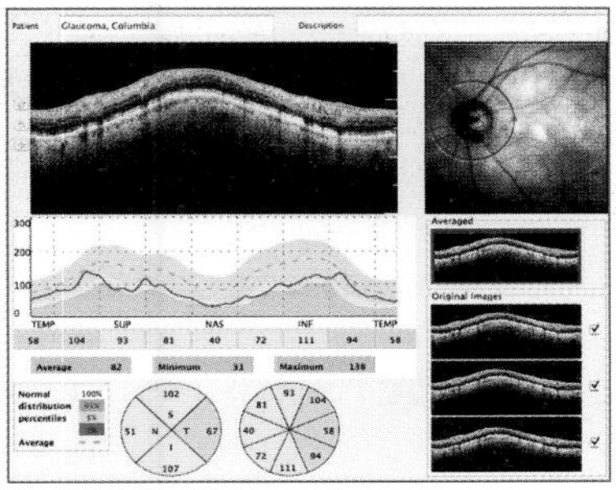

3D topography / tomography optic nerve head analysis

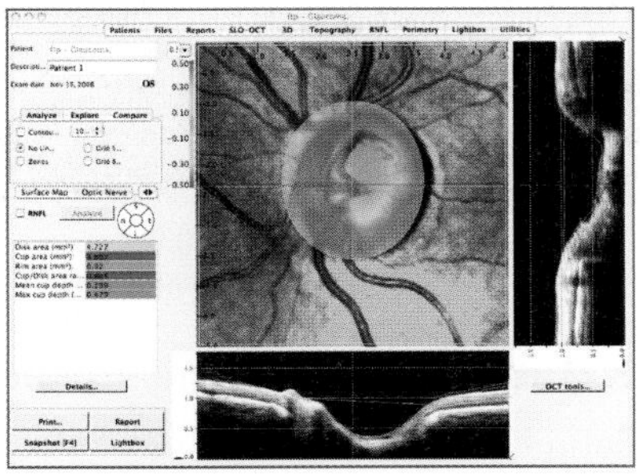

The RNFL program acquires a circular OCT with a 3.4 mm diameter around the Optic Disc to capture Retinal Nerve Fiber Layer Thickness and its ratio to normative values.

Cirrus™ HD-OCT-Carl Zeiss Meditec

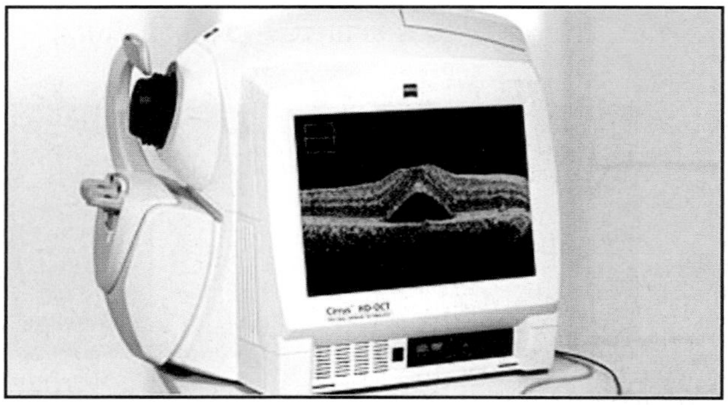

	Spectral-Domain OCT	Stratus Time-Domain OCT	Advantages of Spectral-Domain OCT
Light source	840 nm	820 nm	High resolution
Detector	Spectrometer	Unique detector	Faster acquisition
Axial resolution	5-7 µm	10 µm	Better visualization of retinal layers
Transverse resolution	10 - 20 µm	20 µm	
Number of A-scans per B-scan	4,000 - 8,000	512	Better visualization of lesions
A-scan depth	2 mm	2 mm	Slight improvement of light penetration
Number of A-scans per second	18,000 – 40,000	400	Better registration, 3D analysis

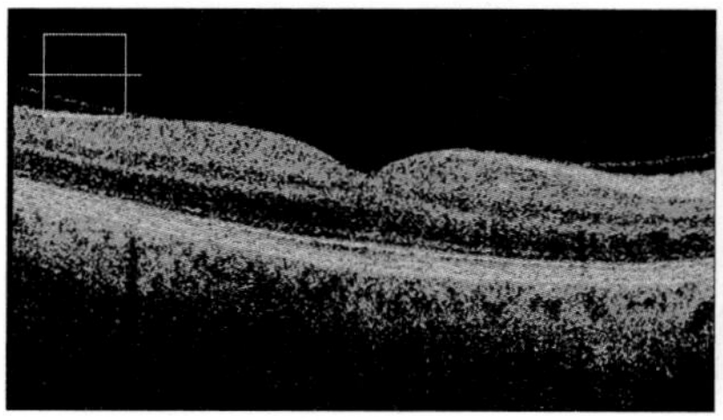

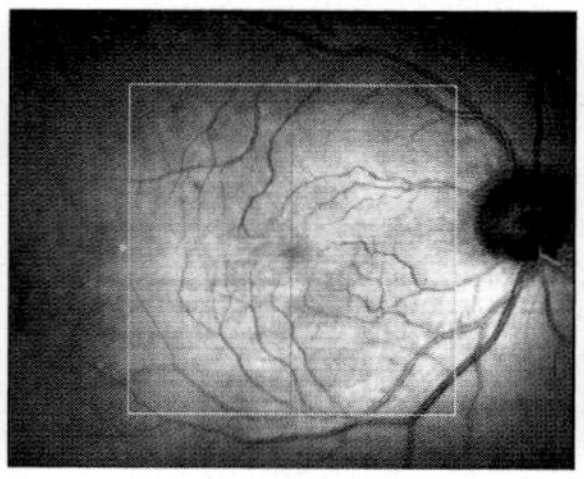

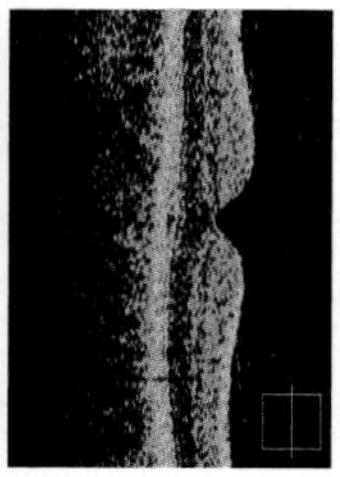

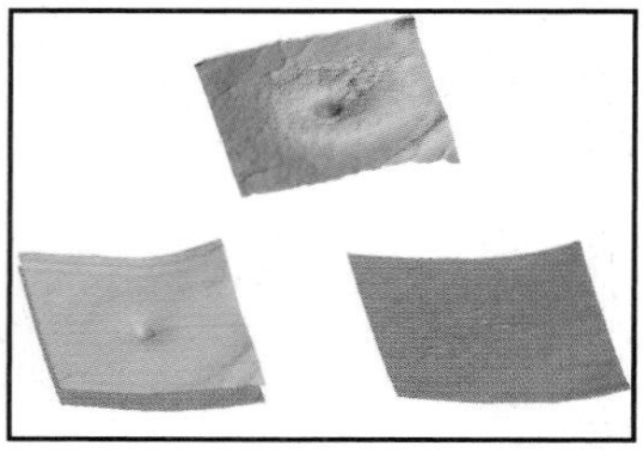

Main technical characteristics

- ***Light source:*** superluminescent diode (SLD), 840 nm
- ***Pupil diameter:*** Minimum: l 2.5 mm / Optimum: 3 mm
- ***Scan speed:*** 27,000 A-scans per second
- ***Field of view:*** 36° x 30°
- ***Axial resolution:*** 5 µm in tissue
- ***Transverse resolution:*** 20 µm in tissue
- ***Fundus imaging***
  Light source: superluminescent diode (SLD), 750 nm
  Live imaging during scanning
  Internal and external fixation
  Focus adjustment range: -20 to +20 D
- **Retinal imaging**
  Retinal thickness mapping
  3D retinal mapping
  3D mapping of certain retinal layers

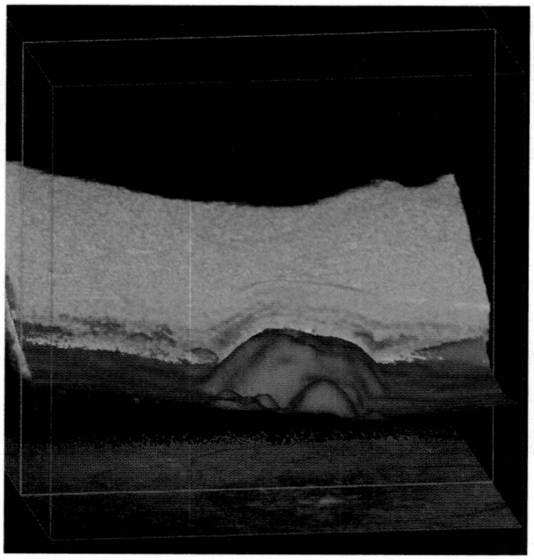

Carl Zeiss Meditec presents the advantages of the Cirrus™ HD-OCT as:

- High definition - High resolution
- Easy image capture
- Compact
- Ergonomic

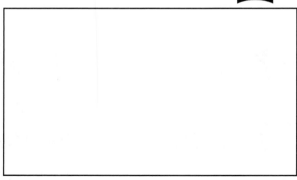

Cirrus™ HD-OCT-Carl Zeiss Meditec

The yellow square on the fundus image represents the limits of the cube analyzed (6 mm x 6 mm)

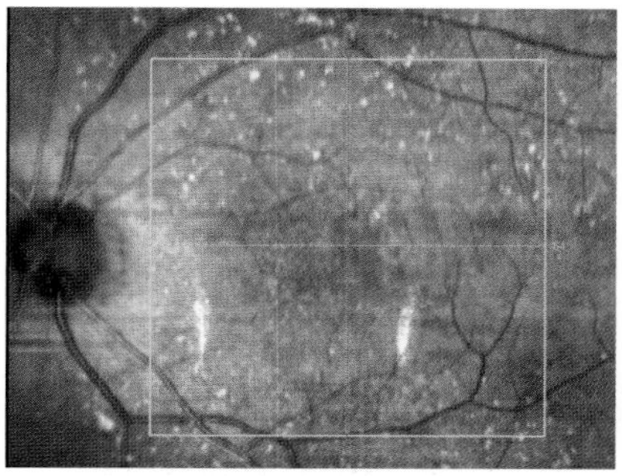

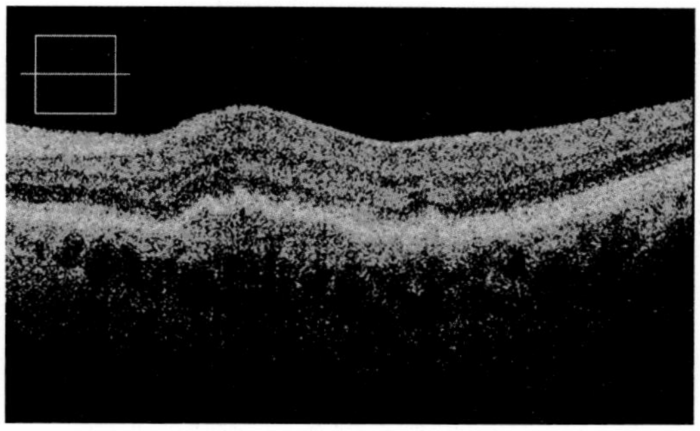

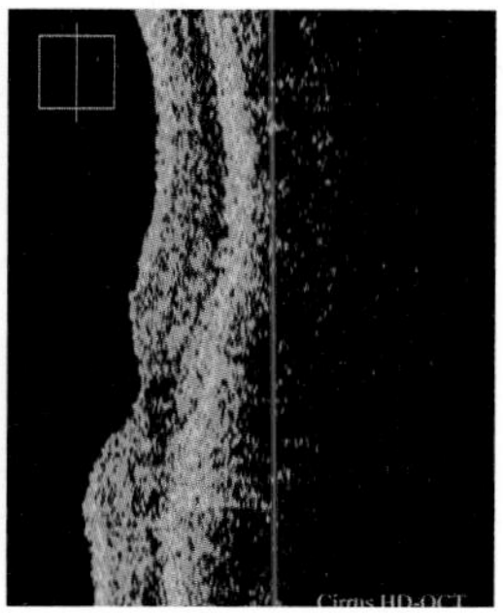

Precise localization of raster lines visible on the fundus image

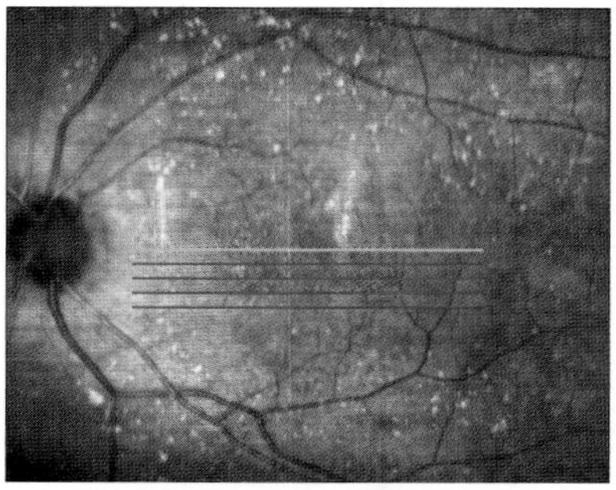

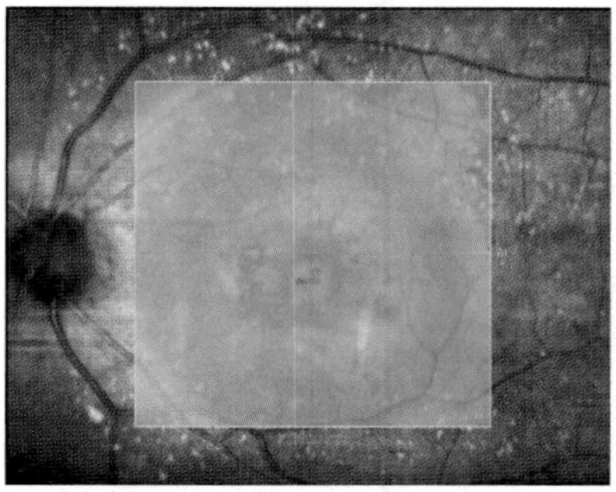

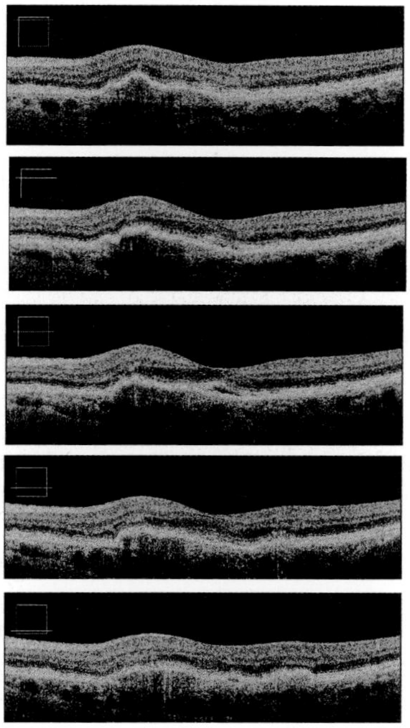

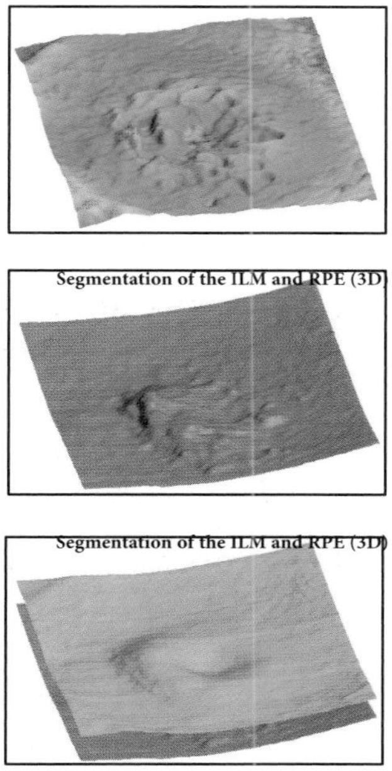

Segmentation of the ILM and RPE (3D)

LSLO fundus image with overlay on retinal thickness maps

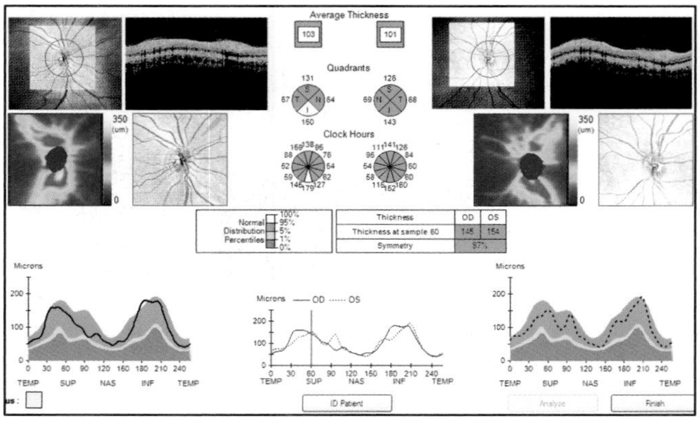

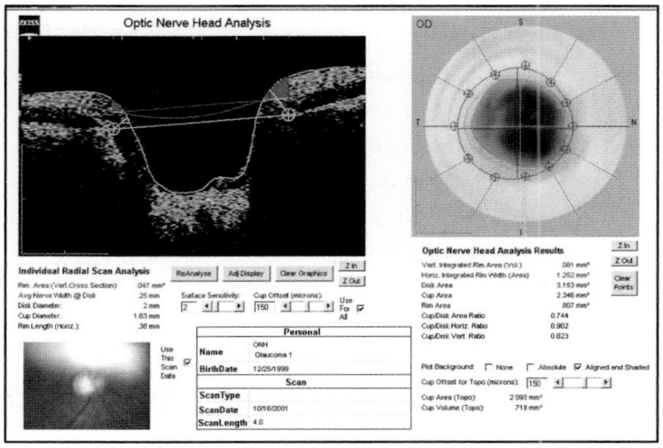

Retinal fiber thickness measurements
Normative database for glaucoma

Detailed optic nerve head analysis

Printing and Binding: Stürtz GmbH, Würzburg